Handbook of

Colorectal Surgery

Third Edition

Handbook of

Colorectal Surgery

Third Edition

David E Beck, MD, FACS, FASCRS
Professor and Chairman
Department of Colon and Rectal Surgery
Ochsner Clinic Foundation
New Orleans, Louisiana

Ochsner Clinical School
University of Queensland School of Medicine
Brisbane, Australia

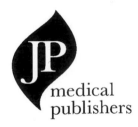

JP
medical
publishers

London • St Louis • Panama City • New Delhi

Foreword to the third edition

A myriad of textbooks have been published with seemingly increased frequency during the last few years, ranging from in-depth treatises of colorectal surgery to specific works focusing on certain areas. Some of these are published in multiple volumes and endeavor to address in precise detail every single nuance of the evaluation and management of patients with diseases of the colon, rectum and anus. Other textbooks focus on certain areas such as laparoscopy, physiologic assessment or imaging. In addition to these are virtual electronic books and surgical atlases.

The *Handbook of Colorectal Surgery* occupies a unique niche within the published literature. Most other textbooks in this area are aimed largely at practicing colorectal and general surgeons and colorectal surgery residents. This book, however, is written with surgical trainees in mind, and will also be of use to nurses and nursing students, medical students, and allied health professionals. The topics are selected from the basic core of colorectal surgery, and deliberately do not delve deeply within each area. Thus, the topics such as anatomy, pathophysiology, history and physical examination, diagnostic imaging, endoscopy, minimally invasive surgery and intestinal stomas all contain very practical and basic instructions for all readers.

The brief outline at the beginning of each chapter and the list of references at the end are an invaluable resource for readers. The illustrations are readily understood and the tables provide quick reference without being overly detailed, cumbersome or unwieldy. This edition contains new information which has been incorporated into each of the chapters.

A unique feature is the Rounds Questions, which highlight the fundamental teaching points of each chapter. These have been expanded upon and provide invaluable material for self assessment.

Finally, the relatively low cost and small size make the *Handbook of Colorectal Surgery* both affordable and portable, allowing the reader to keep this highly useful book in their lab coat or briefcase.

I congratulate my good friend, Dr. David Beck, on having produced this unique, high quality resource. This third edition will occupy a unique and much needed position within the spectrum of colorectal surgery textbooks. I also wish to thank Dr. Beck for giving me the honor of writing this foreword. I will certainly commend this book to all of our trainees, residents, nurses, and other allied health professionals as the textbook for their education, so that they can help us better treat our patients.

Steven D. Wexner, MD, FACS, FASCRS, FRCS
Chairman, Department of Colorectal Surgery
21st Century Oncology Chair in Colorectal Surgery
Cleveland Clinic Florida
Westin, Florida
Clinical Professor
Department of Surgery
University of South Florida College of Medicine
Tampa, Florida
June 2012

Foreword to the second edition

Despite the increasing number of texts in colorectal surgery over the past few years, reflecting the importance of teaching and learning the essentials of care for patients with diseases of the colon, rectum and anus, the Handbook of Colorectal Surgery is being released in its second edition just five years from its first publication. In the original preface, Dr. Beck indicated that the book was an 'ideal portable reference' for nurses, students and residents; time has proven this to be correct.

Organizational aspects of the book include a brief outline at the outset of each chapter and a list of classic references at the end. Tables are succinct and uniformly helpful, as are the illustrations. Although the line-up of chapters is exactly the same, nearly each has been rewritten by Dr. Beck, with updating of information to incorporate new advances where appropriate. Rounds Questions, a list of often-asked questions that highlight the essential teaching points of each topic, have been continued and expanded in the new edition.

Other unique aspects of this book, in addition to its format, include its size and cost. It is indeed portable and affordable – in contradistinction to the usual comprehensive volumes most often encountered on colorectal topics. The book is not portrayed as a reference book but rather a basic useful guide to the care of patients which will be used repeatedly in daily practice.

Experienced surgeons will find this a most useful adjunct to training medical students and residents of all levels, including colon and rectal residents. Physician extenders involved in colorectal and general surgery practices, as well as nurses, should find this book invaluable.

Dr. Beck should be congratulated for devoting considerable precious time to updating this singular contribution to the colorectal literature. Educators should not omit this book from their lists of required reading and should, in fact, consider providing copies of it to all of their trainees.

David J. Schoetz, Jr, MD
Chairman, Department of Colon and Rectal Surgery
Lahey Clinic
Burlington, MA
Professor of Surgery
Tufts University School of Medicine
Boston, Massachusetts
2003

Preface

- How do you evaluate and treat constipation?
- What do we get a patient ready for an operative procedure?
- What is the follow-up for colorectal cancer?
- What are the indications for colonoscopy?
- What are the options for treating hemorrhoids?

Questions such as these continue to be asked by residents, students, and nurses working in our colorectal surgery program. It was the number and range of these questions that provided the initial impetus for writing the first two editions of this book. Despite the availability of several outstanding texts covering our specialty, there remains a need for an affordable manual to recommend to residents, nurses, and other members of our health care team seeking this kind of information. The answers to the questions posed above, and many more, were covered in the first and second editions of Handbook of Colorectal Surgery. Each medical specialty, and Colon and Rectal Surgery is no exception, has seen new developments and knowledge.

The third edition continues to serve as a basic guide to the management of patients with colorectal diseases. Each chapter was reviewed, updated and rewritten to present current concepts and recommendations. Outlines are provided at the beginning of each chapter to assist the reader in organizing his or her thoughts and to facilitate quick access to important information. In addition, key elements throughout the book are reinforced by the Rounds Questions following each chapter, and extensive updated references provide options for further study. Newer concepts in patient care and operative technique, such as laparoscopic surgery and fistula management are covered and profusely illustrated. The third edition of this handbook remains an ideal portable reference for residents, students, and nurses. Experienced surgeons will find this manual helpful in their training of residents and fellows, and it may serve as a stimulus for additional thought and research.

This book incorporates the collaborative efforts of many individuals. The contributors to the first and second edition did an excellent job, and their contributions served as a foundation for the updated third edition. Two of the original contributors have been retained and additional experts in specialized fields have lent their expertise. These talented and dedicated individuals are active in teaching medical students and residents and continue to shape the future of colorectal surgery. The illustrations used in this text were produced by or reviewed by Barbara Siede, Director of Ochsner Medical Illustrations, whose exceptional ability has clarified many difficult concepts. Finally, my thanks to the staff of JP Medical, who worked hard to make this third edition a reality.

David E. Beck, MD
June 2012

Contents

Appendixes

Contributors to the 3rd edition

Kevin P Lally, MD, FACS
University of Texas Health Science Center
at Houston, Houston, Texas, USA

Francis R Rodwig, Jr, MD, MPH
Ochsner Clinic Foundation,
New Orleans, Louisiana, USA

Shinil K Shah, DO
University of Texas Health Science Center
at Houston, Houston, Texas, USA

Barbara Siede
Director of Ochsner Medical Illustrations,
Louisiana, USA

Steven D Wexner, MD, FACS, FASCRS
Cleveland Clinic Florida,
Weston, Florida, USA

Contributors to 1st and 2nd editions

Chapter 2
First and second edition chapters:
**Thomas E Read, MD and Patricia L
Roberts, MD**

Chapter 3
First and second edition chapters:
Dr W Brian Perry

Chapter 13
Second edition chapter coauthored by:
Frank G Opelka, MD

Chapter 14
Second edition chapter
Steven D Wexner, MD

Chapter 15
Second edition chapter coauthored by:
Charles B Whitlow, MD

Chapter 17
First edition chapter:
Carol-Ann Vasilevsky, MD

Chapter 18
First edition chapter:
Alan E. Timmcke, MD

Chapter 19
First edition chapter:
Richard E Karulf, MD

Chapter 23
First edition chapter :
Terry C Hicks, MD

Section 1

Basic Principles and Skills

Anatomy

Knowledge of intra-abdominal anatomy is essential to understand and treat intestinal diseases. This chapter briefly summarizes anatomic features and principles that are important to the colorectal surgeon. Discussions in greater depth are available in comprehensive anatomy and colon and rectal surgery books [1–6]. Although study and experience increases a surgeon's knowledge of expected anatomic findings, it must be remembered that variability is the rule in human anatomy. The abdominal cavity contains many structures (**Figure 1.1**). The abdominal portion of the intestinal tract starts with the esophagus which connects to the stomach. Structures of major importance to the colorectal surgeon include the small bowel, colon, rectum, and anus.

Macroscopic anatomy

Small bowel

The small bowel starts at the stomach and connects to the large bowel or colon at the ileocecal valve. The small bowel has three parts, the duodenum, jejunum, and ileum. The proximal portion, the duodenum is approximately 25 cm in length. The bile duct from the liver passes through the head of the pancreas and enters into the second part of the duodenum. The duodenum ends at a fibrous band called the ligament of Treitz. Two-fifths of the remaining small bowel is called the jejunum and the distal three-fifths is called the ileum.

The total length of the small bowel varies from 250 to 800 cm with a mean of 500 cm. It is folded in a variable fashion to accommodate the length of bowel in the abdomen. The major function of the small bowel is digestion and absorption of fluid and nutrients. The diameter of the small bowel is greatest at the duodenum and gradually narrows to the ileum.

Colon

The colon (large intestine) starts from the cecum (usually located in the right lower quadrant) and continues through all portions of the abdomen to the colorectal junction in the pelvis. The colon is about 1.5 m long and classically has been divided into segments based on the vascular supply and location of each segment within the abdomen, as shown in **Figure 1.2** [1]. The **cecum, right colon** (supplied by the right and ileocolic artery), and **left colon** (supplied by the left colic artery) are usually retroperitoneal and fixed. The **transverse colon** (supplied by the middle colic artery) and sigmoid colon (supplied by branches

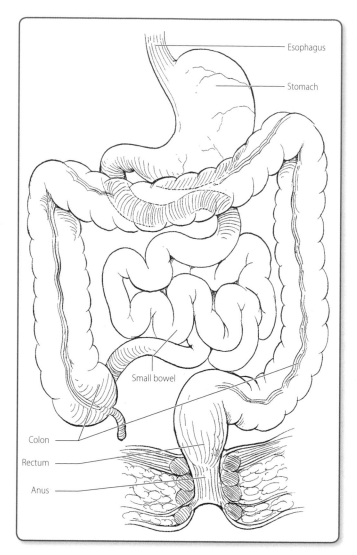

Figure 1.1 Normal gastrointestinal anatomy (mid-coronal view).

of the inferior mesenteric artery) are intraperitoneal and relatively mobile. The colon contains two **flexures** (or bends) in the right upper quadrant (hepatic) and left upper quadrant (splenic). When the colon is not unduly distended with feces, its diameter is largest at the cecum and gradually narrows to the distal sigmoid colon (the narrowest part of the colon).

The external wall of the colon is unique because of the presence of several **appendages** (taeniae, omentum, appendices epiploicae, and diverticula). The outer longitudinal muscle is thickened into three longitudinal bands called **taeniae.** These average 8 mm in width and are named in reference to their relationship to the bowel mesentery or omentum. Thus there is a taenia mesocolica (associated with the mesentery), a taenia omentalis (associated with the omentum), and

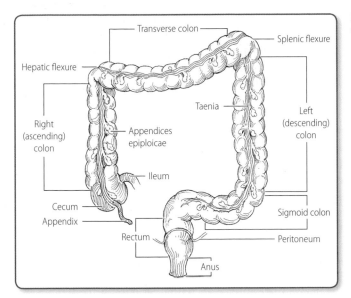

Figure 1.2 Topographic anatomy of the colon.

a taenia libera (not related to either the mesentery or omentum). The three taeniae meet at the appendiceal orifice and continue to the colorectal junction, where they expand to form a solid layer. Intermittent contractions of the inner circular muscle result in formation of semicircular folds called haustra, which are thought to aid in mixing the stool. The haustra are visible on the exterior surface of the colon.

The omentum is a sheet of fat and fibrous tissue that is well vascularized.

It starts at the greater curvature of the stomach, attaches to the transverse colon at the taenia omentalis, and extends into the abdomen. It doubles back on itself and attaches again to the colon, dividing the abdomen into several spaces (**Figure 1.3**). This arrangement allows it to be detached from the colon with minimal dissection in an almost bloodless plane. It has been theorized that the omentum functions

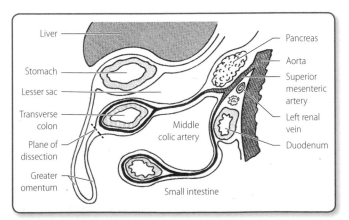

Figure 1.3 Sagittal section of the abdomen, demonstrating attachments of the greater omentum.

to localize inflammatory processes and to assist in healing. This is supported by clinical experience and the frequent finding of omental adhesions to other portions of the bowel. Because of its multiple important functions, I prefer to preserve the omentum in operations on patients in whom neoplastic lesions are not present. This is easily accomplished by elevating the omentum superiorly and dividing the thin avascular tissues that attach the omentum to the colon. With care, the omentum can be detached intact.

The **appendices epiploicae** are subserous pockets of fat that occur in two rows on the right and the sigmoid colon and in a single row on the transverse colon. Their only recognized role is to act as a storage site for fat cells. Many adults also have colonic diverticula (mucosal herniations) located adjacent to the taeniae (see Chapter 13).

The colon connects to the small bowel at the ileocecal valve. Although lacking an anatomic sphincter, this functional valve is responsible for several physiologic actions: it allows the digested contents of the small bowel to pass into the cecum at a controlled rate and acts as a relative barrier to prevent the large number of bacteria (concentration of 10^{10}) in the colon from moving to the distal small intestine (concentration of 10^3). Approximately 15% of patients have an incompetent ileocecal valve as demonstrated on barium enema studies.

Rectum

The rectum (**Figure 1.4**) is 12–15 cm long and can be divided into thirds based on its **peritoneal relations.** The upper third is intraperitoneal and covered anteriorly and laterally by peritoneum. At its middle portion, the rectum passes through the peritoneal floor and is covered by peritoneum on the anterior surface. The lower third is extraperitoneal

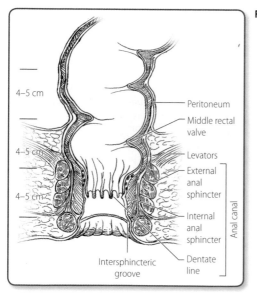

4–5 cm

4–5 cm

4–5 cm

Peritoneum

Middle rectal valve

Levators

External anal sphincter

Internal anal sphincter

Anal canal

Intersphincteric groove

Dentate line

Figure 1.4 Rectum and anus (coronal section).

as it travels through the levators to the anus. The lower rectum is enveloped by visceral pelvic fascia. Anteriorly, Denonvilliers' fascia (**Figure 1.5**) separates the rectum from the seminal vesicles, prostate, and bladder trigone in males and the posterior vaginal wall in women. Posteriorly, Waldeyer's fascia separates the rectum from the presacral venous plexus.

The rectum can be differentiated from the colon by its lack of a posterior mesentery, sacculations, and appendices epiploicae. The outer longitudinal muscle layer of the rectum diffuses to form a solid, thick layer. Thus there are no taeniae or diverticula. The rectum is also larger in diameter than the sigmoid colon.

The inner rectum contains three indentations or **valves of Houston.** These are composed of circular muscle only. The superior valve is located 4 cm below the rectosigmoid junction on the left side; the middle valve is located at the peritoneal reflection on the right side; the inferior valve is located 2–3 cm above the dentate line on the left side. These valves aid the surgeon in localizing lesions with respect to the peritoneal location.

Anus

The **anal canal** starts at the anorectal junction located at the palpable upper edge of the anal sphincter mechanism (junction of the puborectalis and the anal sphincter). The anal canal ends at the intersphincteric groove (approximately 2 cm distal to the dentate line). The anal margin is that portion of the perineum from the intersphincteric groove to approximately 5 cm out from the dentate line (**Figure 1.4**). The surface of the anal margin is skin that lacks appendages such as hair follicles. The surface outside the anal margin is referred to as perianal skin and contains all appendages of skin elsewhere.

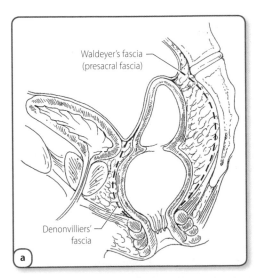
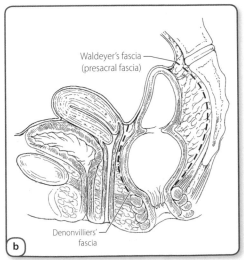

Figure 1.5 Sagittal section of the pelvis demonstrating anterior and posterior rectal fascia. (a) Male, (b) female.

The complex **musculature** of the anal canal can be thought of as composed of two tubes: the outer tube is funnel shaped, composed of skeletal muscle, and innervated by somatic nerves; the upper portion of this funnel is formed by the levator ani muscles. This sheet of muscle originates from the pelvic side wall (laterally), the sacrum (posteriorly), and the pubis (anteriorly) to the upper anus. Fibers of the levators can be grouped into three sections: the puborectalis (inner), pubococcygeus, and ileococcygeus muscles (posterolateral).

The lower portion of this outer cylinder of muscle is composed of the **external anal sphincter.** Although this voluntary muscle has been divided into three portions, clinically and physiologically it acts as a unit. Contraction of this muscle and the puborectalis produces the anal squeeze examined during the digital examination described in Chapters 2 and 3.

The inner tube of the anal canal is composed of visceral smooth muscle that is controlled by autonomic nerves. At the anus the inner circular muscle of the rectum thickens to become the **internal anal sphincter.** The longitudinal muscles of the rectum pass through the internal sphincter and attach to the perianal skin. The inner muscles of the anus are controlled by branches of the inferior rectal nerve and the perineal branch of the fourth sacral nerve. The internal anal sphincter is normally contracted and provides the resting anal tone felt during a digital anal examination. At rest, the lateral walls of the anal canal are opposed to form an anteroposterior slit [7].

The pelvic musculature and its attachments divide the pelvis into several spaces; these are described in Chapter 17.

Vascular anatomy

The colon receives its blood supply from branches of two major vessels, the superior and inferior mesenteric arteries (**Figure 1.6**). The **superior mesenteric artery (SMA)** originates on the anterior surface of the aorta, at the level of the first lumbar vertebrae, 1.25 cm caudal to the celiac artery, superior to the duodenum and pancreas [1]. Its first major branch is the middle colic artery. The middle colic artery divides close to its origin into an ascending and descending branch. After further branching it connects to the marginal artery and supplies the transverse colon. Distal to the marginal artery, end vessels travel in the mesentery to connect the marginal artery to the bowel (**Figure 1.6**).

The **inferior mesenteric artery (IMA)** originates 2–3 cm caudal to the SMA (inferior to the duodenum and pancreas). Its first major branch is the left colic artery. The left colic artery usually divides into two branches within 4–5 cm of its origin. This area is important in colonic operations. The next branches off the IMA are three to six sigmoid arteries. As branches of the artery approach the bowel, they communicate with the marginal artery.

The IMA continues to the upper rectum, where it becomes the superior hemorrhoidal artery. As it courses distally it splits into multiple branches that enter the rectum laterally.

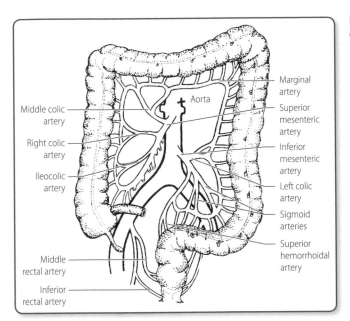

Figure 1.6 Arterial supply to the colon.

Middle colic artery

Right colic artery

Ileocolic artery

Middle rectal artery

Inferior rectal artery

Aorta

Marginal artery

Superior mesenteric artery

Inferior mesenteric artery

Left colic artery

Sigmoid arteries

Superior hemorrhoidal artery

The venous drainage of the colon (**Figure 1.7**) goes to the portal system and tends to follow the arterial system. The ileocolic vein attaches to the **superior mesenteric vein (SMV)** approximately 3 cm before the SMV joins to the splenic vein (inferior to the pancreas). The left colic vein enters the **inferior mesenteric vein (IMV)** at the level of the IMA origin. The IMV travels to the left of the IMA and continues to enter the splenic vein beneath the pancreas.

The lymphatic drainage of the colon follows the arterial supply. Major lymphatic chains are located along and named after the major named veins. The lymph nodes along these chains are important in colorectal cancer recurrence and prognosis.

The upper rectum receives blood from branches of the IMA. At the upper rectum this vessel is called the **superior hemorrhoidal (rectal) artery**. As it continues down the rectum the vessel splits, and branches move laterally and communicate with branches of the middle hemorrhoidal arteries. The distal rectum and anus are supplied by branches of **middle and inferior hemorrhoidal arteries.** As these vessels approach the internal iliac arteries and the bowel, they split into multiple communicating vessels.

The anus receives blood from two sources: branches of the lower hemorrhoidal plexus (inferior hemorrhoidal arteries) communicate with the middle hemorrhoidal arteries (as described previously) and with branches from the pudendal arteries. The pudendal arteries branch from the internal iliac arteries. Venous and lymphatic drainage goes to both mesenteric and systemic veins.

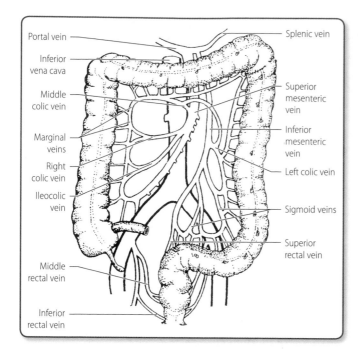

Portal vein

Inferior
vena cava

Middle
colic vein

Marginal
veins

Right
colic vein

Ileocolic
vein

Middle
rectal vein

Inferior
rectal vein

Splenic vein

Superior
mesenteric
vein

Inferior
mesenteric
vein

Left colic vein

Sigmoid veins

Superior
rectal vein

Figure 1.7 Venous drainage of the colon.

Nervous supply

The colon and rectum are richly innervated by multiple nerves whose function is poorly understood. The majority of efferent fibers to the intestine originate in the hypothalamus. The **parasympathetic efferent fibers** exit the central nervous system in two areas (cranial and sacral). The foregut is supplied via the **vagus nerves** and the hindgut fibers exit the sacral cord via the dorsal columns at sacral roots 2 through 4. Fibers from S3 and S4 are called the nervi erigentes [8]. After exiting the spinal cord, the fibers pass through a sacral plexus and then join with the hypogastric nerves (sympathetic nerves) to form the pelvic plexus. Parasympathetic nerves then pass upward in the inferior mesenteric plexus to be distributed to the superior hemorrhoidal artery and left colonic arteries. Other sacral fibers (S2–4) supply fibers to the levators, then enter the perineum via Alcock's canal as the pudendal nerve. At the anus the pudendal nerve becomes the hemorrhoidal nerve, perianal and dorsal penile nerve, or clitoral nerve.

The **sympathetic efferent nerves** exit the spinal cord at the thoracic and lumbar segments. The fibers pass through the splanchnic nerves to the mesenteric ganglia. Fibers then travel along the superior and inferior mesenteric arteries to reach the intestine. Additional fibers pass through the inferior hypogastric (pelvic) plexus, as previously described, to supply the rectum.

Afferent fibers from the intestine carry sensations of stretch, distention, and pain (anoxia or chemical damage) to the brain. The intestines are also affected by intrinsic innervation via the enteric plexus. These nerve cells and fibers are grouped into the **myenteric (Auerbach) plexus** and the **submucosal (Meissner) plexus**.

Bowel wall

The colon wall is composed of several layers (**Figure 1.8**). The innermost layer is the **mucosa**, a single layer of columnar cells with a cuticular border; it contains tubular pits and goblet cells. The **submucosa** is the strength layer of the bowel; this layer also contains blood vessels, lymphatics, Meissner's plexus, and solitary lymphatic nodules. There are two muscular layers: the inner layer, composed of muscle cells oriented in a circular fashion, and the outer layer of muscle, oriented in a linear fashion. In three areas the muscle fibers are thickened and fused to form the taeniae. The outermost layer is the **serosa**, which is composed of fibrous tissue.

The rectum contains layers similar to those of the colon, with two exceptions. The upper rectum contains a serosal covering on the anterior and lateral surface; however, this is lost as the rectum becomes extraperitoneal. The outer longitudinal muscle layer is thickened and diffused to form a solid sheet. The inner muscles are circular and, as described earlier, form three semicircular valves. The inner and outer muscles contribute fibers to the formation of the internal anal sphincter, as described previously.

The lining of the **anus** is composed of a transitional zone, where the mucosa changes from a columnar cell layer to a squamous cell layer at the dentate line. The area distal to the anal canal is lined by modified

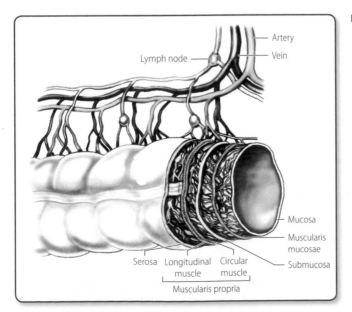

Figure 1.8 Bowel wall anatomy.

squamous epithelium without hair or glands [7]. Further caudally, the lining changes to squamous epithelium, with hair and glands at the anal verge.

The submucosa of the anal canal contains three bundles of vascular sinusoids, called hemorrhoidal tissue [9]. (For additional discussion of these structures, see Chapter 16.)

Rounds questions

1. How many taeniae does the colon have and what are their names?
2. How do you identify where the colon ends and the rectum starts?
3. Define the cranial and caudal boundaries of the anal canal.
4. What is the blood supply to the cecum?
5. The inferior mesenteric vein empties into what vessel?
6. What type of mucosa does the colon contain?
7. Which layer of the bowel is the strongest?
8. Which nerve roots supply the distal bowel?

References

1. Gray H, Goss CM. Anatomy of the Human Body. Philadelphia: Lea & Febiger 1974;1233.
2. Hollinshead WH. Anatomy for Surgeons: The thorax, abdomen, and pelvis. New York: Harper & Row 1971;676–718.
3. Goligher JC. Surgery of the Anus, Rectum, and Colon 5th ed. London: Baillière Tindall, 1984;1–47.
4. Netter F. Ciba Collection of Medical Illustrations, vol 3, part 11. Summit, NJ: Ciba-Geigy Corp 1962.
5. Gordon PH, Nivatvongs S (eds). Principles and Practice of Surgery for the Colon, Rectum, and Anus. St. Louis: Quality Medical Publishing 1992;3–38.
6. Jorge JMN, Habr-Gama A. Anatomy and embryology of the colon, rectum, and anus. In: Wolff BG, Fleshman JW. Beck DE, Pemberton JH, Wexner SD (eds). ASCRS Textbook of Colorectal Surgery. Springer-Verlag, New York 2007;1–22.
7. Phillips SF, Edwards DAW. Some aspects of anal continence and defecation. Gut 1965;6:396–406.
8. Pemberton JH. Anatomy and physiology of the anus and rectum. In: Beck DE, Wexner SD (eds). Fundamentals of Anorectal Surgery. New York:McGraw-Hill 1992;1–24.
9. Corman ML. Colon and Rectal Surgery 3rd ed. Philadelphia: JB Lippincott 1984;1–48.

Pathophysiology

Diseases related to bowel physiology are increasing in incidence. Effective treatment of these and other colorectal disorders depends on a sound understanding of basic physiology. In recent years, our knowledge of the physiology of the colon and anorectum has increased substantially. They are responsible for the storage, transport, processing, and timely expulsion of intestinal contents exiting the ileocecal valve. These functions depend on coordination of neural, hormonal, and muscular interactions both locally and centrally. This chapter reviews basic concepts in the physiology of the colon, rectum, and anus in a normal individual and briefly discusses the altered physiology of several disease states.

Colonic motility

Motility is of central importance when discussing colonic function. Although laypersons tend to categorize colonic motility as 'too fast,' 'too slow,' or 'just right,' the actual study of colonic motility physiology is more complex. Colonic motility is more difficult to study than small bowel motility because of the great regional heterogeneity in the colon and the intermittent and unpredictable nature of colonic contractile waves. Even the normal pattern of motility remains the subject of debate. This review of colonic motility is divided into sections on motor activity and myoelectric activity, although these functions are inextricably woven together in vivo. The coordinated process of defecation will be discussed later in the chapter.

Colonic motor activity

Our understanding of human colonic contractile activity was initially inferred from in vivo animal studies and then based on radiographic observations of ingested barium and radiopaque markers in the human colon and on manometric studies using balloon- or open-tipped catheters. To simplify a complex field of often conflicting evidence, it is helpful to refer to the work of Cannon [1] and Elliot and Barclay [2, 3] at the turn of the century, much of which has been confirmed by later investigators [4].

Contractions in the proximal colon are characterized by **antiperi-staltic waves** traveling from the midtransverse colon toward the cecum. These waves were initially described as having a fundamental frequency of 5.5 cycles/min, lasting for 2–8 minutes, with 10–15 minutes of inactivity between episodes [1]. These waves are more prominent in herbivores than omnivores and are thus thought to allow for return of complex polysaccharides toward the cecum for fermentation. They may also function to improve the efficiency of water and salt absorption in the proximal colon. The region extending from the midtransverse colon to the proximal rectosigmoid is characterized by **intermittent contractile waves** causing primarily segmental, nonpropulsive movement. There is, however, a slow net distal progression of feces toward the rectum. The proposed function of these segmental contractions is to mix the colonic contents to improve absorption.

The rectosigmoid and descending colon have been observed to have strong, organized contraction waves that propel a stool bolus distally through a long segment of colon. These so-called mass movements occur a few times daily and are associated with meals.

Colonic transit studies using radiopaque nonabsorbable markers reveal two areas of delayed colonic transit: the midtransverse colon and the rectosigmoid colon. The midtransverse colon is the area of transition where the proximal pattern of retrograde peristalsis changes to the distal pattern of antegrade peristalsis. For this reason, the midtransverse colon has been proposed to be the site of the **colonic pacemaker** [5]. The second area of transit delay is the rectosigmoid, referred to as the rectosigmoid sphincter of O'Beirne [6]. In the 19th century, O'Beirne and others proposed that the thickened muscularis of the sigmoid functioned as an anatomic sphincter and was the major determinant of fecal continence. Although there is not a true sphincter in the rectosigmoid, the delay in stool transit at this level may serve a purpose, since it enables more complete water and sodium absorption by the left colon [7].

Many factors affect colonic motility. Emotions such as hostility, anger, and resentment are associated with hypermotility, whereas anxiety and fear are associated with hypomotility. Exercise has been shown to increase both segmental and peristaltic colonic activity; sleep is a depressant of colonic motility. Mechanical colonic distention stimulates motility and is the basis for the effect of bulking laxatives. Nondigestible polysaccharides and cellulose derivatives absorb water and increase fecal mass, thus stimulating colonic propulsion [8].

As anyone who has hurried to the toilet after breakfast can attest, eating is a potent colonic stimulant. This **gastrocolic reflex,** as described by Hertz and Newton [9], involves increased motor and electrical activity in the colon and causes the urge to defecate after a meal. The exact mechanism of this response is not known, but various neural and hormonal mediators have been implicated [10,11]. Fatty meals appear to have a greater effect on colonic motility than carbohydrate or protein meals.

Colonic myoelectric activity

Although the electrical activity of gastric and small intestinal smooth muscle has been well documented, that of colonic smooth muscle remains less well defined. As in the stomach and small intestine, two types of electrical signals are generated in the colon: slow waves or slow electrical transients and spikes or rapid transients. Because of the difficulties in measuring electrical activity in the human colon, much controversy exists regarding the origin, frequency, and incidence of slow waves [9,12]. It is thought that several **slow wave pacemaker sites** are present in the colon, one being in the midtransverse colon corresponding to the site of origin of retrograde peristalsis (as discussed earlier) [5]. Although **slow wave activity** often leads to uncoordinated smooth muscle cell depolarization (phase unlocked), it may propagate in such a way that depolarization proceeds with a constant time lag along a directional gradient causing coordinated colonic contractions (phase locked) [8].

Colonic spike activity occurs either as short or long bursts. Clusters of spike bursts may migrate in either direction in the colon. Long spike bursts that migrate rapidly in a distal direction are associated with passing flatus or defecating [12]. The relationship of slow waves to spike activity is unclear.

Marker and scintigraphic studies

Measurement of colonic motor and myoelectric activity does not always correlate with **colonic transit,** because electrical and contractile waves do not always propagate distally. Thus measurement of colonic transit time does not involve measurement of colonic motor or myoelectric activity directly. The most common method involves ingestion of several radiopaque markers and sequential plain abdominal radiography. In individuals with normal gastrointestinal transit, the first markers are excreted at 36–48 hours, and 80% of the markers are excreted within 5 days. An alternate method involves ingestion of three different shaped radiopaque markers on 3 successive days, followed by plain abdominal radiography on the fourth day. If 24 markers are ingested on 3 successive days, the number of markers corresponds to the colonic transit time in hours. This method also permits the evaluation of transit through different areas of the colon [5].

Colonic transit has also been studied with nuclear scanning (scintigraphic) techniques. In one method, the patient ingests a capsule coated with pH-sensitive polymer containing indium 111 (^{111}In)-labeled isotope. The coating dissolves in the distal ileum and the radioactive material passes into the colon [13,14]. In another technique the patient ingests ^{111}In-labeled material with water and serial images are obtained with a gamma camera. Segmental transit is usually calculated for the right, left, and rectosigmoid portions of the colon. Results are expressed as the percentage of the total amount of isotope ingested in each segment at a point in time. The total percentage retained compared to normal is also calculated.

Colonic motility disorders

Perturbations in **colonic motility** are associated with a number of clinical disorders, including irritable bowel syndrome, diverticular disease, idiopathic megacolon, constipation, diarrhea, postoperative ileus, and colonic pseudo-obstruction. Some of these topics are covered in more detail elsewhere in this book.

Irritable bowel syndrome and diverticular disease

Irritable bowel syndrome is a disorder manifested by altered bowel habits and abdominal pain in the absence of other pathologic findings. Patients with a diagnosis of irritable bowel syndrome have been shown to have increased slow wave activity (3 cycles/min) in the rectosigmoid, corresponding to increased contractile activity at the same frequency [15,16]. A similar motility pattern has been noted in patients with diverticular disease, and some authors [8,17] have suggested that the underlying mechanism producing diverticula and irritable bowel syndrome is the same. Uncoordinated smooth muscle activity, followed by increased intraluminal pressure, may in part contribute to the pathogenesis of colonic diverticula [17].

It should be noted, however, that irritable bowel syndrome is a diagnosis of exclusion and has many different presentations. Thus caution should be exercised when interpreting studies of patients who carry the diagnosis, because these patients may have different causes of their symptoms.

Postoperative ileus

Postoperative ileus is a temporary impairment of intestinal motility after operation. Ileus is most commonly seen after laparotomy, but it may follow thoracotomy or other extraperitoneal procedures. In the past, the duration of postoperative ileus has been said to be proportional to the severity and duration of the surgical procedure. However, experimental evidence exists showing that the recovery of coordinated intestinal function is not influenced by either the magnitude or the length of an operative procedure [18,19]. The shorter period of ileus noted after laparoscopic gastrointestinal procedures has lent further credence to this concept.

A growing body of evidence implicates the colon, primarily the distal colon, as the most persistent site of postoperative ileus. Studies by Condon et al [19, 20] in monkeys and humans have shown that recovery from ileus is faster in the stomach and small bowel than in the colon and that the right colon recovers more rapidly than the left colon. The sequential return of motility in different segments of the gastrointestinal tract after operation may explain why a patient may have active bowel sounds postoperatively and yet have persistent colonic ileus, and a trial of oral feeding fails (see Chapter 10).

The pathogenesis of postoperative ileus is unclear. Several theories exist that attempt to explain the mechanism of ileus, including sympathetic hyperactivity inhibiting bowel motility, peritoneal irritation caused by foreign material, electrolyte imbalance, and the effects of anesthetics and narcotic analgesics. The traditional view of the effect of the autonomic nervous system on the intestine consisted of a prokinetic, secretagogue action of the parasympathetic system and an inhibitory, antisecretory action of the sympathetic system. Using this concept, investigators have tried to shorten the duration of ileus with adrenergic blockade and parasympathetic stimulation [21–23]. The results have been mixed. Although the treatment has simple physiologic appeal, part of the lack of consistent success can be attributed to the complexity of the body's control of intestinal motility, which includes the effects of a plethora of intestinal hormones, such as vasoactive inhibitory peptide, motilin, peptide YY, cholecystokinin, and neuropeptide Y [5].

Electrolyte imbalances are thought to play a role in the prolongation of ileus. Hypokalemia, in particular, has been shown to reduce colonic contractile activity in monkeys [24]. Anesthesia was once thought to cause postoperative ileus. Although inhaled anesthetics, specifically enflurane and halothane, have been shown to reduce contractions in the colon, the effect is short lived and is rapidly reversed by cessation of the anesthetic [25]. Nitrous oxide has no effect on colonic contractile activity [25]. Narcotics have been shown to depress colonic motility, although not in a uniform fashion. Low doses of morphine increase the number of non-migrating random colonic contractions. Higher doses of morphine, however, inhibit colonic electrical and contractile activity [19, 26, 27]. This narcotic effect may play a major role in the postoperative ileus seen after major laparotomies. The use of colonic μ receptor agonists (alvimopan [Entereg] Adolor, Eaton, PA, USA) has been shown to reduce the incidence and duration of postoperative ileus [14]. Epidural morphine does not directly affect colonic motility, suggesting that the opioid receptors in the spinal cord do not control intestinal motility [26].

Colonic pseudo-obstruction (Ogilvie's syndrome)

Intestinal pseudo-obstruction, a profound ileus without evidence of mechanical obstruction, was first described by Ingelfinger in 1943 [28]. The first description of the colonic variant of pseudo-obstruction is thought to be Sir Heneage Ogilvie's 1948 report of two cases associated with malignant infiltration of the celiac plexus [29]. Colonic pseudo-obstruction is associated with neuroleptic medications, opiates, malignancy, and severe metabolic illness. One mechanism thought to play a role in its pathogenesis is sympathetic overactivity overriding the parasympathetic system. This concept is supported by anecdotal reports of success with epidural anesthesia [30], which paralyzes the sympathetic afferent and efferent nerve fibers to the colon, and with neostigmine [31], which increases parasympathetic tone by its anticholinesterase effect. Colonoscopic decompression remains a primary treatment modality [5].

Water and electrolyte transport

Absorption

The major absorptive function of the colon is the final regulation of water and electrolyte balance in the intestine, deemed colonic salvage.

The colon reduces the volume of enteric contents by absorbing greater than 90% of the water and electrolytes presented to it. On average, this accounts for 1 or 2 L of fluid and 200 mEq of sodium and chloride per day. During a 24-hour period, 8 L of fluid enters the jejunum. In healthy individuals, the small bowel absorbs about 6.5 L and the colon 1.4 L, leaving 0.1 L of normal **fecal water** content. Under maximum conditions, the colon can absorb 5–6 L of fluid a day. Only if small bowel absorption is reduced to less than 2 L a day is colonic salvage overwhelmed, and the resultant increase in fecal water content manifested as diarrhea [5].

The colon is able to absorb **sodium** against high concentration gradients, especially in the distal colon, which shares many basic cellular mechanisms of sodium and water transport with the distal convoluted tubule of the kidney [32]. The colonic response to aldosterone stimulation may be an important compensatory mechanism during dehydration.

Although active absorption of nutrients is minimal, the colon can passively absorb short-chain fatty acids formed by intraluminal bacterial fermentation of unabsorbed carbohydrates. This can account for up to 540 kcal per day of assimilated calories. The absorbed **short-chain fatty acids,** principally butyrate, are the major fuel sources of the colonic epithelium [33–35]. Evidence exists that short-chain fatty acid metabolism is impaired in patients with ulcerative colitis [36–41] and that intraluminal infusion of short-chain fatty acids can be of benefit in patients with colitis [42]. Short-chain fatty acids have also been shown to be effective in treating diversion colitis, implicating colonocyte nutritional deficiency as the cause of this disorder [43–44].

Secretion

In healthy persons the colon absorbs water, sodium, and chloride while secreting potassium and bicarbonate. Potassium transport in the colon is mainly passive along an electrochemical gradient generated by the active transport of sodium. Bicarbonate is exchanged with chloride by an electroneutral mechanism [45].

A number of agents can stimulate fluid and electrolyte secretion in the colon, including bacteria, enterotoxins, hormones, neurotransmitters, and laxatives. The diarrhea associated with *Shigella* and *Salmonella* infection is caused by diminished absorption or increased secretion of water, sodium, and chloride. Intestinal hormones, particularly vasoactive intestinal polypeptide (VIP), have been shown to have significant effects on colonic absorption and secretion. Prostaglandins play a role in the pathogenesis of diarrhea associated with ulcerative colitis and several laxatives [8].

Any sort of irritation to the colon can cause increased secretion, which results in diarrhea. Common causes of this sort of diarrhea include bile salt malabsorption after resection of the terminal ileum and long-chain fatty acid malabsorption in steatorrhea. The induced colonic mucus and fluid are high in potassium and may result in potassium depletion in chronic cases.

Bacterial barrier

The human colon is sterile at birth, but within a matter of hours the intestine is colonized from the environment in an oral to anal direction. Bacteroides, destined to be the dominant bacteria in the colon, is first noted at about 10 days after birth. By 3–4 weeks after birth, the characteristic stool flora is established and persists into adult life. An individual's pattern of bacterial flora most closely resembles that of his or her mother.

The bacterial population of the colon is a complex collection of aerobic and anaerobic microorganisms. Nearly one third of the fecal dry weight consists of viable bacteria, with as many as 10^{10}–10^{12} bacteria present per gram of feces. Anaerobic bacteria dominate the flora by as much as 10,000 : 1 over aerobic organisms, but the mixture is diverse, with as many as 400 different species cultured from the stool of one individual. Knowledge of the types of normal colonic bacteria is of paramount importance to the surgeon who must use this information to guide the selection of antibiotic therapy, both for prophylaxis and treatment.

Intestinal gas

Nitrogen, oxygen, carbon dioxide, hydrogen, and methane make up 99% of all the gas in the intestine [42]. Nitrogen and oxygen are found in the atmosphere and appear in the colon by means of swallowing air. Hydrogen, methane, and carbon dioxide are produced by bacterial fermentation of carbohydrates and proteins in the colon. An eminent flatologist, Levitt [46], has shown that most patients who complain of excessive flatus have high concentrations of hydrogen and carbon dioxide in their intestinal gas. Since carbon dioxide is an end-product of bacterial fermentation, therapy consists of diet manipulation to decrease the amount of ingested carbohydrates, especially lactose, wheat, and potatoes.

One of the most important points for the surgeon to remember is the explosive nature of hydrogen and methane. Opening unprepared colon with an electrocautery device can have dramatic and disastrous consequences.

Anorectal physiology

Fecal continence is the ability to defer the urge to defecate until a socially convenient time and place can be found. Many factors are involved in fecal continence, including anal canal pressures generated by the sphincter mechanism, anorectal angle formed by the pelvic floor musculature, anorectal sensation, rectal compliance, anorectal reflexes, colonic transit, and stool volume and consistency. This section focuses on the anorectal mechanisms that contribute to fecal continence.

Anal canal pressures and anal sphincters

The internal and external anal sphincters surround the anal canal and are responsible for maintaining resting pressure and generating squeeze pressures. The internal anal sphincter is composed of smooth muscle and is tonically contracted at rest. It contributes about 85% of the **resting tone** of the anal canal. Dividing the internal anal sphincter in the presence of an intact external anal sphincter weakens anal tone but does not abolish it [47]. The external anal sphincter is one of the only striated muscles in the body that maintains a constant tone. External anal sphincter tone is maintained during the day and, to a lesser extent, during sleep.

Anal canal squeeze pressures are generated by the puborectalis muscle and the external anal sphincter, which are under voluntary control. Squeeze pressures are more than twice the resting pressure during maximum effort. Maximum squeeze pressure can be maintained for less than 1 minute; the sphincter rapidly fatigues after that time.

The sphincter mechanism is not symmetric. Anal manometric measurements have shown that resting pressures posteriorly are highest proximally and lowest near the anal verge [48]. Anterior resting pressures vary between the sexes, being highest distally in women and highest proximally in men [49]. Squeeze pressures are also asymmetric. The high-pressure zone of the anal sphincter is located distal to the midpoint of the sphincter (**Figure 2.1**). A transition from posterior predominance to anterior predominance occurs as one travels from proximal to distal in the anal canal [50].

The relative contributions of the internal and external anal sphincters to maintaining continence has been the subject of some debate. At one

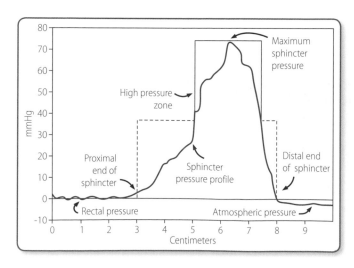

Figure 2.1 Characteristics of a typical longitudinal pressure profile of the resting anorectal sphincter. Pressures have been equated to a zero rectal pressure. The pressures from an eight-channel multilumen probe during continuous resting pullout have been averaged at each point along the sphincter by microcomputer. (From Coller JA. Clinical application of anorectal manometry. Gastroenterol Clin North Am 1987;16:20. With permission.)

time, it was thought that the internal anal sphincter was not important in continence because of the reflex relaxation of the internal sphincter that occurs with rectal distention, the **rectoanal inhibitory reflex** [51] (see p. 23). However, after surgeons found that complete division of the internal sphincter for treatment of anal fissure resulted in a 40% risk of soiling or incontinence for flatus or liquid stool [52], this view was modified. Loss of internal anal sphincter function can he compensated for by intact and well-functioning external anal sphincter and puborectalis muscles. However, if these muscles weaken with age or are subsequently injured, incontinence may result [53].

The external anal sphincter is important in maintaining continence. In one study [54], a persistent defect of the external anal sphincter by ultrasonography was associated with a 50% prevalence of incontinence to flatus or stool in patients who underwent primary suture repair of obstetric sphincter injuries. Further evidence of the role of the external sphincter in continence comes from the good results achieved by direct sphincteroplasty in incontinent patients with simple defects of the external anal sphincter [55].

Anorectal angle

Another mechanism that helps to maintain fecal continence is the configuration of the pelvic floor, formed predominantly by the anterior pull of the **puborectalis muscle** at the level of the anorectal ring, producing the anorectal angle (**Figure 2.2**). The angle is between 60° and 105° at rest and becomes more acute during squeeze and more obtuse during defecation. The **flap valve theory,** proposed by Parks et al [56], suggests that the puborectalis pulls the anorectal junction anteriorly and that increases in abdominal pressure seal the anterior wall to the posterior wall of the anal canal (**Figure 2.3**). A Valsalva maneuver

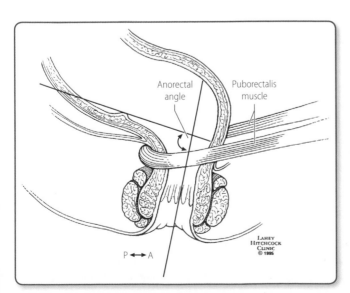

Anorectal angle

Puborectalis muscle

P ←→ A

LAHEY
HITCHCOCK
CLINIC
© 1995

Figure 2.2 The anorectal angle is formed by the anterior pull of the puborectalis muscle. The angle is measured at the intersection of lines drawn through the center of the anal canal and along the posterior wall of the rectum. The angle is 60–105° at rest and becomes more acute during squeeze and more obtuse during defecation. (Courtesy of the Lahey Hitchcock Clinic.)

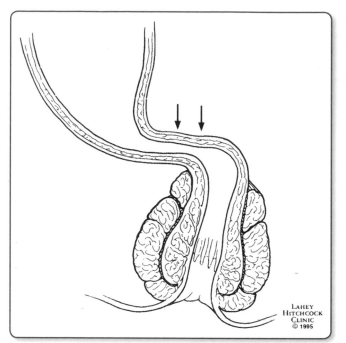

Figure 2.3 The 'flap valve' effect: the effect of the of the puborectalis pulling the rectum anteriorly during squeeze, thereby permitting intra-abdominal pressures during the Valsalva maneuver to close off the rectum. (Courtesy of the Lahey Hitchcock Clinic.)

Lahey
Hitchcock
Clinic
© 1995

would thus occlude the lumen and protect the lower anal canal from the transmission of pressure and leakage of stool. The flap valve theory and the contribution of the anorectal angle to maintaining continence are controversial, however. Bartolo et al [57] demonstrated that during maximum Valsalva maneuver, the anterior wall remains separate from the posterior wall and the lumen remains patent in normal subjects. Although the flap valve theory may not be entirely accurate, the puborectalis is an important part of the continence mechanism. This is illustrated by the fact that division of the puborectalis in the treatment of constipation is associated with a high degree of incontinence of flatus and liquid stool [58].

The **flutter valve theory,** proposed by Phillips and Edwards [59], suggests that the puborectalis flattens the walls of the rectum from side to side and creates a slitlike opening in the pelvic floor. They proposed that sudden increases in abdominal pressure force the opposing walls of the proximal anorectal canal together, thus helping to maintain fecal continence (**Figure 2.4**). Anteroposterior and lateral images of the barium paste-coated rectum tend to support this view.

Anorectal sensation

Sensory mechanisms exist that permit discrimination of the character of rectal contents (stool, liquid, or gas) and of the need to expel that content. These sensory receptors are located in the rectal muscularis, in the surrounding muscles of the pelvic floor, and/or in the anal canal mucosa [47]. A **sampling response** occurs in which transient relaxation

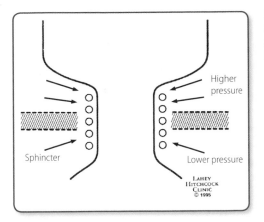

Figure 2.4 The 'flutter valve' effect: the effect of increasing intra-abdominal pressure causes the walls of the anorectum to flatten together. (Courtesy Lahey Hitchcock Clinic.)

of the upper part of the internal sphincter permits rectal contents to come into contact with the sensory epithelium of the proximal anal canal (the anal transition zone) for assessment of the nature of rectal content [60, 61]. The ultimate importance of the sampling response is a matter of debate, however, since patients undergoing proctectomy and ileoanal anastomosis retain the ability to discriminate gas from stool, yet do not show evidence of a sampling response [62]. Furthermore, anesthetizing the anal canal mucosa has been shown not to affect continence to large-volume saline solution enemas [63].

Rectal compliance

The rectum accommodates passively to distention. As intraluminal volume increases, intraluminal pressure remains low. In healthy individuals the rectum can accommodate a maximum tolerable volume of 400 mL while pressure remains low, less than 20 mmHg [47]. The rectum is also thought to have an accommodation response, which consists of receptive relaxation of the rectal ampulla to accommodate a fecal bolus [45]. Disease states that alter rectal compliance, such as inflammatory bowel disease and radiation proctitis, may result in frequency, urgency, tenesmus, and incontinence as the rectum loses its ability to distend and becomes a stiff conduit.

Reflexes

A number of involuntary reflexes involve the anal sphincters. Testing of these reflexes may assist in evaluation of pelvic floor innervation. As mentioned earlier, the **rectoanal inhibitory reflex** is relaxation of the internal anal sphincter and brief contraction of the external anal sphincter with distention of the rectum. Rapid intermittent rectal distention causes prolonged relaxation of the internal anal sphincter, whereas continuous rectal distention initially causes internal anal sphincter relaxation, but the muscle gradually returns to its resting tone over time [64]. First described by Gowers in 1877 [66], this reflex is probably mediated by means of intramural nerve plexuses as it persists in patients with spinal cord and sacral nerve root lesions. The reflex is absent in patients with Hirschsprung's disease and may be used as an adjunct to rectal biopsy to make this diagnosis [64].

The **anocutaneous reflex** consists of a visible contraction, the so-called anal wink, with stimulation of the perianal skin. The pudendal nerve supplies both the afferent and efferent pathways through sacral segments S1–S4. Testing of this reflex is useful when evaluating a patient for fecal incontinence, because it can give information about pudendal nerve function. The bulbocavernosus reflex consists of contraction of the bulbocavernosus muscle, external anal sphincter, and urethral sphincter with stimulation of the glans penis or clitoris. The **vesicoanal reflex** is inhibition of external anal sphincter activity and increased internal anal sphincter activity during micturition.

Defecation

Defecation commonly begins with distention of the left colon by stool. Although the individual may not be aware of any discomfort, the colon responds to this distention by generating mass movement waves that carry the stool from the descending and sigmoid colon into the rectum. The rectal distention may or may not be sensed by the individual if the amount of stool entering the rectum is small. The reflex response to rectal distention is inhibition of the internal anal sphincter and contraction of the external anal sphincter.

If it is a socially acceptable time for defecation, the individual assumes a squatting or seated position. This action straightens the anorectal angle and facilitates passage of stool. Intrarectal and intra-abdominal pressures then rise, resulting in reflex relaxation of the external and internal anal sphincters and puborectalis muscles. A conscious relaxation of the external anal sphincter also occurs. Some individuals may pass stool without straining. Others, however, must strain to initiate rectal emptying. Straining causes the external and internal anal sphincters and puborectalis muscles to relax further. If mass movement peristalsis occurs simultaneously with rectal emptying, the entire left colon may be emptied. If not, the bowel is evacuated in piecemeal fashion. At the end of defecation, the pelvic floor musculature, sphincters, and anorectal angle return to their normal configuration.

If rectal distention occurs at an inopportune time, the rectoanal inhibitory reflex provides brief automatic protection by means of contraction of the external anal sphincter. Continued voluntary squeeze of the external sphincter permits further deferment of defecation. This mechanism alone would soon fail because of the rapid fatigue of skeletal muscle were it not for the rapid, receptive relaxation of the rectum. The accommodation response of the rectum permits the external sphincter to relax after the pressure in the rectum has decreased. At this point both the awareness of stool in the rectum and the urge to defecate decrease. The accommodation response can be overwhelmed, however, if the volume of stool coming into the rectum is great or if the rectum is already near maximum distention, as in the case of fecal impaction.

Rounds questions

1. What is the function of segmental colonic contractions?
2. Where is the proposed site of the colonic pacemaker?
3. What is postoperative ileus?
4. What is intestinal pseudo-obstruction (Ogilvie's syndrome)?
5. What does the colon absorb and secrete?
6. Which muscle is mainly responsible for the resting tone of the anal sphincter?
7. What is the sampling response?
8. What disease is associated with an absence of the rectoanal inhibitory reflex?

References

1. Cannon W. The movements of the intestine studied by means of roentgen rays. Am J Physiol 1902;6:251–77.
2. Barclay A. Radiological studies of the large intestine. Br J Surg 1915;2:638–52.
3. Elliot T, Barclay S. Antiperistalsis and other activities of the colon. J Physiol 1904;31:272–303.
4. Ritchie J. Colonic motor activity and bowel function. Gut 1968;9:442–56.
5. Armstrong D, Ballantyne G. Physiology of the small and large intestines. In: Mazier W, Luchtefeld M, Levien D, Senagore A (eds). Surgery of the Colon, Rectum, and Anus. Philadelphia: WB Saunders, 1995;40–65.
6. Ballantyne G. Rectosigmoid sphincter of O'Beirne. Dis Colon Rectum 1986;29:525–31.
7. Debongnie J, Phillips S. Capacity of the human colon to absorb fluid. Gastroenterology 1978;74:698–703.
8. Frantzides CT. Physiology of the colon. In: Condon R (ed). Colon, vol 4. In: Zuidema G (ed). Shackelford's Surgery of the Alimentary Tract, 4th ed. Philadelphia: WB Saunders, 1995;17–22.
9. Hertz A, Newton A. The normal movements of the colon in man. J Physiol 1913;45:57.
10. Snape W, Matarazzo S, Cohen S. Effect of eating and gastrointestinal hormones on human colonic myoelectric and motor activity. Gastroenterology 1978;75:373–8.
11. Strom J, Condon R, Schulte W, Cowles V, Go V. Glucagon, gastric inhibitory polypeptide and the gastrocolic response. Am J Surg 1982;143:155–9.
12. Frantzides C, Condon R, Cowles V. Early postoperative colon electrical response activity. Surg Forum 1985;36:163–5.
13. Hull TL. Physiology: colonic. In: Wolff BG, Fleshman JW, Beck DE, Pemberton JH, Wexner SD (eds). ASCRS Textbook of Colorectal Surgery. New York, Springer-Verlag 2007:23–32.
14. Scott SM, Knowles CH, Newell M, et al. Scintigraphic assessment of colonic transit in women with slow-transit constipation arising de novo following pelvic surgery or childbirth. Br J Surg 2001;88:405–11.
15. Snape W, Carlson G, Matarazzo S, Cohen S. Evidence that abnormal myoelectrical activity produces colonic motor dysfunction in the irritable bowel syndrome. Gastroenterology 1977;72:383–7.
16. Taylor I, Darby C, Hammond P. Comparison of rectosigmoid myoelectriccal activity in the irritable colon syndrome during relapses and remissions. Gut 1978;19:923–29.
17. Painter N, Truelove S, Ardran G, Tuckey M. Segmentation and the localization of intraluminal pressures in the human colon, with special reference to the pathogenesis of colonic diverticula. Gastroenterology 1965;49:169–77.
18. Graber J, Schulte W, Condon R, Cowles V. Relationship of duration of postoperative ileus to

extent and site of operative dissection. Surgery 1982;92:87–92.

19. Condon R, Cowles V, Schulte W, et al. Resolution of postoperative ileus in humans. Ann Surg 1986;203:574–81.

20. Woods J, Erickson L, Condon R, Schulte W, Sillin L. Postoperative ileus: a colonic problem? Surgery 1978;54:527–33.

21. Heimbeck D, Crout J. Treatment of paralytic ileus with adrenergic neuronal blocking drugs. Surgery 1971;69:582–87.

22. Neely J, Catchpole B. The restoration of alimentary tract motility by pharmacological means. Br J Surg 1971;58:21–8.

23. Catchpole B. Ileus: Use of sympathetic blocking agents in its treatment. Surgery 1969;66:811–20.

24. Schulte W, Cowles V, Condon R. Hypokalemia and the gastrocolic response [abst]. Dig Dis Sci 1984;29:551.

25. Condon R, Cowles V, Ekbom G, Schulte W, Hess G. Effects of halothane, enflurane and nitrous oxide on colon motility. Surgery 1987;101:61–85.

26. Frantzides C, Cowles V, Salaymeh B, Tekin E, Condon R. Morphine effects on human colonic myoelectric activity in the postoperative period. Am J Surg 1992;163:144–9.

27. Frantzides C, Condon R, Schulte W, Cowles V. Effects of morphine on colonic myoelectric activity in subhuman primates. Am J Physiol 1990;21:247–52.

28. Ingelfinger E. The diagnosis of sprue in nontropical cases. N Engl J Med 1943;228:180–4.

29. Ogilvie H. Large intestinal colic due to sympathetic deprivation: a new clinical syndrome. Br Med J 1948;2:671–3.

30. Lee J, Taylor B, Singleton B. Epidural anesthesia for acute pseudo-obstruction of the colon (Ogilvie's syndrome). Dis Colon Rectum 1988;31:666–91.

31. Stephenson B, Morgan A, Salaman J, Wheeler M. Ogilvie's syndrome: a new approach to an old problem. Dis Colon Rectum 1995;38:424–7.

32. Frizzel R, Schults S. Effect of aldosterone on ion transport by rabbit colon in vitro. J Membr Biol 1978;39:1–26.

33. Cummings J. Short chain fatty acids in the human colon. Gut 1981;22:763–9.

34. Clausen M, Mortensen P. Kinetic studies on the metabolism of short chain fatty acids and glucose by isolated rat colonocytes. Gastroenterology 1994;108:423–32.

35. Roediger W. Role of anaerobic bacteria in the metabolic welfare of the colonic mucosa in man. Gut 1980;21:793–8.

36. Chapman M, Grahn M, Boyle M. Butyrate oxidation is impaired in the colonic mucosa of sufferers of quiescent ulcerative colitis. Gut 1994;35:73–6.

37. Chapman M, Grahn M, Hutton M, Williams N. Butyrate metabolism in the terminal ileal mucosa of patients with ulcerative colitis. Br J Surg 1995;82:36–8.

38. Roediger W. The colonic epithelium in ulcerative colitis: an energy-deficient disease? Lancet 1980;2:712–5.

39. Roediger W. The starved colon-diminished mucosal nutrition, diminished absorption, and colitis. Dis Colon Rectum 1990;33:858–62.

40. Vernia P, Gnaedinger A, Hauck W, Breuer R. Organic anions and the diarrhea of inflammatory bowel disease. Dig Dis Sci 1988;33:1353–8.

41. Vernia P, Caprilli R, Latella G, Fecal lactate and ulcerative colitis. Gastroenterology 1988;95:1564–8.

42. Senagore A, MacKeigan J, Scheider M, Ehrom S. Short-chain fatty acid enemas: A cost-effective alternative in the treatment of nonspecific proctosigmoiditis. Dis Colon Rectum 1992;35:923–7.

43. Harig J, Soergel K, Komorowski R, Wood C. Treatment of diversion colitis with short chain fatty acid irrigation. N Engl J Med 1989;320: 23–8.

44. Kissmeyer-Nielsen P, Mortensen F, Laurherg S, Hessov I. Transmural trophic effect of short chain fatty acid infusions on atrophic, defunctioned rat colon. Dis Colon Rectum 1995;38:946–51.

45. Schouten W, Gordon PH. Physiology. In: Gordon PH, Navatvongs S (eds). Principles and Practice of Surgery for the Colon, Rectum, and Anus. St. Louis: Quality Medical Publishing, 1992;39–79.

46. Levitt M. Intestinal gas production - recent advances in flatology. N Engl J Med 1980;302:1474–5.

47. Pemherton J, Meagher A. Anatomy and physiology of the anus and rectum. In: Condon R: (ed). Colon, vol 4. In: Zuidema G (ed). Shackelford's Surgery of the Alimentary Tract, 4th ed. Philadelphia: WB Saunders, 1995;275–309.

48. Coller J. Clinical application of anorectal manometry. Gastroenterol Clin North Am 1987;16:17–33.

49. McHugh S, Diamant N. Anal canal pressure profile: a reappraisal as determined by rapid pullthrough technique. Gut 1987;28:1234–41.

50. Taylor B, Beart RJ, Phillips S. Longitudinal and radial variations of pressure in the human anal sphincter. Gastroenterology 1984;86:693–7.

51. Goligher J, Hughes E. Sensibility of the rectum and colon: its role in the mechanism of anal continence. Lancet 1951;1:543–8.

52. Bennett R, Goligher J. Results of internal sphincterotomy for anal fissure. Br Med J 1962;2:1500–3.

53. Rasmussen O. Anorectal function. Dis Colon Rectum 1994;37:386–403.

54. Nielsen M, Hauge C, Rasmussen O, Pedersen J, Christiansen J. Anal endosonographic findings in the follow-up of primarily sutured sphincteric ruptures. Br J Surg 1992;79:104–6.

55. Jorge J, Wexner S. Etiology and management of fecal incontinence. Dis Colon Rectum 1993;36:77–97.

56. Parks A, Porter N, Hardcastle J. The syndrome of the descending perineum, Proc R Soc Med 1966;59:477–82.

57. Bartolo D, Roe A, Locke-Edwards J, Virjee J, Mortensen N. Flap-valve theory of anorectal continence. Br J Surg 1986;73:1012–4.

58. Barnes P, Hawley P, Preston D, Lennard-Jones J. Experience of posterior division of the puborectalis muscle in the management of chronic constipation. Br J Surg 1985;72:475–7.

59. Phillips S, Edwards D. Some aspects of anal incontinence and defecation. Gut 1965;6:396–406.

60. Duthie H, Bennett R. The relation of sensation in the anal canal to the functional anal sphincter. A possible factor in anal continence. Gut 1963;4:179–82.

61. Miller R, Bartolo D, Cervero F, Mortensen N. Anorectal temperature sensation: a comparison of normal and incontinent patients. Br J Surg 1987;74:511–5.

62. Beart RJ, Dozois R, Wolff B, Pemberton J. Mechanisms of rectal continence: lessons from the ileoanal procedure. Am J Surg 1985;149:31–4.

63. Read M, Read N. The role of anorectal sensation in preserving continence. Gut 1982;23:345–7.

64. Burleigh D, D'Mello A. Physiology and pharmacology of the internal anal sphincter. In: Henry M, Swash M (eds). Coloproctology and the Pelvic Floor. Cambridge: Cambridge University Press, 1985;22–41.

65. Gowers W. The autonomic action of the sphincter ani. Proc R Soc Med 1877;26:77–84.

3 History and physical examination

A compassionately taken and thorough history, complemented by a directed but gentle physical examination, is usually more revealing than a battery of sophisticated diagnostic tests in evaluating the patient with colorectal and anal complaints. Disorders of this 'unmentionable' part of the body are often embarrassing for the patient to discuss and require great tact on the part of the examiner. This chapter focuses on features of the patient encounter that are unique to the colorectal patient.

History

The value of a carefully taken history cannot be overemphasized. It often uncovers pieces of the puzzle that allow for proper diagnosis. One of the rewards in medicine is finding on physical examination the problem that was suspected on taking the history [1].

Present illness

The patient should first be asked to describe the problem in his or her own words. Duration of symptoms is important; incontinence may date to the birth of a child, possibly signifying an obstetric sphincter injury. When did the patient first notice his or her symptom? Exacerbating or alleviating circumstances should be sought, as should prior treatment attempts. Is this the first episode, or is it a recurring problem? Questions need to direct the patient to the present circumstance and should be tailored to the age and educational level of the patient.

Pain is the presenting symptom of many disorders. Abdominal complaints are often nonspecific; colonic distention causes hypogastric pain, whereas rectal conditions may be felt in the sacral or perineal areas. Crampy, colicky pain usually accompanies obstruction, possibly from a tumor, or excessive contraction of the colon, seen with diarrheal illnesses. Inflammatory conditions such as diverticulitis may cause peritoneal irritation, which is more readily localized, since this type of pain is carried by the somatic inervation. Discomfort that is worsened by hitting bumps during the car ride to the examination often signifies peritoneal irritation. It is important to uncover associated initiating or relieving factors such as relief with passage of stool or flatus and changes in symptoms with posture or medication. In women, pain that is cyclical with menses may be caused by endometriosis. Finally, the character of the pain (sharp, dull), any movement (radiation), and intensity are explored.

To many patients, any anorectal condition is caused by 'hemorrhoids'. The nature of the discomfort should be elicited. Sharp pain that follows a bowel movement is indicative of a fissure, whereas a throbbing pain often accompanies an abscess. Tenesmus, the urge to defecate, is found in inflammatory or neoplastic conditions. Swelling may represent hemorrhoids or rectal prolapse [2]. Bleeding is often quite worrisome to patients but usually represents benign disease. Is the blood bright red, dark blue, accompanied by clots, mixed with stool, or is it on the toilet tissue only (denoting an anal source)? Melena usually denotes a proximal source but may come from the right colon. Bloody diarrhea is seen in inflammatory or ischemic colitis; a combination of blood and mucus suggests neoplasia.

No evaluation of colorectal complaints is complete without an inquiry into bowel habits. Consistency, frequency, and size of stool as well as recent changes should be noted. What is the patient's normal bowel pattern? What has changed? Constipation, the infrequent bowel movement, should be distinguished from regular bowel movements that are hard to pass. Any maneuvers that the patient performs, such as abdominal or vaginal pressure or digitalization, need to be sought out. The degree of incontinence is assessed and one should determine whether the patient is incontinent of flatus or liquid or solid stool as well as the number of incontinent episodes per day. The ability to sense stool in the rectum but inability to reach the toilet in time is differentiated from incontinence without warning. The relation of any changes to events such as childbirth, pelvic surgery, or irradiation or conditions such as diabetes is also important [3].

Review of systems

A brief systems review is useful in evaluating the colorectal patient. Unexpected weight loss may herald an underlying malignancy. Inflammatory bowel disease can manifest itself by a number of extraintestinal complaints – arthritis, uveitis, skin lesions, or jaundice. Recent travel to areas of poor sanitation could explain new-onset diarrhea. A tactful exploration of sexual contacts and practices may be warranted. Dietary practices and any recent changes are documented. Symptoms of systemic diseases that may have an intestinal component are also reviewed. Weight gain, letheragy, and constipation might suggest hypothyroidism, whereas weight loss, rapid heart rate, skin changes, and diarrhea could result from hyperthyroidism.

Past medical history

A survey of the patient's medical history should he included, with particular attention to prior colorectal problems, previous abdominal and anorectal operations, difficult labor or childbirth, and prior infections. Current prescription and over-the-counter medications must be reviewed. Laxative use or abuse is important to ascertain. Previous radiation therapy to the pelvis for gynecologic, prostatic, or rectal malignancy may explain certain symptoms, such as tenesmus. A recent course of antibiotic therapy could he the cause of diarrhea.

Immunosuppression from steroidal medications or antirejection medications, chemotherapy, or AIDS can make conditions that are usually easily managed life threatening [4]. Medical conditions such as diabetes or thyroid abnormalities can produce intestinal problems.

Family history

A pertinent family history must be included in the patient interview. Familial adenomatous polyposis (FAP) is an inherited condition of colonic polyps that leads to early colorectal carcinoma. It is inherited in an autosomal dominant pattern; screening of family members should begin at age 10. Sporadic colorectal carcinomas (those without an inherited or identified cause) also show a familial tendency, especially for first-degree relatives (parents, siblings, or children) [5]. Periodic colonoscopic screening is currently recommended for patients beginning at the age of 50 years, or 10 years before the age at which their relative was diagnosed with colorectal cancer (whichever comes first). When a positive family history involves multiple family members over two or more generations, the possibility of an inherited cancer syndrome must be considered [6].

The two inherited colorectal cancer syndromes are FAP (previously desribed) and the much more common hereditary non-polyposis colorectal cancer (HNPCC). As many as 9% of patients with colorectal cancer may have HNPCC [6]. While FAP has the diagnostic findings of colonic polyposis, HNPCC is usually diagnosed on the basis of the family history using the Amsterdam or Bethesda criteria [7, 9]. Patients with HNPCC also have an associated increased risk of gynecologic and urinary tract cancers. Patients with HNPCC have a 70% lifetime risk of developing colorectal cancer and a 90% risk of developing one of the HNPCC-related cancers [6]. First-degree relatives (parents, siblings, and children) of patients with HNPCC have a 50% risk of also having the syndrome. Patients with HNPCC and their at-risk relatives need frequent screening for colorectal and associated malignancies. Some patients may also choose prophylactic surgery.

A history of more distant relatives with colorectal cancer or a history of sporadic polyps in a close relative does add risk but it is not as high as that with a first degree relative. Inflammatory bowel disease may also show a tendency to run in families. Do other family members or close associates have similar symptoms?

Physical examination

Physical assessment begins as soon as the patient is seen. Is the patient uncomfortable walking or sitting? Are the clothes too loose, from recent weight loss, or too tight, from abdominal distention? Is the skin discolored from jaundice or renal failure? Does the face show the effects of long-term steroid use? Much about the patient's overall state of health can be gleaned from careful observation during the interview.

Abdominal examination

A complete abdominal examination is indicated in all patients with new complaints and as part of routine cancer follow-up. It should consist of inspection, auscultation, percussion, and palpation. This section will not describe examination techniques in detail but will focus on key points for the evaluation of colorectal patients. The patient is positioned flat on the examination table, with the entire abdomen and the inguinal region accessible. The contour of the abdomen as well as any surgical scars and stomas should be noted. Auscultation may assess the timbre and vigor of bowel sounds. Bowel sounds result from muscular contraction of bowel that contains air and fluid. Shaking a water bottle that is completely filled produces no sound; however, if the bottle is half filled, sound will be produced. Some patients with ileus may have no sounds, while some patients with an obstruction may have hyperactive sounds. Abdominal auscultation is subjective and appears to be more useful in determining an ileus [9]. However, the value of other findings has questioned the usefulness of auscultation (Thomas Read, personal communication).

The patient is asked to identify the location of any abdominal pain. Gentle percussion should always precede vigorous palpation. The skilled examiner can elicit signs of peritoneal irritation through gentle percussion with ease; aggressive, deep palpation to find rebound tenderness only hurts the patient and makes subsequent examinations difficult. If no significant tenderness or tympany is found on percussion, the abdomen may be palpated for masses and organomegaly. Each incision should be carefully palpated with the patient straining to check for incisional hernias. Appliances should be removed from stomas and a gentle digital examination performed to assess for stenosis or parastomal hernia. Finally, the inguinal region should be examined for hernia or adenopathy [10].

Anorectal examination

Examination of the perineal region consists of inspection and digital palpation, complemented by anoscopy, proctoscopy, or biopsy as indicated by findings. Before touching the perineal region, the examiner should warn the patient that the lubricant feels wet and cool and that the digital examination may produce mild pressure or a sensation similar to having a bowel movement.

Patient positioning

Several positions can be used for the examination and should take into account patient and examiner comfort, the equipment available, and exposure (**Figure 3.1**). The prone jackknife position is usually used with a moveable procedure table. Patients wearing slacks are asked to kneel on the table platform (shelf) before dropping their slacks and underwear to prevent their trousers from dragging the floor, loss of pocket contents, and to avoid unnecessary undressing. After kneeling on the shelf, the patient bends forward and places his or her chest on

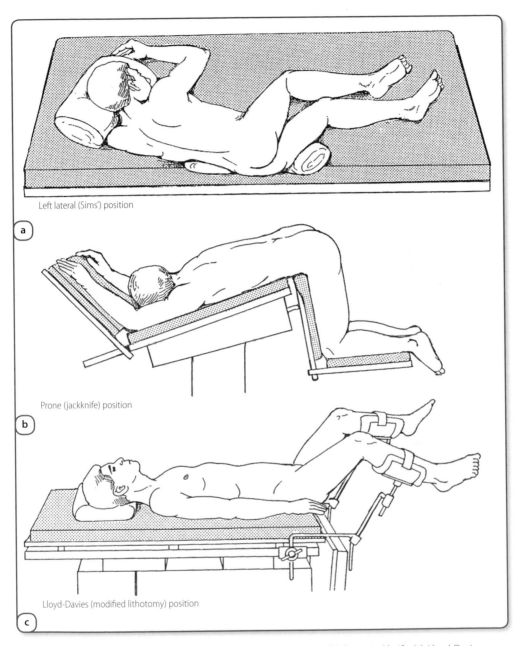

Left lateral (Sims') position

a

Prone (jackknife) position

b

Lloyd-Davies (modified lithotomy) position

c

Figure 3.1 Patient positions for the anorectal examination. (a) Sims'; (b), Prone jackknife; (c), Lloyd-Davies (modified lithotomy).

the table with the elbows forward, palms on the table, and the back in a slight swayback position. The shelf is positioned to allow the abdomen to remain slightly off the table (**Figure 3.1b**). A sheet drapes the back and upper legs, preserving modesty and keeping the patient warm and comfortable.

After the patient is warned, the table is raised and tipped forward. Patients are asked not to straighten their legs, because this might cause them to slip off the table. The prone position allows better access to the perineum. For patients who have difficulty with the prone position (e.g. those who have undergone recent joint replacement surgery or who have arthritis or cardiovascular disease), other positions (such as the Sims' or modified left lateral decubitus) are used.

The Sims' or modified left lateral decubitus position (**Figure 3.1a**) is used if a moveable procedure table is not available or if the patient cannot tolerate the prone position. The patient's head is placed on the opposite corner with the back angling across the table and the buttocks extending off the table. The hips are flexed and the knees are bent. This position is comfortable and prevents the patient from falling off the table. Having the buttocks extend off the table allows the buttocks to be easily spread and the end of an instrument such as a proctoscope, if it is to be used, to be manipulated in any direction. The end of the scope or the examiner's head (when looking through the end piece) is not hindered by the bed. Finally, this positioning allows any anal discharge to drop to the floor and not pool on the table, where it could contaminate the examiner's head or face. If the patient's back is placed parallel to the side of the table, the patient has a tendency to slip and the exposure to the perineum is limited. The modified lithotomy position (**Figure 3.1c**) is rarely used in the office setting because the exposure of the perineum is limited. This position is helpful, however, if a pelvic examination must also be performed and in the operating room if abdominal exposure is required.

Physical inspection

The buttocks should be inspected first for scars from prior abscess drainage, skin lesions, or sinus openings. The sacrococcygeal region is searched for signs of pilonidal disease: pits, cysts, or scars. Next the buttocks are gently retracted and the perianal skin inspected. Is there evidence of dermatitis or excoriation and linear scratches from pruritis (see Figure 18.1)? Is there fecal or mucous soiling, indicating incontinence or prolapse? Swellings and protrusions are noted and characterized:

- condyloma (see Figure 20.1)
- hypertrophied anal papillae (see Figure 18.5)
- sentinel piles
- external hemorrhoids (see Figure 16.6)
- prolapsed internal hemorrhoids
- skin tags (**Figure 3.2**)
- fissures.

Fissures can be seen by gentle distraction on the anus while the patient strains. They are usually found on the posterior midline; fissures found off the midline and accompanied by abscesses raise the suspicion of Crohn's disease. External openings of fistulas should be noted, as should scars and any muscular asymmetry from prior anorectal surgery. These findings can be elicited by having the patient squeeze and strain. Sensation is assessed by light stroking or pinprick.

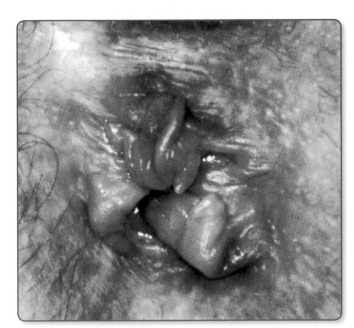

Figure 3.2 Anal skin tags.

To avoid confusion for subsequent examiners, the position of significant findings is recorded by using left, right, anterior, and posterior, not by the face of a clock. A mass felt at 2 o'clock in the prone jackknife position becomes 8 o'clock when the patient is in the lithotomy position. A sketch in the patient's chart is also helpful.

Prolapsing conditions suggested by the patient's history may not be evident on initial inspection, especially when the patient is in the prone jackknife position. A patient with a prolapsing condition is asked to sit on the toilet and strain and is re-examined with the patient leaning forward before he or she rises. Other options include the use of an extendable mirror or a flexible endoscope that can be passed into the toilet to visualize the prolapse (see Chapter 15).

Digital palpation

Digital palpation of the anus and rectum is performed carefully with a gloved hand; finger cots are no longer recommended. The well lubricated index finger is placed on the anal opening and gradually advanced. Having the patient bear down, which relaxes the external sphincters somewhat, may make this easier. The tone and symmetry of the sphincter complex is noted as the anal canal and dentate line are examined for masses, stenosis, scarring, or areas of tenderness. A fissure can often be palpated in the posterior midline as a rough region in the otherwise smooth anal canal. The anorectal junction is identified by the puborectalis sling posteriorly. Once the rectum is entered, palpation begins anteriorly. In men the prostate is examined; in women the cervix may be felt, or the defect of a rectocele may be appreciated. The examination continues circumferentially within the rectum to assess for any pathologic condition both within and outside the rectum. The position, consistency, and fixity of masses should be noted. Laterally, extrarectal adenopathy or pelvic abscesses can sometimes be felt. Posteriorly, sacral masses may be detected. The cul-de-sac is searched for a tumor shelf. Before the examiner withdraws the finger, the patient is asked to repeat a squeeze and strain to assess the function and symmetry of the sphincter once more.

Anoscopy

Anoscopy completes the examination. It allows assessment of the anal canal and distal rectum and requires no special preparation. Several styles of anoscopes are available (**Figure 3.3**). The anoscope is lubricated generously and advanced slowly with the patient bearing down, which facilitates insertion by relaxing the anal canal. The anus is examined circumferentially. Some anoscopes allow this without having to be withdrawn; others need to be reinserted with an obturator to avoid pinching the sensitive anoderm. The anoderm is inspected for fissures, which usually lie on the posterior or anterior midline. Odd-appearing lateral fissures, especially those associated with edematous skin tags or abscess, are hallmarks of Crohn's disease. Hemorrhoids are typically found in three bundles: right posterior, right anterior, and left lateral. They should be graded with respect to the dentate line. If a fistula or abscess is encountered, the offending anal gland may sometimes be apparent by drainage or with gentle probing. Aggressive probing of fistulas is contraindicated, because false passages can be created. Other lesions that may be seen include condylomata involving the anal canal, epidermoid carcinoma, or melanoma [11].

To complete the anorectal examination, additional endoscopy is usually required. These important diagnostic and therapeutic procedures are covered in Chapter 5.

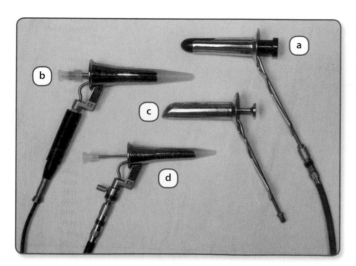

Figure 3.3 Anoscopes. (a) Fansler-Ives. (b) Welch-Allyn, slotted medium with light source attached. (c) Modified Buie-Hirchmann. (d) Welch-Allyn, slotted pediatric with fiber-optic light source attached.

Rounds questions

Explain why the following statements are true or false.

1. Abdominal pain is usually quite specific, and the location of the pain is seldom referred to other areas.
2. Tenesmus, the feeling of the urge to defecate, may accompany rectal cancer.
3. Melena always comes from an upper or proximal source, whereas bright red blood is always from benign anal conditions.
4. A 44-year-old patient whose mother had a cancer diagnosed on a recent colonscopy and whose uncle was diagnosed with colon cancer at the age of 54 years needs full colonoscopic screening.
5. Findings of peritoneal irritation must be confirmed by eliciting rebound tenderness.
6. Typical anal fissures cause painful bleeding that follows bowel movements and are found in the posterior midline by gently spreading the buttocks.
7. The only contraindications to properly performing a digital anorectal examination are (1) no finger, (2) no anus, and (3) no glove.

References

1. Nivatvongs S. Diagnosis. In: Gordon PH, Nivatvongs S (eds). Principles and Practice of Surgery of the Colon, Rectum, and Anus. St. Louis: Quality Medical Publishing 1992;82–93.
2. Veidenheimer MC. Clinical evaluation of the anorectum, perineum, and pelvic floor. In; Henry MM, Swash M (eds). Coloproctology and the Pelvic Floor. Oxford: Butterworth-Heinnmann, 1992;115–8.
3. Roberts PL. Patient evaluation. In Beck DE, Wexner SD (eds). Fundamentals of Surgery of the Alimentary Tract, vol 4. Philadelphia: WB Saunders 1996;310–5.
4. Hicks TC, Opelka FG. Diagnosis of anorectal disease. In: Condon R (ed). Shackelford's Anorectal Surgery. New York: McGraw-Hill 1992;25–35.
5. Ellis CN. Is family history really contributory? Clinics in Colon Rect Surg 2001;14:301.
6. Giardiello FM. Genetic testing in hereditary colorectal cancer. JAMA 1997;278:1278–81.
7. Vasen HF, Mecklin JP, Khan PM, Lynch HT. The International Collaborative Group on Hereditary Non-Polyposis Colorectal Cancer (ICG-HNPCC). Dis Colon Rectum 1991;34:424–5.
8. Rodriguez-Bigas MA, Boland CR, Hamilton SR, et al. A National Cancer Institute Workshop on Hereditary Nonpolyposis Colorectal Cancer Syndrome: meeting highlights and Bethesda guidelines. J Natl Cancer Inst 1997; 89:1758–62.
9. Gu Y, Lim HJ, Moser MAJ. How useful are bowel sounds in assessing the abdomen? Digestive Surgery 2010;27:422–6.
10. Silen W. Cope's Early Diagnosis of the Acute Abdomen 18th ed. New York: Oxford University Press 1991;19–56.
11. Corman ML. Colon and Rectal Surgery 3rd ed. Philadelphia: JB Lippincott 1993;11–13.

In recent years there have been numerous technologic developments in radiology that help physicians in their evaluations of colorectal patients [1]. Radiologic studies include plain and contrast radiographs, ultrasonography, computed tomography, magnetic resonance imaging and nuclear medicine studies. With all this diversity of choice, an understanding of the benefits and limitations of the varying radiologic procedures is helpful in determining which is the most useful examination for a particular problem. This chapter presents a brief analysis of the strengths and weaknesses of the various radiologic procedures so that, in consultation with a diagnostic radiologist, one can select the appropriate imaging study and interpret the findings.

Plain radiographs

In the setting of acute abdominal pain, plain films of the abdomen remain an important radiographic imaging study [2–5]. These examinations are relatively inexpensive, can be performed on virtually all patients (since they can be obtained with portable equipment) and can be evaluated with relative ease by both radiologists and non-radiologists. The standard views for a patient with acute abdominal pain consist of a supine and erect film of the abdomen and an erect film of the chest, centering on the hemidiaphragms. Primarily in this acute abdominal series the physician will be attempting to exclude the presence of free air, evaluating for the presence of radiopaque densities (including gallstones and kidney stones), looking for masses and for deformity of the normal viscous structures (such as the kidney and the liver) and, in particular, assessing the bowel pattern to see whether there is any distention.

As little as 1 or 2 mL of free air can be appreciated on an upright chest or lateral decubitus film (**Figure 4.1a and b**). Larger quantities of free air can be identified on supine films as air inside and outside the bowel produces a 'double lumen' sign (**Figure 4.1c**). Free intra-abdominal air is frequently seen in the initial postoperative films of a laparotomy patient. This usually resolves in 5–7 days. Serial postoperative films should show a reduction in free air. Cholelithiasis and urolithiasis as well as other calcified masses and radiopaque foreign bodies may be visible on a plain film of the abdomen (**Figure 4.2**). However, other imaging modalities such as ultrasonography, computed tomography (CT) or an intravenous urogram (IVU) are often needed for definitive evaluation [6]. The bony structures of the lumbosacral spine, lower

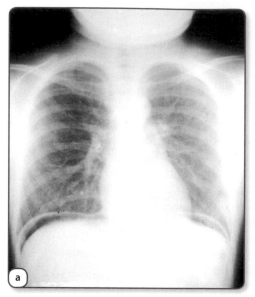

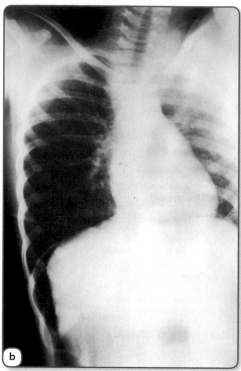

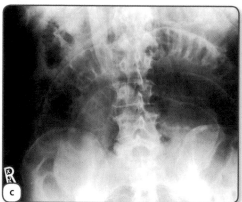

Figure 4.1 Radiographs showing free air. (a) Erect film of chest demonstrating free air beneath the diaphragm. (b) Left decubitus film (left side down) demonstrating free air rising above the liver in a patient with a large bowel perforation. (c) Abdominal film demonstrating double lumen sign.

thoracic spine, the ribs, pelvis, and femoral head are also visualized on these plain films and should be carefully evaluated for sclerotic as well as lytic lesions. Fractures and lesions of the bony structures may frequently present with abdominal pain when ileus is a secondary complicating factor.

Radio-opaque foreign bodies can also be demonstrated on plain films (**Figure 4.3**). In addition to identifying and localizing the foreign body, an acute abdominal series can exclude free air, which suggests a bowel perforation.

Plain films of the abdomen also allow the examiner to evaluate the visceral structures of the liver, spleen, kidneys, and bladder. The outlines of these structures should be assessed for deformity or displacement. The sensitivity of this examination will vary, depending on the patient's body habitus, ability to cooperate, hold his breath, and remain still. Of particular interest to those concerned with colorectal surgery is evaluation of the bowel gas pattern. Gas, which is a product of both swallowed air and bacteria production, is normally seen within the colon and stomach and, to a lesser extent, within the small bowel. The small bowel is considered abnormal if it measures more than 3 cm in diameter and the wall abnormal if it is greater than 3 mm. The transverse colon is considered abnormal if it measures more than 5.5 cm in diameter. The extent and pattern of the bowel gas is important as well. If there is distention both of the small bowel and large bowel, including the rectum, then consideration should be given that an ileus may be present. Similarly, if the patient has recently undergone surgery, the possibility of an ileus must be considered as well. Clinical setting and change over time are important factors that help determine the significance of radiographic findings. Serial films at

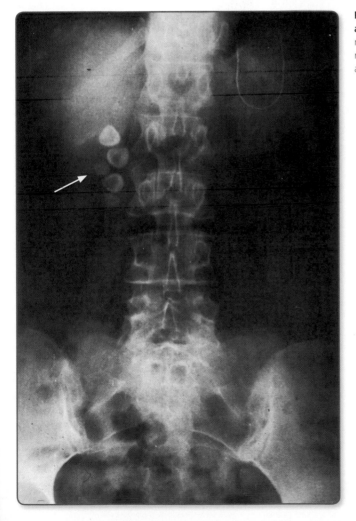

Figure 4.2 Plain film of the abdomen reveals four calcified masses in the right upper quadrant, representing cholelithiasis (white arrow).

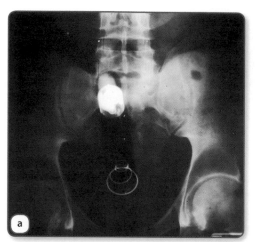

Figure 4.3 Posterior and lateral radiographs.
(a) Posterior to anterior radiograph demonstrating rectal foreign body. (b) Lateral radiograph of rectal foreign body. (c) Plain radiogram demonstrating a retained laparotomy sponge.

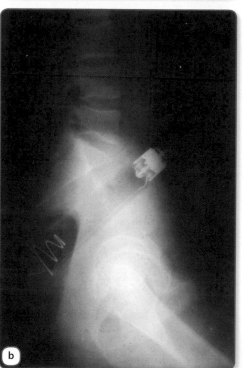

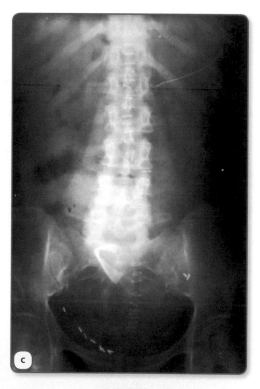

regular intervals provide important clinical information and help the examiner determine the significance of radiographic findings.

Volvulus or twisting of the large bowel can be identified on plain films (**Figures 4.4** and **4.5**, and see Figures 23.1 and 23.2). In some circumstances a contrast study as described below may assist in confirming the location of the volvulus. This study may also reduce the volvulus and excludes other colonic pathology.

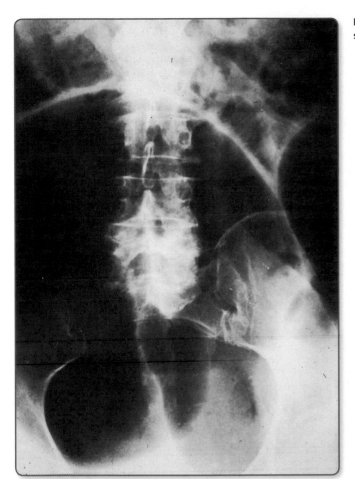

Figure 4.4 Radiograph of sigmoid volvulus.

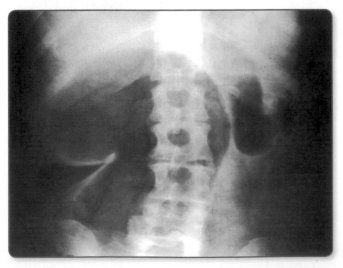

Figure 4.5 Radiograph of cecal volvulus.

Barium enema

Barium enemas are performed to evaluate patients with heme-positive stools, a family history of colon carcinoma, inflammatory bowel disease, change in bowel habits, and abdominal pain [7, 8]. Contrast enemas employ a single- or double-contrast technique. The indications for single- versus double-contrast barium enema are controversial. Double-contrast studies are generally considered superior, particularly for the detection of small polyps and the mucosal changes of inflammatory bowel disease.

In a **single-contrast barium enema,** the colon is slowly filled with barium and compressed manually or mechanically. The examination is monitored by live fluoroscopy. 'Spot' images are acquired in multiple projections as the colon is being distended. Each portion of the colon must be examined free from overlapping bowel. Once the colon is completely filled, as demonstrated by visualization of the terminal ileum, appendix, or ileocecal valve, films of the entire colon are obtained (**Figures 4.6 and 4.7**).

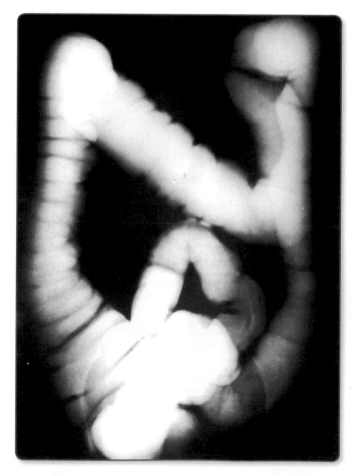

Figure 4.6 Single-contrast barium overhead film demonstrating a normal 'filled' colon.

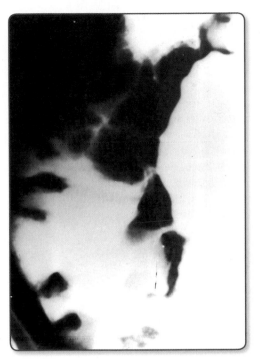

Figure 4.7 Constricting lesion (adenocarcinoma) of the ascending colon on a single-contrast barium enema spot film.

With a **double-contrast barium enema,** a higher viscosity, more dense barium suspension is introduced into the colon, then the colon is distended by air insufflation. Fluoroscopic examination is performed as the colon fills and then a series of overhead films is taken (**Figures 4.8** and **4.9**). The patient must retain the barium and air during these overhead films. A double-contrast barium enema is more time consuming and often not as well tolerated by the patient. Contrast enemas have a sensitivity of 50–80% for lesions <1 cm and 70–90% for lesions >1 cm [2]. A contrast study tends to be less accurate in the rectosigmoid area.

Rigorous cleansing of the colon is required before a barium enema, especially with the double-contrast technique. Even a small amount of retained stool can obscure mucosal detail, leading to inconclusive results or even misinterpretation. Regimens to prepare the colon often include clear liquid diet and laxatives the day before the examination and a suppository the morning of the study. An additional 24-hour preparation or stronger laxatives are necessary in a small number of patients (see Chapter 8).

Incompetence of the ileocecal valve can also degrade the quality of barium enemas by preventing full colonic distention and obscuring segments of colon. An incompetent ileocecal valve causes greater difficulty in a double-contrast barium enema, where there is less control of the contrast column. Colonic spasm can interfere with single- and double-contrast barium enemas. Spasm causes patient discomfort and

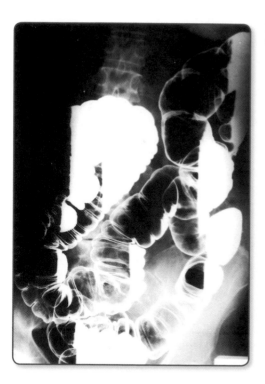

Figure 4.8 Left lateral decubitus overhead film of a normal double-contrast barium enema.

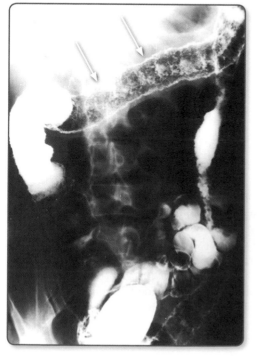

Figure 4.9 Diffuse colonic ulceration, best seen in the transverse colon (arrows) from a double-contrast barium enema in a patient with ulcerative colitis.

makes full distention of the colon impossible. Intravenous glucagon is commonly administered to combat spasm. In some institutions, glucagon is given prophylactically before all double-contrast barium enemas.

Because of its imaging characteristics, barium is the agent of choice for most contrast enemas. If intestinal perforation is suspected or emergency surgery is anticipated, water-soluble, iodine-based, single-column contrast agents (Gastrografin, Oral Hypaque) are often preferred. These types of contrast medium are considerably more expensive and can have a high osmolality. These high-osmolar agents may cause fluid shifts and act as cathartics.

Small bowel examination

Effective examination of the small bowel requires a thorough knowledge of the disease processes that can affect it. Methods of study include standard barium small bowel follow-through and enteroclysis [9]. Standard barium **small bowel follow-through (SBFT)** is usually combined with an upper gastrointestinal (UGI) barium examination (**Figure 4.10**). 480–600 mL of medium-density barium is given orally at a delivery speed that depends on patient toleration and gut and small bowel motility as observed by fluoroscopy. Intermittent supine abdominal radiographs are taken at intervals, depending on observed

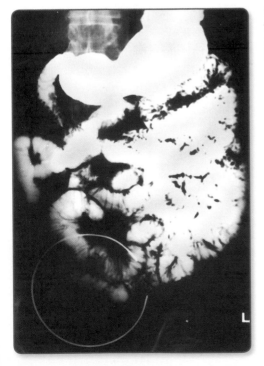

Figure 4.10 Overhead film from a small bowel follow-through shows a normal small-bowel loop and mucosal fold patterns. External compression device (white ring) helps to isolate single loops of small bowel.

small bowel motility (usually every 30 minutes) until barium reaches the large bowel. During the course of the examination, manual examination of the small bowel is performed, paying careful attention to small bowel caliber and mucosal pattern. When the terminal ileum is reached, it is thoroughly examined manually using compression and spot images taken fluoroscopically. Several films are necessary for a complete examination to image the small bowel in various stages of the passage of the barium meal.

Standard **enteroclysis** examination can provide increased sensitivity to the barium examination of the small bowel; however, it is more expensive, more invasive and less tolerated by patients (**Figure 4.11**) [10]. Medium-density barium followed by methylcellulose is injected through a nasal-intestinal tube at a rapid rate (100 mL/min), either manually or with an infusion device. This provides excellent distention of the small bowel and a double-contrast effect that may show partially obstructing lesions that might have been less well seen by conventional SBFT. The examination is monitored fluoroscopically with intermittent manual examination and supine abdomen filming. Various disease states can change the mucosal fold pattern, cause complete or partial obstruction through mass effect, stricture, or kinking of small bowel loops. Small bowel studies can characterize these clinically suspected lesions or show the likely location of lesions, allowing directed surgical exploration for diagnosis and therapy. Differential diagnosis is then offered by the radiologist after carefully correlating the radiologic data with the clinical data provided by the referring physician.

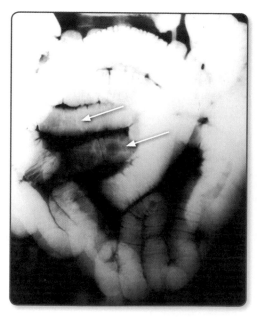

Figure 4.11 Overhead film from normal enteroclysis reveals multiple nonpersistent filling defects (arrows), which are air bubbles.

Ultrasonography

Diagnostic

Diagnostic ultrasonography is of great value in diagnosing abnormalities of the gastrointestinal tract [11]. This modality is not invasive and uses sound waves to provide rapid and inexpensive multiplanar images of the major abdominal organs [12,13]. Examinations can be performed at the patient's bedside, and therefore virtually all patients can undergo evaluation. The structures that can be studied include the liver, spleen, pancreas, kidneys, aorta and periaortic areas, and pelvis. Abnormal loops of bowel can be identified as well. Persistent loops of noncompressible bowel, similar to the sonographic appearance of the kidney, have been called the **pseudokidney** and indicate bowel wall thickening [14]. These abnormalities can be seen in conditions that produce bowel wall thickening, including neoplasms, inflammatory bowel disease, inflammatory processes such as diverticulitis, infectious processes such as tuberculosis, and acute appendicitis (**Figure 4.12**) [15–17].

Inflammatory processes such as abscesses can be visualized and separated from normal structures. Under ultrasound guidance, these can also be percutaneously aspirated and drained.

Masses, particularly in the liver, can be appropriately visualized with ultrasonography. Although CT portography has a greater sensitivity and specificity than diagnostic ultrasound, most sensitive of all appears to be intraoperative ultrasound in identifying focal liver lesions. Patients with mucinous adenocarcinoma metastatic to the liver frequently have a characteristic pattern of calcified liver masses causing posterior shadowing. Once a liver mass is identified with ultrasound, a diagnostic

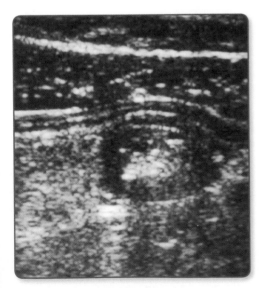

Figure 4.12 Ultrasound showing 'pseudokidney' sign in the right lower quadrant, indicating acute appendicitis.

percutaneous biopsy can be performed. Ultrasonography is also helpful intraoperatively when segmental resections of the liver are being planned.

Intraluminal

Ultrasonography is also of increasing value in evaluating the extent of anal and rectal cancer [18–20]. Intra-anal ultrasound is extremely helpful in evaluating the anal sphincter to confirm defects in the incontinent patient (**Figures 4.13** and **4.14**) [21]. It can be helpful in evaluating complex anorectal fistulas or abscesses. Hydrogen peroxide injected into the fistula serves as an ecogenic contrast. Rectal cancers can be staged using **transrectal ultrasound**, not only to determine the extent of wall penetration (**Figure 4.15**), but also to visualize the presence of nodal enlargement. Intrarectal ultrasound of the normal rectum produces five rings, three hyperecoic (white) and two hypoecoic (black), which correspond to the interfaces demonstrated in **Figure 4.16**. An ultrasound staging system is described in **Table 4.1**. Intra-anal ultrasonography produces images slightly different from those taken in the rectum. In the upper anal canal the puborectalis

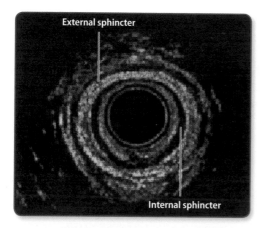

Figure 4.13 Normal intra-anal ultrasound.

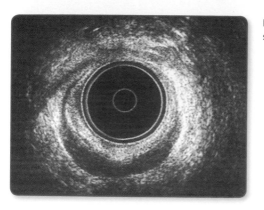

Figure 4.14 Intra-anal ultrasound demonstrating sphincter defect.

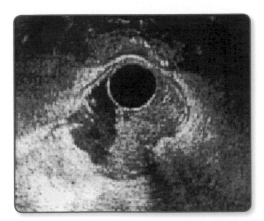

Figure 4.15 Intrarectal ultrasound demonstrating a uT3 lesion.

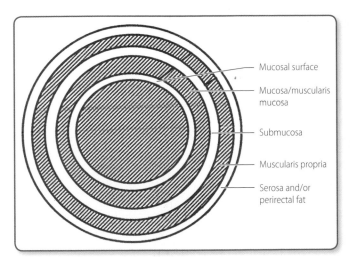

Figure 4.16 Graphic representation of intrarectal ultrasound.

Mucosal surface

Mucosa/muscularis mucosa

Submucosa

Muscularis propria

Serosa and/or perirectal fat

Table 4.1 Intrarectal ultrasound staging system	
Level	Description
uT1	Malignant lesion confined to mucosa and submucosa
uT2	Invasion into, but not through, the muscularis propria
uT3	Invasion into perirectal fat
uT4	Invasion into adjacent organ (e.g. prostrate, vagina, bladder)
N0	No evidence of regional nodal metastases
N1	Involvement of perirectal nodes with metastatic disease

muscle appears as a U-shaped structure with the open anterior end (**Figure 4.17**). The lower anal canal is presented in **Figure 4.18**.

Retained stool in the rectum will degrade or produce false images. Patient preparation includes enemas and a proctoscopic examination

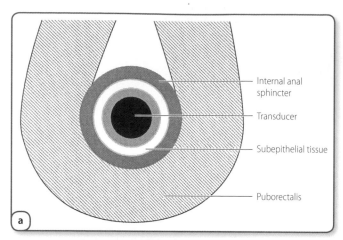

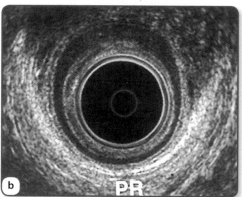

Figure 4.17 Anatomy of the upper anal canal. (a) Diagramatic representation of normal anatomy of the upper anal canal. (b) Corresponding endoanal ultrasound image demonstrating the hypsechoic internal anal sphincter and the hyperechoic 'U' shaped puborectalis as denoted by PR. From Wong DW. Endoscongraphy of the anal canal. Persp Colon Rectal Surg 1998;10:1–21. With permission.

to confirm the adequacy of the preparation and if necessary to suction any residual stool. This need for proctoscopy along with a superior knowledge of anorectal anatomy explains the superior results obtained by colorectal surgeons performing intraluminal ultrasound. Impediments to abdominal ultrasound include bowel gas as well as barium. Preparation for abdominal ultrasonographic examination requires that the patient be NPO for at least 4–8 hours before the examination. Since this examination is operator dependent, it is absolutely necessary to have highly qualified individuals performing and interpreting these examinations.

Computed tomography

Computed tomography imaging is a useful modality for the evaluation of pathologic conditions of the abdomen, including colon carcinoma (**Figure 4.19**) [22]. As X-rays course through the patient, they are attenuated. The CT scanner's detectors sum up the transmitted attenuated X-ray energies and use a computer to process the information to produce an image. The original concept for CT was introduced in 1972 by G.N.

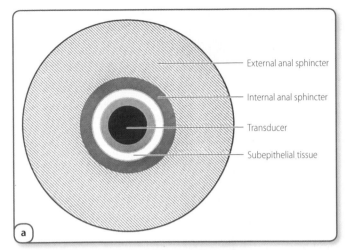

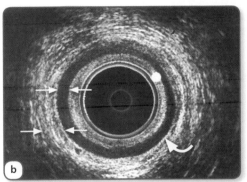

Figure 4.18 Anatomy of the mid anal canal. (a) Diagramatic representation of normal anatomy of the mid anal canal. (b) Corresponding endoanal ultrasound image demonstrating the inner hyperechoic subepithelial tissues (white dot), the thin circular hypoechoic ring of the internal anal sphincter marked by the two opposing solid arrows, a portion of the thin longitudinal muscle denoted by the curved arrow, and the mixed echogenicity ring of the external anal sphincter seen between the two opposing open arrows. From Wong DW. Endoscongraphy of the anal canal. Persp Colon Rectal Surg 1998;10:1-21. With permission.

Hounsfield. Today, higher heat capacity tubes have made CT scanning much faster. The modern spiral multi-detector CT units have increased resolution, reduced radiation exposure and dramatically decreased scan time.

Patient preparation before CT imaging should be discussed with the consulting radiologist. In general, the use of an oral gastrointestinal contrast medium is crucial, whereas intravenous contrast is not. Oral contrast medium is administered to outline the intestinal wall, which should not exceed 5 mm in thickness (includes large and small bowel). An oral suspension of 2% barium sulfate or 2% water-soluble contrast medium (Hypaque or Gastrografin) should be given before any scanning. The use of barium should be avoided if one suspects a bowel perforation. If this is a concern, then Hypaque (less expensive) or Gastrografin (more expensive) can be given. Water-soluble contrast should be avoided in patients with intestinal obstruction. Intravenous contrast medium should be administered when details of vascular structures or vascular lesions are needed unless contraindicated by prior allergic reaction or renal insufficiency. Rectal contrast allows better

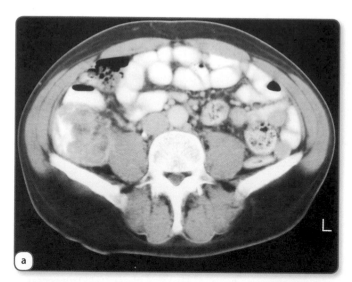

Figure 4.19 Selected images from an abdominal CT study using both intravenous and oral contrast media. (a) There is large (4.5 cm) enhancing soft tissue mass obliterating the cecal lumen. (b) Same patient 47 months later with multiple calcified liver masses. The patient had a known adenocarcinoma of the colon with metastasis.

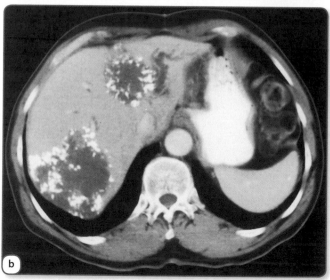

visualization of the distal bowel and may highlight an anastomotic leak or abscess.

Abdominal CT imaging is commonly used in the evaluation of trauma, abscess, diverticulitis, and tumors and can aid in interventional biopsy and drainage procedures. It plays a major role in the preoperative and postoperative evaluation of colon carcinoma [23,24]. CT imaging helps in the staging (especially of metastasis [see **Figure 4.19b**]) and detection of recurrence of colon carcinoma. It has limited sensitivity and accuracy for the detection of local extension of colon cancer.

Spiral CT scanning is currently the procedure of choice to diagnose pulmonary emboli (**Figure 4.20**) [25].

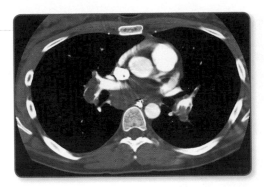

Figure 4.20 Spiral CT scan of chest demonstrating pulmonary emboli.

Magnetic resonance imaging

Magnetic resonance imaging (MRI) is performed by placing the patient in a strong magnetic field. Ionizing radiation and iodinated contrast are not used.

Ferromagnetic materials, including monitoring equipment for critically ill patients and many biopsy and interventional devices, cannot be taken into the magnetic field.

First generation equipment had long image acquisition times which made MRI susceptible to motion artifacts. Respiratory and cardiac activity and intestinal peristalsis degraded the images, precluding the application of MRI to intestinal imaging. The sigmoid colon and rectum, however, are reasonably well evaluated by MRI because they are somewhat fixed in position. Newer generation equipment has resolved many of these problems. Endorectal and surface arrayed coils allow greater assessment of the depth of tumor invasion into the bowel wall and evaluation of lymph nodes.

MRI, with its multiplanar images, is valuable in examining the solid abdominal viscera [26]. In some studies, MRI is more sensitive in detecting liver metastases than can be determined by dynamic CT (**Figures 4.21** and **4.22**) [27]. At this time, MRI does not approach the sensitivity of intraoperative ultrasound and CT arterial portography in identifying liver metastases. New superparamagnetic contrast agents, higher field strength magnets, and shorter imaging times are being used to improve the sensitivity of MRI in evaluating hepatic disease and rectal tumors. In Europe, MRI is preferred over endoluminal ultrasound in staging rectal cancer [28]. Advantages of MRI for initial rectal cancer staging include accuracy that does not vary with the height of the rectal lesion and visualization of the entire pelvis. This allows surgeons to assess of the radial margin and pelvic sidewall prior to surgery.

Positron emission tomography

Positron emission tomography (PET) uses positron-emitting isotope-labeled compounds to image tissue [29]. Functional images of colorectal

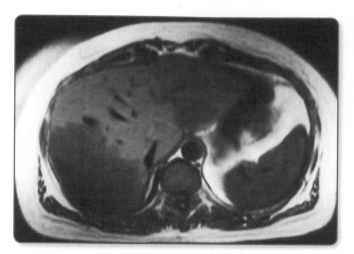

Figure 4.21 T1-weighted axial MRI demonstrating two hepatic metastases.

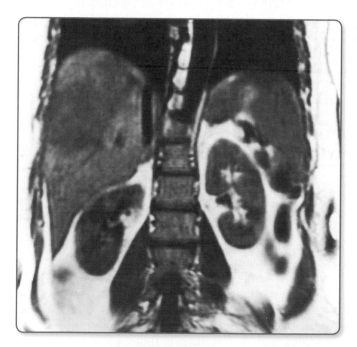

Figure 4.22 T1-weighted coronal MRI of a large liver metastasis.

neoplasms are obtained by taking advantage of the increased anaerobic glycolysis that occurs in malignant cells. Intravenous fluorine-18 deoxyglucose (FDG), like glucose, is variably absorbed and metabolized by cells. An emission image is then obtained and oriented into sagittal, coronal, and transverse views (**Figure 4.23**). Qualitative image anaylsis is performed for each of the views. Limitations of this procedure include limited resolution, and cost. PET scans are currently used in cancer staging for metastatic and recurrent colorectal cancer [30]. Additional experience, availability, and reduced cost will help establish its role in colon and rectal surgery.

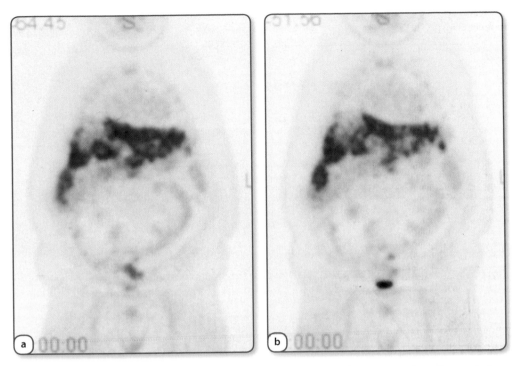

Figure 4.23 Positron emission tomogram. (a) Early and (b) delayed images demonstrating increasing uptake in liver and rectum.

Colography and wireless capsule

Colography may be performed using computed tomography or magnetic resonance [32]. Both modalities look at two-dimensional (2D) and three-dimensional (3D) images of the colon and rectum (**Figure 4.24**). The 3D form most closely simulates the endoscopic view and is referred to by some people as virtual colonoscopy. The wide spread adoption of the term virtual colonoscopy is unfortunate as it is misleading. Colography is a radiologic study that indirectly visualizes the colon and rectum. It is virtual but, as described in this book, it is not colonoscopy. Currently, the patient must undergo a complete mechanical bowel preparation as residual stool may produce false lesions. No sedation is required, the study takes only a few minutes to perform, and instillation of air into the colon is required for CT colography. A significant amount of computer time and storage is required to process the images. The radiation dose for CT colography approximates that received with a barium enema.

The ability of colography to detect neoplasms of the bowel continues to be investigated. Data regarding the sensitivity and specificity of this technique has been variable. The best results have been obtained from specialized centers with interest in the techniques. Advantages include patient compliance and minimal risk of complications. Disadvantages

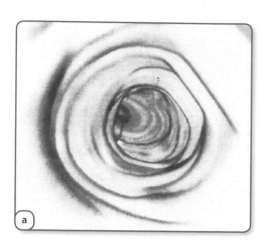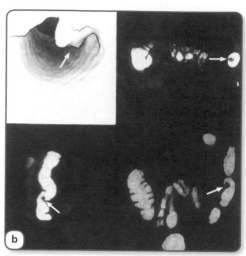

Figure 4.24 Three-dimesional colograms. (a) Three-dimensional computed tomography colonogram. (b) Three-dimensional magnetic resonance colonogram.

include the need for a full bowel preparation and inconclusive data regarding accuracy and cost.

The wireless capsule (**Figure 4.25**) is swallowed and painlessly propelled by peristalsis throughout the bowel. Photographic images are obtained by the capsule and transmitted via radiowaves to a receiver that the patient wears around their waist. The capsule has the ability to look at the small bowel as well as the colon and rectum. Localization of the images obtained can be challenging.

Angiography

Interventional radiologic diagnostic and interventional procedures play an important role in the assessment of visceral disease processes and traumatic injury [31,32]. Intravenous iodinated contrast medium is injected from percutaneously, selectively placed catheters to opacify visceral vessels (**Figure 4.26a**) and end organs yielding important diagnostic information. Various interventional techniques can then be employed to provide therapy, definitive in many cases.

Diseases involving the mesenteric vessels, e.g. arteriosclerosis-causing conditions such as acute mesenteric ischemia, intestinal angina, aneurysms of the aorta and its abdominal branches, and thrombo-embolism, can be readily diagnosed and treated angiographically with angioplasty, metallic stent placement, or site-selective infusion of clot-dissolving medicines. Angiographic evaluation of gastrointestinal hemorrhage is indicated to locate bleeding sites identified by nuclear medicine scans and potentially treat them with selective arterial infusion of vasoconstricting agents or injection of thromboembolic material. (**Figure 4.26b**) [34].

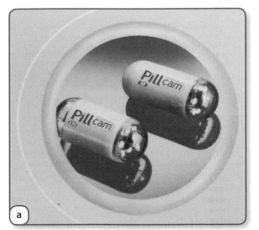

Figure 4.25 M2A wireless capsule. (a) Low power view 11 mm x 26 mm (Given Imaging Inc, Yogneam, Israel and Norcross, GA, USA). (b) Inside the M2A capsule: 1. Optical dome, 2. Lens holder, 3. Lens, 4. Illuminating light emitting diode, 5. Complementary metal oxide semiconductor imager, 6. Battery, 7. Application specific integrated circuit transmitter, 8. Antenna.

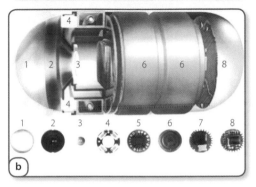

Diagnosis and nonsurgical intervention in neoplastic disease of the abdomen has become increasingly more important. Many vascular tumors, especially those within the liver, are well seen with contrast enhancement of their feeding vessels. Selective arterial infusion of the superior mesenteric artery with contrast agents during CT of the liver can reveal sites of metastatic disease not seen on conventional contrast-enhanced CT, enabling more accurate staging and preoperative planning. Arterial catheters placed percutaneously or surgically can also be used to selectively infuse chemotherapeutic agents. Endocrine tumors escaping imaging with CT can sometimes be located angiographically. Sampling veins draining regions where these endocrine tumors arise can reveal high concentrations of tumor-produced hormones and thus direct the surgeon in exploration.

Usually patient preparation includes baseline laboratory studies, such as a complete blood count (CBC), prothrombin time (PT), anorectal reflexes partial thromboplastin time (PTT), and fasting. The surgeon obtains a directed history and reviews the patient's chart, performs a limited physical examination, and ascertains that informed consent has been obtained. It is always helpful if the patient has been told what to expect by his referring physician, because considerable planning may be required.

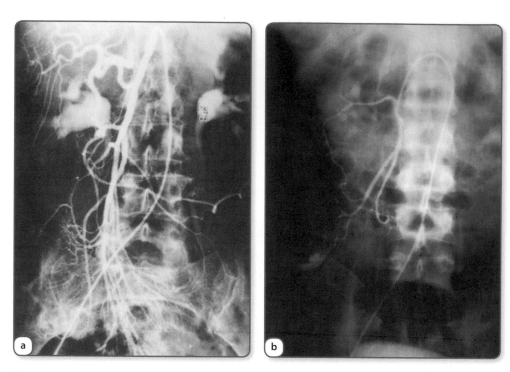

Figure 4.26 Angiograms. (a) Angiogram of normal arterial anatomy. (b) Angiogram demonstrating extravasion (hemorrhage) in cecum.

Bleeding complications such as hematomas account for the majority of postangiographic complications. They are usually self-limited and rarely require further therapy, unless there is a vascular injury such as pseudoaneurysm formation or arteriovenous fistula. Patients taking aspirin prophylaxis must cease 36 hours before the procedure. Patients receiving heparin or warfarin sodium (Coumadin) are prepared according to their PT and PTT. After the procedure is completed, pressure is held at the puncture site until hemostasis is achieved (15–30 minutes). A period of strict bed rest (4–6 hours) is then required to ensure adequate hemostasis. Patient hydration is important to limit any nephrotoxicity from the contrast agent. Uncommon to rare complications include infection, an allergic reaction to the contrast agent, distal embolization, or vascular injuries, such as creation of an intimal flap.

Interventional and diagnostic angiography has proved to be an invaluable tool in the diagnosis and treatment of abdominal diseases. Care must be taken to individualize the use of these invasive, sometimes difficult, procedures to minimize the risks of complications and maximize possible benefits.

Nuclear medicine/scintigraphy

Certain colonic disorders can be diagnosed with radioisotopic imaging [35, 36]. The radioisotope of choice for most nuclear medicine imaging examinations is technetium 99 m (^{99m}Tc) because of its relative low cost and ideal imaging characteristics. This radioactive material is labeled to a substance (the patient's own RBCs, sulfur colloid, etc.) in an in vivo, in vitro, or modified in vitro fashion. It is administered intravenously, taken up by a target organ (usually the organ of interest) where it decays and is imaged with a gamma (scintillation) camera. Usually, there is little or no patient preparation for such studies. However, any concerns should be discussed with the consulting radiologist.

A ^{99m}Tc RBC bleeding study, ^{99m}Tc sulfur colloid liver/spleen study, mebrofenin/HIDA biliary study, and ^{111}In white blood cell abscess study are some of the commonly performed examinations [37]. The noninvasive RBC bleeding study can be used to evaluate lower GI bleeding (**Figure 4.27**) and hyperemic colon (**Figure 4.28**). A hyperemic colon would include disorders such as colitis and angiodysplasia. Nuclear medicine is more sensitive than conventional angiography in detecting GI bleeding. Nuclear medicine can detect bleeding rates as low as 0.2 mL/min compared to 1.0 mL/min for angiography. When used in conjunction with angiography, nuclear medicine bleeding studies can help localize the bleeding site (SMA or IMA distribution) for faster surgical or percutaneous interventional treatment.

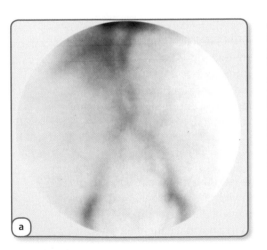 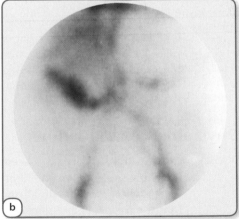

Figure 4.27 Selected images from a ^{99m} Tc-labeled RBC GI bleeding study. These images were acquired (a) at 1 minute and (b) at 14 minutes into the sequential static imaging phase. Abnormal increased isotopic activity developed in the proximal transverse colon, which *progressed* antegrade to the descending colon. This was confirmed angiographically. The patient had known diverticulosis.

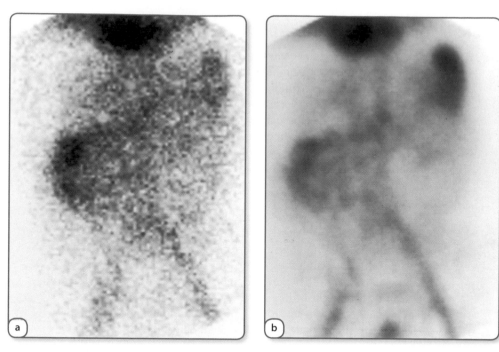

Figure 4.28 Selected images from a ⁹⁹ᵐ Tc-labeled RBC GI bleeding study. These images were acquired (a) during the dynamic blood flow phase and (b) 53 minutes into the sequential static imaging phase. There is similar abnormal increased isotopic activity in the colon on both the flow and static images. The isotopic activity did not progress on static imaging, consistent with a hyperemic colon. The patient had known panulcerative colitis.

Gastrointestinal tumor imaging with nuclear scintigraphy has a limited role. Colonoscopy, barium enema, and CT scans play crucial roles. Gallium-67 is used in tumor imaging but is excreted into the bowel after 24 hours, thus decreasing sensitivity for tumor detection. It is to be hoped that investigational monoclonal antibodies for detecting colorectal tumor will produce better imaging in the future [38].

Physiologic examinations

Colonic transit may be assessed by several methods [39]. Simply obtaining serial abdominal films following a barium meal will document transit time. Virtually all orally ingested barium should be cleared from the colon four days after ingestion in a normal patient on a normal diet.

A more accurate transit time can be obtained by having the patient ingest radiopaque markers and by documenting the marker location with plain abdominal radiographs. The method described by Eastwood requires ingestion of 20–80 markers (available commercially, Sitzmark radiopaque markers, or 2–4 mm cut segments of a nasogastric tube) and daily abdominal radiographs until the markers are passed (**Figure 4.29**).

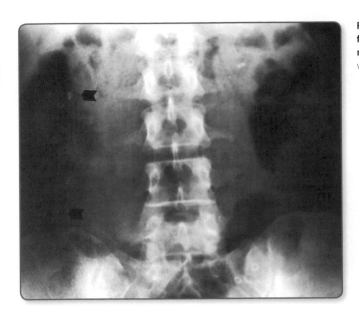

Figure 4.29 Plain abdominal film demonstrating multiple radiopaque markers predominant within the right colon (arrowheads).

Normal subjects will pass 80% of the markers by 5 days and all markers by 7 days. Several modifications of this technique have recently been described that reduce X-ray exposure. One technique entails ingestion of distinctively shaped markers on 3 successive days, and an abdominal film is taken on days 4 and 7. The location and number of the markers are used in calculations to assess the rate of segmental and total colonic transit. A second technique involves the ingestion of 24 markers a day for 7 days. An abdominal radiograph is taken on day 7. The number of markers remaining in the colon equals the colonic transit time in hours.

Cinedefecograms have been used to visualize the anal canal and rectum at rest and during defecation (**Figure 4.30**). A contrast medium placed into the rectum is used to simulate stool. Radiographs are taken under fluoroscopic control with the patient at rest, with voluntary anal contraction, and during defecation. The films demonstrate several important features. First, the anorectal angle at rest and during maneuvers can be measured. During defecation the anal canal descends, and the anorectal angle widens (i.e. straightens). In patients with outlet obstruction, the angle may not widen, and the contrast agent is not totally expelled. This may be the result of failure of the puborectalis muscle to relax. A normal test excludes perineal descent syndrome, intussusception, or a nonrelaxing puborectalis as a cause of constipation. This study also documents the presence of a rectocele and the amount of contrast remaining during evacuation. Although much information is obtained by this study, it is embarrassing and unpleasant for patients and complicated for radiologists to perform. In addition, the patient receives a significant radiation exposure.

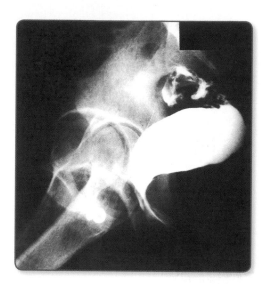

Figure 4.30 Cinedefecogram.

Because no single test provides all the information necessary, a combination of tests is used to assist the clinician to make an objective diagnosis of colonic inertia or outlet dysfunction. The selection of tests will depend on the clinical experience of the physician and availability of the test.

Rounds questions

1. The small bowel is considered abnormal when it is greater than what size?
2. The transverse colon is considered abnormal when it is greater than what size?
3. Double-contrast barium enema is generally considered superior to single-contrast, particularly in the detection of what two abnormalities?
4. Why is the preparatory regimen to cleanse the colon important?
5. How can one prevent or relieve colonic spasm during a barium enema?
6. Double-contrast effect can be used in which of the following examinations? (a) Upper GI series, (b) small bowel follow-through, (c) enteroclysis, or (d) Gastrografin enema.
7. Diseases such as sprue that change the mucosal fold pattern in the small bowel are best demonstrated by which diagnostic tests? (a) Abdominal CT with oral contrast (b) mesenteric angiogram with delayed venous phase images (c) enteroclysis, or (d) abdominal ultrasound.

8. What preparation is required for an abdominal ultrasound examination? An intrarectal ultrasound?
9. What is the pseudokidney sign?
10. True or false: prior allergic reaction to intravenous contrast and renal insufficiency are relative contraindications to IV contrast administration for CT scanning.
11. Which oral GI contrast suspension should be used in scanning a patient suspected of having bowel perforation?
12. True or false: a patient who is allergic to iodine can undergo MRI, but only without an intravenous contrast agent.
13. True or false: MRI with intravenous contrast is the most sensitive test to evaluate suspected hepatic metastases.
14. Gastrointestinal hemorrhage can be evaluated by which of the following modalities? (a) Endoscopy (b) nuclear medicine bleeding scan (c) mesenteric angiography or (d) exploratory laparotomy.
15. Typical clinical scenarios in which angiography may be useful are: (a) Evaluation of metastatic disease in the liver (b) treatment of gastrointestinal hemorrhage (c) diagnosis and treatment of acute mesenteric ischemia or (d) all of the above.
16. Which is more sensitive in detecting lower GI bleeding: a nuclear medicine bleeding study or conventional angiography?
17. Nuclear medicine can detect lower GI bleeding rates as low as ____ mL/min compared with _____ mL/min for conventional angiography.
18. In a normal patient on a normal diet, how long should it take for orally ingested barium to be cleared from the colon?
19. How long does it take for Sitzmark radiopaque markers to be passed from the colon?

References

1. Blanchard TJ, Altmeyer WB, Matthews CC. Limitations of colorectal imaging studies. In: Whitlow CB, Beck DE, Margolin DA, Hicks TC, Timmcke AE (eds). Improved Outcomes in Colon and Rectal Surgery. London: Informa Healthcare 2010;97–131.
2. Eisenberg RL. Diagnostic Imaging in Surgery. New York: McGraw-Hill 1987.
3. Margulis AR, Burhenne HJ (eds). Alimentary Tract Radiology, 4th ed. St. Louis: Mosby, 1989.
4. Meyers MA. Dynamic Radiology of the Abdomen: Normal and Pathologic Anatomy 3rd ed. New York: Springer-Verlag 1988.
5. Teplick JG, Haskin ME (eds). Surgical Radiology. Philadelphia: WB Saunders 1981.
6. Bluth E. Ultrasound evaluation of the gastrointestinal tract. In: Brascho T, Schawker T (eds). Diagnostic Ultrasound in Oncology. New York: John Wiley & Sons 1980;347–67.
7. Beck DE. Constipation. In: Fazio VW (ed). Current Therapy in Colon and Rectal Surgery. Philadelphia: BC Decker 1990;339–43.
8. Ott DJ. Role of the barium enema in colorectal carcinoma. Radiol Clin North Am 1993;31:1293–312.
9. Herlinger H, Maglinte D. Clinical Radiology of the Small Intestine. Philadelphia:WB Saunders 1989.

10. Sellink J, Miller RE. Radiology of the Small Bowel. The Hague: Mortinus Nijhoff 1982.

11. Bluth E, Merritt C, Sullivan M. Ultrasound evaluation of the stomach, small bowel, and colon. Radiology 1979;133:667–80.

12. Merritt C, Bluth E, Sullivan M, et al. Efficacy of abdominal ultrasound and the incidence and relevance of incidental findings. J Ultrasound Med 1984;3:11.

13. Mittelstaedt CA, Vincent LM. Abdominal Ultrasound. New York: Churchill Livingstone 1987.

14. Bluth E, Merritt C, Sullivan M. Ultrasound of small bowel abnormalities. Gastroenterology 1981;80:1114.

15. Bluth E. Ultrasonic detection of colonic carcinoma in emergency. Dis Colon Rectum 1984;27:693.

16. Bluth E. Ultrasound evaluation of small bowel abnormalities. Am J Gastroenterol 1983;78:788–92.

17. Kurchin A, Ray JE, Bluth EI, et al. Cholelithiasis in ileostomy patients. Dis Colon Rectum 1984;27:585–88.

18. Beynon J. An evaluation of the role of rectal endosonography in rectal cancer. Ann R Coll Surg Engl 1989;71:131–9.

19. Sentovich SM, Wong WD, Blatchford GJ. Accuracy and reliability of transanal ultrasound for anterior anal sphincter injury. Dis Colon Rectum 1998;41:1000–04.

20. Kim D, Wong WD, Bleday R. Rectal carcinoma: etiology and evaluation. In: Beck DE, Wexner SD (eds). Fundamentals of Anorectal Surgery. London: WB Saunders 2nd ed. 1998:278–300.

21. Wong DW. Endoscongraphy of the anal canal. Persp Colon Rectal Surg 1998;10:1–21.

22. Balthazar EJ. CT of the gastrointestinal tract: principles and integration. Am J Radiol 1991;156:23–32.

23. Ferrucci JT. Liver tumor imaging: current concepts. Radiol Clin North Am 1994;32:39–54.

24. Dreyfuss JR, Janower ML. Radiology of the Colon (No. 21). Baltimore: Williams & Wilkins 1980.

25. Garg K. CT of pulmonary thromboembolic disease. Radiol Clin North Am 2002;40:111–22.

26. Edelman RR, Hesselink JR. Clinical Magnetic Resonance Imaging. Philadelphia: WB Saunders 1990.

27. Hagspiel KD, Neidl KF, Eichenberger AC, et al. Detection of liver metastases: comparison of superparamagnetic iron-oxide enhanced and unenhanced MR imaging at 1.5 T with dynamic CT, intraoperative US, and percutaneous US. Radiology 1995;196:471–78.

28. Bohl JL, Timmcke AE. Radiology. In: Beck DE, Wexner SD, Roberts PL, Senagore A, Stamos M (eds). ASCRS Textbook of Colorectal Surgery 2nd ed. New York: Springer-Verlag. 2010.

29. Nivatvongs S. Diagnosis. In: Gordon PH, Nivatvongs S (eds). Principles and Practice of Surgery for the Colon, Rectum, and Anus. St. Louis: Quality Medical Publishing 1999;87–131.

30. Ruhlman J, Schomburg A, Bender H, et al. Fluorodeoxyglucose whole-body positron emission tomography in colorectal cancer patients studied in routine daily practice. Dis Colon Rectum 1997;40:1195–204.

31. Weinstein LS, Timmcke AE. Colography and the wireless capsule. Clinics Colon Rectum Surg 2001;14:393–400.

32. Wojtowycz M. Handbook of Interventional Radiology and Angiography. St. Louis: Mosby 1995.

33. Reuter SR, Redman HC, Cho KJ. Gastrointestinal Angiography, 3rd ed. Philadelphia: WB Saunders 1986.

34. Ng DA, Opelka FG, Beck DE, et al. Predictive value of Tc99m-labeled red blood cell scintigraphy for positive angiogram in massive lower gastrointestinal hemorrhage. Dis Colon Rectum. 1997;40:471–7.

35. Stark DD, Bradley WG. Magnetic Resonance Imaging. St. Louis: Mosby 1988.

36. Mettler FA Jr, Guiberteau MJ. Essentials of Nuclear Medicine Imaging 2nd ed. Philadelphia: WB Saunders 1986.

37. Faingold R, Zwas ST, Lorberboym M. Technetium ^{99m} dynamic and static red blood cell bleeding study showing increased blood flow to the entire colon. Semin Nucl Med 1994;24:248–50.

38. Goldenberg DM, Wlodkowski TJ, Sharket RM, et al. Colorectal cancer imaging with iodine-123- labeled CEA monoclonal antibody fragments. J Nucl Med 1993;34:61–70.

39. Eastwood HDH. Bowel transit studies in the elderly: radio-opaque markers in the investigation of constipation. Gerontol Clin 1972;14:154–9.

Endoscopy is a natural extension of the colorectal physical examination and is essential to the proper diagnosis and treatment of colorectal disease. Anoscopy was discussed in Chapter 2. This chapter discusses the other types and techniques of endoscopy used by colorectal surgeons.

Proctoscopy

Proctoscopy allows visualization of the rectum and anus. The examination has traditionally been performed with a 25 cm rigid scope (**Figure 5.1**). Although this examination has an inappropriately negative reputation among the general public, with proper technique it can be accomplished in a quick, relatively painless manner [1]. Despite the use of fiberoptic scopes described later in this chapter, the rigid proctoscope maintains a role in the colorectal surgeon's armentarium [2].

Patient preparation

One or two Fleet enemas given within 1 hour of the examination are usually sufficient to empty the rectum and distal colon. If administered before this time, the enemas may stimulate movement of stool from proximal (right and transverse) colon to move into the distal colon and rectum, making proctoscopy difficult.

The patient is reassured that the examination will not hurt and that each phase of the examination will be explained as it proceeds. The patient is asked to take slow, even breaths, to refrain from bearing down and forcing the scope out, and is informed that he or she may experience a mild sensation of cramping or 'gas' during insufflation.

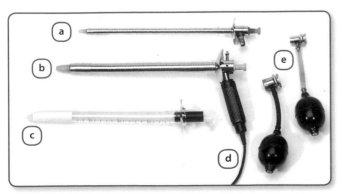

Figure 5.1 Rigid proctoscopes.
(a), Pediatric (11 mm x 25 cm);
(b), adult (19 mm x 25 cm);
(c), disposable (19 mm x 25 cm);
(d), light source; (e), insufflators.

Finally, the patient is told when the limits of the examination have been reached and that 'things will feel better now' as the scope is withdrawn. Remember the merits of 'vocal anesthesia'.

One of the reasons patients fear rigid proctoscopy is the zealous physicians who pride themselves on always inserting the scope to 25 cm. It is inappropriate to demand a 25 cm examination in every case; many patients have had pelvic surgery, prior radiation, or pelvic infections and have relatively fixed rectums or looped sigmoid colons. The experienced examiner knows how far the scope can humanely be inserted and will stop before unforgettable discomfort occurs. Inserting the scope to only 14–16 cm does not demonstrate a lack of skill. A large review of proctoscopic examinations found that the average length of scope inserted was 17–20 cm [3,4]. Patients who have an extremely painful experience because of an excessive examination will understandably be reluctant to repeat it later. Although the incidence of perforation is low, patient discomfort is a significant warning sign.

Proctoscopes come in a variety of sizes and shapes (**Figure 5.1**). For many adult examinations, the disposable plastic scopes give adequate visibility and avoid the fuss and possible disease exposure of reusable scopes. An adult proctoscope can usually be used in most patients including children; 'pediatric' proctoscopes are useful in cases of narrowed lumina, tight stomas, and in some children. Children will often cooperate with the examiner and tolerate an examination without anesthesia if the procedure is explained in a calm and understanding manner. However, selected patients may require sedation or even general anesthesia.

The typical plastic disposable proctoscope is 25 cm in length and 19 mm in diameter. Some special operating proctoscopes are as large as 40 mm in diameter and up to 50 cm in length. These larger scopes usually require general or regional anesthesia and are designed for resecting large villous adenomas or fulgurating rectal cancers in poor-risk patients. Proctoscopes are available in proximal and distal lighted versions. Each type works equally well, and a preference is usually based on operator experience.

Diagnostic technique

Several positions can be used for the examination. I prefer the prone position (described in Chapter 3), with the Sims' position as an acceptable alternative. In either position the patient's head is positioned below the buttocks. The procedure starts with a perineal and digital examination (see Chapter 3). Using a three-glove technique (two gloves on the right hand and one on the left), the examiner performs a careful digital examination with the right index finger (lubricated with water-soluble jelly), checking especially the posterior rectum, an area that is potentially blind to the endoscope. The outer right glove is then discarded.

The scope is introduced initially toward the umbilicus (**Figure 5.2**), with the thumb of the right hand firmly pressed against the handle

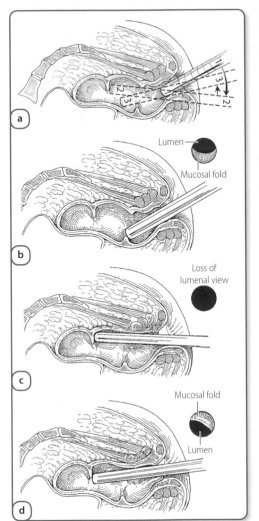

Figure 5.2 Insertion of a proctoscope (a). Note the various angles required to negotiate the rectum as it conforms to the sacral curve. (b–d) Advancement of a proctoscope. Views are through the advancing proctoscope, straightening out a mucosal fold. The lumen is always at least partially in view when the scope is advanced.

Lumen

Mucosal fold

Loss of lumenal view

Mucosal fold

Lumen

of the obturator. The obturator is withdrawn and discarded after the scope is inserted beyond the sphincters. The examiner's left hand grasps the light source at the end of the scope, and the right hand uses the suction wand to aspirate rectal contents as the scope is advanced, keeping the lumen in view at all times. When the scope reaches 6–8 cm, the lumen takes a sharp turn posteriorly, following the curvature of the sacrum. At the 14–16 cm depth, the scope is directed in an anterior direction, often angling slightly to the right. At this point the lumen may become difficult to follow. One technique is to withdraw the suction wand, shut the lens end of the scope, and administer gentle insufflation to distend the bowel lumen. Insufflation, however, may cause discomfort and ought to be minimized; it is also unnecessary in the lower part of the rectum in most patients. Occasionally one encounters stool in the upper rectum, which is difficult to remove with suction and which obscures the mucosa. The rectum can be cleaned by instilling about 50 mL of tap water into the proctoscope, closing the lens cap, and insufflating air. The air will often flush the stool and water down into the more proximal bowel, allowing a more complete examination of the distal colon and rectum. For obvious reasons, all advancement is performed under direct vision with the lumen in view, and any significant discomfort is countered with partial withdrawal of the scope and redirection (**Figure 5.2**).

Obvious lesions will be identified during insertion, but the most important part of the examination occurs while withdrawing the scope. After the rectum has been cleaned using the suction wand, the examiner should study all areas of the wall as the proctoscope is withdrawn in a spiral motion, inspecting for polyps, vascular abnormalities, and signs of inflammatory bowel disease or tumors. Care is taken to look behind valves and to clean all areas, where pooling of fluid may occur, to ensure that all the mucosa is inspected.

Therapy

For patients requiring therapeutic procedures, use of aspirin products, clopidogrel bisulfate (Plavix, Sanofi Pharmaceuticals, New York, NY, USA), and anticoagulants should be discontinued 3–14 days before the procedure [5]. A history of bleeding merits evaluation and possibly therapy. Biopsies are obtained as indicated and are performed at readily accessible areas. The size of the biopsied tissue depends on the forceps used and the indication for the biopsy. For cancer or amyloidosis, a large piece is useful. The edge of a valve of Houston is usually a safe area for a deep biopsy. In proctitis or inflammatory bowel disease, a small piece is adequate. Biopsy forceps from a flexible scope work very well for these small samples.

If the biopsy site bleeds, it may be controlled by several methods. The best technique for cauterization is to trap the targeted mucosa in the end of the proctoscope, thus walling out gas or liquid from the lumen of the bowel, and then to aspirate any residual gas or liquid remaining inside the scope. This minimizes the chances of a cautery explosion through the proctoscope [6]. If cautery is unavailable, a long epinephrine-soaked swab can be held against the biopsy site for several minutes. Almost all biopsy sites will stop bleeding after a few minutes of pressure. Small hyperplastic-appearing polyps can be cauterized using a long electrocautery pencil.

Snare excision of rectal polyps via a proctoscope is a useful technique. Polyps that are two large to excise with a fiberoptic scope can often be excised in one or multiple pieces [7]. The open nature of the procedure allows it to be performed with a limited bowel preparation.

After the scope is withdrawn, the table is returned to a horizontal position and allowed to settle toward the floor. The patient is warned about getting up too quickly, because there is a risk of syncope after having been in the exaggerated jackknife position. The patient is helped to a bathroom and observed for a few moments. The procedure is documented by recording the:

- insertion depth
- the appearance of the mucosa
- the size, location, and appearance of any lesions
- the location of any biopsies taken
- the adequacy of the preparation.

Before leaving the office, the patient is informed of the findings and any need for further examinations or tests. Postprocedure discussions include the possibility of gas, cramping pains, and if biopsies were taken, the passage of small amounts of blood with the first bowel movement. The patient is also instructed to seek immediate medical attention for the development of pelvic pain, fever, difficult urination, or passage of a large amount of blood.

Complications

An occasional patient has difficulty tolerating the position or discomfort of proctoscopy and may hyperventilate or have a vasovagal reaction. Usually, reminding the patient to breathe slowly is enough to combat hyperventilation. Vasovagal reactions can be more serious. The patient may report a faint feeling or might suddenly stop talking and become cool and diaphoretic to the touch. Since it is difficult to manage such a patient in the prone jackknife position, the first response is to remove the proctoscope and bring the patient's head back up by tilting the table to the horizontal position. If the patient remains unresponsive, he or she is quickly lifted off the table, placed in the supine position, and oxygen is administered. Recovery is usually quick and uneventful, and little harm occurs from such a reaction. However, the potential exists for a serious arrhythmia or even a full cardiopulmonary arrest. Thus oxygen, a crash cart, intravenous fluid, and other resuscitation equipment should be readily available in the proctoscopy clinic.

Rigid proctosigmoidoscopy was the standard for inspecting the rectum and lower sigmoid colon before the introduction of fiberoptic colonoscopy. At the Mayo Clinic some 350,000 proctoscopies over 20 years were performed, with four injuries to the bowel (three mucosal tears and one perforation) [1]. Corman [5] reported more than 70,000 examinations without a perforation but had one case of ventricular fibrillation resulting in death. Other large series confirm the low incidence of perforation and bleeding after proctoscopy [8–10].

An additional use for the rigid proctoscope is to aid in transrectal ultrasonography. The scope allows the examiner to insure the absence of feces or to remove any residual intralumenal material and to aid insertion of the ultrasound probe above rectal lesions.

Flexible fiberoptic sigmoidoscopy

Fiberoptic technology became available in the late 1960s. Flexible fiberoptic sigmoidoscopes (**Figure 5.3**) are 35–65 cm in length. The

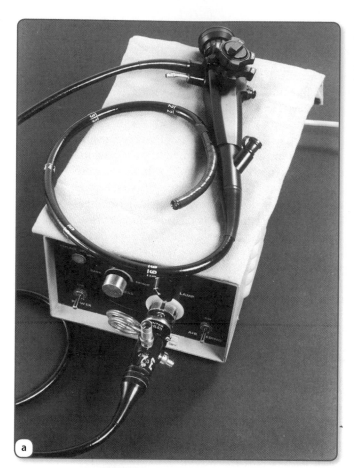

Figure 5.3 Typical 65 cm flexible fiberoptic sigmoidoscope and light source (a). (b) Close-up demonstrating control handle and flexible tip.

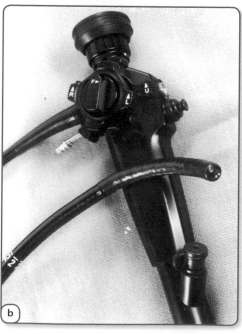

advantages of these instruments are obvious: more bowel length is examined, greatly increasing the chances of finding a pathologic condition, and the patient is generally more comfortable because of the flexible nature of the scope. More recently, video technology has been incorporated into sigmoidoscopy. Videosigmoidoscopy allows the entire health care team to view the procedure, but is more expensive than an optic scope. In defense of the rigid scope, flexible instruments are very expensive, tend to break periodically, and are not disposable and thus need to be cleaned after each use (which may spread disease if improperly cleaned). In addition, cautery should not be used with flexible sigmoidoscopes if the bowel has not been completely prepared with a bowel-cleansing agent, whereas cautery is safer with a rigid scope (because of its open end) if used after a less-thorough preparation. Another concern is that flexible sigmoidoscopes cannot replace full length colonoscopy.

Patient preparation

The cleansing preparation for flexible sigmoidoscopy is similar to that described for proctoscopy (e.g. two Fleet enemas).

Diagnostic technique

The flexible scope is inspected to ensure that it is in perfect working order before insertion. This entails looking through the lens to confirm that it is in focus and not cloudy (suggestive of water leakage), checking the light source for adequate brightness and testing the suction, insufflation, and irrigation valves for movability and function.

The perianal and digital examinations are performed as described previously. The distal 10 cm of the scope is lubricated and inserted using firm, gentle pressure to overcome sphincter resistance. The shaft of the scope is grasped with the right hand (a dry gauze pad can be used to provide a secure grip) and the control handle is held with the left hand. Once the scope is in the distal rectum, any residual enema fluid or mucus is aspirated. The flexible fiberoptic sigmoidoscope is advanced with the right hand while the left hand controls insufflation, suction, irrigation, and the vertical and horizontal tip controls. Occasionally, it is necessary to have a helper hold the scope at the anus, while the horizontal control is manipulated with the right hand. Air insufflation distends the bowel and the lumen is kept in sight by use of the tip controls or torsion (axial rotation of the scope shaft) of the scope. The goal is to visualize the entire colorectal mucosa without injuring the patient. As in proctoscopy, it is not always possible to insert the scope completely. Limitations occur when the bowel is incompletely prepared, is strictured, or angulated in a fixed position because of prior pelvic infection, surgery, or radiotherapy. As in rigid proctoscopy, it is always better to abort or shorten the examination rather than cause the patient undue discomfort or complications.

During the procedure the scope is advanced as far as possible. When it is withdrawn, the bowel wall mucosa is inspected. Air is aspirated as the withdrawal progresses. Mucosal characteristics such as friability, easy bleeding, loss of vascularity, polyps, strictures, or ulcers are noted. Lesion location is described as being a certain distance along the scope. This distance will vary according to the amount of bowel telescoped on the scope, stretch of bowel, and whether the scope was entering or exiting the bowel. If indicated, cold biopsies of suspicious lesions may be obtained. Patients rarely experience discomfort during examination of the distal 25–30 cm; however, examination of the proximal bowel may be uncomfortable and this part of the examination should be expedited.

Techniques used to assist in advancing the scope through the sigmoid colon include 'dithering', the 'alpha maneuver', torquing, hooking, external compression, and the 'slide-by' maneuver [11]. Each examiner develops personal techniques; there is not one correct way to conduct the examination. The skill and experience of the examiner play a key role in the successful outcome of flexible fiberoptic sigmoidoscopy. Certainly the seasoned endoscopist can do this procedure quickly and with minimal discomfort. Becoming facile in endoscopy follows a learning curve, and the beginner should do this procedure under the supervision of a patient teacher. The following are useful endoscopic maneuvers [12].

Dithering

It is possible to sit on a chair and, without having the feet touch the floor, move the chair about by jerking the body; similarly, one can advance the scope within the bowel by a series of rapid, back-and-forth movements. This oscillating, jerking movement is called 'dithering'. One advances the scope a few inches in a rapid forward motion, and then withdraws the scope more slowly. This has the effect of pleating the bowel onto the scope and is less painful than simply pushing ahead. The examiner should remember that stretch of the mesentery or excess distention of the bowel will cause pain to the patient.

Alpha maneuver

The occasional sigmoid colon will be very redundant, with fixed points proximal and distal. The alpha maneuver is the deliberate formation of an alpha-shaped loop in the sigmoid, followed by the withdrawal and clockwise torque of the scope to straighten out the sigmoid. This maneuver demonstrates the important principle that generally any counterclockwise rotation or torque will generate a sigmoid loop and will stretch the bowel anteriorly along the abdominal wall, whereas clockwise rotation will tend to eliminate the sigmoid loop and will pull the bowel posteriorly, avoiding stretch and pain. Usually the alpha maneuver will allow examination up to the descending colon with the flexible sigmoidoscope but will not get to the splenic flexure.

Torquing

A mark of a truly skilled endoscopist is how the right hand is used and how torque is applied to the shaft of the scope to aid advancement. Clockwise rotation of the scope seems to be a key feature in comfortable and successful examination. The right hand interprets the feel of the scope and the amount of resistance to passage of the scope. Often the novice endoscopist forgets to concentrate on this area of the examination.

Hooking

One can negotiate sharp turns in the colon by flexing the tip of the scope, 'hooking' the fold in the mucosa, then advancing the scope after the lumen comes into view.

External compression

At times the sigmoid colon simply cannot be traversed without applying external compression. The patient is usually rolled into a supine position, and an assistant applies left lower quadrant pressure, thus splinting the bowel from the exterior and facilitating passage.

Slide-by maneuver

At times it is impossible to see the lumen of the bowel, but as the scope is advanced, one sees the mucosal wall 'sliding by'. The lumen is usually seen soon after, and the examination continues. This maneuver is potentially dangerous and can lead to perforation if done too vigorously. If performed in an area of diverticula, there is danger that the tip of the scope might lodge in a diverticulum and cause a perforation. Thus the presence of diverticula is a relative contraindication to the slide-by maneuver.

Often a simultaneous combination of multiple techniques is used to advance the scope [11]. A good rule is to partially withdraw the scope when it does not appear to be advancing properly and to reinsert it using a more clockwise torque. If a large amount of stool is encountered, the patient becomes too uncomfortable, the scope simply cannot be passed higher, or the scope is passed to its limit, the procedure is terminated by a slow withdrawal and inspection of all the bowel mucosa. Lesions are biopsied and their location documented according to the distance from the anal verge or the anatomic location of the colon. The distance from the anal verge is variable when measured with a flexible scope because of the amount of bowel stretched by the scope; it is not a reproducible or reliable measurement above the rectum. One can determine the location in the colon by internal landmarks and by observation of transilluminated light or palpation as described earlier. As in proctoscopy, it is not always possible to insert the scope to its full length. The important point is to see as much as possible without hurting the patient.

Complications

Complications with flexible sigmoidoscopy are similar to those with proctoscopy [13]. The greater amount of bowel examined, however, does slightly increase the perforation rate. Other problems associated with this closed system are discussed in the colonoscopy section.

Colonoscopy

Colonoscopy uses a flexible fibroscopic scope of 120–160 cm in length (**Figure 5.4**). The procedure is not comparable to flexible sigmoidoscopy, because the flexibility and feel of the scope is different, the examination is more uncomfortable for the patient, the preparation is more extensive, and the techniques involved are more difficult to learn [11,12]. Some capable physicians who are expert at flexible sigmoidoscopy cannot do or have never learned colonoscopy. There is no one correct way to perform colonoscopy. The acknowledged experts each seem to have individual techniques and tricks to passing the scope [11]. The student who wants to become a colonoscopist needs to work with a competent teacher and participate in the care of a number of patients before achieving credentialed status [13]. The exact number of colonoscopies that should be required is problematic; certainly one should examine 50–75 patients to feel comfortable with the technique. Maneuvers similar to that described for flexible sigmoidoscopy are used with the colonoscope. However, loops in the sigmoid colon need to be straightened to successfully advance the colonoscope to the cecum, and several barriers to advancement exist beyond the sigmoid colon.

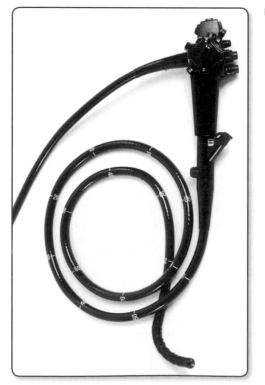

Figure 5.4 Typical flexible videocolonoscope.

Patient preparation

The bowel should be subjected to a rigorous, formal preparation, resulting in an absence of hydrogen or methane gas and intraluminal particulate matter. Common cleansing methods use an oral electrolyte lavage solution (PEG lavage), hypertonic solutions, stimulate laxatives or combinations of these as described in Chapter 6.

Not every patient requires sedative medication for a successful examination. Using gentle and careful technique, it is possible in selected patients to advance the scope with a fully awake patient. Discomfort is anticipated and scope configuration is corrected before pain is perceived. For most situations, however, intravenous sedation facilitates the procedure [14]. Medications usually administered include meperidine (Demerol), 25–100 mg, given slowly in 25 mg increments intravenously or fentanyl, 25–150 mg intravenously, and midazolam (Versed), 0.5–10 mg intravenously, depending on the age and general state of the patient. Meperidine and fentanyl are analgesics, while midazolam is a sedative with amnesic effects. It is convenient to have an intravenous catheter started before the patient is brought to the endoscopy suite. Each medication is given, then flushed with normal saline solution. The goal of conscious sedation is to have the patient awake enough to be able to respond to painful stimuli, yet relaxed enough to allow for easy passage of the scope [15]. Having the patient responsive is thought to reduce the risk of perforation. Because there is a risk of respiratory arrest with these agents, proper resuscitation equipment must be within easy reach in the endoscopy suite. The effects of meperidine can be reversed with administration of naloxone (Narcan), 0.2 mg IV along with 0.2 mg IM, whereas midazolam is reversed with flumazenil (Romazicon), a benzodiazepine-receptor antagonist, 0.2–1.0 mg IV.

Rarely, it will be necessary to perform colonoscopy with the patient under general anesthesia. The risks of perforation increase, and there is a small but finite risk associated with general anesthesia itself. However, in a pediatric patient or in the rare adult who cannot undergo colonoscopy while sedated, general anesthesia is an option. Most colonoscopies are performed in a clinic setting, with the patient arriving the morning of the procedure, having accomplished most of the bowel preparation at home the day or night before. A heparin lock or intravenous catheter is started, and the patient is taken to the endoscopy suite. During the examination the patient is monitored and observed using a pulse oximeter, automated blood pressure monitoring, and in selected patients, with electrocardiac (ECG) monitoring [15,16]. After completion of colonoscopy, patients are observed until they are awake and stable. Any patient who has received sedation is not allowed to drive home and needs to be accompanied by someone else. Colonoscopy is a major procedure, and patients must be properly informed of potential risks, including perforation, bleeding, ileus, reactions to medications, and respiratory or cardiac arrest.

Informed consent is obtained before the procedure and should include the possibility of overlooking a polyp or other lesion and an incomplete examination (failure to reach the cecum) because of unusual anatomy, prior surgery, or disease activity. The patient is also informed that some polyps are impossible to remove endoscopically and that occasionally a laparotomy will be required for complete removal.

Diagnostic technique

The initial positioning and insertion techniques described for flexible sigmoidoscopy are similar for colonoscopy. The examination begins with the patient in the left lateral decubitus position. After the scope is inserted past the splenic flexure, it is often helpful to rotate the patient to the supine position for further advancement of the scope around the flexure (often the dark bluish color of the spleen can be seen at the flexure and serves as a landmark.) External pressure in the left lower quadrant often facilitates passage of the scope. The transverse colon characteristically has a triangular lumen which, along with transilluminated light seen in the epigastric area, serves as a landmark. The bluish color of the liver is often seen through the colon at the hepatic flexure. To facilitate passage of the scope at the hepatic flexure, the patient is asked to inhale deeply to lower the hepatic flexure and lessen the acuity of the angle or acuity of the bowel. After entering the ascending colon, the scope is advanced with aspiration and slight withdrawal. The cecum is entered and inspected. Confirmatory landmarks include the ileocecal valve, the appendiceal lumen, and the convergence of the three taeniae coli. Indirect evidence of cecal intubation includes transillumination of light in the right lower quadrant and abdominal wall percussion (seen as movement of the cecal wall).

While the colonoscope is slowly withdrawn, the luminal wall is inspected. New technology allows easy photographic documentation, and biopsies are performed as indicated. All findings are documented, with special attention to location, size, appearance, and feel during biopsy. As the scope is withdrawn, some of the insufflated air is aspirated to make the patient more comfortable.

Therapy

In preparation for the use of cautery (hot biopsy forceps or snare polypectomy), a grounding pad is attached to the patient. The assistant passes the snare or biopsy forceps (**Figure 5.5**) to the colonoscopist and controls the handle to open and close the instrument [17]. It is important to manipulate the snare in a controlled manner. Tightening the snare too rapidly or vigorously can detach the polyp before hemostasis is achieved. Videoendoscopy allows both the endoscopist and assistant to view the scope image and coordinate these actions.

Most polypectomies should be performed with the polyp in the 6 o'clock position [17]. In this location the snare comes out of the scope in the bottom field of view. The snare is opened and with a combination

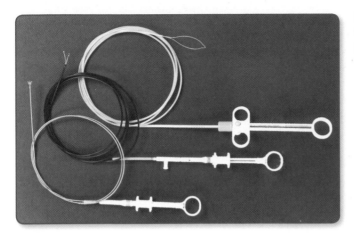

Figure 5.5 Top to bottom: colonoscopic snare, tripod grasper, and biopsy forceps.

of scope manipulation and back-and-forth movement of the snare, the wire loop encircles the polyp. The plastic sheath is advanced forward to the base of the polyp, pinning the stalk in one place as the snare is tightened. The goal is to transect the stalk near the neck of the polyp, leaving some stalk behind. Before applying cautery through the snare, the examiner aspirates and insufflates the colon to minimize the risk of an explosion. If preparation is inadequate, the polypectomy should not proceed. The amount of electrical current used should be tailored to the size and configuration of the polyp, and it is important to check the cautery settings before each application. Cutting current is used sparingly because of its risk of perforation. If hemorrhage occurs after the stalk is transected, it may be regrasped with the snare, recauterized carefully with forceps, or controlled with endoscopic placed clips or a detachable snare (loop). Irrigation with an epinephrine solution is also helpful. If no bleeding is observed on inspection of the polypectomy site, the polyp is grasped with retrieval forceps or a basket (**Figure 5.5**) and removed with the scope. Care is taken to ensure that the polyp is not lost during retrieval. After removal, the specimen is rapidly placed in a fixative solution and sent for pathologic review.

Complications

The major complications of colonoscopy are bleeding, perforation, and transmural burn. Infrequent complications include reaction to medications given at the time of the procedure, cardiac and pulmonary difficulties as a result of the preparation, explosions, contraction of communicable diseases via the scope, injury of the mucosa from cleaning solution left on or in the scope, phlebitis, ileus, Ogilvie's syndrome, retained polypectomy snare, volvulus, and splenic rupture [13,18].

Bleeding

Bleeding is the most common complication reported, with an incidence ranging from 0.5–3% [13,18–20]. Risk factors for bleeding include anticoagulation (secondary to ingestion of aspirin products or warfarin sodium before the procedure) and the performance of therapeutic procedures (polypectomy or biopsy). Patients with postpolypectomy bleeding are managed in the following manner. After resuscitation with intravenous fluid, a tagged RBC scan is obtained. If evidence of bleeding is documented on this examination, an angiogram is obtained. If ongoing bleeding is observed, a pitressin infusion is started (0.4 µg/min). A review from the Ochsner Clinic of 13 patients with postpolypectomy hemorrhage demonstrated that most patients with angiographic bleeding can be controlled with a pitressin drip [19]. More recently, the bleeding is controlled with angiographic microembolozation of the bleeding vessel using sterile gelatin (Gelfoam) or coils.

Transmural burn

Transmural burn or postpolypectomy syndrome is heralded by a presentation similar to that of diverticulitis. If the abdominal pain and tenderness remains localized, the patient can be managed with intravenous fluids, antibiotics, and bowel rest. Usually this complication occurs in thin, right-sided bowel after removal of a sessile polyp or performance of a hot biopsy. It is also possible for the electrical current to injure the mucosa opposite the polyp if the tip of the polyp is allowed to touch the opposing wall during application of the cautery. Moving the polyp back and forth during cautery dissipates any current.

Perforation

Perforation results from mechanical forces during colonoscopic insertion or from barotrauma during colonic insufflation. The incidence after diagnostic procedures ranges from 0.06–0.8%, whereas after therapeutic procedures the incidence is 0.5–3.0%. Perforation is diagnosed during the procedure by observation of extraluminal fat or other intra-abdominal contents (e.g. small bowel, liver) via the colonoscope. Patients with this complication usually report immediate pain and demonstrate signs of peritoneal irritation. Postprocedure presentations vary from asymptomatic free intra-abdominal air to fluid peritonitis and sepsis. Patients with localized to absent symptoms can be observed and treated with intravenous fluids, antibiotics, and bowel rest [18]. If signs of peritoneal irritation develop, laparotomy is mandated, and repair of the perforation performed. The most common site of perforation is the sigmoid colon, probably because of pre-existing disease. Nivatvongs [20] stated that overinsufflation of the bowel is not only painful for the patient, but also thins the wall and predisposes to perforation.

Besides the routine diagnostic and therapeutic colonoscopy procedures, the colonoscope is useful for a variety of other conditions including the retrieval of foreign bodies, the application of laser energy to cauterize vascular malformations and core out unresectable malignancies for palliation, the reduction of sigmoid or cecal volvulus, the intraoperative localization of prior polypectomy sites to aid in performing appropriate colonic resections, the diagnosis of ileal Crohn's disease, and the decompression of the distended colon in Ogilvie's syndrome [21, 22].

Scope cleaning and disinfection

Endoscopes are complex and fragile pieces of equipment, and because of their repeated use on different patients they may transmit infection. The care and maintenance of endoscopes are therefore of prime importance. Each endoscopy unit should have established written guidelines on the cleaning and disinfection of their endoscopes. In general, after each procedure the scope and its channels are irrigated with water and an enzymatic detergent solution. The scope is then mechanically cleaned and rinsed. This is followed by disinfection with a solution such as glutearaldehyde [23]. Finally the scope is rinsed and dried. Many of the procedures can be accomplished by an automated cleaner.

Rounds questions

1. What is the average depth of insertion during a proctoscopy?
2. When is the best look at the bowel mucosa obtained?
3. What are the symptoms of a vasovagal reaction?
4. Is it safe to use cautery after a bowel preparation consisting of one or two Fleet enemas?
5. What are the risks of a 'slide-by' maneuver?
6. What medications are used to reverse the pain and sedative medications used during colonoscopy?
7. What monitors should be used in a patient who is receiving conscious sedation?
8. A polypectomy is best performed when the lesion is positioned in what relationship to the colonoscopic field of view?
9. What are the major complications of colonoscopy?

References

1. Welling DR. Endoscopy. In: Beck DE, Welling DR, (eds). Patient Care in Colorectal Surgery. Boston: Little, Brown 1991;49–63.
2. Hicks TC. Transanal endoscopy. In: Whitlow CB, Beck DE, Margolin DA, Hicks TC, Timmcke AE (eds). Improved Outcomes in Colon and Rectal Surgery London: Informa Healthcare, London 2010;132–9.
3. Nivatvongs S, Fryd DS. How far does the proctosigmoidoscope reach? N Engl J Med 1980;303:380–2.
4. Mazier WP, Levin DH, Lutchtefeld MA, Senagore AJ. Surgery of the Colon, Rectum, and Anus. Philadelphia: WB Saunders 1995;70–71.
5. Timothy SKC, Timmcke AE, Hicks TC, Beck DE, Opelka FG. Colonoscopy in the anticoagulated patient. Dis Colon Rectum 2001;44:1845–8.
6. Corman MD. Colon and Rectal Surgery, 2nd ed. Philadelphia: JB Lippincott 1989;10.
7. Whitlow CW, Beck DE, Gathright JB, Jr. Surgical excision of large rectal villous adenomas. Surg Onc Clin N Am 1996;5:723–34.
8. Goldberg SM, Gordon PH, Nivatvongs S. Essentials of Anorectal Surgery. Philadelphia: JB Lippincott 1980.
9. Goligher J. Surgery of the Anus, Rectum, and Colon, 5th ed. London: Baillière Tindall, 1984; 64–8.

10. Gilhertson VA. Proctosigmoidoscopy and polypectomy in reducing the incidence of rectal cancer. Cancer 34(Suppl): 1974;936–9.

11. Church JM. Technical pearls. Clinics Colon Rectal Surg 2001;14:331–6.

12. Nivatvongs S. How to teach colonoscopy. Clinics Colon Rectal Surg 2001;14:387–92.

13. Opelka FG. Transanal endoscopy. In Hicks TC, Beck DE, Opelka FG, Timmcke AE (eds) Complications of Colon & Rectal Surgery. Baltimore: Williams & Wilkins, 1996;143–52.

14. Bigard MA, Gaucher P, Lassalle C. Fatal colonic explosion during colonoscopic polypectomy. Gastroenterology 1979;77:1307–10.

15. Larach SW, Neto JS, Gentry GL. Sedation, analgesia, and monitoring. Clinics Colon Rectal Surg 2001;14:325–30.

16. Sedation and monitoring of patients undergoing gastrointestinal endoscopic procedures. American Society for Gastrointestinal Endoscopy. Gastrointest Endosc 1995;42:626–9.

17. Khurrum M, Weiss EG. Therapeutic colonoscopy. Clinics Colon Rectal Surg 2001;14:347–58.

18. Reickert CA, Beck DE. Complications of colonoscopy. Clinics Colon Rectal Surg 2001;14:379–86.

19. Gibbs DG, Opelka FG, Beck DE, Hicks TC, Timmcke AE, Gathright JB. Post-polypectomy hemorrhage of the lower gastrointestine. Dis Colon Rectum 1996;39:806–10.

20. Nivatvongs S. Complications in colonoscopic polypectomy: An experience with 1555 polypectomies. Dis Colon Rectum 1986;29:825–30.

21. Roberts PL. Patient evaluation. In: Beck DE, Wexner SD (eds). Fundamentals of anorectal surgery. New York: McGraw-Hill 1992;25–35.

22. Shinya H. Colonoscopy. New York: Igaku-Shoin 1982.

23. Pishori T, Efron J. Scope cleaning and disinfection. Clinics Colon Rectal Surg 2001;14:317–23.

Minimally invasive surgery

Laparoscopy has a long history and recent technologic advancements, such as videolaparoscopy, and economic inducements have encouraged general and colorectal surgeons to adopt this technology [1]. For frequently performed procedures that are less demanding, such as cholecystectomy, laparoscopic methods have rapidly become the method of choice for most patients. However, colon and rectal procedures are significantly more difficult, and, despite almost 20 years of experience, minimally invasive techniques have had a slower and less significant impact on patient care [2].

The colon is a large, hollow organ located in all four abdominal quadrants. Colorectal procedures require extensive mobilization of the colon, with ligation of numerous large blood vessels, extraction of a large specimen, and restoration of bowel continuity. These additional challenges have required special instruments and techniques. Potential advantages of laparoscopic techniques over open approaches include less pain and disability, shorter postoperative ileus, a shorter hospital stay, and improved cosmesis. Unfortunately, with the exception of cosmesis, few of these advantages have been consistently demonstrated by prospective controlled trials. Disadvantages of laparoscopy are its additional cost, reduction or loss of tactile information for the surgeon, and limited data on cancer recurrence and survival rates after laparoscopic procedures.

This chapter briefly reviews the expanding status of laparoscopy in colorectal surgery.

Equipment

Laparoscopic procedures require considerable equipment and personnel. These are frequently arranged in the operating room as shown in **Figure 6.1**. The video monitors must be positioned to allow direct viewing by the surgeon and assistant.

Table

The primary mode of retraction during laparoscopic surgery is gravity [3]; therefore the operating table must be able to move maximally in all positions: Trendelenburg, reverse Trendelenburg, airplane right and left (axial rotation to place the patient's right side or left side down). In addition, the patient must remain securely attached to the table by a bean bag (with Velcro attachments), tape, straps, or table rests. The patient is positioned in the supine or low lithotomy position

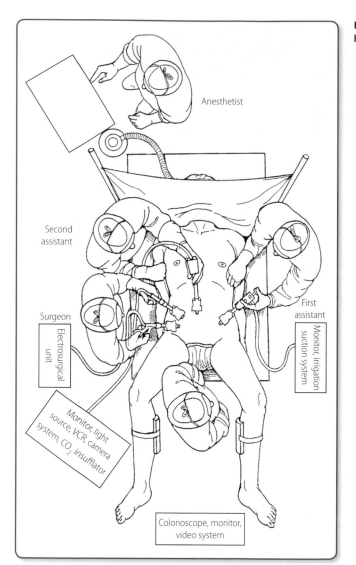

Figure 6.1 Room setup for laparoscopic surgery.

Anesthetist

Second assistant

Surgeon

Electrosurgical unit

Monitor, light source, VCR, camera system, CO_2 insufflator

First assistant

Monitor, irrigation suction system

Colonoscope, monitor, video system

(**Figure 6.2**). This prevents the patient's thighs from limiting instrument manipulation and allows a surgeon or assistant to stand between the patient's legs. Tucking one or both of the patient's arms to their sides allows two members of the surgical team to stand on a patient's side.

Laparoscopic tower

The tower contains the video camera, light source, high-flow volume-regulated insufflator, and monitors (two or three) with or without recording capability. This type of tower may be mounted on a wheeled cart or suspended from the ceiling (**Figure 6.3**). Suction, irrigation, and electrocautery equipment may be included or available as stand-alone

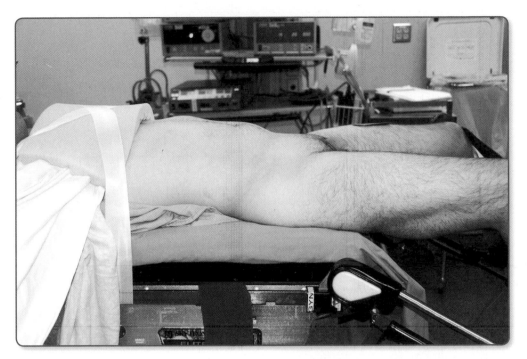

Figure 6.2 Low lithotomy position. Legs supported by stirrups with minimal flexure of hips. The patient is secured to the table with tape.

units. Current state of the art video uses a high definition camera that is attached to a laparoscopic wand. Current wands incorporate end viewing (0°), angle viewing (30° or 45°), or flexible tip lenses and are illuminated with a xenon light source.

Instruments for pneumoperitoneum and access

Gas (CO_2) with a pressure of 12–15 mmHg is instilled into the abdomen to distend the abdominal wall and allow adequate visualization. This pneumoperitoneum is established with a blunt-tipped (Hasson) cannula, placed in the peritoneal cavity under direct vision using a small incision, as in an open technique for peritoneal lavage. An alternative method uses a Veress needle placed through a small infraumbilical incision. A wide variety of cannulas and trocars is available to provide access to the peritoneal cavity while the pneumoperitoneum is maintained (**Figure 6.4**).

Another variation is the use of a Handport (**Figure 6.5**). This device uses a small incision (6.5–8.0 cm) that allows insertion of a surgeon's hand into the abdomen while maintaining a pneumoperitoneum. The device shown (gel port, Applied Medical, Rancho Santa Margarita, CA) allows hand exchange while maintaining pneumoperitoneum. This hand-assisted laparoscopy shortens operating time, allows completion of some procedures that might not be possible with standard laparoscopy, and may lessen costs.

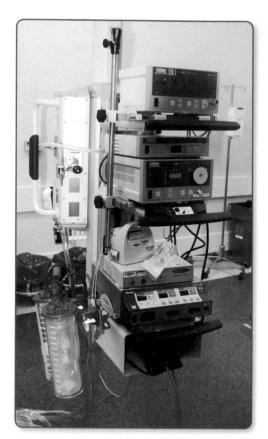

Figure 6.3 Ceiling mounted laparoscopic tower.

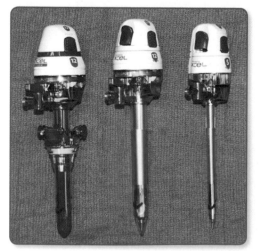

Figure 6.4 Laparoscopic trocars. Left to right: 12 mm blunt trocar, 12 mm trocar, 5 mm trocar.

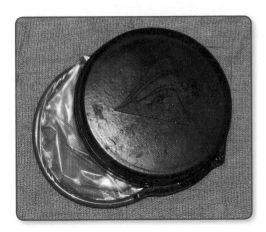

Figure 6.5 Hand port.

Laparoscopic instruments

Laparoscopic instruments must be of adequate length. The most frequently used instruments for dissection are graspers (e.g. Babcock's) and scissors. A selection of instruments is shown in **Figure 6.6**. Rotation of the instrument shaft and insulation are useful characteristics. To perform advanced techniques the surgeon must operate with both hands and instruments should be designed with this in mind.

Vascular control remains a difficult problem. Currently available options include cautery for small vessels, clips (placed with laparoscopic clip applier), endoscopic looped ligatures (e.g. EndoLoops, Ethicon), ligatures (tied intracorporeally or extracorporeally), and alternate energy instruments: Harmonic scalpel (Ethicon Endo-Surgery), Ligasure (Valley Lab, Boulder, CO, USA), Enseal (Ethicon Endo-Surgery,) and vascular staples. Laparoscopic staplers include linear cutters of 30–60 mm in length, circular intraluminal staplers, and linear staplers for vascular control. Surgical experience and preference play a major role in instrument selection.

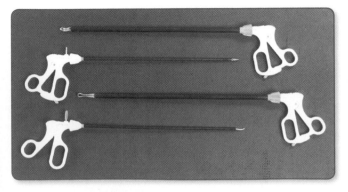

Figure 6.6 Laparoscopic instruments. Top to bottom: anvil grasper, 5 mm grasper, 10 mm Endo-Babcock grasper, and 5 mm curved scissors. (Courtesy of Ethicon Endo-Surgery, Cincinnati, OH, USA)

Patient selection and indications

Theoretically, all abdominal procedures are amenable to laparoscopic techniques. However, relative contraindications to laparoscopy include contraindications to general anesthesia, severe chronic obstructive pulmonary disease, dense adhesions, significant fecal peritonitis, massive abdominal wall hernias, late stage pregnancy, aortic or iliac aneurysms, and uncorrected coagulopathy. Other less significant contraindications include another indication for an open procedure, previous abdominal procedures, obesity, and redundant bowel.

The next section discusses colon and rectal procedures that are most successful, as well as current equipment and techniques.

Procedures

When discussing laparoscopic procedures it is critical to define terms and explain what each author or surgeon means by 'laparoscopically assisted'; this can vary from laparoscopically assisted mobilization, intracorporeal or extracorporeal vessel division, to how the specimen is removed (through either an enlarged incision, a trocar site after specimen morcellation, or the anus), and intracorporeal or extracorporeal anastomosis. Additional options include a hand assisted technique [4].

For a laparoscopic colorectal procedure, patient preparation is similar to that for an open procedure. As described in Chapter 8, the patient receives a mechanical and an antibiotic preparation. Informed consent for the procedure includes the developmental nature of laparoscopic procedures and the potential need for conversion to an open procedure. The operations are performed with the patient under general anesthesia and positioned in the modified Lloyd-Davies (using Lloyd-Davies or Allen stirrups) or supine position with one or both arms tucked. The patient's hips are minimally flexed to provide maximal abdominal exposure and prevent hindrance of the instrument handles or cameras (**Figure 6.2**). A Foley catheter and an orogastric tube are placed to decompress the bladder and stomach.

Stomas

Modern surgical procedures (as described elsewhere in this book) are being used with increased frequency to minimize the need for permanent intestinal stomas. However, many current operations use temporary stomas, and despite advances, a small number of patients will still require a permanent stoma. Many stoma procedures are well suited to laparoscopic techniques [2, 5].

Creation of the stoma

Indications for laparoscopic stomal creation are similar to those for open surgery. These include proximal diversion to protect an anastomosis or distal leak and to provide an intestinal outlet after a resection of the anus or in patients whose intra-abdominal condition would make an anastomosis inappropriate [6]. A sigmoid colostomy is also an option in patients with incontinence and patients who require intestinal diversion (e.g. massive decubitus ulcers, perineal injuries, or obstructing cancers). The patient is counseled by an experienced stoma therapist, and appropriate locations for potential ostomies are marked preoperatively.

Loop ileostomy

In patients who are not expected to require adhesiolysis, a two-trocar technique is used to create a **loop ileostomy**. This method creates the stomal opening before the pneumoperitoneum is established [5]. The stoma opening is created in a standard fashion by removing a 2.5 cm circular disk of skin at the preoperatively marked ileostomy site [5] The subcutaneous fat of the stomal site is divided in a vertical direction with electrocautery. Right-angle retractors are used to hold the divided subcutaneous tissue apart, which exposes the anterior rectus fascia. A traction suture (e.g. 2-0 Vicryl, Ethicon, Inc., Somerville, NJ, USA) is placed through each rectus fascial edge. This fascia is incised with an electrocautery device in a vertical direction, exposing the fibers of the rectus muscle. The muscle fibers are spread in a vertical direction with a straight clamp or scissors. The retractors are repositioned one at a time to retract the muscle and expose the posterior fascia. Two additional traction sutures or a pursestring suture are placed and the fascia is incised in a vertical direction with the electrocautery. Entrance into the peritoneal cavity is confirmed, and the previously placed traction sutures are used to secure a 10/12 mm Hasson trocar, which is placed through the stomal opening. A pneumoperitoneum is established, a camera is inserted, and the abdomen is explored.

Under direct vision a second 10/12 mm trocar is placed in one of two locations (**Figure 6.7a**). If the midline is clear of adhesions, the trocar can be placed near the umbilicus. If midline adhesions are present, the second trocar is placed in the right upper quadrant. This positioning conforms to the basic laparoscopic principles of placing trocars at least a handsbreadth apart and allowing the working trocars to remain between the camera and the work area. The camera is moved to this second port and the table is positioned to a head down, left side down position. This causes the small bowel to move out of the right lower abdominal quadrant and exposes the cecum and terminal ileum.

An atraumatic clamp is inserted in the ostomy port. If there are no adhesions, the most distal portion of the ileum that will reach the abdominal wall is identified. The Babcock clamp then grasps the distal ileum at the anticipated ostomy site. Under direct vision the bowel is manipulated to the stomal site (**Figure 6.8**). If the ileum easily reaches the posterior abdominal wall at the stomal site with an intact pneumoperitoneum, enough mobility is present to construct a stoma after the pneumoperitoneum is released in all but a massively obese patient. If the bowel does not easily reach, the clamp is moved to a

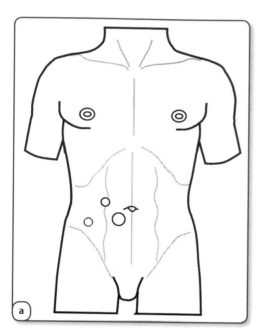

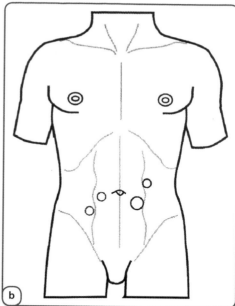

Figure 6.7 Port placement for laparoscopically assisted stoma creation. (a) Ileostomy. (b) Colostomy.

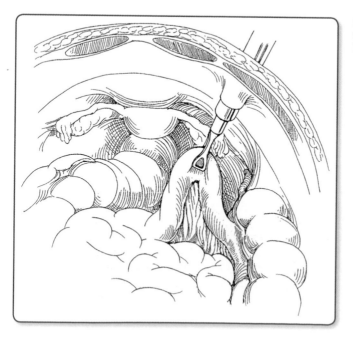

Figure 6.8 Bowel manipulated to the stomal opening using the laparoscopic Babcock grasper.

more proximal portion of the bowel or additional bowel is mobilized. In manipulating the bowel to the stomal site, one must ensure that the bowel is not inappropriately twisted and that there is no hemorrhage.

At this point the pneumoperitoneum is released through the camera port to allow the abdominal wall to relax and reduce tension on the mesentery. The Hasson trocar containing the Babcock clamp holding the bowel is slid up the Babcock shaft and advanced out the stomal site. The stomal opening is enlarged by lateral traction on two right-angle retractors placed along the Babcock shaft while the fascia is divided using electrocautery. The muscle split is adequate when the surgeon's finger has room to easily pass along the Babcock shaft into the abdomen. The Babcock clamp is then manipulated to bring the grasped loop of ileum out the stoma site. The bowel is then regrasped with regular Babcock clamps and, if desired, a stoma rod may be passed through the mesentery. The loop of ileum is opened and matured in the usual manner (see Figure 7.4). If an end loop stoma is preferred, the loop of bowel outside the abdomen may be divided with a linear cutting stapler. The nonfunctional end is then returned to a subcutaneous or intra-abdominal position. Care is taken to ensure that the functional (proximal) end is matured and the nonfunctional end is left closed.

After the stoma is matured, the remaining trocar sites are closed by approximating the anterior fascia with 2-0 Vicryl sutures (or Endo Judge, Synergistic Medical Technologies, FL, USA) and the skin is closed with 4-0 Vicryl sutures and Steri-Strips (3M Corporation, St. Paul, MN, USA). If division of adhesions is required or if the surgeon prefers to loop the bowel with an umbilical tape or Penrose drain to elevate the bowel rather than elevating it with a clamp, additional ports will be needed. Surgeon preference, experience, and intra-abdominal findings will determine the number, size, and location of additional trocars.

In an alternative method for creating a loop ileostomy, the pneumoperitoneum is established first with a Veress needle or blunt trocar (using the Hasson technique) placed in the supraumbilical area. Through this periumbilical or supraumbilical catheter (10/12 mm), a 10 mm camera is inserted. After the patient is positioned head down, left side down, an exploration is performed. Additional trocars are inserted at the stomal site and in the suprapubic area. After the bowel is grasped with a Babcock clamp passed through the port (trocar) placed at the stomal site, a circular piece of skin around the trocar is excised. The cannula is elevated along the clamp, and the pneumoperitoneum is released. The subcutaneous fat and rectus fascia are incised and stretched to two fingerbreadths to allow easy passage of the loop of ileum. The Babcock clamp and loop of ileum are withdrawn through this opening. The bowel is matured and the ports are closed as previously described.

Loop sigmoid colostomy

A loop sigmoid colostomy is accomplished in a manner similar to that described for a loop ileostomy, except for the location of the stoma and trocar sites, which are moved to the left side (**Figure 6.7b**). After the stoma opening in the left lower quadrant is created and trocars are inserted as described previously, the patient is positioned head down, right side down to expose the left lower quadrant and sigmoid colon. The distal portion of the sigmoid colon that will reach the abdominal wall is identified. It is often necessary to incise the lateral retroperitoneal attachments to create extra length and allow the sigmoid colon to easily reach the abdominal wall [8]. This requires placement of additional ports. Electrocautery scissors or Enseal are used to divide these attachments. An adequate amount of bowel is mobilized and brought through the stomal opening as described for ileostomies. A stoma rod is inserted and the bowel is opened and matured. The remaining trocar sites are closed as previously described.

End ileostomy

To create an end ileostomy, three to five ports are required. The number and location will depend on whether the bowel will be divided extracorporeally or intracorporeally or be resected. Intracorporeal division produces a distal stoma and minimizes colonic mobilization; however, it requires ileal mesentery division. To divide the ileum it is placed on traction between two clamps. A mesenteric window is created with cautery scissors or Enseal adjacent to the anticipated line of division. Depending on the bowel size, a 45 or 60 mm linear cutting stapler is inserted into the abdomen through a lower quadrant port and placed across the bowel. After the stapler is fired, the proximal divided end is grasped and elevated, which should place the associated mesentery on traction. The mesentery is divided with an Enseal or other energy device. Adequate mesentery is divided to provide enough mobilized bowel to easily reach 5 cm above the skin level (the length required to produce adequate extension for the ileostomy spout). A grasping clamp is inserted in the trocar placed at the stomal site, and the proximal end of the ileum is grasped. The stomal opening is enlarged as described previously, and under direct vision the end of the ileum is manipulated out the ostomy opening. Release of the pneumoperitoneum during this stage lowers the abdominal wall and minimizes mesenteric tension. The end ileostomy is opened and matured (see Figure 7.3).

End colostomy

Creation of an end colostomy is accomplished in a manner similar to that described for an ileostomy. The locations of the stoma and trocar site are moved to the left side. The patient is also positioned head down, right side down to expose the left lower quadrant and sigmoid colon [9]. The bowel and mesentery are mobilized and divided. The divided end of the stoma is brought out the ostomy opening and matured [10].

Takedown or closure of the stoma

Loop stomas can be closed without the need for laparoscopy. End stomas, especially end sigmoid colostomies with a Hartmann's pouch, are ideally suited to laparoscopic techniques. A laparoscopic colostomy takedown (or closure) is facilitated if several actions are taken at the initial operation [5]. These include performing an adequate resection and mobilization of the remaining colon. Removal of all diseased bowel and the distal sigmoid colon results in creation of the Hartmann's pouch in the upper rectum. Closure at the upper rectum ensures a good blood supply at the level of the future anastomosis. This portion of the rectum has a diameter and compliance that are adequate to accommodate a transanally placed circular intraluminal stapler and eliminates the need for a bowel resection at the time of the colostomy takedown. Previous mobilization of the left colon (e.g. takedown of the splenic flexure and division of the inferior mesenteric artery at the aorta) minimizes the need for additional laparoscopic mobilization or major vessel division. If the end of the colon to be used for the stoma can easily reach the end of the Hartmann's pouch in the pelvis, adequate length is available for an easy closure at a future operation. I also place an omental pedicle flap along the left gutter into pelvic raw surfaces and place an antiadhesion product such as Seprafilm (Genzyme Surgical Products, Cambridge, MA, USA) in the pelvis and below the abdominal wound to minimize small bowel adhesions.

Before any reconstructive bowel surgery it is imperative to clear the proximal and distal bowel to exclude any neoplasms or disease processes that would alter the planned surgery and to assess the location and condition of the distal bowel. This knowledge is especially important if laparoscopically assisted surgery is considered. The inability to palpate the remaining bowel during laparoscopy severely limits the surgeon's ability to evaluate the remaining bowel. Preoperative evaluation of the bowel is often performed with colonoscopy and proctoscopy. However, a barium study can occasionally provide more information on the bowel's condition. As mentioned previously, it is important to confirm that distal bowel closure was accomplished in the rectum. A colorectal anastomosis is technically easier and safer than a colosigmoid anastomosis.

The stoma is mobilized by dividing the stomal mucocutaneous junction at the skin level with a scalpel. Four Allis clamps are used to elevate the bowel end and provide traction. With sharp dissection, the bowel is mobilized in the avascular plane between the bowel serosa and the abdominal wall down to the anterior fascia. Retractors assist with the exposure. The fascial attachments are divided to completely free the bowel. A finger inserted in the fascial opening confirms that all peristomal adhesions have been divided. The end of the bowel is cleansed or excised and a purse-string suture is placed. This is accomplished with a 2-0 or 0-Prolene suture (Ethicon) placed with a whipstitch or using a fenestrated purse-string clamp. After the purse-string suture is placed, an appropriate-sized detached anvil (from an intraluminal circular stapler) is inserted into the bowel (**Figure 6.9**). The size of the stapler is determined by the size of the bowel at the stoma and in the rectum. The pursestring is closed and tied around the anvil shaft. The suture is left long, because it assists in locating the anvil after it is placed back in the abdomen. With retractors on the fascia, the bowel containing the anvil is carefully manipulated into the abdomen. It is often necessary to enlarge the opening in the skin or fascia to allow the bowel containing the anvil to return to the abdomen, taking care to prevent the purse-string suture from tearing.

Two or three figure-of-eight fascial sutures (No. 2 Prolene or PDS, Ethicon) are placed at the fascial edges of the stoma and are used to secure a Hasson trocar placed through the stomal opening. A pneumoperitoneum is established and a 10 mm camera is inserted through this trocar. The patient is moved to a head down, right side down position and the abdomen is examined, with attention to small bowel adhesions to the pelvis and the location of the bowel containing the anvil. The long ends of the purse-string suture assist in this maneuver. Under direct vision, additional trocars are placed.

Any small bowel adhesions to the pelvis are divided with cautery scissors or entergy devices. Extensive or dense adhesions or hemorrhage may necessitate conversion to an open operation. With the pelvis

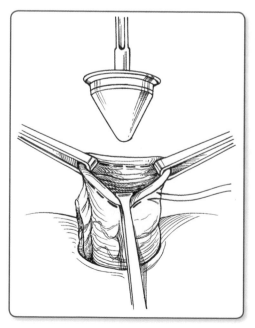

Figure 6.9 Placement of anvil into the proximal bowel. (From Beck DE. Creation and takedown of intestinal stomas by laparoscopy. Semin Colon Rectal Surg 1994;5:244–50. With permission.)

cleared, the end of the Hartmann's pouch is identified. A proctoscope inserted through the anus helps to identify the end of the rectum.

An intraluminal stapler (e.g. CDH-29, Ethicon) is inserted into the anus; under laparoscopic observation, it is advanced to the apex of the Hartmann's pouch. After the surgeon ensures that the apex of the Hartmann's pouch is free of adhesions and adjacent organs, the stapler trocar is extended through the apex of the rectal pouch. The end of a clamp assists by providing counterpressure against the bowel wall to ease advancement of the stapler trocar as it passes through the rectal wall. It is important to ensure that other structures, such as the back wall of the vagina, are free of the rectal pouch. Elevation of the uterus or bladder with Babcock clamps will often provide the required exposure.

The end of the anvil shaft is grasped with an anvil grasper or Babcock clamp and positioned toward the stapler trocar (**Figure 6.10**). After the anvil shaft is connected to the stapler trocar, the stapler is closed under direct vision. Care is taken to prevent any tissue or organs from being caught between the stapler as it is closed. After closure, the stapler is fired, opened, and removed from the bowel via the anus.

After removal of the stapler, the anastomosis should be tested. This is more accurate than looking at the 'doughnuts' from the stapler – a large leak can occur with complete doughnuts, and a secure anastomosis is possible with incomplete doughnuts. The anastomosis can be tested in a number of ways. With the bowel proximal to the anastomosis occluded with an atraumatic clamp, a dilute povidone-iodine solution is instilled into the rectum via the anus with a bulb syringe. Under laparoscopic observation the rectum can be seen to distend. Any anastomotic leakage is readily visible. Another option is to fill the pelvis with saline and instill

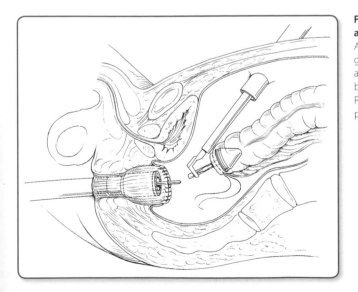

Figure 6.10 Manipulating the anvil toward the stapler trocar. Anvil shaft is held by an anvil grasper. (From Beck DE. Creation and takedown of intestinal stomas by laparoscopy. Semin Colon Rectal Surg 1994;5:244-50. With permission.)

air into the rectum. Anastomotic leaks result in bubbles of air escaping from the anastomosis. If no leaks are identified, the residual povidone-iodine or air is released from the anus by inserting a finger into the anus and providing posterior pressure. Small anastomotic leaks can be repaired with laparoscopic suture techniques. Major leaks are best managed by redoing the anastomosis or by conversion to an open procedure.

Patients are treated according to their individual requirements. Pain control is provided by low-dose patient-controlled analgesia or oral medications. Patients are offered liquids when they are hungry and a regular diet when flatus is passed. After diet toleration and bowel function are confirmed, the patient may be discharged.

Laparoscopically assisted procedures

Polyps

In any large practice, a few patients will be identified with polyps that are too large to remove safely with a colonoscope alone, but without clinical features suggestive of the need for a colectomy (e.g. ulceration, fixation, or hardness). Biopsy of the lesion should demonstrate benign histology, and there should be no other indication for abdominal surgery. In the past, this select group of patients was managed with a laparoscopically assisted colonoscopic polypectomy [11]. However, with increased laparoscopic experience most surgeons now perform a segmental colectomy in these patents. One group that may also benefit from laparoscopically assisted colonoscopic polypectomy are the patients with intra-abdominal adhesions that prevent complete colonoscopy. Limitations of this procedure involve the associated length of operating time and cost. The costs associated with these procedures include the operating room, general anesthesia, endoscopy, and laparoscopic equipment, which must be balanced against the costs associated with a major colonic resection. If the laparoscopically assisted technique is successful, the bowel is never opened, and the patient is spared the morbidity associated with a major resection.

Diverticular disease

Treatment of **diverticular disease** would seem to be suited to laparoscopic techniques, because it is a benign process. Unfortunately, the intense inflammatory processes associated with severe disease and the limitations of identifying thickened, diseased bowel with a laparoscope have hindered widespread adoption of laparoscopic techniques [12]. Many patients require emergency surgery for perforations, and the significant intra-abdominal contamination is often difficult to remove with laparoscopic techniques. Indications for surgery and patient preparation are discussed in Chapter 13. The goal of surgical therapy is to perform an operation to safely remove the diseased bowel, which usually requires a sigmoid colectomy. Hand ports have increased the number of laparoscopic assisted procedures performed for diverticular disease. The ability to insert the surgeon's hand into the abdomen to palpate the bowel and bluntly divide inflammatory adhesions makes the operation easier, shorter, and less stressful.

A laparoscopic **sigmoid colectomy** is performed with trocars at the umbilicus, right and left lower quadrant, and suprapubic locations. The colon is mobilized, divided distally at the proximal rectum with a linear cutting stapler. Sigmoid vessels are identified and divided. An abdominal incision is created, by extending one of the trocar sites. I prefer to extend the suprapubic site, making a small lower midline incision. After a small wound protector is placed, the diseased colon is exteriorized through this incision. The proximal line of resection is identified and the bowel divided. A purse-string suture is placed with 0 or 2–0 monofilament suture. As described in the section on Hartmann's closure (pages 93–96), an intraluminal anvil is inserted into the bowel and replaced into the abdomen. The circular stapler is inserted into the rectum and the trocar is advanced through the previously placed staple line. The anvil is attached to the trocar, and the stapler is closed, fired, and removed. Testing of the anastomosis confirms a secure anastomosis. The trocar sites and incision are closed. If a hand port is used, it is placed in the midline 3–4 cm above the pubis.

Inflammatory bowel disease

Laparoscopy has been used successfully in inflammatory bowel disease [13]. In Crohn's disease, laparoscopically assisted resections have been very helpful in patients with limited disease who are undergoing their first abdominal operation [14]. Most of these patients need a limited ileocolic resection. Port placement includes an initial port at the umbilicus and three or four additional ports (suprapubic and left and right lower quadrant or left lower, suprapubic, and upper abdomen). After a pneumoperitoneum is established, the small intestine is examined for areas of hyperemia, thickening, or fibrosis. A complete assessment of the small bowel is time consuming but possible, with careful persistence. For ileocolic disease, the lateral and posterior peritoneal attachments of the right colon are divided with scissors, cautery, or energy devices. This mobilization allows the right colon sufficient mobility to reach the midline. The ileocolic mesentery can be divided intracorporeally or the bowel can be exteriorized through a small (3–6 cm) midline or right upper quadrant muscle-splitting incision. After exteriorization, the bowel and (if not divided previously) the mesentery are divided. An ileocolic anastomosis is created (see Figure 22.2). Closure of the mesenteric defect is optional. The reconstituted bowel is returned to the abdomen and the incisions and trocar sites are closed.

Segmental sections of ileal disease are managed in a similar fashion with resections or strictureplasty (see Chapter 14). Any adherent loops of intestine are carefully dissected and examined, and if fistulization to normal intestine is present, these fistulas are divided, and the normal intestine is sutured with intracorporeal or extracorporeal techniques.

Patients with refractory ulcerative colitis can be treated with a total abdominal colectomy, mucosal proctectomy, and ileoanal pouch anastomosis using laparoscopic technique [15]. The colon and rectum are mobilized as described in other sections, the mesentery is divided (intracorporeally or extracorporeally), and the colon is exteriorized through a small lower midline or Pfannenstiel incision. An ileal pouch is created (Chapter 14) and the distal rectum is divided at the anorectal ring with a stapler. The ileal pouch anastomosis is created with a circular stapler inserted through the anus. A loop ileostomy is created and the incisions are closed. This laparoscopically assisted procedure provides improved cosmetic results, but the operative times are longer [16]. The use of hand ports has significantly reduced the operative times to ranges similar to open procedures [2].

Colorectal carcinoma

The role of laparoscopy in curative resections for **colorectal carcinoma** has progressed with increasing experience [2,17,18]. The feasibility of laparoscopically assisted colorectal procedures has been established and several prospective randomized trials have demonstrated equivalent local control and medium term survival for colon caner [19–21]. The role of laparoscopy in rectal cancer is currently being evaluated.

Of special concern is the potential for metastatic tumor recurrence or dissemination to trocar sites. Some early reports described port site recurrences [22,23]. Later reports using proper technique documented the rate of port site recurrence to be the same as open procedures [24].

Procedures used for colorectal cancer include right and left hemicolectomies and abdominoperineal resection (APR) [17–26]. An APR is well suited for laparoscopic techniques, because the specimen can usually be removed through the perineal wound [27]. Technique involved in this procedure uses either four or five trocars. The inferior mesenteric artery (IMA) and vein are identified and divided proximally at the aorta or just distal to the takeoff of the left colic artery. With care to protect the ureters, the sigmoid and rectal mesentery is mobilized inferior to the IMA. The left colon is divided at a level at which a good supply and enough mobilization are provided to reach the skin as a colostomy. The rectum is mobilized by posterior, lateral, and anterior dissection to the level of the anal levators. Use of a Harmonic scalpel or Ligasure eases the laparoscopic division of the lateral rectal mesentery. The operation then moves to the perineum, where the anal sphincters are excised (as described in Chapter 22) and the specimen is removed through the perineum. The perineal wound is closed and the colostomy is matured.

Miscellaneous conditions

A number of surgical procedures have been performed using laparoscopic techniques. These include rectal fixation procedures for prolapse [28,29], colectomies for colonic inertia [30], volvulus [31], and other procedures. The small number of each procedure performed by even the most experienced surgeons limits definitive statements; although the feasibility of the procedures has been established, questions about cost effectiveness and appropriateness remain.

Complications

Laparoscopy, like any invasive procedure, has associated complications [32]. The rapid adoption of this technology by general surgeons and those of the surgical subspecialties (e.g. colorectal surgeons) and expansion to new procedures have produced a unique situation. Surgeons initially adopted this new technology without the benefit of traditional training, such as residency and fellowships. An interim lack of organized progressive experience in colorectal laparoscopic surgery and the challenges of advanced procedures have contributed to the rate of complications. Complications are inversely related to the operating surgeon's experience, with multiple reports documenting a higher complication rate during a surgeon's early laparoscopic experience [33, 34]. Laparoscopic colon and rectal surgical procedures, as described previously, are more difficult than other advanced laparoscopic procedures. Complications of laparoscopic procedures can be divided into those related to trocars, the pneumoperitoneum, and the procedure itself.

Trocar-related complications

Although relatively safe, the placement and use of trocars and pneumoperitoneum needles (e.g. Veress needles) have been associated with complications. During trocar and needle insertion, there is the potential for injury of any organ and structure in the abdomen. Knowledge of vascular anatomy (e.g. the location of the epigastric arteries) is helpful in avoiding abdominal wall vascular injuries. Several extensive reviews of diagnostic laparoscopic procedures described a morbidity rate of 0.15–0.6% and a mortality rate of 0.04–0.13% [35]. Identification of an injury is important in minimizing associated morbidity.

To eliminate the potential complications from use of a Veress needle and the initial trocar insertion, some surgeons avoid the use of an insufflation needle and insert the first trocar with an open or Hasson technique [36]. However, the open technique has associated complications, such as avulsion of adhesions. Comparison of complications using an open versus a closed technique has shown fewer complications with the open method, but little prospective randomized data are available [37].

The major risk with trocars is related to the initial trocar insertion. Because this is often a blind procedure, organs adhered to the abdominal wall may be inadvertently injured. Secondary trocars that are inserted under direct vision from the laparoscopic camera, which is placed through the initial trocar, have a lower potential for injury. Bleeding can result from injury to abdominal wall vessels, such as the epigastric artery or vein. Bleeding will stop with compression in most cases, but transfusion or ligation may be required. Abdominal wall nerve injury is minimized by avoiding areas of the abdomen in which major nerve trunks are located (e.g. the inguinal area, areas medial and superior to the iliac spine, and close to the ribs). Complete transection of nerves will manifest as an area of anesthesia distal to the transected nerve trunk, whereas partial transection or injury to a nerve trunk injury may result in causalgia.

Most trocar injuries result from technical problems, such as inappropriate placement, an inadequate skin incision (which causes increased insertion force), extraperitoneal location of the trocar (usually from failure to penetrate a loose peritoneal layer), excessive depth of insertion (usually from excessive force), and faulty instruments [38]. An adequate pneumoperitoneum moves the abdominal wall away from the intraperitoneal organs and lessens the chances of organ injury. Trocar site hernias are rare; their occurrence is related to the location and size of the trocar (or cannula) wound. To minimize the occurrence of a hernia, the fascia on all trocar wounds that are 10 mm or larger requires closure [32].

Wound infection of trocar sites has also been uncommon, with a reported incidence of 0.1–3% [39]. Most of these infections have been associated with intra-abdominal contamination (e.g. ruptured appendix) or with specimen removal (e.g. in appendicitis or cholecystitis). These small, deep wounds, if not appropriately managed, have the potential to progress to necrotizing fasciitis, an uncommon but potentially lethal problem. Because many laparoscopic patients are discharged from the hospital in the early postoperative period, it is important to instruct them on the signs and symptoms of wound infections. Development of wound erythema, drainage, or increasing pain should prompt the patient to seek medical attention. Any suspected wound infection requires exploration (opening), debridement, and drainage of fluid collection.

Pneumoperitoneum-related complications

A carbon dioxide (CO_2) pneumoperitoneum results in several physiologic changes, including alterations in acid-base balance, pulmonary mechanics, and cardiopulmonary physiology [34]. Transperitoneal absorption of CO_2 results in elevation of arterial pCO_2, and all patients should have continuous monitoring of end-tidal CO_2. While most patients can be managed by increasing the ventilation rate, patients with cardiovascular diseases may develop hypercarbia and acidemia. Treatment of severe hypercarbia and acidosis requires prompt evacuation of the intraperitoneal CO_2, and mechanical hyperventilation [40, 41].

Hemodynamic and pulmonary complications resulting from increased intra-abdominal pressure have also been described [42, 43]. The magnitude of these alterations is related to the amount of intra-abdominal pressure, baseline hemodynamic function, and volume status. It is recommended that the intra-abdominal pressure remain lower than 15 mmHg to minimize these effects. The increased intra-abdominal pressure used in laparoscopy also raises the diaphragm and decreases pulmonary compliance. This can be compensated for by increasing the ventilator's inflation presure [42, 43]. Severe bradycardia can occur during intraperitoneal insufflation of CO_2, because the peritoneal distention increases vagal tone. Careful monitoring will identify these changes, and appropriate measures can be instituted.

Subcutaneous emphysema results from failure of an insufflating Veress needle to reach the peritoneal cavity or from CO_2 being forced into the abdominal wall during accidental withdrawal of a trocar and its subsequent replacement. Minimal subcutaneous emphysema will resolve spontaneously. The presence of significant subcutaneous gas may lead to a pneumothorax or a pneumomediastinum, which requires prompt diagnosis and treatment. A large amount of sequestrated CO_2 can also overwhelm the endogenous clearance mechanisms and lead to hypercarbia and acidosis [44].

The high flow and volume of gas used to obtain and maintain the pneumoperitoneum can cause problems. The temperature of CO_2 used to inflate the abdomen is generally 16 to 17°C when it comes in contact with the peritoneum [10]. Prolonged exposure to unheated gas (more than 3–4 hours) leads to hypothermia. Hypothermia is minimized by the use of air or water warming blankets; warming intravenous fluids, irrigating fluids, and anesthesia gases; and limiting laparoscopic operating time. An extremely rare and potentially lethal complication is a gas embolus. Direct injection of CO_2 into a blood vessel results in the characteristic 'mill wheel' murmur that prompts initial treatment (administration of 100% oxygen, movement of the patient to left lateral and head down position, and attempted aspiration of gas from the ventricle) [45].

A potential secondary problem associated with use of a pneumoperitoneum is venous oozing. The increased intra-abdominal pressure of the pneumoperitoneum acts to compress or tamponade small veins. Thus during the procedure no hemorrhage is observed, but after release of the pneumoperitoneum these vessels may ooze. The drop in hematocrit level occasionally seen after laparoscopic surgery may be caused by this phenomenon. To minimize this problem, surgeons have either lowered the pneumoperitoneum pressure used during the operation or made a special effort to observe the intra-abdominal cavity at the completion of the procedure when the intra-abdominal pressure has been reduced.

Procedure-related complications

Complications related to the procedure can be discussed in terms of those that occur intraoperatively and those that develop postoperatively. The rate of intraoperative complications has ranged from 14–17%, whereas the range for postoperative complications has varied from 8–33% [32]. Early complications include conversion to an open procedure, organ injury, and hemorrhage.

Conversion to an open procedure is not necessarily a complication, but rather may be an indicator of good surgical judgment. For this reason some surgeons describe 'alternating' to an open procedure rather than 'converting'. The reasons for converting or alternatng to an open procedure include unclear anatomy, excessive operating time, intraoperative complications (e.g. hemorrhage or organ injury) or inability to complete the procedure (usually because of adhesions, abscesses, etc.). The reported rates of conversion have varied from 8–50%. The large range reflects differences in patient selection, surgeon's experience, and definitions of what constitutes conversion. Most studies have documented that patients who require converted operations have more frequent complications, higher costs, and longer postoperative hospital stays.

Injury to organs can occur from trocars, as described in the previous section, from use of laser or electrocautery, or trauma can occur from instruments. Laser is used in gynecologic procedures to vaporize endometriomas. However, laser has fewer applications for laparoscopic colon and rectal procedures, and most colorectal laparoscopic surgeons use scissors or electrocautery. The electrosurgical instruments used in laparoscopy are associated with a significant portion of laparoscopic complications. Injuries that occur as a result of energy transfer outside the visual field often go unrecognized. Injuries can also occur from defective insulation on the active electrode, from capacity coupling, or from direct coupling between the active electrode and metal instruments or electrode and the laparoscope itself [32,46].

An unrecognized thermal bowel injury may progress to a transmural perforation and be recognized hours to days after the injury. Patients with this type of injury usually present with an ileus, signs of peritoneal irritation, fever, and leukocytosis [33]. These types of injuries are minimized by ensuring that the active electrodes come in contact with only the intended tissue. A small electrocautery injury of the bowel is managed by imbrication, while more extensive burns usually require a resection. It is often best to evaluate and manage these significant injuries with the abdomen open.

Minor hemorrhage can be dealt with using laparoscopic techniques, such as occlusion with a laparoscopic clamp followed by placement of a ligaclip, EndoLoop, Harmonic scalpel, Ligasure or Enseal. Electrocautery is useful for small vessels; some surgeons prefer bipolar cautery. A useful technique to assist with hemorrhage is to insert a sponge or small pad through a trocar into the abdomen. The gauze absorbs the blood that hinders vision. This technique is more efficient than irrigation and suction. To prevent the loss of the sponge only one should be placed into the abdomen at a time. An additional aid is to attach a long suture to the end of the sponge. Major hemorrhage is appropriately managed by expeditiously opening the abdomen while a clamp or suction wand inserted through a trocar temporarily tamponades the bleeding.

Ureteral injury is the most common urologic complication occurring during laparoscopic surgery [47]. Knowledge of pelvic anatomy, as seen laparoscopically, and good operative technique are essential to avoid this complication. Exposing and visualizing the ureter at all times during the procedure minimizes its potential for injury. Electrocoagulation in the vicinity of the ureter should be avoided to prevent thermal injury. Some surgeons use a preoperative CT scan or intravenous pyelogram to confirm the location of the ureter and identify medial deviation associated with inflammatory or neoplastic conditions [48]. Stenting the ureters with standard or fiberoptic ureteral catheters or use of a laparoscopic Doppler probe may be helpful in difficult cases [10]. An injured ureter identified during laparoscopy has been repaired laparoscopically. The technique involves mobilizing the ureter, placing stents in an antegrade or retrograde manner, and suturing the injury with 4-0 chromic catgut [34]. More extensive repairs such as a ureteroureterostomy or ureterocystostomy are best accomplished after a laparotomy. Unrecognized urinary injuries usually result in fever, abdominal and flank pain, leukocytosis, and peritoneal signs. An aggressive evaluation will identify the cause of the problem, and the patient is best treated through a routine multispecialty approach.

Inability to locate intraluminal lesions such as polyps or small tumors remains a problem with laparoscopic colorectal surgery. Several reports have documented missing the intended lesion after a colectomy. Ideas to improve intraoperative identification of the target lesion include preoperatively tattooing or marking the colon with clips near the lesion, preoperative radiologic verification of lesion location and intraoperative colonoscopy [11,32,49].

Laparoscopic procedures are relatively lengthy, so it is imperative that the patient be positioned correctly [32]. Adequate padding of extremities and pressure areas is necessary to prevent pressure injuries [51]. Sequential compression stockings minimize the venous pooling in the lower extremities associated with operative procedures and the use of a pneumoperitoneum.

Late complications of laparoscopic colorectal surgery result from an anastomotic leak or contamination [33]. Multiple technical maneuvers used to minimize contamination include bowel preparation, wound protectors, specimen bags, and bowel occlusion devices or clamps. Current techniques of performing an intracorporeal anastomosis have a higher potential for contamination. The experience to date has demonstrated equivalent leak rates after comparable open and laparoscopic procedures. The controversy of tumor dissemination was discussed previously.

With any developmental technology and new procedures, complications will occur. Appropriate training and experience, as well as care and objective review of results, will hopefully minimize morbidity to laparoscopic colorectal patients.

Learning curve

Learning and becoming proficient in laparoscopic procedures requires the performance of a certain number of procedures [51,52]. This is the so called 'learning curve'. Analysis of operative times, conversion rates, costs, complications and the quality of instruction, document that performance of 10–20 successful procedures is necessary. Fortunately, current trainees are getting this experience during their formal training.

Current and future role

Laparoscopy has a significant role in colorectal surgery. General and colorectal surgery training programs have incorporated laparoscopy into their curriculum and the respective Boards have made laparoscopic experience a requirement for certification. Thus recent graduates finish their training with formal education in this modality. The role of laparoscopy in an individual surgeon's practice depends on the advantages and disadvantages of the technology, patient factors, and the surgeon's experience.

Rounds questions

1. What advantages of laparoscopic procedures have been confirmed?
2. What is the primary mode of retraction of the small bowel during laparoscopic procedures?
3. What type of bowel preparations are used for laparoscopic colorectal procedures?
4. Are laparoscopic complications related to a surgeon's experience?
5. How does absorbed CO_2 affect arterial pH?
6. How is a large intravascular gas embolus treated?

References

1. Beck DE, Rosenthal D. Introduction to colon and rectal surgery. Semin Colon Rectal Surg 1994;5:217.
2. Fleshman JW, Chun JS. Laparoscopic colorectal surgery. In Whitlow CB, Beck DE, Margolin DA, Hicks TC, Timmcke AE (eds). Improved Outcomes In Colon And Rectal Surgery. London: Informa Healthcare 2010;140–7.
3. Simmang CL, Rosenthal D. Tools for laparoscopic colectomy. Semin Colon Rectal Surg 1994;5:228–38.
4. Darzi A. Hand-assisted laparoscopic colorectal surgery. Semin Laparosc Surg 2001;8:153–60.
5. Beck DE. Creation and takedown of intestinal stomas by laparoscopy. Semin Colon Rectal Surg 1994;5:244–50.
6. Fleshman JW. Loop ileostomy. Surg Rounds 1992;15:129–40.
7. Khoo RE, Montrey J, Cohen MM. Laparoscopic loop ileostomy for temporary fecal diversion. Dis Colon Rectum 1993;36:966–8.
8. Lange V, Meyer G, Schardey HM, et al. Laparoscopic creation of a loop colostomy. J Laparoendosc Surg 1991;1:307–12.
9. Luchtefeld MA, MacKeigan JM. Laparoscopic-assisted colostomy. In: MacKeigan JM, Cataldo P, (eds). Intestinal Stomas: Principles, Techniques, and Management. St. Louis: Quality Medical Publishing 1993;228–33.
10. Beck DE. End sigmoid colostomy. In: MacKeigan JM, Cataldo P, (eds). Intestinal Stomas: Principles, Techniques, and Management. St. Louis: Quality Medical Publishing 1993;97–106.
11. Beck DE. Laparoscopic assisted colonoscopic polypectomy. Sure Oncol Clin North Am 1994;3:679–86.

12. Puente I, Sosa JL, Sleeman D, et al. Laparoscopic assisted colorectal surgery. J Laparoendosc Surg 1994;4:1–7.

13. Jager RM. Laparoscopic right colectomy. In: Jager RM, Wexner SD, (eds). New York: Churchhill Livingstone 1995;229–41.

14. Bauer JJ, Harris MT, Gmmbach NM, et al. Laparoscopic-assisted intestinal resection for Crohn's disease. Dis Colon Rectum 1995;38:712–5.

15. Schmitt SL, Cohen SM, Wexner SD, et al. Does laparoscopic-assisted ileal pouch anal anastomosis reduce the length of hospitalization? Int J Colorectal Dis 1994;9:134–7.

16. Wexner SD, Johansen OB, Nogueras JJ, Jagelman DG. Laparoscopic total abdominal colectomy: A prospective trial. Dis Colon Rectum 1992;35:651–5.

17. Ota DM. Laparoscopic colectomy for colonic inertia. In: Cohen Am, Winawer ST, (eds). Cancer of the colon, Rectum, and Anus. New York: McGraw-Hill 1995;455–64.

18. Lacy L, Garcia-Valdecasas C, Pique JM, et al. Short-term outcome analysis of a randomized study comparing laparoscopic vs open colectomy for colon cancer. Surg Endosc 1995;9:1101–5.

19. Fleshman JW, Sargent DJ, Green E et al. Laparoscopic colectomy for cancer is not inferior to open surgery based on 5-year data from the COST Study Group trial. Ann Surg 2007;246: 655–62.

20. Guillou, PJ, Quirke P, Thorpe H, et al. Short-term endpoints of conventional versus laparoscopic-assisted surgery in patients with colorectal cancer (MRC CLASICC trial): multicentre, randomised controlled trial. Lancet 2005;365:1718–26.

21. Hazebroek EJ and the Color study group. COLOR. A randomized clinical trial laparoscopic and open resection for colon cancer. Surg Endoscopy 2001;16:949–53.

22. Wexner SD, Cohen SM. Port site metastases after laparoscopic colorectal surgery for cure of malignancy. Br J Surg 1995;82:295–8.

23. Hughes ES, McDermott FT, Polglase AL, Johnson WR. Tumor recurrence in the abdominal wall scar tissue after large-bowel cancer surgery. Dis Coon Rectum 1983;26:571–2.

24. Bonjer, HJ, Hop WC, Nelson H, et al. Laparoscopically assisted vs open colectomy for colon cancer: a meta-analysis. Arch Surg 2007;142:298–303.

25. Fleshman JW, Nelson H, Peters WR, et al. Early results of laparoscopic surgery for colorectal cancer. Retrospective analysis of 372 patients treated by Clinical Outcomes of Surgical Therapy (COST) Study Group. Dis Colon Rectum 1996;39:S53–8.

26. Decanini C, Milsom JW, Bohn B, et al. Laparoscopic oncologic abdominoperineal resection. Dis Colon Rectum 1994;37:552–8.

27. Jones DB, Fleshman JW. Laparoscopic approaches to rectal cancer. Prob Gen Surg 1996;12:135–45.

28. Berman IR. Sutureless laparoscopic rectopexy for procidentia. Techniques and implications. Dis Colon Rectum 1992;36:689–93.

29. Darzi A, Monson JRT. Laparoscopic rectopexy for rectal prolapse. In: Jager RM, Wexner SD, (eds). Laparoscopic Colorectal Surgery. New York: Churchhill Livingstone 1995;179–85.

30. Rhodes M, Stitz RW. Laparoscopic subtotal colectomy. Semin Colon Rectal Surg 1994;5:244–50.

31. Fingerhut A. Laparoscopic-assisted colonic resection: The French experience. In: Jager RM, Wexner SD, (eds). Laparoscopic Colorectal Surgery. New York: Churchhill Livingstone 1995;253–7.

32. Beck DE, Opelka FG. Laparoscopic complications. In: Jager RM, Wexner SD, (eds). Laparoscopic Colorectal Surgery. New York: Churchhill Livingstone, 1995:267–71.

33. See WA, Cooper CS, Fisher RJ. Predictors of laparoscopic complications after formal training in laparoscopic surgery. JAMA 1993;270:2689–92.

34. Ramos R. Complications in laparoscopic colon surgery. Semin Colon Rectal Surg 1994;5:239–43.

35. Lightdale CJ. Indications, contraindications and complications of laparoscopy. In: Sivak M, (ed). Gastroenterologic Endoscopy. Philadelphia: WB Saunders 1987;1039–44.

36. Hasson HM. Window for open laparoscopy. Am J Obstet Gynecol 1980;137:869–70.

37. Hasson HM. Open laparoscopy versus closed laparoscopy: A comparison of complication rates. Adv Planned Parent 1978;13:41–50.

38. Borten M. Complications of trocar insertion. In: Fredman EA, (ed). Laparoscopic Complications: Prevention and Management. Philadelphia: BC Decker 1986;286–95.

39. Crist WD, Gadacz RT. Complications of laparoscopic surgery. Surg Clin North Am 1993;3:269–70.

40. Hall D, Goldstein A, Tynan E, et al. Profound hypercarbia late in the course of laparoscopic cholecystectomy: Detection by continuous capnometry. Anesthesiology 1993;79:173–4.

41. Fitzgerald SD, Andrus CH, Baudendistel LJ, et al. Hypercarbia during carbon dioxide pneumoperitoneum. Am J Surg 1992;163:186–90.

42. Safran DB, Orlando R. Physiological effects of pneumoperitoneum. Am J Surg 1994;167:281–6.

43. Wittgen CM, Andrus CH, Fitzgerald SD, et al. Analysis of hemodynamic and ventilatory effects of laparoscopic cholecystectomy. Arch Surg 1991;126:997–1000.

44. Kent RB III. Subcutaneous emphysema and hypercarbia following laparoscopic cholecystectomy. Arch Surg 1991;126:1154–6.

45. Au-Yeung P. Gas embolism during attempted laparoscopic vagotomy [letter]. Anes-thesiology 1992;47:817.

46. Voyles CR, Tucker RD. Education and engineering solutions for potential problems with laparoscopic monopolar electrosurgery. Am J Surg 1992;164:57–62.

47. Evans RM, Hulbert JC, Reddy PK. Complications of laparoscopy. Semin Urol 1992;10:164–8.

48. Grainger DA, Soderstrom RM, Schiff SF, et al. Ureteral injuries at laparoscopy: Insights into diagnosis, management and prevention. Obstet Gynecol 1990;75:839–43.

49. Beck DE. Colonoscopy and laparoscopy. In: Jager RM, Wexner SD, (eds). Laparoscopic Colorectal Surgery. New York: Churchill Livingstone 1994;143–8.

50. Senagore AJ, Luchtefeld MA, MacKeigan JM. What is the learning curve for laparoscopic colectomy? Am Surgeon 1995;61:681–4.

51. Simons AJ, Anthone GJ, Ortega AE, et al. Laparoscopic-assisted colectomy learning curve. Dis Colon Rectum 1995;38:600–3.

Intestinal stomas

An intestinal stoma is an artificial opening between a portion of the gastrointestinal tract and the skin surface. An ileostomy is created by bringing the ileum to the skin; a colostomy uses colon. Creation of an intestinal stoma is often but a small part of an extensive operative procedure. It is, however, a part of the operation that the patient will have to deal with on a daily basis and, as such, deserves the surgeon's full attention. Small differences in technique may make the difference between a well-functioning stoma and one that is at best a daily inconvenience for the patient and at worst a source of major morbidity [1].

Selecting the stoma site

The first step in the construction of an enterocutaneous stoma is the selection of an appropriate site. Stomas should be located within the rectus muscle, because the rate of parastomal hernia appears to be higher when the stoma is brought out through the abdominal wall lateral edge of the rectus sheaf [2]. There are some situations where a midline colostomy is the best placement option.

The surgeon should bring the stoma through a scar-free part of the abdominal wall, because a scar might make it difficult to get a good seal with the faceplate of the ostomy equipment. The site should be chosen so that the appliance can be placed without abutting on bony prominences such as the iliac crest or the rib cage. Most people have a fat roll just below the umbilicus; in most patients, the optimal site for stoma placement is on the crest of that roll on the outer third of the rectus sheath (**Figure 7.1**). Except in dire emergencies, before the patient is taken to the operating room, a template of the faceplate or the faceplate itself should be used to pick a site so that there is maximal contact between the faceplate and the skin. The site is chosen with the patient supine, then it is checked with the patient sitting up and standing. Often the crest of the fat roll changes position when the patient is sitting or a crease appears that was not apparent with the patient supine. The type of clothing that the patient is accustomed to wearing should also be considered. If the patient has had several previous operations or if there is intra-abdominal sepsis or the possibility of edematous bowel and foreshortened mesentery, several alternate sites should be chosen. The stoma site is indicated with an indelible marker, silver nitrate, gentian violet, or a small subcuticular tattoo created with methylene blue dye. If

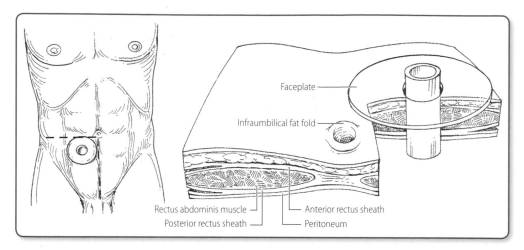

Figure 7.1 **Stomal placement.** The site is selected to bring the stoma through the lower rectus abdominis muscle. (From Fleshman JW Jr. Ostomies. In: Hicks TC, Beck DE, Opelka FG, Timmcke AE, (eds). Complications in Colorectal Surgery. Baltimore: Williams & Wilkins 1996; 357–381. With permission.)

an indelible marker is used, a mark is scratched on the skin after the patient has been anesthetized so that the mark is not removed during the abdominal wall preparation.

Laparscopic methods of stomal creation and closure were briefly described in Chapter 5. The remainder of this chapter will concentrate on traditional techniques and general principles.

Ileostomy

Creation

The ileostomy may be an end ileostomy, a loop ileostomy, a loop-end ileostomy, or a double-barrel type of stoma. When the stoma site has been chosen, a disk of skin approximately 2 cm in diameter is excised and a longitudinal (vertical) incision made in the subcutaneous fat. When the anterior rectus sheath is reached, the subcutaneous fat is retracted and the anterior rectus sheath incised vertically with a cautery device. To protect the viscera from injury, a laparotomy pad is placed underneath the rectus muscle and supported firmly with the left hand while the rectus muscle is split in the direction of its fibers. Retractors are inserted to hold the muscle apart and the posterior rectus sheath and peritoneum are incised in a longitudinal direction with cautery. The aperture should easily admit two fingers. Five to 6 cm of ileum is pulled through the cutaneous opening so that when the bowel is inverted, the ileostomy will be 2–3 cm long. Once the ileum is pulled through, the mesentery of the protruding bowel is trimmed. This can safely be done for a length of 6 cm, because the submucosal circulation will be sufficient to prevent ischemia. One should be more circumspect about trimming the mesentery if the bowel has been previously radiated or in a critically ill patient in whom a low-flow state might be anticipated. In such a case, the mesentery is secured to the posterior rectus sheath, taking care not to interfere with the vessels within the mesentery. A few sutures may be placed between the seromuscular layer of the ileum and the anterior rectus sheath or Scarpa's fascia to prevent any retraction. This is helpful in obese patients, but is not necessary if there is no tension on the bowel. At this point, the ileostomy gutter is closed. One can do this with a purse-string suture by sewing the cut edge of the right colon mesentery to the anterior abdominal wall up to the ligamentum teres. Alternatively, the ileal mesentery can be placed in a retroperitoneal tunnel, as described by Goligher (**Figure 7.2c**) [3]. Any one of these three methods will prevent a loop of small bowel from becoming entrapped between the ileum and the lateral abdominal wall. Some surgeons prefer to leave the lateral gutter wide open. It is felt that a wide open gutter is unlikely

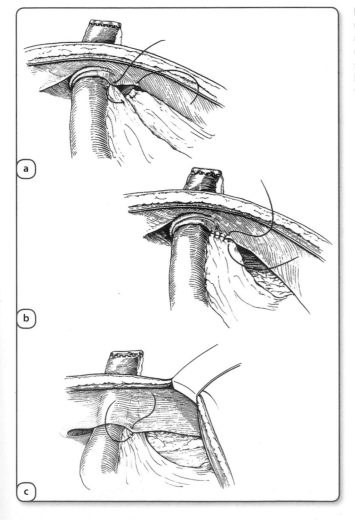

Figure 7.2 Ileostomy fixation.
(a) Purse-string suture joining the mesentery and abdominal wall.
(b) Cut edge of the ileal mesentery sewn to abdominal wall. (c) Ileum brought through a retroperitoneal tunnel.

to trap the small bowel. This has gained wider acceptance with the increase in laparoscopic experience.

After the ileum is secured and the lateral gutter obliterated, the laparotomy wound is closed. Absorbable sutures are placed through the full thickness of ileum and the subcuticular layer of skin to mature the ileostomy. Some surgeons also take a bite of ileum at the skin level to ensure that the stoma everts (**Figure 7.3**). This suture must be placed carefully (not full thickness and not tied too tightly) to prevent creation of a fistula.

A loop ileostomy is sometimes indicated for colonic obstruction or to protect a distal anastomosis. The aperture in the abdominal wall should be made in exactly the same way as previously described. A loop of ileum should be selected that appears to have the greatest length and can be most easily brought through the abdominal wall. A small aperture is made in the mesentery and a small Penrose drain or umbilical tape is passed through to help bring the bowel through the abdominal wall. When making the loop ileostomy, some surgeons rotate the bowel loops to bring the bowel out so that the proximal part of the ileum is in the caudad position and the distal ileum in the cephalad

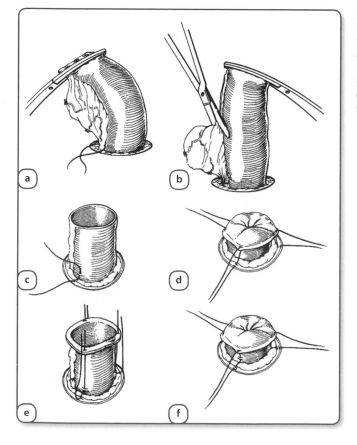

a

b

c

d

e

f

Figure 7.3 Ileostomy maturation.
(a) Ligation and (b) trimming of the ileal mesentery. (c & d) Serosa attached to Scarpa's fascia and mucosal edge sutured to dermis. (e & f) Triangular stitch from ileal end to serosa to dermis. Tying sutures inverts the ileum to the skin.

position. A study of this rotational technique in patients receiving temporary loop ileostomies as part of a restorative proctocolectomy found a higher incidence of post-operative small bowel obstruction [4]. Due to this finding, many surgeons will not rotate the bowel loops or partially rotate the loops to place the functional end in a lateral position. If the stoma is a temporary one, many surgeons will wrap the bowel brought through the abdominal wall with an antiadhesive product such as Seprafilm (Genzyme Corporation, Cambridge, MA, USA). Use of this product may ease the closure of temporary ileostomies [5].

Once the loop is brought through the abdominal wall, the Penrose drain or umbilical tape may be replaced with a small plastic ileostomy rod. The rod is fastened to the skin with a suture so it does not become displaced. A rod is helpful if the bowel is under tension and is left in place for 1–7 days. The length of time the rod is retained will depend on a number of factors: tension on the bowel and mesentery, size of skin incision, patients' body habitus, and surgeon and wound ostomy continence nurse (WOCN) or enterostomal (ET) nurse experience. The proximal and distal bowel can be identified relative to the aperture in the mesentery by using a silk and a chromic suture so that the proper orientation is maintained when the bowel is brought through the orifice (functional end in inferior or lateral position). Once the rod is in, these identifying sutures are removed and a transverse incision is made at the skin level in the cephalad part of the loop (**Figure 7.4**).

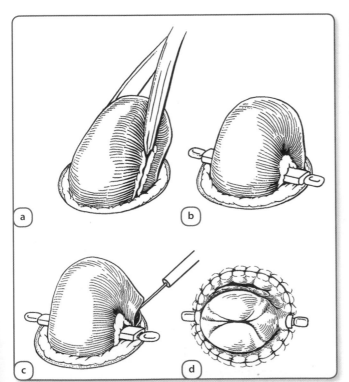

Figure 7.4 Loop ileostomy.
(a) Loop brought through the abdominal wall with a Penrose drain or umbilical tape. (b) Loop secured with a plastic ileostomy rod. (c) Incision made at the skin level through the distal (cephalad) aspect of loop. (d) Matured stoma.

Sutures are placed between the distal cut edge of the bowel and the subcuticular layer of skin. Eight to ten sutures are placed to evert the bowel and create a spout. It is important that the transverse incision in the ileum be made to be more than 80% of the circumference of the ileum; if it is not, the proximal part of the loop will not evert easily.

A modified loop ileostomy (loop-end ileostomy) can be used even when the colon has been excised. The last several centimeters of ileum are used for the loop, with the short oversewn non-functional end of the ileum allowed to lie inside the abdomen (**Figure 7.4**). This technique is useful when, because of a foreshortened mesentery and a thick abdominal wall, an end ileostomy cannot easily be fashioned. A loop-end ileostomy in this circumstance affords greater length, and the stoma can be constructed with less tension and better blood supply.

A loop ileostomy, constructed correctly, should be totally diverting. Placing the proximal part of the loop in the dependent caudad or lateral position allows the effluent to drain into the appliance without passing over the distal limb, at least while the patient is in the erect position. Another strategy for complete diversion is to bring up a loop of ileum, transect the bowel, and oversew the distal loop while tacking it to the proximal loop at the level of the fascia with several sutures, leaving the proximal limb 4–5 cm above the fascia, which is matured as a standard end ileostomy (end-loop ileostomy) [6]. If there is a need for a mucous fistula, such as in a patient with a distal obstruction, a corner of the distal suture line can be excised and this brought up to the skin level and sutured next to the proximal stoma (**Figure 7.5**). This ileostomy can

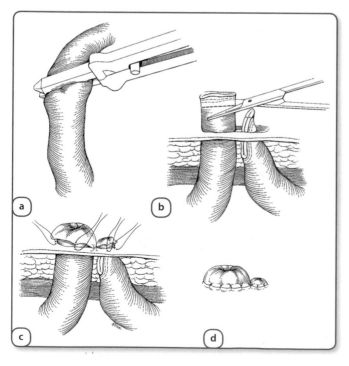

Figure 7.5 Divided loop ileostomy. (a) Bowel divided with linear stapler. (b) Functional end of ileum is brought through the abdominal wall and opened. The comer of the non-functional distal ileum is brought through the stomal opening. (c) Both ends of bowel matured. (d) Completed stomas.

usually be taken down and the ileum reanastomosed without a formal laparotomy, just as one can do with the loop ileostomy.

Closure

There are several alternative methods for closing loop ileostomies. Common to all these methods is the necessity of completely mobilizing both limbs of the ileum down to the peritoneal cavity so that the anastomosed bowel can be returned to the abdominal cavity. The simplest method of closing the loop ileostomy is to simply trim the bowel of all attached skin and then close the antimesenteric aspect of the bowel, just as one would close the anterior aspect of any bowel anastomosis. If the distal loop is very small, an antimesenteric slit should be made so that the diameter of the anastomosis is satisfactory. An alternative method is to do a side-to-side anastomosis using sutures or a linear stapling device inserted through the stomal ends. The residual opening is then closed with sutures (I use a two layer running closure) or with a stapler. This type of closure can be performed with or without incising the distal limbs of the stoma proximal to the ileocutaneous junction. Once completed, the anastomosis is placed in the peritoneal cavity, and the fascia is closed. The superficial wound is managed by closing or partially closing the skin with sutures or by packing the wound open to allow healing by secondary intention (granulation). I partially close the skin with interrupted absorbable sutures to leave a small opening which heals quickly with minimal wound care (**Figure 7.6**). If one chooses to close the skin, the wound may be extended somewhat laterally and medially so that a linear closure can be made. If this option is chosen, it can be expected that a certain number of these wounds will have to be opened because of wound infection.

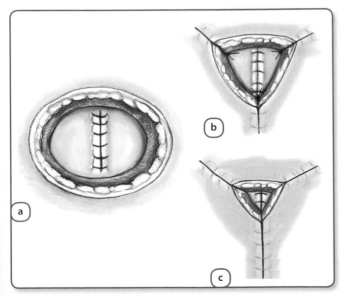

Figure 7.6 Closure of ostomy wound. (a) Stoma site with fascia closed. (b) Initial approximation of skin and subcutaneous fat. (c) Completed closure with small area in center left open for drainage and secondary healing.

Complications

The most common complication of an ileostomy is leakage. This is usually secondary to bad placement, which is the result of poor planning by the surgeon. Remedial management of leakage and treatment of resultant dermatitis will be discussed later. Stenosis of the ileostomy secondary to contraction of the incision may occur occasionally. Stenosis can usually be remedied by taking down the mucocutaneous junction and enlarging the skin orifice under local anesthesia.

Ileostomy retraction may occur, usually as a consequence of bringing up an inadequate length of bowel at the initial operation or bringing it up under tension. Ileostomy retraction may also occur if the patient gains excessive weight after the initial surgery. This can sometimes be remedied with mobilization of the ileum through a peristomal incision. However, a laparotomy may be necessary to free up enough ileum to bring an adequate length of ileum through the stoma site without tension. Prolapse of the ileostomy is much less common than prolapse of a colostomy; however, it does occur. It can be treated effectively by amputating the excessive ileum and reconstructing the ileostomy.

Peristomal abscesses may occur in the early postoperative period or later on. Those occurring as late complications are very often associated with Crohn's disease. Usually, these abscesses can be drained adequately by making an incision in the mucocutaneous junction and inserting a drain. If the abscess is pointing at some distance from the stoma, it can be drained lateral to the stomal appliance. Paraileostomy fistula can occur as the end result of a peristomal abscess, as a result of injury to the ileum with the faceplate of the appliance, from a suture placed too deeply in the ileum at the fascial level, or as a result of recurrent Crohn's disease. These fistulas must be treated surgically, very often with transposition or relocation of the stoma to a different site.

Paraileostomy hernia is a less frequent complication than is paracolostomy hernia, occurring in 3–10% of cases. Some authors have advocated local repair, whereas others suggest that stomal transposition is the best approach. A local repair involves closure of the fascial defect with sutures. An additional option is to reinforce the suture repair with mesh [7]. Recently, the use of biologic mesh to reinforce hernia repair or prophictically to prevent hernias has been advocated [8].

Occasionally a patient who has undergone proctocolectomy for ulcerative colitis will develop hepatic cirrhosis and portal hypertension. Varices can develop at the mucocutaneous junction of the ileostomy, forming a caput medusae. These varices are easily traumatized, and impressive bleeding may result. Direct pressure or ligation can usually control the immediate hemorhage [9]. The problem can be treated more definitively through interruption of the portosystemic shunt by incising the stoma at the mucocutaneous junction and carefully ligating all the large venous vessels [9]. The procedure may be repeated as necessary. A longer-lasting remedy is to reduce portal pressure. A transcutaneous intrahepatic portosystemic shunt (TIPS) to accomplish this yields the least morbidity. Because of its success, the TIPS has replaced splenorenal or portocaval shunts for most patients. The definitive option is a hepatic transplant, but all these major operative procedures have a significant morbidity and mortality.

Continent ileostomy

Creation

In 1967 Dr. Nils Kock [10] designed a reservoir constructed from the terminal ileum whose purpose was to make the patient continent of feces. As the technique evolved, he added a nipple valve by intussuscepting the efferent loop of the pouch. This addition proved to be the key element in preservation of continence. He and others have made various modifications that include enlargement of the pouch with a third loop, creation of a mesenteric window to facilitate the intussusception of the efferent loop, scarification of the ileum in the intussuscepted segment, and stabilization of the nipple valve with staples (**Figure 7.7**) [12–16]. Prosthetic material has been used to reinforce the intussusception, and the efferent limb and valve have been fashioned from the antiperistaltic segment of ileum instead of the isoperistaltic design of the 'original pouch.' More recently the valve has been stapled to the side of the reservoir [15]. A modification by Barnett [16] used an ileal cuff instead of prosthetic material to pass through the mesentery once the efferent limb has been intussuscepted to form the nipple valve; he then constructed the pouch so that the efferent limb is an antiperistaltic segment of ileum. This method of continent ileostomy construction has been called a Barnett Continent Ileostomy Reservoir (BCIR). Another modification of a continent ileostomy is the 'T pouch.' This type of pouch is similar to a type of urostomy in which an isolated segment of ileum is invaginated into the wall of the pouch [17]. This type of pouch is complicated to construct and is not widely offered.

The nipple valve is the key to the maintenance of continence; however, it is the Achilles heel of the procedure because most complications are related to the valve. Discussion of the technical details of this procedure is beyond the scope of this book; however, the references at the end of this chapter include a number of articles on the procedure [11,14–17].

Complications

Early complications include leakage from the suture lines, common necrosis of the intussuscepted valve, and hemorrhage from the various sutures lines [18]. Minor hemorrhage can be managed with irrigation of the pouch with saline or saline with epinephrine or endoscopic fulguration. Major hemorrhage, perforation, or valve necrosis usually requires surgical repair.

Late complications include valve slippage, prolapse, fistulas, volvulus, perforation or pouchitis.

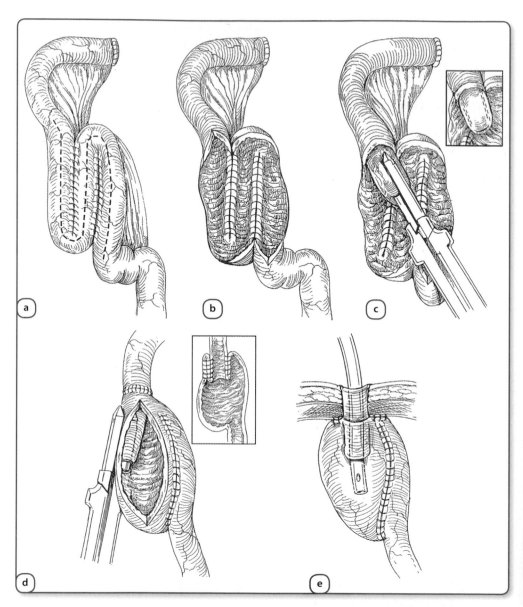

Figure 7.7 Continent ileostomy. (a) Three limbs of small bowel are measured. (b) After opening the bowel (see the dotted lines in (a), the edges are sewn together in two layers. (c) A valve is created by intussuscepting the efferent limb into the pouch and fixing it in place with a linear noncutting stapler. (Inset: staples in place on valve) (d) The valve is attached to the pouch sidewall with the linear noncutting stapler (a cross section of the finished pouch is shown). (e) After closure of the last suture line, the pouch is attached to the abdominal wall and a catheter is inserted to keep the pouch decompressed during healing.

Valve slippage

Valve slippage, when it occurs, usually does so in the first 3 months postoperatively and is uncommon after 12 months. The symptoms are either incontinence to gas or feces or difficulty in intubating the pouch.

When the valve cannot be intubated but remains totally continent, a pediatric or flexible endoscope is inserted through the stoma into the pouch. A guide wire or stylet is passed through the scope channel and using this as a guide a catheter is inserted into the pouch to relieve the small-bowel obstruction. The tube should then remain in the pouch until it can be revised.

Valve prolapse

Valve prolapse occurs when the fascial defect, which is made to bring out the efferent loop, is too large. This can be remedied merely by narrowing the opening in the fascia.

Fistula formation

Fistulas can form at the base of the valve and cause incontinence by allowing the fecal stream to bypass the valve. In these situations, the patient will notice incontinence, but will not have difficulty intubating, as is the case with valve slippage. Fistulas can occur anytime after the operation. Valve fistulas are the result of sutures being placed through the walls of the valve and tied too tightly, overzealous use of electrocautery in the scarification of the bowel, or erosion of prosthetic material. Fistulas can also form between the pouch and the abdominal wall. They commonly present as a parastomal abscess, which then drains and matures as an enterocutaneous fistula. Selected fistulas have been repaired with fibrin glue or collagen plugs, but most require valve revision.

Volvulus

Dislocation and volvulus of the pouch are caused by inadequate fixation on the reservoir to the abdominal wall. If volvulus occurs, it can result in necrosis of the entire pouch.

Perforation

Catheter perforation occurs but is a very rare complication. It will usually require operative repair.

Pouchitis

The incidence of mucosal inflammation in the pouch (pouchitis) varies from 10–40% in various series. It is manifested clinically by an increase in volume of the effluent. The succus entericus becomes watery, foul smelling, and sometimes bloody. Patients may also develop abdominal pain, distention, fever, and nausea. The complication is thought to be secondary to overgrowth of bacteria and is usually treated successfully with metronidazole or probiotics and continuous catheter drainage to avoid stasis.

Crohn's disease

There were some early disastrous experiences with patients who developed recurrence of Crohn's disease in continent ileostomy pouches. Most authors strongly advise against this procedure in Crohn's disease. A few groups, however, continue to construct continent ileostomies in patients who have had Crohn's colitis without any small bowel involvement. Barnett [16] and colleagues have done a small number of operations using a jejunum for construction of the pouch and anastomosing the terminal ileum to the jejunal pouch. Unfortunately, follow-up on these patients has not been reported.

Revision

The overall revision rate for continent ileostomy was as high as 43% in some of the early experiences. Subsequent studies have reported an overall revision rate of 7–15%. It is noteworthy that patients generally will opt for multiple revisions if necessary, rather than conversion to a conventional ileostomy.

Colostomy

Creation

An end colostomy using the sigmoid or descending colon is made after an abdominoperineal resection or a Hartmann procedure [19]. The site is selected just as one would select a site for an ileostomy. If it is anticipated that the patient will have frequent or loose bowel movements after the colostomy (i.e. someone in whom postoperative chemotherapy or radiotherapy is anticipated), the stoma should be made to protrude for 1 or 2 cm above the skin level to prevent pouching problems if the stoma output is liquid. On the other hand, if the patient has a constipated bowel habit preoperatively, there is no reason to believe that this will change; a skin-level colostomy will suffice and will be more convenient for the patient, especially if he or she can irrigate and will not have to wear an appliance.

The aperture in the abdominal wall for end colostomy is made in the same manner as that for ileostomy. However, the opening for a colostomy is usually slightly larger than an ileostomy. When the colon is brought out through the abdominal wall, the gutter can be closed using either a purse-string suture technique or a retroperitoneal tunnel. The colon may be secured, like the ileum, to the anterior rectus sheath or Scarpa's fascia with several interrupted sutures and the edge of the colon sewn to the subcuticular layer of skin. An end colostomy can also be brought out through the midline. Proponents of this technique claim that the strength of the linea alba prevents parastomal herniation [20]. If the colon may be brought out through the midline, the entire left colon should be mobilized so the mesentery can be easily brought up to abdominal wall, and no mesenteric sling is formed in the left upper quadrant.

A loop colostomy may be constructed as an independent procedure or in conjunction with a low anterior resection or coloanal anastomosis when the surgeon wishes to divert the fecal stream proximal to the anastomosis. A transverse loop colostomy may be brought out through the right rectus muscle or, as described by Turnbull and Weakley [21], through the midline laparotomy wound. When the loop of transverse colon is identified, it is freed of its omental attachment and the gastrocolic ligament is incised. If the loop is to be brought through the rectus muscle, a transverse incision is made on the anterior and posterior rectus sheath, the muscle is split, and a Penrose drain is passed through to the mesentery of the colon loop to aid in guiding the bowel through the aperture. This incision should be made wide enough to accommodate both the loop of bowel and an index finger. Once the bowel loop is brought out to the skin level, the Penrose drain is replaced with a plastic colostomy rod. Next an incision is made on the antimesenteric surface of the colon (**Figure 7.8**); this incision should be about 5 cm long to ensure that the orifices of the proximal and distal limbs will be far enough apart to divert the fecal stream. The same method is used to secure the colostomy if it is brought out through the midline.

The efficacy of fecal diversion in a loop colostomy constructed in such a fashion has been demonstrated. Eventually loop colostomies invariably retract somewhat and then fail to completely divert the fecal stream. This usually does not pose a clinical problem, because most of these stomas are temporary. One method of ensuring that the stoma remains permanently diverting is to staple across the distal loop just below the skin line. As described later, prolapse is a common long term problem with loop colostomies.

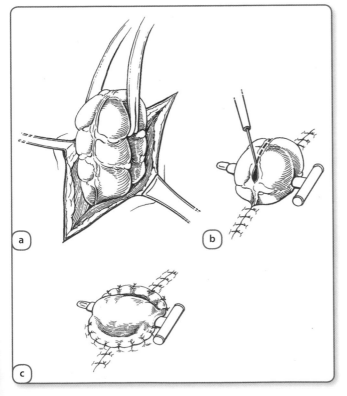

Figure 7.8 Loop colostomy.
(a) A loop of colon is brought out through an adequate fascial opening. (b) A rod is placed through the mesentery and the colon is incised for 5 cm on the antimesenteric surface. (c) The colon edges are sewn to the skin.

A blowhole colostomy or cecostomy can be used in the presence of colonic obstruction, either mechanical or functional, when the colon is markedly distended and the wall quite thin [22,23]. Using the blowhole stoma avoids having to bring a loop of distended colon out through the abdominal wall and reduces the risk of rupture and fecal contamination. An incision is made in the abdominal wall over a prominent distended loop of colon. In the case of a cecostomy, a McBurney incision in the right lower quadrant is used. Once the peritoneum is incised, the distended loop will be readily apparent. The wall of the colon is carefully sutured to the fascial edges of the incision before the colon is opened. Once the suture line is completed and the peritoneum is thus protected from any fecal contamination, the colon is carefully opened, with suction used to prevent contamination in the wound. The edge of the opened bowel is then sewn to the skin edges (**Figure 7.9**). These stomas are very effective in decompressing the bowel but do not divert feces at all. These are all temporary measures, and prolapse of the very large and redundant colon through the stoma is often a problem.

Several methods have been described for rendering a colostomy continent by use of external devices. These include the insertion of a magnetic ring under the skin and use of a magnetized plug as a cap over the colostomy, a silicone sleeve with a plug that is inserted through the stoma to block the opening, and subcutaneous pneumatic compression devices. Problems of extrusion and infection

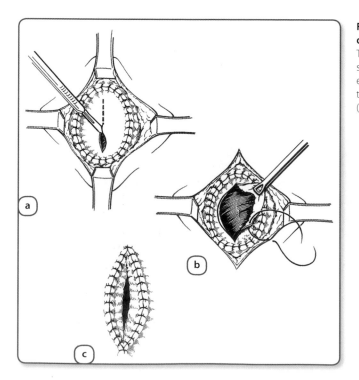

Figure 7.9 Skin-level decompressing colostomy. (a) The colon is incised after the wall is sutured to the fascia edges. (b) The edge of the colonic mucosa is sewn to the skin. (c) Completed blowhole (tangential) colostomy.

have plagued all these methods, which must still be considered experimental. Schmidt [24] has described a technique using a free graft of colonic muscle that is attached just proximal to the stoma; 80% of his patients were reported not to require the use of an appliance. It is unclear how many of those patients would have been able to irrigate successfully without this implanted muscular cuff, but the patients who had the procedure performed as a secondary procedure reported improved function. A new option for selected colostomy patients is the Vitala Continence Control Device (CCD; Convatec, Inc, NJ, USA). This is a noninvasive pouchless Ostomy Device that allows individuals to manage their colostomy without a belt or irrigation. Indicated for use up to 12 hours, Vitala CCD functions by sealing against the stoma to prevent the release of stool while permitting gasses to vent through an integrated, deodorizing filter. Vitala CCD is recommended for use 6–12 weeks after surgery. Research continues on new devices to provide stomal continence.

Closure

Loop colostomies can be closed by detaching the colon from the skin and closing the antimesenteric aspect of the colon or by excising the loop completely and doing an end-to-end or side-by-side anastomosis either with sutures or staples. If a loop colostomy is constructed to protect a distal anastomosis, it is important to test the integrity of that anastomosis with a contrast study before colostomy closure.

An end colostomy closure is a colocolostomy or coloproctostomy; in the cases of patients who have previously undergone a Hartmann procedure, it involves a laparotomy or it can be done as a laparoscopically assisted procedure in many cases (see Chapter 6). In this situation, the coloproctostomy is most easily accomplished by using an end-to-end stapling device inserted through the anus.

Surgical complications of colostomy closure include wound infection, anastomotic leak, and intestinal obstruction [25]. Many studies have investigated the relationship between techniques of closure and the timing of closure with these complications. No clear-cut relationship between technique and postoperative morbidity has been established [26]. The timing of the colostomy closure should be individualized, waiting longer in those patients who have had peritonitis at the time of the first surgery or who had complications following the colostomy. It is prudent to wait at least 3 months in patients who have these complicating factors; however, it appears that if these factors are not present, closure can be done earlier (6–8 weeks) without any increased morbidity. Use of anti-adhesion products (such as Seprafilm, Genzyme, Cambridge, MA, USA) may allow even earlier closure of stomas [27].

Complications

Many of the complications occurring after ileostomy are also seen after colostomy formation [28]. Leakage of fecal material is less common with a colostomy than with an ileostomy, because the stool is usually solid.

However, in patients with liquid colostomy output this can be a very troublesome problem. As with ileostomy, meticulous attention must be paid to the placement of the stoma. Stenosis of the colostomy, like that of an ileostomy, usually results from an inadequate skin or fascial incision or as a result of contraction secondary to ischemia. In this situation, it is usually associated with stoma retraction. However, stoma retraction in a colostomy patient may not need to be revised if the stool is solid and the patient is having no problems with leakage of fecal material.

Parastomal abscesses that occur around the colostomy are treated in the same way as those found with an ileostomy. Parastomal fistulas in colostomies may sometimes be treated by just laying open the fistulous tract as one would do with a fistula-in-ano. This is usually satisfactory, especially if the patient has a solid stool.

Prolapse following colostomy is much more common than after ileostomy. A prolapse is most commonly seen with loop transverse colostomies, especially those done in the presence of distal obstruction. Prolapsing of the distal limb is more common. Some techniques of tacking the distal bowel wall to the abdominal wall have been described; however, very often these measures are only transiently successful. The most definitive treatment of prolapse is amputation and reconstruction of the distal part of the stoma. Prolapse can also occur with an end colostomy and is treated with an amputative procedure, just as one would do with an ileostomy prolapse.

Parastomal hernia is a much more common problem after a colostomy than after an ileostomy and are more common if the colostomy is brought out lateral to the rectus muscle. These hernias are troublesome in that they may interfere with proper fitting of the appliance. They are also dangerous in patients who irrigate, increasing the risk of perforation. These hernias may be repaired locally through a parastomal incision if they are small. However, recurrence is common after this technique is used and transposition is usually necessary, especially if the stoma was not placed through the rectus muscle. As described previously mesh reinforcement is being increasingly used. Occasionally parastomal hernias may become extremely large, and prosthetic mesh must be used to repair the large defect in the fascia and the stoma relocated to a different site on the anterior abdominal wall [29]. Prospective trials are also underway to evaluate the value of prophylactic placement of biologic mesh to reduce the incidence of peristomal hernias.

Enterostomal therapy

General principles

Ostomy appliances are adhered to the skin in the operating room. There are numerous products available, many manufacturers supplying sterile pouches for operating room use [30].

Pouching systems vary from one-piece, presized stoma openings to a separate wafer with a flange and a snap-on pouch. The latter must be cut to fit the size and shape of the stoma. Whichever type is used, proper fit is imperative. The appliance opening should be no more than 3 mm larger than the stoma, because parastomal skin exposed to effluent will very quickly become excoriated.

Immediately postoperatively, if the vascular integrity of the stoma is the least bit suspect, the pouch should be removed to allow inspection of the stoma and its site. After inspection a new appliance is reapplied. All stomas will have a serosanguinous output in the immediate post-operative period. The stoma made in an unprepared bowel may have drainage of stool during this time, but one should not consider bowel function to have been re-established until flatus is present in the pouch.

Before discharge, the patient is fitted with an appliance based on his or her physical ability and mental awareness. One of the most popular products consists of a pectin-based wafer with a flange, to which a snap-on pouch is attached. These wafers must be cut individually to fit stoma size and shape. Severely arthritic patients or those with poor coordination may prefer a presized, one-piece appliance.

Whatever equipment is chosen, there must be proper size and adherence, no leakage or odor, and no skin irritation. The system should have a minimum wearing time of 24 hours. Most adhere from 4–7 days without leakage. Each week the patient must examine the peristomal skin for signs of irritation.

The stoma will shrink dramatically in the first 6–8 weeks postop-eratively and may continue to do so for as long as 8 months. The patient should be alerted to this fact and taught to adjust the appliance opening as needed. Ostomates should be seen in the clinic and their stoma size remeasured at 1 month, 3 months, 6 months, and 1 year after their hospital discharge. At these outpatient visits the physician should always remove the appliance and inspect the stoma and surrounding skin. Irritation is most commonly caused by an improperly fitted appliance, leakage, or allergies to skin barriers, appliance adhesive, or tape. Careful observation and questioning the patient will almost always provide the answer.

Many patients do not adjust appliance size as the stoma shrinks. The skin immediately surrounding the stoma, exposed to effluent, will become irritated. Adjusting the appliance size to 3 mm larger than the stoma should solve the problem. If the patient complains of leakage, the area should be inspected with the patient in a sitting position. Skin irritation will denote the area of leakage. Any indentation from scars, skinfolds, or retraction should be noted and these areas filled with a pectin-based paste before an appliance is applied.

Allergic reactions to the skin barriers, adhesive, or tape manifest themselves by skin irritation only over the area with which they come in contact [31]. Use of the present brand should be discontinued. When moisture is trapped under an appliance, a monilial rash may develop. Small amounts of antifungal powder can be dusted on the involved skin before applying an appliance. Excess powder should be wiped or blown off to prevent it from preventing adherence of the applicance. Severe skin irritation may require treatment with a steroid in spray form. Ointments and creams should not be used on peristomal skin because they interfere with proper adherence.

One of the greatest concerns to the ostomate is odor. Almost all products on the market today are made from odor-proof materials. There should never be odors unless the patient has emptied the appliance. If odor is a problem, one should look for holes in the pouch, leakage, a pouch not properly snapped onto the wafer's flange, or poor hygiene. If none of these factors is identified, the patient should be offered pouch deodorants or nonprescription oral medication such as bismuth subgallate (Devrom chewable tablets) or chlorophyll (Derifil tablets). Certain foods, including fish, eggs, garlic, onions, and cruciferous vegetables may contribute to odor problems. Another common problem of ileostomates or colostomates is flatus. This is frequently audible, especially in the early postoperative period when the stoma is edematous and the lumen narrowed to some degree. As the stoma matures, this becomes less of a problem. Patients should be advised that chewing gum, drinking through straws, smoking and drinking carbonated beverages will increase flatus, as will ingesting foods that contain poorly digestible carbohydrates.

Patients with permanent ostomies should be encouraged to eat anything they like. Some foods may cause more odor, diarrhea, or constipation, but these will generally follow patterns that were present preoperatively. A colostomate who is using irrigation for self-management will want to avoid food known to have a laxative effect so that he or she is continent between irrigations. Patients with ileostomies may have problems with food obstruction; they will need more stringent dietary guidelines. For the first 6–8 weeks, they should avoid all foods that may cause obstruction: popcorn, nuts, coconut, dried fruit (all swell after ingestion). Food must be chewed well, and potato skins, beans, celery, corn, grapes, apple skins, and Chinese vegetables should be avoided in the immediate postoperative period.

After 6–8 weeks, when stomal edema has decreased, patients can add restricted items to their diets in small amounts. If abdominal cramping occurs, they should discontinue that food for 2–3 weeks and then introduce it again. Patients will soon learn which foods they cannot tolerate. If a patient with an ileostomy presents with a bowel obstruction, a thorough history should be taken regarding which particular foods the patient has ingested recently. Irrigations with normal saline solution through the stoma in volumes of 60–150 mL, repeated many times, may relieve a food obstruction.

Colostomy irrigation is used to cleanse the bowel before surgery, relieve constipation on occasion, or as an everyday management technique for the ostomate. Not all colostomy patients are good candidates for irrigation management; it is appropriate only for patients whose frequency of bowel movement preoperatively was less than 2 per day, with a formed stool. Patients who are undergoing radiotherapy or chemotherapy might have a liquid stool and may not be candidates for irrigation. Patients who have a colostomy formed from the transverse colon or more proximal to that are usually not good candidates, because their stools are frequently liquid. The patient who does successfully irrigate his or her colostomy will usually do so on a daily or every-other-day basis. Ideally, the stoma will then be free of stool until the next irrigation, and pouching is no longer required. A small dressing or stoma cap applied over the stoma absorbs any mucus or flatus. Patients can be taught irrigation about 6–8 weeks postoperatively in the clinic when their diet and bowel habits are near normal. It may take several weeks to establish a routine that is ideal for the individual patient. Occasionally medications such as loperamide (Imodium) can be used to constipate the patient if this is necessary.

Colostomy irrigation

Irrigation is normally done in the bathroom. There are sets of equipment specifically designed for colostomy irrigation, consisting of an irrigation sleeve, an enema bag with tubing, and a cone tip. The cone is preferred to an irrigating catheter because it reduces the chance of perforation and serves as a dam for the irrigation solution.

Patients can be taught the following procedure for at-home colostomy irrigation. Research is underway to develop mechanical methods to ease and shorten the irrigation process.

Instructions for at-home colostomy irrigation

Sit on the commode or on a chair in front of the commode. Attach the irrigation sleeve to the faceplate of the colostomy appliance and put the bottom of the sleeve into the bowl. With the control valve in the off position, fill the irrigation bag with lukewarm tap water and then clear the tubing of air by running the water slowly through it. Gently insert the cone into the stoma, applying enough pressure so that the water does not leak out around the cone. Most patients with a descending or sigmoid colostomy can tolerate 700–1000 mL of water. If cramping occurs during the procedure, it is usually because the water is running too quickly or is too cold. If this should happen, stop the flow of water until the cramping subsides. When it has subsided, continue the irrigation. After all the fluid is infused, remove the cone slowly, being sure that the irrigation sleeve covers the stoma. Most of the irrigation fluid will return in the first 15 minutes, and you may leave the bathroom at this time. Leave the sleeve in place for another 30–40 minutes, however, because the colon may continue to expel water and stool. With experience, you will come to know how long this will take. Once the fluid has stopped flowing, replace the irrigation sleeve with a small safety pouch or just a dressing, depending on whether any further leakage of fluid during the day is anticipated.

Rounds questions

1. Where should stomas be located?
2. What is the most common complication of an ileostomy?
3. What are the major complications of a stoma?
4. What is the most difficult problem with a continent ileostomy?
5. Is a patient with Crohn's disease a candidate for a continent ileostomy?
6. Is a parastomal hernia more common after an ileostomy or a colostomy?
7. Why must a stomal appliance be remeasured in the postoperative period?
8. Which colostomy patients are good candidates for irrigation?

References

1. Barker WF, Benfield JR, deKernion JB, Fonkalsrud EW, Fowler E. The creation and care of enterocutaneous stomas. Curr Probl Surg 1975;12:1–62.
2. Corman ML. Colon & Rectal Surgery. Philadelphia: JB Lippincott, 1989.
3. Goligher J. Surgery of the Anus, Rectum and Colon, 5th ed. London: Ballibre Tindall, 1984.
4. Marcello PW, Roberts PL, Schoetz DJ Jr, Coller JA, Murray JJ, Veidenheimer MC. Obstruction after ileal pouch-anal anastomosis: A preventable complication? Dis Colon Rectum 1993;36:1105–11.
5. Kawamura YJ, Kakizawa N, Tan KY, et al. Sushi-roll wrap of Seprafilm for ileostomy limbs facilitates ileostomy closure. Tech Coloproctol 2009;13:211–14.
6. Sitzmann JV. A new alternative to diverting double barreled ileostomy. Surg Gynecol Obstet 1987;165:461–4.
7. Bayer I, Kyzer S, Chaimoff C. A new approach to primary strengthening of colostomy with Marlex mesh to prevent paracolostomy hernia. Surg Gynecol Obstet 1986;163:579–80.
8. Slater NJ, Hansson BME, Buyne OR, Hendriks T, Bleichrodt RP. Repair of parastomal hernias with biologic grafts: A systemic review. J Gastroint Surg 2011;15:1252–58.
9. Beck DE, Fazio VW, Grundfest-Broniatowski SG. Surgical management of bleeding stomal varices. Dis Colon Rectum 1988;31:343–6.
10. Kock NG. Intra-abdominal 'reservoir' in patients with permanent ileostomy: Preliminary observations on a procedure resulting in fecal 'continence' in five ileostomy patients. Arch Surg 1969;99:223–31.
11. Cranley B. The Kock reservoir ileostomy: A review of its development problems and role in modern surgical practice. Br J Surg 1983;70:94–9.
12. Dozois RR, Kelly KA, Beart RW, Beahrs OH. Improved results with continent ileostomy. Ann Surg 1980;19:2319–24.
13. Kock NG, Darle N, Hulten L, Kewenter J, Myrvoid H, Philipson B. Ileostomy. Curr Probl Surg 1977;14:1–52.
14. McLeod RS. Fazio VW. The continent ileostomy: An acceptable alternative. J Enterostom Ther 1984;11:140–6.
15. Fazio VW, Tjandra JJ. Technique for nipple valve fixation to prevent valve slippage in continent ileostomy. Dis Colon Rectum 1992;35:1177–9.
16. Barnett WO. Current experiences with the continent intestinal reservoir. Surg Gynecol Obstet 1989;168:1–5.
17. Kaiser AM, Stein JP, Beart RW. T-pouch: a new valve design for a continent ileostomy. Dis Colon Rectum 2002;45:411–5.
18. Gorfine, SR, Bauer JJ, Gelernt IM. Continent stomas. In MacKeigan J, Cataldo PA, (eds). Intestinal Stomas. St. Louis: Quality Medical Publishing 1993;154–87.
19. Beck DE. End sigmoid colostomy. In MacKeigan J, Cataldo PA (eds). Intestinal Stomas. St. Louis: Quality Medical Publishing, 1993;97–106.
20. Raza SD, Portin BA, Bernhoft WH. Umbilical colostomy: A better intestinal stoma. Dis Colon Rectum 1977;20:223–30.

21. Turnhull RB, Weakley FL. Atlas of Intestinal Stomas. St. Louis: CV Mosby, 1967.

22. Gierson ED, Storm FK. Blowhole cecostomy for cecal decompression. Arch Surg 1975;110:444–5.

23. Rombeau JL, Wilk PJ, Turnhull RB, Fazio VW. Total fecal diversion by the temporary skin-level loop transverse colostomy. Dis Colon Rectum 1978;21:223–6.

24. Schmidt E. The continent colostomy. World J Surg 1982;6:805–9.

25. Pittman DM, Smith LE. Complications of colostomy closure. Dis Colon Rectum 1985;28:836–43.

26. Khoury D, Beck DE, Opelka FG, Hicks TC, Timmcke AE, Gathright JB. Colostomy closure: Ochsner Clinic experience. Dis Colon Rectum 1996;39:605–9.

27. Salum M, Wexner SD, Nogueras JJ, et al. Does sodium, hyaluronate- and carboxymethylcellulose-based bioresorbable membrane (Seprafilm) decrease operative time to loop ileostomy closure? Tech Coloproctol 2006;10:187–90.

28. Fleshman JW Jr. Ostomies. In Hicks TC, Beck DE, Opelka FG, Timmcke AE (eds). Complications of Colon & Rectal Surgery. Baltimore: Williams & Wilkins 1996;357–81.

29. Sugarbaker PH. Peritoneal approach to prosthetic mesh repair of paraostomy hernias. Ann Surg 1985;201:344–6.

30. Daniel N, Porrett T. Nursing considerations. In Beck DE, Wexner SD. Fundamentals of anorectal surgery, 2nd ed. London: WB Saunders Ltd 1992;533–45.

31. Fry RD, Swatske ME. Skin problems in stoma management. MacKeigan J, Cataldo PA (eds). Intestinal Stomas. St. Louis: Quality Medical Publishing 1993;329–38.

Section 2

Perioperative Management

Preoperative preparation

Preparing patients for colorectal surgery is extremely important because it reduces morbidity and mortality and improves chances of a good outcome [1]. This chapter describes methods of nutritional management and bowel preparation and reviews other important aspects of preoperative preparation.

Nutrition and fluid management

Goals

The goals of nutritional management include prevention of nutritional and fluid defects, identification of patients needing nutritional support (nutritional assessment), and providing adequate nutrition and fluids in a safe and cost-effective manner. Prevention of malnutrition is best accomplished when nutrition has a high priority. Hospitalized patients should receive adequate nutrition, and the quality and quantity of administered nutrients should be monitored. Intervention should occur before problems develop.

Nutritional assessment

Malnutrition is common among colorectal patients and is associated with significant morbidity and mortality [2, 3]. Many colorectal diseases produce nutritional defects by direct activity against the gastrointestinal tract or indirectly by increasing metabolic requirements and losses and reducing the patient's appetite. Each patient should therefore undergo a nutritional evaluation tailored to his or her individual situation. Our knowledge of nutrition is increasing, but no ideal assessment method is currently available. The components of nutritional assessment currently used by most clinicians are listed in **Table 8.1** [4]. Of these, the most useful is the weight history: an assessment of current weight, how that weight relates to ideal body weight (from standard tables), and any history of recent weight loss. The amount of weight lost and the time period over which it was lost are also important. The medication and dietary histories also provide insight into potential problems and corroborate the weight history.

Anthropometric characteristics such as the triceps skinfold and midarm circumference can be determined by a nurse or dietician. These measurements assist in assessing fat stores and skeletal muscle mass.

Biochemical measurements of blood and urine are obtained. Albumin, a visceral and serum protein with a long biologic half-life, is

Table 8.1 Nutritional assessment components

Assessment	Components
Medical history and physical examination	Weight history (body weight) Medical history
Diet history	–
Anthropometric measurements	Triceps skinfold Midarm circumference Midarm muscle circumference

Biochemical measurements	Plasma proteins
	  Albumin
	  Transferrin
	  Prealbumin
	  Retinol-binding protein
	Urinary measurements
	  Creatinine height index
	  3-Methylhistadine

Immunologic markers	Total lymphocyte count Delayed cutaneous hypersensitivity

From Kirby DF, DeLegge MH. Nutritional assessment: the high tech and low tech tour. In: Kirby OF, Dudrick SJ: (eds). Practical Handbook of Nutrition in Clinical Practice. Boca Raton: CRC Press 1994;1–18. With permission.

frequently measured through automated biochemical screening and is a good indicator of long-term protein status. Serum transferrin, a protein with a short biologic half-life, measures the recent protein status. Other shorter half-life proteins such as prealbumin and retinol-binding protein are becoming more available. The creatinine height index, a measure of muscle turnover, can be calculated with measurements from a timed urine collection along with a serum creatinine level. A 2-hour urine collection is a reasonable screening measurement, but a 24-hour collection is more accurate. This calculation provides additional information about protein status. The total lymphocyte count and delayed cutaneous hypersensitivity measure the body's ability to respond to infections. Their values are not affected until malnutrition becomes severe.

Several attempts have been made to quantify some of these values for prognostic purposes. Dr. Mullen and colleagues have devised a formula called the **prognostic nutritional index (PNI)** [5].

$$PNI = 150 - 16.6\,(Alb) - 0.78\,(TSF) - 0.2\,(TFN) - 5.8\,(DH)$$

Where *Alb* is the serum albumin (g/dL), *TSF* is the triceps skinfold (mm), *TFN* is the serum transferrin level (mg/dL), and *DH* is the grade of skin reaction to injected antigens (e.g. Dermatophytid, *Candida*, mumps). Patients with a high PNI have a high risk of complications [2]. This formula is often used by nutritional support teams but is difficult for the busy clinician to use.

An alternative to the PNI is the **subjective global assessment** proposed by Detsky et al [6]. This method divides patients into three categories: well nourished, moderately malnourished, and severely malnourished. This is accomplished by making a subjective assessment of the patient's medical history (weight change, dietary intake, and gastrointestinal symptoms), physical examination (subcutaneous fat, muscle mass, edema, and ascites), and serum albumin [7]. The values associated with each category are listed in **Table 8.2**.

Requirements

Each patient has daily requirements for water, electrolytes, carbohydrates, protein, and fat. When deficiencies occur, the human body can compensate to different degrees and for variable periods of time. Water is critical and a daily supply is essential for health. Maintenance requirements for water are related to energy expenditure. An estimate for water requirements for children was devised by Holliday and Segar [8]. Using body weight, this formula (the Holliday or kilogram method) suggests providing 100 mL/kg/24 h for the first 10 kg of body weight, 50 mL/kg/24 h for the next 10 kg of body weight, and 10 mL/kg/24 h for the remainder of body weight [9]. Although devised for children, this method has been widely used for all age groups. Based on this formula, a 70 kg man would receive 2,000 mL/day:

$$(100 \times 10) + (50 \times 10) + (10 \times 50) = 2000 \, mL/day$$

A variation of this method is often used to calculate an hourly rate. It recommends 4 mL/kg/h for the first 10 kg of body weight, 2 mL/kg/h for the next 10 kg of body weight, and 1 mL/kg/h for the remainder of body weight. Thus the same 70 kg man would receive 2,640 mL/day using this formula:

$$(4 \times 10) + (2 \times 10) + (1 \times 50) = 110 \, mL/h \text{ or } 2{,}640 \, mL/day$$

These estimates are just that, and the clinician is reminded that fluid management must be individualized for each patient and modified as the clinical status changes.

It is important to provide this maintenance fluid as well as to correct previous deficiencies (e.g. dehydration) and to replace ongoing

Table 8.2 Subjective global assessment			
Criteria	Well nourished	Moderately malnourished	Severely malnourished
Medical history			
Body weight change in last 6 months	Loss < 5%	Loss 5–10%	Loss > 10%
Dietary intake	Balanced diet that meets requirements	70–90% of requirements	< 70% of requirements
GI symptoms (vomiting, diarrhea)	None	Intermittent	Daily for > 2 weeks
Functional capacity	Full capacity	Reduced	Bedridden
Physical examination			
Subcutaneous fat	Normal	Decreased	Markedly decreased
Muscle mass (quadriceps, deltoids)	Normal	Decreased	Markedly decreased
Edema (ankle, sacral)	None	Present	Marked
Ascites	None	Present	Marked
Serum albumin	> 4.0 g/dL	3.0–4.0 g/dL	< 3.0 g/dL

losses (e.g. from nasogastric suction, excess ileostomy losses, etc.) [9]. Characteristics of commonly used intravenous fluids are presented in **Table 8.3**. Additional information on determining these requirements is available in major texts on perioperative management [10–12]. To compensate for having nothing by mouth before surgery, patients should receive intravenous fluid whenever possible the evening before or the morning of a major operation.

An estimation of daily needs for electrolytes, carbohydrates, protein, fat, and calories is presented in **Table 8.4**. The electrolytes and carbohydrates should be provided on a daily basis. Most patients can tolerate the absence of the other requirements for 5–7 days. After this time, nutritional supplementation should be instituted. When additional nutritional support is indicated, it may be delivered by several routes.

Methods of support

Enteral

The enteral route is the preferred method for its beneficial physiologic effects, its safety, and its reduced costs [13]. Nutrients in the intestinal lumen preserve the normal physiology of nutrient metabolism and maintain intestinal integrity and hormonal balance. Metabolic complications are reduced with enteral nutrition, and mechanical and infectious complications associated with central lines (required

Table 8.3 Intravenous fluids							
Solution	Na^+	K^+	Ca^{++}	Cl^-	HCO_3^-	Glucose	Replacement
0.9% Sodium chloride (normal saline solution)	154			154			Fluid losses
0.45% Sodium chloride (1/2 normal saline solution)	77			77			Nasogastric output or diarrhea mL for mL with 20 mEq KCl/L added to fluid
Lactated Ringer's solution	130	4	2.7	109	28		Duodenal output or proximal fistula
Dextrose 5% in water						50 g	Carbohydrate requirement
Electrolyte content in mEq/L.							

Table 8.4 Estimated daily nutritional requirements	
Carbohydrates	50–100 g/day
Protein	1 g/kg/day
Fat (linoleic acid)	500 mL intralipid/week
Calories (energy)	30 kcal/kg/day
Electrolytes	
Sodium	1–3 mEq/kg/day
Potassium	0.5–1 mEq/kg/day
Chloride	1–3 mEq/kg/day

for parenteral nutrition) are avoided. All studies comparing methods of support have demonstrated lower costs with enteral nutrition. If the gut can be used, enteral nutrition is preferred.

Many enteral solutions are available. Elemental (monomeric) solutions such as Vivonex T.E.N. (Nestle Nutrition, Florham Park, NJ) and Vital HN (Abbott Nutrition, Columbus, OH, USA) are totally absorbed in the small intestine and thus no residue reaches the colon. These solutions provide complete nutrition and glutamine (an amino acid whose importance is increasingly being documented). With their low viscosity, these solutions can be used with small-diameter tubes. A disadvantage of elemental solutions is their relatively high osmolality (600–1200 mOsm/L). This requires either dilution or gradual advancement of rate when these solutions are used in the small intestine.

Low-residue or polymeric solutions are composed of complete proteins or small peptides. Their osmolality is lower (approximating serum osmolality) and they cost less than elemental solutions. Information on the advantages of one solution over another is confusing and limited; therefore most clinicians choose the least expensive solution that fits the patient's needs.

Enteral nutrition is contraindicated when the gut cannot be used (e.g. because of intestinal obstruction, ileus, distal enteric anastomosis, high-output fistulas, bowel inflammation). In addition, the metabolic needs of some patients cannot be met using the gut alone (pancreatitis, inflammatory bowel disease, hypercatabolic states, sepsis, and trauma). In these conditions parenteral nutrition is indicated to supplement enteral nutrition or to provide total needs.

Parenteral

Parenteral solutions use a high dextrose concentration (i.e. 25% dextrose), electrolytes, amino acids, and lipids [14]. Currently available solutions can provide complete nutrition, but their high osmolality requires central venous access. The disadvantages of parenteral nutrition are cost and safety. There is a risk with central line placement and infectious complications associated with the invasive line. Potential metabolic complications can be reduced by gradual advancement of the solution infusion rate and frequent laboratory monitoring.

Role in specific diseases

Preoperative preparation

Malnourished patients have a higher morbidity than well-nourished patients do. While intuitively it would seem that taking malnourished patients and providing them with nutrition before surgery would improve results, this has been difficult to verify with prospective studies. Nutritional support for less than 4 days provides no alteration in complication rates, and therapy for longer than 14 days is difficult to justify on a cost basis. I recommend a minimum of 5–10 days of therapy. This will allow most patients to become anabolic, the cost is reasonable, and this does not delay surgery for too long.

Ulcerative colitis

Nutritional support has a role in ulcerative colitis and may assist patients in recovering from acute attacks. However, nutritional support provides no long-term benefit with respect to future flares. Nutritional support can prevent patients from developing malnutrition and seems to improve their ability to tolerate surgery (see Chapter 14). Parenteral nutrition is therefore adjunctive for severely ill patients with ulcerative colitis. It does not appear to alter the natural history of ulcerative colitis or induce remissions [15].

Crohn's disease

Temporary remissions have been obtained in 70–80% of patients with active Crohn's disease using parenteral nutrition [15,16] Long-term results have been questionable (see Chapter 14). The enteral fistulas and potential for shortened gut associated with Crohn's disease provide additional indications for parenteral nutrition [17].

Malignancies

Nutritional support is indicated in patients who are undergoing treatment for a malignancy to improve tolerance to chemotherapy and/or radiotherapy [17]. Advantages of preoperative support were discussed previously. Nutritional supplementation is difficult to justify in terminal patients who are not receiving treatment for their malignancy. The risks and costs of the nutrition must be weighed against the expected benefit. It often comes to an ethical question of whether the therapy is prolonging life.

Postoperative use

Postoperative nutritional support is indicated when a delay in postoperative oral intake is anticipated or if the patient has severe preoperative malnutrition or excessive metabolic needs.

Bowel preparation

Preoperative preparation of the bowel has been standard practice in colon and rectal surgery [18]. Accomplishing this involves two components: mechanical cleansing and antibiotic preparation. The relative importance of each of these components has been questioned [19–21]. Five randomized trials have found that mechanical cleansing adds little for colon cases [24–26]. In contrast, a recent study from Europe suggests that mechanical cleansing is useful for rectal cases [27]. Colonic cleansing is required for colonoscopy.

A clean colon is aesthetically pleasing to the surgeon and is necessary for intraoperative endoscopy which may be needed or for laparoscopic cases. The ideal mechanical bowel preparation would be safe, cost effective, and rapid, provide good cleansing, and cause minimal patient discomfort and inconvenience. Furthermore, it should be easy to administer so it could be used effectively in both inpatient and outpatient situations. No single method has yet fulfilled all these criteria, and most regimens use a combination of methods.

Mechanical preparation options

Dietary restriction

One to 5 days on a clear liquid or low residue diet reduces the amount of stool. However, this method by itself is insufficient to adequately cleanse the colon. It is helpful in cases of partial bowel obstruction.

Cathartics

Cathartics stimulate bowel evacuation. Regimens using these medications usually require 2–3 days to empty the colon of stool and are frequently combined with enemas and dietary restrictions. Cathartics have been associated with dehydration and electrolyte changes. In controlled trials using cathartics, adequate cleansing occurs in only 75–80% of patients [18]. Medications commonly used along with their mechanism of action are listed in **Table 8.5**. Sodium phosphate solutions (Fleet Phospho-soda, Fleet Laboratories, Lynchburg, VA, USA) are concentrated, low volume hyperosmotic solutions that exert an osmotic effect to draw fluid into the bowel lumen to assist in transit of contents [18, 28–31]. These solutions are administered as two 15 mL dispensations that are diluted and ingested by the patient at pre-set times, the day prior to elective colorectal surgery or colonoscopy. Electrolyte alterations that may occur include hyperphosphatemia, hypocalcemia, hypernatremia, and hypokalemia, which in most patients was minimal and or transient in nature.

A tablet form of NaP, developed in 2000, showed equal or improved efficacy and/or improved tolerance when compared to both liquid NaP, PEG, and PEG plus bisacodyl regimens [32–34]. These tablet preparations (OsmoPrep and Visicol, Salix Pharmaceuticals, Morrisville, NC, USA) offered an alternative to the solution-type NaP formulation. The tablet preparation regimen consists of 28–40 tablets given the day prior to the elective procedure or in a split dose manner, similar to the fluid formulation.

Patients with impaired renal function, dehydration, hypercalcemia, hyperphosphatemia, congestive heart failure, or advanced liver disease could experience severe complications with NaP administration including phosphate nephropathy [35, 36]. This is especially true in hypertensive patients taking certain medications, namely angiotensin converting enzyme (ACE) inhibitors or angiotensin receptor blockers (ARB). This led the Federal Drug Administration to issue a black box warning for the over-the-counter version of this preparation and the

Table 8.5 Cathartic preparations

Agent	Mechanism of action
Castor oil	Whole-gut irritant
Magnesium citrate	Nonabsorbed cation (osmotic diarrheic)
Sodium phosphate (Fleet Phospho-soda, Visacol)	Osmotic cathartic
Extract of senna (X-Prep)	Works predominately in the colon by an unknown mechanism
Bisacodyl (Dulcolax)	Contact irritant (oral or rectal use)

manufacturer to voluntarily remove the preparation from the market. As this preparation is hypertonic, significant fluid and electrolyte shifts can occur and it is necessary to maintain adequate hydration while undergoing the preparation [36,37]. Absolute contraindications to any bowel preparation include obstruction, ileus, perforation, diverticulitis, severe colitis, toxic megacolon, gastric retention, and gastric paresis.

Enemas

Enemas (saline solution, soapsuds, tap water) work by dilution or irritation. They are messy and uncomfortable for patients and the nursing staff. They rarely provide adequate cleansing when used alone but may be helpful in patients with obstructing lesions to remove stool from the distal bowel.

Oral lavage

Oral lavage methods had been developed to reduce the time required for mechanical cleansing (usually only 2–4 hours are required). Three solutions have been described. The first was **saline solution,** infused at 1.5–2 L/h through a small (10 Fr) nasogastric tube. Seven to 10 L of fluid are usually required to obtain good cleansing [38]. This preparation has been associated with fluid and electrolyte disturbances and weight gain. It should not be used in patients with compromised renal or cardiovascular status. It provides good to excellent cleansing in approximately 90% of patients, but it is rarely used in current clinical practice [18,39].

Polyethylene glycol electrolyte gastrointestinal lavage solution (PEG lavage) is an isosmotic solution composed of polyethylene glycol 3350 and an electrolyte solution (sodium 125 mmol/L, sulfate 40 mmol/L, chloride 35 mmol/L, bicarbonate 20 mmol/L, and potassium 10 mmol/L). This solution is available commercially as **GoLytely** (Braintree Laboratories) and **Colyte** (Reed and Carnrick). This preparation provides excellent cleansing (in 90–100% of patients) and is associated with no fluid or electrolyte problems. It has a mildly salty taste, is well tolerated by patients, and multiple clinical trials have demonstrated its superiority over other methods [18,40,41]. This solution is now available in several flavors (e.g. pineapple, cherry). A slightly modified solution (NuLytely, Braintree Laboratories) is also available [42]. The PEG lavage solutions rapidly became a popular choice for colonoscopy and colon surgery [18,39]. Since then several other lavage solutions have been developed and marketed. A reduced volume solution (Halflightly, Braintree Laboratories) was combined with a stimulate (bisacodyl) [43]. MoviPrep (Salix) is a 2 L hypertonic solution that contains PEG, electrolytes and ascorbic acid which can be used as a single or split dosing regimen [44].

Several alternate dosage schemes have been described. One includes bisacodyl (Dulcolax, Boehringer Ingelheim, Ridgefield, CT, USA) 20 mg PO on the morning before the procedure, followed by 2 L of PEG lavage 4–5 hours later ingested at the rate described above.

Another, often referred to as a 'split dosing', administers half the preparation the afternoon prior to the procedure and the remainder of the preparation the morning of the procedure [45]. The timing of the morning dosage is adjusted so that the preparation is completed 4 hours to the scheduled procedure starting time. For early morning cases, this often requires the patient to start the morning portion at 3–4 am. These additional options provide physicians with flexibility in preparation selection.

Intraoperative lavage methods have been described for patients who require emergency operations [18]. Proponents of these techniques suggest that their use may allow safe primary anastomosis after resection [46]. The transrectal method involves placing a large Malecot or Pezzer latex catheter (32 or 34 Fr) into the rectum through the anus. This allows irrigation of the left colon, which may be accomplished before or during the operation. At laparotomy, fluid may be inserted into the proximal colon or distal ileum through an operatively placed tube and drained out through a large tube placed into the distal colon. Although cumbersome, these methods may adequately cleanse the colon, permitting a primary anastomosis in selected cases (**Figure 8.1**) [18].

As discussed previously, at least five randomized prospective trials have look at the importance of preoperative mechanical bowel cleansing [22–26]. Although these studies have limitations (small numbers of patients, high infection rates in both groups, etc.), they do challenge the current surgical dogma of the absolute requirement for a mechanical preparation with the appropriate use of modern antibiotics. The results of these studies are bolstered by the increasing experience with colorectal trauma. Currently, almost all surgeons continue to use preoperative **mechanical bowel preparation** (**MBP**), however some

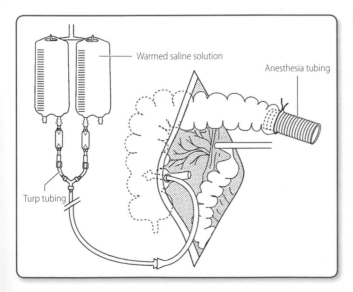

Figure 8.1 Intraoperative lavage.

Warmed saline solution

Anesthesia tubing

Turp tubing

surgeons (including the author) are beginning to reduce the rigor of their mechanical preparations. Additional experience will hopefully provide additional information to guide clinical decisions.

Summary of trials and meta-analyses

Over the past few years, and as recently as mid-2008, numerous clinical trials and meta-analyses have been performed in an attempt to understand the role of MBP in elective colorectal surgery [47,48]. These studies are summarized in **Table 8.6**. This issue of MBP versus no MBP was reviewed in a Cochrane Database review published in 2005 [49]. This comprehensive meta-analysis included nine clinical trials and a total of 1592 patients. The authors reiterated a belief raised in other studies, that the use of MBP frequently resulted in a 'semi prepared' colon full of liquid feces that was difficult to control, often leading to spillage and peritoneal contamination and thus explaining the higher rates of complications found in the MBP group.

The most thorough and current meta-analysis on the subject was recently published by Pineda and colleagues from Stanford, who completed a systematic review of the literature through early 2008 and found 13 prospective trials available with a total of 4601 patients, the greatest number of patients available to date [50]. In this meta-analysis, the authors analyzed two primary outcomes – anastomotic leaks and wound infections. They found no statistically significant difference between 2304 patients receiving MBP compared to 2297 patients receiving no MBP in either outcome. Anastomotic leaks

Table 8.6 Randomized bowel preparation studies					
	Zmora (2003)	Fa-Si-Oen (2005)	Ram (2005)	Bucher (2005)	Miettinen (2000)
Patients (n)	415	250	329	153	267
Patients (MBP/no MBP)	187/193	125/125	164/165	78/75	138/129
Mean age (MBP/no MBP)	68/68	68/70	68/68	63/63	61/64
Cancer, % (MBP/no MBP)	78/78	90/92	75/88	32/28	46/55
Left colon surgery, % (MBP/no MBP)	68/72	48/58	89/85	100/100	45/47
Type of prep	PEG	PEG	$NaPO_4$	PEG	PEG
Anastomotic leak, % (MBP/no MBP)	3.7/2.1 (NS)	5.6/4.8 (NS)	0.6/1.2 (NS)	6/1 (NS)	4/2 (NS)
Wound infection, % (MBP/no MBP)	6.4/5.7 (NS)	7.2/5.6 (NS)	9.8/6.1 (NS)	13/4 (NS)	4/2 (NS)
Intra-abdominal abscess % (MBP/no MBP)	1.1/1 (NS)	Not given	0.6/0.6 (NS)	1/3 (NS)	2/3 (NS)

NS, non-significant; MBP, mechanical bowel preparation; PEG, polyethelene glycol

were reported in 97 patients (4.2%) with MBP and 81 patients (3.5%) without MBP ($p = 0.206$). Wound infections occurred in 9.9% vs. 8.8% ($p = 0.155$). This lack of any statistically significant difference between the two arms in the largest meta-analysis yet performed prompted the authors to conclude that MBP is of no benefit to patients undergoing elective colorectal resection. Though the authors acknowledge certain scenarios when the use of MBP is warranted, such as the anticipated need for intraoperative colonoscopy, they propose that routine MBP need not be considered a 'prerequisite of safe colorectal surgery.' Despite this data, a 2003 survey of practicing colorectal surgeons revealed that 99% of respondents continue to employ MBP, though 10% did question its role in elective surgery [51].

Antibiotic preparation options

Rationale

Mechanical cleansing of the bowel reduces the amount of stool and bacteria but does not alter the concentration of bacteria remaining in the colon [18,52]. Usage of appropriate prophylactic antibiotics in several prospective studies has reduced the incidence of infectious complications associated with colonic resections from 40–50% to approximately 5–10% [53]. To be effective, the drugs must adequately cover the spectrum of bacteria encountered in the colon (e.g., gram negative bacteria and anaerobes) and be administered before bacterial contamination to provide adequate intraluminal and tissue levels. In addition, to reduce the development of resistant bacterial strains, the duration of use must be short (less than 24 hours) [54].

Bowel flora

The colon contains a large number of bacteria [55]. The species of bacteria and their average concentration in stool are listed in **Table 8.7**. Bacteriologic studies have demonstrated a wide variation in the bacterial species between individuals, but the flora of each person remains relatively stable over time [56].

Methods

Luminal antibiotics are inexpensive and effective. Overgrowth of resistant bacteria is avoided if these agents are used for less than 24 hours [55]. The systemic absorption of these agents is variable, and there is controversy about the importance of luminal and tissue concentrations. These medications may cause GI upset or diarrhea. Appropriate agents are listed in **Table 8.8**.

Systemic antibiotics produce results that are equal to luminal medications if the appropriate drugs are used and they are administered before surgery (adequate tissue levels are needed at the time of contamination). Appropriate agents are described in **Table 8.9**.

Topical antibiotics are used at surgery [53]. In prospective studies they have been found to be equivalent to other methods of prophylactic antibiotic administration. Use of **combination methods** is difficult to justify because of the additional cost. When single methods have

Table 8.7 Colonic bacteria

Organisms	Concentration in stool (log counts/g of stool)	Organisms	Concentration in stool (log counts/g of stool)
Anaerobes		*Aerobes*	
Gram negative bacilli		Gram negative bacilli	
Bactmoides pagilis	10^9	*Escherichia coli*	10^8
Bacteroides spp.	10^8	*Klebsiella* spp.	10^6
Gram positive cocci	10^7	Gram positive cocci	
		Streptococcus faecalis	10^6
		Staphylococcus aureus	10^6
Gram positive bacilli			
Clostridia	10^7		

Table 8.8 Oral antibiotic agents

Medication	Bacterial coverage	Dosage
Erythromycin	Gram positive organisms, anaerobes	1 g orally
Neomycin	Gram negative organisms	1 g orally
Metronidazole	Anaerobes	250–500 mg orally

Table 8.9 Parenteral antibiotic agents

Medication	Spectrum of coverage	Dosage
Cefotetan	Gram positive and negative organisms, anaerobes	1–2 g (every 12 h)
Cefoxitin	Gram positive and negative organisms, anaerobes	1–2 g (every 6 h)
Gentamicin	Gram negative organisms, aerobes	80 mg (every 8 h)
Cleocin	Aerobes, anaerobes	150 mg (every 6 h)
Metronidazole	Anaerobes	500 mg (every 6 h)
Ciprofloxin	Gram positive and negative organisms	400 mg (every 8–12 h)
Ampicillin and sulbactam	Gram positive and negative organisms	3 g (every 6–8 h)

been compared with a combination of methods in prospective trials, a statistical improvement has not been demonstrated unless the single method had an unusually large infection rate. However, despite the lack of consistent scientific support, a majority of surgeons surveyed use a combination of methods (usually oral and systemic agents) [39, 57, 58].

Recommendations are shown in **Table 8.10**; a 1-day preparation provides good cleansing, and its short duration makes it cost effective. Sample preoperative orders are provided in Appendix 1.

Miscellaneous preoperative evaluations and management

Deep venous thrombosis prophylaxis

Thrombosis of the veins of the lower extremity is a potentially serious complication following abdominal and pelvic surgery [60]. Many

Table 8.10 Recommended bowel preparation regimen

Mechanical cleansing	
PEG lavage preparation	
Preoperative day 1	Clear liquid diet
10:00 hours	Bisacodyl 5–10 mg orally
16:00 hours	**Full preparation:** PEG lavage, 240 mL orally every 10 min (1.5 L/h) until rectal effluent becomes clear and free of particulate matter
	Limited preparation: 17 g of PEG 3350 in 120 mL of water every 30 min × 3
Antibiotics	
Oral antibiotics	
Preoperative day 1	
13:00 hours	
14:00 hours	Neomycin, 1 g orally
23:00 hours	Erythromycin, 1 g orally
Metronidazole, 250–500 mg, may be substituted for the erythromycin	
Parenteral antibiotics: *Second-generation cephalosporin or broad spectrum antibiotic*	
Cefotetan, 1 g intravenously, when patient is on call to the operating room or	
Cefoxitin, 1 g intravenously, when patient is on call to the operating room, and every 6 h for three doses after surgery or	
Unasyn, 3 g intravenously, when patient is on call to the operating room, and every 6–8 h for three to four doses after surgery	
Topical antibiotic: *First-generation cephalosporin*	
Cefadyl, 1 g/L of saline solution: irrigate abdomen and wound at the end of the operation	
From Kirby DF, DeLegge MH. Nutritional assessment: the high tech and low tech tour. In: Kirby OF, Dudrick SJ, (eds). Practical Handbook of Nutrition in Clinical Practice. Boca Raton: CRC Press, 1994;1–18. With permission.	

of these deep venous thrombi (DVT) are asymptomatic, but some progress to proximal veins and break free and migrate to produce pulmonary emboli (PE) with potentially fatal results. The numerous risk factors for DVT are listed in **Table 8.11**.

Prevention of DVT is accomplished by pharmacologic and non-pharmacologic measures. Pharmacologic options include sub-cutaneous heparin, low-dose aspirin, warfarin, low molecular weight heparin, and dextran. Subcutaneous heparin (5000 units twice daily) is the most popular method [59]. Nonpharmacologic measures include graduated elastic stockings, sequential compression stockings, and early ambulation. I prefer elastic compression and intermittent compression stockings and early ambulation in almost all patients. In patients with additional serious risk factors, such as a history of previous DVT or pulmonary emboli, subcutaneous heparin is also administered.

Diagnosis of DVT or pulmonary emboli can be subtle and requires a high index of suspicion. Classic findings of DVT include calf swelling and discomfort, distal venous engorgement, and pain on passive dorsiflexion of the foot (Homan's sign). Confirmatory diagnostic tests include

Table 8.11 Risk factors for deep vein thrombosis	
Clinical risk factors	**Operative risk factors**
Age >40 years	Duration of surgery >1 h
Prior DVT or pulmonary emboli	Pelvic surgery
Malignancy	Major orthopedic surgery
Obesity	General (versus regional) anesthesia
Congestive heart failure/cardiomyopathy	Use of stirrups (lithotomy position)
History of stroke or myocardial infarction	
Estrogen use (high dose)	
Pelvic/hip fracture	
Paraplegia/quadriplegia	
Prolonged immobility	
Hypercoagulable state	
Varicose veins	
Sepsis	
Polycythemia rubra vera	
Inflammatory bowel disease	
Dehydration	
Postpartum state	
Preoperative hospitalization >5 days	

From Stamos MJ, Theuer CP, Headrick CN. General postoperative complications. In: Hicks TC, Beck DE, Opelka FG, Timmcke AE, (eds). Complications of Colon & Rectal Surgery. Baltimore: Williams & Wilkins, 1996.

duplex scanning (with or without color flow Doppler), impedance plethysmography, phlebography, V/Q scanning, CT angiography, and pulmonary angiography.

Using recent prospective and outcome-based studies, Worsley and Alavi [60] have published the following conclusions on the diagnostic evaluation of patients with suspected PE.

1. A normal V/Q scan excludes the diagnosis of clinically significant PE.
2. Patients with a low-probability V/Q scan and a low clinical likelihood of PE do not require angiography or anticoagulation.
3. Patients with a low-probability V/Q scan and a moderate to high clinical likelihood of PE and negative noninvasive venous studies of the lower extremity do not require anticoagulation or treatment. If serial noninvasive venous studies are positive, the patient should be treated.
4. High probable V/Q scan and high clinical likelihood should be treated.
5. High probable V/Q scan, low clinical likelihood, and negative noninvasive studies of the legs often require CT angiography or pulmonary CT for a definitive diagnosis (see Figure 4.20).

Treatment options include anticoagulation and vena caval interruption (e.g. Greenfield filter). Initial anticoagulation is started with intravenous heparin and continued with warfarin.

Laboratory requirements

Before a surgical procedure, screening laboratory studies should be considered. In the past, multiple studies were routinely ordered. Recent critical evaluation of this policy has resulted in significantly fewer studies being performed. Unneeded tests result in unnecessary cost and morbidity. Many of these result from the workup suggested by an abnormal value obtained on 'screening tests.' Currently, in the absence of symptoms or disease processes that require evaluation, the evaluations listed in **Table 8.12** are recommended.

Informed consent

An important component of any invasive procedure involves providing the patient with information and knowledge about the intended procedure, its indications, inherent risks, benefits, and alternatives. With this information the patient can give informed consent. It is the physician's duty to disclose all the associated risks that are significant or material [62–64]. For medicolegal reasons, this exchange of information and consent is documented in the medical record.

Table 8.12 Preoperative laboratory evaluations		
Age (years)	Men	Women
<40	No laboratory tests required	Hemoglobin and hematocrit
>40	ECG	ECG

Rounds questions

1. What is the 24-hour maintenance fluid total for a 60 kg man?
2. What fluid total is recommended for replacement of excess nasogastric tube output?
3. What are the daily requirements for protein and carbohydrates?
4. Does a mechanical bowel preparation alter the concentration of bacteria in the colon?
5. Are the postoperative wound infection rates different with oral versus intravenous antibiotics?
6. What are the clinical findings of deep vein thrombosis?

References

1. Beck DE. Preoperative preparation. In: Beck DE, Welling DN (eds). Patient Care in Colorectal Surgery. Boston: Little, Brown, 1991;67–75.
2. Buzby GP, Mullen JL, Matthews DC, et al. Prognostic nutritional index in gastrointestinal surgery. Am J Surg 1980;139:160–7.
3. Dudrick SJ. Parenteral nutrition. In: Dudrick SJ, Baue AE, Eiseman B, et al. (eds). Manual of Preoperative and Postoperative Care, 3rd ed. Philadelphia: WB Saunders 1983;86–105.
4. Kirby DF, DeLegge MH. Nutritional assessment: The high tech and low tech tour. In: Kirby DF, Dudrick SJ (eds). Practical Handbook of Nutrition in Clinical Practice. Boca Raton: CRC Press 1994;1–18.
5. Mullen JL, Buzby GP, Waldman MT, et al. Prediction of operative morbidity by preoperative nutritional assessment. Surg Forum 1979;30:80–2.
6. Detsky AS, McLaughlin JR, Baker JP, et al. What is subjective global assessment of nutritional status? J Parenter Enteral Nutr 1987;11:8–13.
7. Palacio JC, Rombeau JL. Nutritional support. In: Fazio VW, (ed). Current Therapy in Colon and Rectal Surgery. Philadelphia: BC Decker, 1990;391–6.
8. Holliday MA, Segar WE. The maintenance need for water in parenteral fluid therapy. Pediatrics 1957;19:823–32.
9. Filsto HC, Edwards CH, Chitwood WR, et al. Estimation of postoperative fluid requirements in infants and children. Ann Surg 1982;196:76–81.
10. Fakhry SM, Sheldon GF. Postoperative management. In: Wilmore DW, Brennan MF, Harken AH, et al. (eds). Care of the Surgical Patient, vol 2. New York: Scientific American, 1989;1–23.
11. Miller TA, Duke JH. Fluid and electrolyte management. In Dudrick SJ, Baue AE, Eiseman B, et al. (eds). Manual of Preoperative and Postoperative Care, 3rd ed. Philadelphia: WB Saunders, 1983;38–67.
12. Shires GT, Shires GT III, Lowry SF. Fluid, electrolyte, and nutritional management of the surgical patient. In: Schwartz SI, Shires GT, Spencer FC, et al. (eds). Principles of Surgery, 6th ed. New York: McGraw-Hill, 1994;61–94.
13. Daly JM. Malnutrition. In: Wilmore OW, Brennan MF, Harken AH, et al. (eds). Care of the Surgical Patient, vol 2. New York: Scientific American 1991;1–18.
14. LaFrance RJ, Miyagawa CI. Pharmaceutical considerations in total parenteral nutrition. In: Fischer JE, (ed). Total Parenteral Nutrition. Boston: Little, Brown, 1991;57–97.
15. Haubrich WS, Schaffner F, Berk JE. Gastroenterology. Philadelphia: WB Saunders 1995;1378–513.
16. Levine GM. Nutritional support in gastrointestinal disease. Surg Clin North Am 1981;61:701–8.
17. Sax HC, Hasselgren P. Indications. In Fischer JE, (ed). Total Parenteral Nutrition. Boston: Little, Brown 1991;3–12.
18. Beck DE. Mechanical bowel cleansing for surgery. Perspect Colon Rectal Surg 1994;7:97–114.
19. Patell C, Hall J. What is the role of mechanical bowel preparation in patients undergoing colorectal surgery. Dis Colon rectum 1998;41:875–83.
20. Miettinen RPJ, Laiteben ST, Makela JT, Paakkonen ME. Bowel preparation with oral polyethylene glycol electrolyte solution vs. no preparation in elective open colorectal surgery. Dis Colon Rectum 2000;43:669–77.
21. van Gekdere D, Fa-Si-Oen P, Noach LA, et al. Complications after colorectal surgery without mechanical bowel preparation. J AM Coll Surg 2002;194:40–7.
22. Zmora O, Mahajna A, Bar-Zakai B, et al. Colon and rectal surgery without mechanical bowel preparation: a randomized prospective trial. Ann Surg 2003;237:363–7.
23. Fa-Si-Oen P, Roumen R, Buitenweg J, et al. Mechanical bowel preparation or not? Outcome of a multicenter, randomized trial in elective open colon surgery. Dis Colon Rectum. 2005;48:1509–16.
24. Ram E, Sherman Y, Weil R, et al. Is mechanical bowel preparation mandatory for elective colon surgery? A prospective randomized study. Arch Surg 2005;140:285–8.
25. Bucher P, Gervaz P, Soravia C, et al. Randomized clinical trial of mechanical bowel preparation versus no preparation before elective left-sided colorectal surgery. Br J Surg. 2005;92:409–14. Erratum in: Br J Surg. 2005;92:1051.
26. Miettinen RP, Laitinen ST, Mäkelä JT, Pääkkönen ME. Bowel preparation with oral polyethylene glycol electrolyte solution vs. no preparation in elective open colorectal surgery: prospective, randomized study. Dis

Colon Rectum. 2000;43:669–75; discussion 675–7.

27. Bretagnol F; PanisY, Rullier E, et al. Rectal Cancer Surgery With or Without Bowel Preparation: The French Greccar III Multicenter Single-Blinded Randomized Trial. Ann Surg 2010;252:863–8.

28. Vanner SJ, MacDonald PH, Paterson WG, et al. Randomized prospective trial comparing oral sodium phosphate with standard polyethylene glycol-based lavage solution (Golytely) in the preparation of patients for colonoscopy. Am J Gastroenterol 1990;85:422–7.

29. Lieberman DA, Ghormley J, Flora K. Effect of oral sodium phosphate colon preparation on serum electrolytes in patients with normal serum creatinine. Gastrointestinal Endoscopy 1996;43:467–9.

30. Cohen SM, Wexner SD, Binderow SR, Nogueras JJ, et al. Prospective, randomized, endoscopic-blinded trial comparing precolonoscopy bowel cleansing methods. Dis Colon Rectum 1994;37:689–96.

31. Zmora O, Wexner SD. Bowel preparation for colonoscopy. Clinics Colon Rect Surg 2001;14:309–15.

32. Aronchick CA, Lipshutz WH, Wright SH, et al. A novel tableted purgative for colonoscopic preparation: efficacy and safety comparisons with Colyte and Fleet Phospho-Soda. Gastrointest Endosc 2000;52:346–52.

33. Lichtenstein GR, Grandhi N, Schmalz M, et al. Clinical trial: sodium phosphate tablets are preferred and better tolerated by patients compared to polyethylene glycol solution plus bisacodyl tablets for bowel preparation. Alimentary Pharmacology & Therapeutics 2007;26:1361–70.

34. Johanson JF, Popp JW, Cohen LB, et al. Randomized, multicenter study comparing the safety and efficacy of sodium phosphate tablets with 2L polyethylene glycol solution plus bisacodyl tablets for colon cleansing. Am J Gastroenterol 2007;102:2238–46.

35. Markowitz GS, Stokes MB, Radhakrishnan, J, D'Agati, VD. Acute phosphate nephropathy following oral sodium phosphate bowel purgative: an underrecognized cause of chronic renal failure. J Am Soc Nephrology 2005;16:3389–96.

36. Carl DE, Sica DA. Acute Phosphate Nephropathy Following Colonoscopy Preparation. Am J Medical Sciences 2007;334:151–4.

37. Bucher P, Gervaz P, Egger JF, et al. Morphologic alterations associated with mechanical bowel preparation before elective colorectal surgery: a randomized trial. Dis Colon Rectum 2006;49:109–12.

38. Chung RS, Gurill NJ, Berglund EM. A controlled clinical trial of whole gut lavage as a method of bowel preparation for colonic operations. Am J Surg 1979;137:75–81.

39. Beck DE, Fazio VW. Current preoperative bowel cleansing methods: A survey of American Society of Colon and Rectal Surgeons members. Dis Colon Rectum 1990;33:12–5.

40. Beck DE, Fazio VW, Jagelman DG. Comparison of lavage methods for preoperative colonic cleansing. Dis Colon Rectum 1986;29:699–703.

41. Beck DE, Harford FJ, DiPalma JA, et al. Colon cleansing with polyethylene glycol electrolyte lavage solution. South Med J 1985;78:1414–8.

42. Beck DE, DiPalma JA. Comparison of a new oral lavage solution (Nulytely) to a cathartic and enema method for preoperative colonic cleansing. Arch Surg 1991;126:552–5.

43. DiPalma JA, Wolff BG, Meagher A, Cleveland M. Comparison of reduced volume versus four liters sulfate-free electrolyte lavage solutions for colonoscopy colon cleansing. Am J Gastroenterol. 2003;98:2187–91.

44. Kastenberg D, Lottes SR, Forbes WP. An Effective 2 L Polyethylene Glycol (PEG) Electrolyte Lavage Solution for Bowel Cleansing. Am J Gastroenterol 2006;101;S532.

45. Pelham RW, Alcorn H Jr, Cleveland M. A pharmacokinetics evaluation of a new, low-volume, oral sulfate colon cleansing preparation in patients with renal or hepatic impairment and healthy volunteers. J Clin Pharmacol. 2010;50:350–4.

46. Koruth NM, Krukowski ZH, Youngson GG, et al. Intra-operative colonic irrigation in the management of left-sided large bowel emergencies. Br J Surg 1985;72:708–11.

47. Raferty JF. Preoperative management. In Beck DE, Wexner SD, Roberts PL, Senagore A, Stamos M (eds). ASCRS Textbook of Colorectal Surgery, 2nd edition. New York: Springer-Verlag 2011. In press.

48. Guenega KF, Matos D, Castro AA, et al. Mechanical bowel preparation for elective colorectal surgery. Cochrane Database Syst Rev 2005, CD001544.

49. Duncan JE, Quietmeyer CM. Bowel preparation: Current status. Clin Colon Rectal Surg 2009;2214–20.

50. Pineda CE, Shelton AA, Hernandez-Boussard T, Morton JM, Welton ML. Mechanical bowel preparation in intestinal surgery: A meta-analysis and review of the literature. J Gastointest Surg 2008;11:2037–2044.

51. Zmora O, Wexner SD, Hajjar L et al. Trends in preparation for colorectal surgery: Survey of members of the American Society of Colon and Rectal Surgeons. Am Surg 2003;69: 150–4.

52. Arabi F, Dimock F, Burdon DW, et al. Influence of bowel preparation and antimicrobials on colonic microflora. Br J Surg 1978;65:555–9.

53. Wilson SE, Sokol T. Antimicrobials in elective colon surgery. Infect Surg 1985;10:609–11.

54. Wexner SD, Beck DE. Sepsis prevention in colorectal surgery. In: Fielding LP, Goldberg SM (eds). Operative Surgery, 5th ed. London: Butterworth-Heinemann, 1993;41–6.

55. Condon RE. Intestinal antisepsis: Rationale and results. World J Surg 1982;6:182–7.

56. Gorbach SL, Nahas L, Lemer PI, et al. Studies of intestinal microflora. Gastroenterology 1967;53:845–55.

57. Bartlett SP. Effects of prophylactic antibiotics on wound infection after elective colon and rectal surgery: 1960 to 1980. Am J Surg 1983;145:300–9.

58. Chapman S, Harford FJ. Perioperative antibiotics. Colon Rect Surg 2001;14:7–14.

59. Stamos MJ, Theuer CP, Headrick CN. General postoperative complications. In Hicks TC, Beck DE, Opelka FG, Timmcke AE, (eds). Complications of Colon & Rectal Surgery. Baltimore: Williams & Wilkins, 1996;118–42.

60. Worsley DF, Alavi A. Radionuclide imaging of acute pulmonary embolism. Radiol Clin North Am 2001;39:1035–52.

61. Gay CF Jr. Medicolegal issues. In: Hicks TC, Beck DE, Opelka FG, Timmcke AE, (eds). Complications of Colon & Rectal Surgery. Baltimore: Williams & Wilkins, 1996;468–77.

62. Gay CF Jr, Hicks TC. Medical legal issues. In: Whitlow CB, Beck DE, Margolin DA, Hicks TC, Timmcke AE (eds). Improved Outcomes in Colon and Rectal Surgery. London: Informa Healthcare 2010;132–9.

63. Meehan MJ. Medical legal. In: Beck DE, Wexzner SD, Roberts PL, Senagore A, Stamos M (eds). ASCRS Textbook of Colorectal Surgery, 2nd edition. New York: Springer-Verlag, 2011. In press.

Anesthetic management

Anesthetic goals are similar in all branches of surgery. The patient's primary concerns are analgesia (freedom from pain), hypnosis (freedom from awareness), and amnesia (freedom from memory of any noxious stimuli). The surgeon's anesthetic goals are safety, paralysis or relaxation, and measured duration. Additional considerations are ease of administration, hemodynamic stability, lack of residual effects, and cost. Although these goals are universal, there are specific requirements unique to colorectal surgery. These objectives are realized through the use of general, regional, or local anesthetic techniques; frequently a combination of two or three may be employed.

In addition to intraoperative care, anesthetic considerations encompass preoperative patient and technique selection as well as postoperative pain management. Improvements in anesthetic techniques and sedation have allowed increasingly invasive surgical procedures to be performed on an outpatient basis.

Preoperative evaluation

Each patient who will receive an anesthetic should undergo a thorough preoperative evaluation. In addition to its importance for surgical considerations, a comprehensive preoperative evaluation averts complications and helps determine the optimal choice of anesthetic. Specific areas for investigation include the patient's previous anesthetic experiences and any family history of anesthetic problems, medications, and allergies. Anesthetic difficulties can often be avoided if they are anticipated.

A history of difficult intubation or previous tracheotomy, tracheal surgery, or trauma may indicate the need for a regional anesthetic or other awake anesthetics. Nitrous oxide and narcotics should be avoided in patients with a previous history of postoperative nausea or vomiting. Transient passage of a nasogastric tube to empty the stomach may also be employed. Similarly, prolonged emergence or postoperative drowsiness should lead to avoidance of benzodiazepines or reduction in dosage. A complete list of medications that might interact with or alter the metabolism of anesthetic agents should be obtained. Any known hypersensitivities or previous organotoxicity should be avoided (e.g. ketamine hallucinations, halothane hepatitis) [1].

Any family history of anesthetic complication or death under anesthesia should he investigated. Particularly if fever was noted, **malignant hyperthermia** should be suspected and an appropriate workup instituted before surgery. Triggered by a number of stimuli, including inhalation agents and succinylcholine, malignant hyperthermia may present with poor relaxation, tachypnea, tachycardia, hyperthermia, cyanosis, and shock. It is treated by administration of dantrolene sodium, 2.5 mg/kg IV, hyperventilation, discontinuance of any provocative agents, and supportive care [2].

Risk factors

A thorough preoperative medical evaluation includes a complete physical examination to evaluate for a recessed chin, poor dentition, decreased cervical or mandibular range of motion, obesity, and poor venous access. Specific considerations such as back deformity or previous back surgery should be reviewed as to the choice of anesthesia and technique if an epidural anesthetic is expected.

Neurologic

Central or peripheral preoperative neurologic compromise should be carefully documented before anesthesia, in the event there is any question of change following the procedure. A normal neurologic examination should be documented before administration of any regional block.

Pulmonary

Patients with a smoking history or long-standing pulmonary or chest wall disease are at increased risk for anesthesia. Preoperative evaluation in these patients should include a chest X-ray evaluation and a baseline arterial blood gas determination. More severe disease should be evaluated with pulmonary function tests and pulmonary medicine consultation for optimization before surgery. In these patients, intubation should be avoided if possible to prevent prolonged postoperative ventilator support. Spinal anesthetic or continuous epidural with sedation can provide adequate anesthesia for intra-abdominal surgery. An attack of reactive airway disease can be precipitated by intubation, beta-blockade, or sodium thiopental.

Cardiac

Several scoring systems have been developed to assess cardiac risk from anesthesia. One of the more notable is from Goldman et al in 1977 [3]. Exertional angina, recent myocardial infarction, a change in ECG, or congestive heart failure should prompt cardiologic evaluation. Use of invasive intraoperative monitoring is justified in patients with severe or unstable cardiac disease.

Hepatic/renal

Many anesthetic medications are eliminated via the renal and hepatic routes. Since nondepolarizing muscle relaxants (D-tubocurarine and pancuronium) are excreted through the kidneys, these agents are used with caution in patients with renal failure. In addition to drug elimination, hepatic insufficiency may lead to coagulopathy, which precludes regional anesthesia. Therefore, any patient with suspected jaundice, increased serum creatinine levels, or recent intravenous administration of a contrast medium should undergo complete laboratory investigation.

Age

With the 'graying of America' we find ourselves operating on a greater number of geriatric patients, defined as 70 years or older. In general, these patients have diminished physiologic reserve and a greater number of advanced comorbid diseases. Independent of other risk factors, elderly patients may have an altered response to anesthesia. The autonomic nervous system will have a blunted response to changes in blood pressure. There is also a decreased end-organ response to circulating catecholamines. Pulmonary changes include a markedly depressed CO_2 response curve in the presence of narcotics. Protective reflexes such as cough and gag are decreased, increasing the risk of aspiration. Decreases in lung elasticity and chest wall compliance lead to increased functional residual capacity, residual volume, and closing volume [4].

ASA Classification

To standardize evaluation for anesthetic risk, the American Society of Anesthesiologists (ASA) has developed the following scale by which all patients are rated before undergoing anesthesia (**Table 9.1**) [5].

Choice of anesthesia

For both intra-abdominal and anorectal procedures many different techniques of anesthesia are available, the major divisions of which are general, regional, and local. The choice is made based on the procedure planned, the patient's medical condition, and the patient's and surgeon's preference. Although these techniques are traditionally used separately, combinations of these techniques are being used to decrease overall anesthetic needs and recovery time.

General anesthesia

General anesthesia is defined as systemic anesthesia that provides the patient with analgesia, amnesia, and unconsciousness. The surgeon

Table 9.1 ASA classification	
ASA I	A healthy patient with no systemic disease, not at either extreme of age, undergoing an elective operation
ASA II	Single system, well-controlled disease, does not affect daily life; this includes smoking, mild obesity, and alcoholism
ASA III	Multisystem disease or well-controlled major system disease that does impact on daily living; patient is not at significant risk of death from disease
ASA IV	Severe incapacitating disease, poorly controlled or end-stage; death due to disease is possible but not likely
ASA V	Patient is at imminent risk of death with or without surgery

is provided a safe, relaxed surgical field. Anesthetic medications are administered systemically through inhalational and intravenous routes.

Contemporary inhalational agents include nitrous oxide (N_2O) and the **halogenated aliphatic compounds:** halothane, enflurane, and isoflurane. Typically, inhaled agents are administered via an endotrachial tube with mechanical ventilation. Mask anesthesia or the newer 'laryngeal mask' device (LMA) is being used more frequently for short, nonintraperitoneal cases.

The principle of inhalational anesthesia is achieving adequate blood levels of agent, given known inhaled vapor concentration and partitioning between gas phase and blood solubility. Clinically, blood solubility is a major determinant of uptake and elimination. Low blood solubility is beneficial, allowing cerebral concentration to closely match alveolar concentration and inspired concentration.

N_2O is a mild anesthetic requiring 80% concentration to induce unconsciousness and hyperbaric levels to produce surgical anesthesia. In addition, a 50% concentration has shown cardiodepressant and vasodilatory effects and increased circulating catecholamines. N_2O is still widely employed because at low concentrations it decreases the requirements for other agents that are stronger cardiodepressants. It is widely held that N_2O should be avoided in open abdominal cases; this is not necessarily true. The concern is based on the fact that N_2O is 30 times more soluble than nitrogen. Nitrogen makes up 80% of swallowed air and thereby bowel gas. In theory, N_2O will enter air-filled spaces faster than N_2 can escape and expand that space (bowel gas) many times over. In practice, however, 50% N_2O will expand an air-filled space only up to 100% and requires many hours. Doubling the bowel gas volume is not of great consequence except in cases of obstruction or megacolon. In these cases prolonged use of N_2O should be avoided [4].

Despite the historical origin of anesthesia from an inhaled substance, many of the mainstays of modern anesthesia are intravenous agents. The anesthetic course often begins in the holding area with the administration of a short-acting benzodiazepine to alleviate the patient's anxiety and permit placement of monitoring devices. Initial general anesthesia is induced by a potent ultra-short-acting barbiturate (thiopental) accompanied by a short-acting paralytic (succinylcholine) to allow tracheal intubation. Barbiturates are potent myocardial depressants and vasodilators. Thus they may cause transient hypotension. Although barbiturates are degraded in the liver and excreted through the kidneys, the pharmacologic effect rapidly dissipates through redistribution into muscle and fat stores. Propofol (Diprivan) is a new injectable sedative hypnotic agent. Extremely fast acting with equally short offset, it is often used as an induction agent or for maintenance of general anesthesia. Propofol is particularly suited to short courses of general anesthesia or heavy sedation.

After induction, general anesthesia is maintained with the addition of inhaled agents and a variety of injectable medications. Ketamine is a dissociative anesthetic chemically related to the illicit drug phencyclidine (PCP). Unlike barbiturates or narcotics, it is a cardiovascular stimulant, which makes it useful in an emergent or mildly unstable patient.

Benzodiazepines (Valium, Ativan) provide tranquilization and amnesia but lack analgesic properties. Used with narcotics, they provide periods of controlled sedation. The use of fast onset/offset midazolam (Versed) is very effective in combination with meperidine or fentanyl for conscious sedation when used for outpatient local procedures or colonoscopy.

Opioids are included in most phases of general anesthesia. They provide strong analgesia as well as sedation. Coupled with this is dose-related suppression of the respiratory response to CO_2. Additional expected effects are nausea and vomiting, mild bradycardia, chest wall rigidity, and systemic histamine release. Whether combined with other general anesthetics or alone, opioids provide a safe, hemodynamically stable effect. They are particularly used in patients with cardiac disease.

Regional anesthesia

Unlike general anesthetics, regional anesthetics are delivered anatomically to the peripheral nervous system to block afferent nerve conduction. Both narcotics and local anesthetics are employed in regional blocks. Local anesthetics produce nondepolarizing blockade. Optimally 1 cm of nerve is bathed in anesthetic to prevent transmission of the action potential. Recovery of function occurs when the agent concentration diminishes as a result of dilution, dissipation, and uptake into the bloodstream. Tetracaine is an **ester-linked anesthetic** that is hydrolyzed to procaine by plasma cholinesterase. It has a prolonged duration of action and is one of the preferred agents for subarachnoid block. The maximal safe dosage is 1 mg/g. Procaine itself is often used for procedures that will last less than 30 minutes. It is a potent vasodilator and myocardial depressant that is inexpensive and safe. The maximal dose in an adult is 1000 mg if it is absorbed slowly. Lidocaine and bupivicaine are **amide-linked compounds;** both are highly stable and are used for all types of regional anesthesia. Lidocaine has excellent penetration and rapid onset. However, it has potent central effects, including sedation and amnesia. The maximal safe dose is 200 mg for a normal-sized adult. Epinephrine is often added, 1:1-200,000, prolonging the effect by decreasing diffusion and increasing the maximal dose to 500 mg. Bupivacaine is four times more potent than lidocaine and highly lipid soluble. With slower onset and longer duration it is a preferred drug for continuous epidural anesthesia. The maximal safe dose is 2 mg/kg (**Table 9.2**).

Ideal for low pelvic and perineal surgery, regional anesthesia is administered into the subarachnoid space (spinal) or the epidural space. A caudal block is an epidural block placed in the caudal canal through the sacral hiatus. These may be administered as a single injection of

Table 9.2 Common local anesthetics			
Agent	Onset (min)	Duration	Maximal dose (mg/kg)
Lidocaine			
Plain	2–5	30–45 min	5
With epinephrine		1–2 h	7
Bupivicaine			
Plain	30	2 h	2
With epinephrine		4 h	4
Procaine	5–10	15–30 min	10

appropriate duration local anesthetic or via catheter as continuous infusion or multiple intraoperative doses. An indwelling catheter may be placed for postoperative pain control. Regional anesthesia may be combined with sedation as an alternative to intubation and general anesthesia in the pulmonary patient. Although often considered less 'stressful' than general anesthesia, a regional anesthetic has no less risk for myocardial infarction than a general anesthetic.

Spinal (subarachnoid) anesthetic is placed directly into the CSF. Usually placed in the L3 or L4 interspace, the agent may diffuse cephalad, producing a T4–T5 level necessary for abdominal surgery. Such a high level is needed to prevent visceral pain from traction. Migration of anesthetic can be controlled by varying the specific gravity of the solution. A well-placed hyperbaric anesthetic may move cephalad, causing respiratory depression when a head down position is used. For this reason a less dense isobaric or hypobaric solution is often used if the prone jackknife (Buie) position is planned. Paralysis of the preganglionic sympathetic fibers of anterior nerve roots of Tl–L2 causes vasodilation and potential hypotension seen with spinal anesthesia. Treatment is volume loading and Trendelenburg positioning until the condition is resolved.

Epidural anesthetic principles are similar to those for spinal anesthetics. Onset of action is slower but anesthetic level is more easily controlled. Hypotension and 'spinal headache' are avoided. A much larger dose of medication is required to achieve the same effect. The site of action of epidural injection is at the nerve root and the spinal cord. Often sensory block can be achieved while preserving motor function. Administration of epidural medication during general anesthesia may block the unconscious perception of pain during abdominal surgery and reduce the requirement for systemic agents and allow lighter anesthesia. Caudal blocks provide dense anesthesia in the perineal region. Their popularity is waning in the adult but increasing in pediatric anesthesia. Anatomic landmarks to the sacral hiatus are more easily palpated in the child.

Narcotics may also be injected in the epidural space creating a local effect similar to the central effect seen with intravenous opiates. Narcotics are of limited usefulness intraoperatively but are frequently used for postoperative pain control. Both anesthetics and narcotics have been used in patient-controlled epidural anesthetics (PCEA), usually placed in the thoracic area [6].

Local anesthesia

A good working knowledge of local anesthesia is particularly important in anal and perineal surgery. Although its use is often limited to 'lumps and bumps,' more involved procedures (e.g. stomal revisions, hernias, and limited bowel surgery) may be performed with local anesthesia with or without light sedation in a high-risk patient. If a patient requires general anesthesia or conscious sedation, effective local anesthesia may greatly diminish the systemic medication needed. Numerous agents are available for local infiltration. The two most commonly used are lidocaine (Xylocaine, 0.5%, 1%, 2%) and bupivacaine (Marcaine, 0.25%, 0.5%). Both are available with or without epinephrine 1:200,000. Epinephrine causes vasoconstriction for hemostasis and prevents diffusion and prolonging blockade. Lidocaine, as described above, is rapidly effective within 2–5 minutes and lasts 1–2 hours. The maximal dose is 5 mg/kg, increasing to 7 mg/kg if epinephrine is added. Bupivacaine may take up to 30 minutes to reach full effect but will last up to 4 hours. The maximal dose is 2 mg/kg or up to 4 mg/kg when combined with epinephrine. Mixing equal volumes of 1–2% lidocaine with 0.5% bupivacaine provides adequate final concentrations of each to allow rapid onset and prolonged anesthesia (**Table 9.2**) [7,8]. Most of these anesthetics come packaged in vials that contain a volume that is equal to or less than the upper safe dose for a 70 kg patient (e.g. 1% Xylocaine – 50 mL). So for most patients using less than one vial will keep the dosage within the safe range.

These anesthetics are provided as sodium salts in a solution of hydrochloric acid so that they will remain in solution. This is the reason for the transient pain associated with infiltration. It is helpful to mix local anesthetic at a ratio of 9 parts to 1 with readily available sodium bicarbonate (10 mEq/mL) solution. If they are combined immediately before infiltration, the pain of injection is reduced. A significant aspect of the pain of infiltration is secondary to rapid expansion of the tissues. Some discomfort can be avoided by very slow injection with a fine needle (25- to 30-gauge) [9]. A field block can be created by infiltrating circumferentially around a site of excision drainage (e.g. perianal abscess).

A perianal block (**Figure 9.1**), easily created with the patient in either the prone or lithotomy position, provides relaxation of the sphincter as well as anesthesia. The anesthetic solution of choice is infiltrated in a fan fashion from the lateral positions to superficially encompass the anal margin. Emphasis should be placed in the posterolateral positions where the greatest concentration of nerves is found. A finger or retractor is placed within the canal. At the anterior, posterior, and lateral positions anesthetic is injected submucosally or intramuscularly through the previously infiltrated tissue. The needle is held parallel to the finger, with care taken to avoid entering the canal.

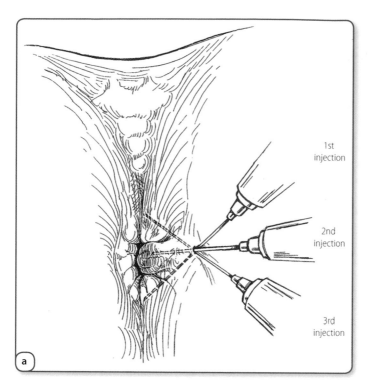

a

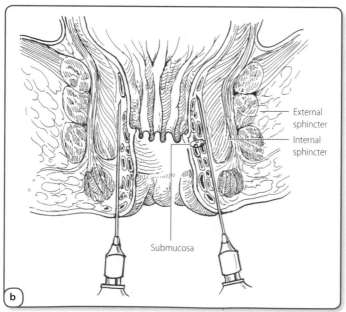

b

Figure 9.1 Technique for anal block. (a) Perianal view of submucosal injection. (b) Sagittal view of injection of anal canal.

A pudendal nerve block can also be created (**Figure 9.2**). The ischial tuberosity is identified by a finger within the rectum. A 22-gauge spinal needle is passed through the infiltrated perianal skin to the tuberosity. Injection of approximately 20 mL of anesthetic bilaterally

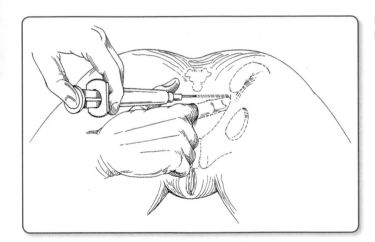

Figure 9.2 Technique for pudendal nerve block.

should provide an adequate result. Care should be taken to aspirate before injection to avoid intravascular dosing of local anesthetic. Signs of toxicity may develop with rapid intravascular injection or with absorption of excessive doses. Early signs are restlessness, vertigo, tinnitus, and perioral paresthesias. More advanced toxicity may lead to CNS depression, seizures, cardiac dysrhythmias, or myocardial depression and hypotension. The ECG may show a prolonged PR interval, widened QRS complex, and AV block. Treatment is 100 % O_2, volume resuscitation, diazepam for seizures, and supportive medications.

Conscious sedation

Colonoscopy and uncomfortable procedures (incision and drainage or examination under anesthesia) can be performed in an outpatient setting with the patient under sedation. This requires adequate personnel and monitoring. Automated pulse and blood pressure monitoring with continuous pulse oximetry are becoming the standard. Exhaled capnography (CO_2) is becoming more available. Dedicated staff must be available for monitoring during the procedure as well as during the recovery period. Adequate intravenous access must be obtained before sedation and maintained until complete recovery. A combination of a fast, short-acting benzodiazepine (midazolam) and a similar narcotic (meperidine or fentanyl) provides safe, effective sedation, analgesia, and amnesia. In the event of overdose, both can be reversed. Naloxone (Narcan) will reverse the effects of narcotics. Given as an initial intravenous dose of 0.4 mg to 2 mg, this may be repeated at 2- to 3-minute intervals, up to a total dose of 10 mg. A dose may also be given intramuscularly (0.2–1 mg) to prolong duration. If increased consciousness and adequate respiratory function have not returned, the diagnosis of narcotic overdose should be questioned. If very high doses or long-acting narcotics are used, repeated doses of naloxone may be required at intervals of 1–2 hours.

Flumazenil (Romazicon) will reverse midazolam and other benzodiazepines. The recommended initial dose of flumazenil is 0.2 mg (2 mL) administered intravenously over 15 seconds. If the desired level of consciousness is not obtained after waiting an additional 45 seconds, a further dose of 0.2 mg (2 mL) can be injected and repeated at 60-second intervals when necessary (up to a maximum of three additional times) to a maximal total dose of 1 mg (10 mL). The dose should be individualized based on the patient's response, with most patients responding to doses of 0.6–1 mg. In the event of resedation, repeated doses may be administered at 20-minute intervals as needed. For repeat treatment, no more than 1 mg (given as 0.2 mg/min) should be administered at any one time, and no more than 3 mg should be given in any 1 hour.

Additional considerations

Urgent/emergent induction

Often patients require urgent surgery and cannot wait the usual 4–8 hours without oral intake. Such patients, as well as those with obstruction, hiatal hernia, gastroesophageal reflux disease, or severe peptic ulcer disease, should be considered to have a full stomach on induction. Before induction an oral antacid and intravenous regional anesthetic should be administered to raise gastric pH, decrease stomach secretion, and lower the risk of aspiration. Patients considered to have a full stomach should undergo a 'rapid sequence' induction. Unlike a normal induction, there is no mask hyperventilation or preoxygenation. General anesthesia is induced with pressure maintained on the anterior aspect of the cricoid cartilage (the Sellick maneuver). This compresses the trachea against the esophagus, reducing reflux of gastric contents.

Invasive monitoring

In patients with advanced cardiac or pulmonary disease the anesthesiologist may desire placement of an intra-arterial pressure monitor, and a pulmonary artery (Swan–Ganz) catheter. An arterial line allows continuous blood pressure monitoring and access for obtaining blood gas levels. Although use of invasive monitoring has never been shown to prevent intraoperative cardiac complications, it may aid the anesthesiologist to recognize events, manage volume, and maintain stability.

Volume management

Overall fluid management is discussed in the chapters on preoperative and postoperative care (see Chapters 8 and 10 respectively). However, many different fluid losses during surgery must be accounted for and replaced by the anesthesia team during the procedure. General maintenance fluids must be given to replace perspiration and respiratory losses and to sustain adequate urine output. This represents approximately 2 mL/kg/h. Respiratory losses may be reduced by use of an in-line heat and moisture exchanger or 'artificial nose' in the anesthesia circuit. Additional losses are attributable to 'third space' losses and increased evaporation during open abdominal cases. An additional 3–4 mL/kg/h are 'lost' during closed or perineal or perianal cases. Seven to 8 mL/kg/h are 'lost' while the abdomen is open. Losses continue to increase with fever and sepsis. Combined requirements can be provided as balanced salt or crystalloid solution. Blood should be replaced with crystalloid solution at three times the volume lost. Colloid solutions with 5% albumin or hetastarch (Hespan) may be used for longer intravascular replacement. Whether a colloid or a crystalloid solution is used, the outcome will be about the same.

Temperature regulation

It is important to remember that patients become poikilothermic (cold blooded) while under general anesthesia. Cooling toward room temperature is accelerated in open abdominal cases. The operating room should be warmed before draping and awakening. Draping should expose as small a field as possible. If possible, a Bair Hugger and/or a warming blanket should be used whenever a case exceeds 1 hour. Inhaled gases and intravenous fluids can be warmed to 40°C. Finally, the room temperature is increased to decrease patient heat loss. These efforts are made to avoid postoperative shivering that can challenge myocardial reserve and increase oxygen demand by up to 400%. Some recent studies have linked hypothermia and surgical infections in colorectal patients [10].

Patient positioning

Patients under general or regional anesthesia lose the ability to protect themselves from injury from pressure or excessive stretch. Pressure injury to soft tissue will begin in as little as 10 minutes after local pressure exceeds capillary perfusion pressure. Peripheral nerves are easily compressed, especially at points crossing bony structures. There are a number of described nerve compression syndromes [11,12]. Nerves can also be injured by excessive stretch. Patients can assume positions under anesthesia and muscle relaxation that would be painful or impossible while awake. Injuries while patients are anesthetized are avoided by taking care in padding and positioning. Preoperative knowledge of orthopedic injuries or limitations is essential. The patient should 'appear comfortable' in the final position. All soft tissue and bony prominences (e.g. breasts, elbows, iliac spines) must be well padded to avoid pressure injury.

Positions used in colon and rectal surgery have particular risks. Patients in the lithotomy and Lloyd-Davies positions run the risk of peroneal nerve compression. The peroneal nerve may be injured if the weight of the leg is allowed to rest on the stirrups only at the lateral point below the knee. When the leg is properly positioned, the weight should rest on the heels and slightly on the posterior calf, as if 'standing in the stirrups.' Patients positioned in stirrups are at increased risk of deep venous thrombosis. This risk is reduced with compression stockings, intermittent pneumatic compression, or subcutaneous administration of low-dose heparin (see Chapter 8).

Similarly, the Buie (prone jackknife) and Sims' (left lateral decubitus) positions create the potential for injury to all dependent points (e.g. breast, penis, shoulder, hip, and knee). The face should be well padded and additional corneal protection is used. If general anesthesia is used, the endotracheal tube must be well secured. Loss of the airway in these positions can be disastrous.

Use of the Trendelenburg position increases pressure on the diaphragm, limiting ventilation, and increases myocardial oxygen demand. Regurgitation of stomach contents and aspiration is more likely. The anesthesiologist should monitor for these problems and limit the use of the head down position in a high-risk patient.

Postoperative pain control

There is an increasing variety of methods to control postoperative pain. The optimal choice will vary with the site and type of procedure, as well as the patient's tolerance and expectations. The mainstay remains narcotics of various forms. As noted by Syndenham in 1680, 'Among the remedies which it has pleased Almighty God to give man to relieve his sufferings, none is so universal and so efficacious as opium.' Traditional pain control is provided by intermittent intramuscular doses of meperidine or the equivalent. Variability in absorption and the dosage schedule provides adequate pain control for 35% of the dosing interval (**Figure 9.3**).

Patient-controlled analgesia (PCA) allows the patient to self-administer smaller doses of narcotic at very short intervals. Continuous infusion of a low-dose narcotic may be added as well. This provides more effective immediate analgesia when needed with less sedation, nausea, and respiratory depression. An additional positive psychologic effect is gained by giving the patient a sense of control over one aspect of his or her environment postoperatively (see Chapter 10).

As described above, regional anesthesia is also employed post-operatively. An epidural catheter, placed before or after a procedure, can provide exceptional pain relief. Continuous or intermittent epidural local anesthetic may provide sensory block and still allow ambulation. However, sympathetic block can cause hypotension. A single epidural injection of morphine can last up to 17 hours. Rostral spread of narcotic may yield many of the expected side effects, including pruritus, nausea and vomiting, and respiratory depression. Many patients receiving epidural anesthesia have urinary retention, requiring a urinary catheter until the epidural is discontinued.

To avoid some of the narcotic effects, including prolonged post-operative ileus, nonsteroidal anti-inflammatory drugs are used to decrease narcotic requirement. Ketorolac (Toradol) may be administered either intravenously or intramuscularly if a patient is receiving nothing

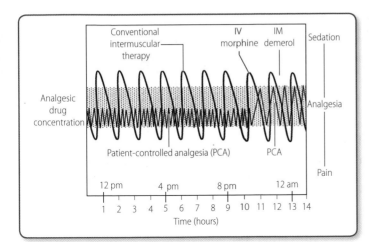

Figure 9.3 Postoperative pain control with different available methods.

by mouth. Once bowel function has returned, both oral narcotics and nonsteroidal anti-inflammatory drugs may be employed. These medications may be contraindicated in patients with peptic ulcer disease or bleeding disorders.

Rounds questions

1. What is the ASA class for a 50-year-old man with mild diabetes and coronary artery disease, who is active but experiences exercise induced angina?
2. Is the use of nitrous oxide contraindicated for intra-abdominal surgery?
3. What is the maximal allowable dose of lidocaine? Of bupivacaine?
4. What is the effect of adding epinephrine to local anesthetic? Of adding bicarbonate?
5. Does use of regional anesthesia have any decreased risk in the patient with cardiac disease? In a patient with pulmonary disease?
6. What alternative anesthetic can be used for a colostomy reversal in a patient with severe pulmonary disease?
7. What medication reverses the effects of opioids? Of benzodiazepines?
8. What effect does intraoperative use of a pulmonary artery catheter have on the incidence of cardiac events?
9. At what rate should isotonic crystalloid be infused during an open abdominal procedure in a 70 kg man?
10. What nerve compression syndrome is seen when the patient has been placed in the Lloyd-Davies position?

References

1. Frost E. Preanesthetic Assessment, 1, 2, and 3 eds. Boston: Birkhauser, 1988, 1989, 1991.
2. Orkin F, Cooperman LH. Complications in Anesthesiology. Philadelphia: JB Lippincott, 1983.
3. Goldman L, Caldera DL, Nussbaum SR, et al. Multifactorial index of cardiac risk in non-cardiac surgical procedures. N Engl J Med 1977;297:845.
4. Camporesi EM, Greeley WJ, Lumb PD, et al. Anesthesia. In: Sabiston DC (ed). Textbook of Surgery, 13th ed. Philadelphia: WB Saunders, 1986;158–77.
5. Dripps RD, Lamont A, Eckenhoff JE. The role of anesthesia in surgical mortality. JAMA 1961;178:261.
6. Liu S, Carpenter RL, Neal JM. Epidural anesthesia and analgesia; their role for postoperative outcome. Anesthesiology 1995;82:1474–506.
7. Thorson AG, Blatchford GJ. Operative and anesthetic techniques. In: Beck DE, Wexner, SD (eds). Fundamentals of Anorectal Surgery. New York: McGraw-Hill 1992;57–67.
8. Nivatvongs S. Local anesthesia in anorectal surgery. In: Gordon PH, Nivatvongs S (eds). Principles and Practice of Surgery for the Colon, Rectum, and Anus. St. Louis: Quality Medical Publishing 1992;139–48.
9. Bernstein M. Reducing the pain of local anesthesia in anal surgery. Selected Topics on Colon and Rectal Surgery, vol 8. Nomalk: United States Surgical Corp 1995;124–6.
10. Kurz A, Sessler D, Lenhardt R. Perioperative normothermia to reduce the incidence of surgical-wound infection and shorten hospitalization N Engl J Med 1996;334:1209–15.
11. Vernava AM, Dean P. Preoperative and postoperative management. In: Beck DE, Wexner SD (eds). Fundamentals of Anorectal Surgery. New York: McGraw-Hill 1992;50–6.
12. Karulf RE. Anesthetic and intraoperative positioning. In Hicks TC, Beck DE, Opelka FG, Timmcke AE (eds). Complications in Colon & Rectal Surgery. Baltimore: Williams & Wilkins 1996;34–49.

Postoperative management of colorectal patients is in many respects similar to that of general surgery patients [1]. Care of patients after perineal procedures is discussed in the appropriate chapters. After intra-abdominal procedures, significant concerns include general care, bowel function, drains, wound care, and fluid management. In order to maximize quality of care and minimize hospital length of stay care paths have been developed. Sample postoperative orders and patient instructions are included in Appendix 1.

General care

Pain management

Adequate pain relief is important. In the postoperative period, a comfortable patient can cooperate with breathing and ambulation instructions to decrease problems with atelectasis and deep vein thrombosis. Analgesia can be obtained by administration of narcotic medications (e.g. morphine, meperidine HCl [Demerol]), patient-controlled analgesia (PCA), intramuscular injections, and epidural infusion. With PCA the patient pushes a button that controls an intravenous pump, which administers small doses of intravenous narcotics within adjustable preset limits. Several studies have demonstrated that patients have less sedation and lower medication usage with PCA compared with intramuscular administration [2,3]. Suggested initial instructions and dosages of these medications are included in Appendixes 1 and 2. However, each patient's analgesic requirements will change during his or her hospitalization and must be evaluated regularly.

Epidural infusion (via a percutaneous epidural catheter) can provide comparable pain relief with less systemic side effects than PCA [2]. However, the additional cost and invasive nature of the epidural method must be evaluated for each patient.

Ambulation

Immobility is a risk factor for pulmonary and thrombotic complications; therefore early mobilization is essential. With assistance and adequate analgesia, almost all patients can stand or ambulate on the first postoperative night and in subsequent days. As the patient recovers from the operation, increased ambulation is encouraged.

Fluid monitoring and laboratory tests

The fluid and electrolyte status of postoperative patients must be monitored. Vital signs (pulse, blood pressure, temperature) and measurements of fluid intake and output provide objective patient status information. The extent and frequency of laboratory tests are determined by the operative procedure, comorbid conditions (e.g. diabetes, renal failure), and the patient's current status. The clinician should be able to justify each study ordered based on the indications listed previously; 'knee-jerk' or routine orders should be avoided. Inappropriate tests are costly and add to morbidity.

Postoperative bowel function

Physiology

After intra-abdominal surgery or a general anesthesia, the bowel usually retains its ability to absorb and/or secrete fluid into or from the lumen [1]. However, this function may be overwhelmed by luminal obstruction or bowel wall edema. By contrast, portions of the gastrointestinal tract commonly lose their normal motility for variable periods of time after surgery. The most significant problem associated with this altered motility is management of solids and gases. Intraluminal gas results from swallowed air and gas produced by intraluminal bacteria. With the exception of hydrogen, this intraluminal gas is not absorbed from the colon. To eliminate this gas, the body must move it through the gastrointestinal tract.

The recovery of intestinal motor function is not influenced by the operative procedure itself but is organ specific [3,4]. The inhibition of bowel motility is referred to as **adynamic ileus,** which generally occurs for the following intervals:

Stomach	Averages 1–2 days
Small bowel	Averages 0–1 day
Colon	Averages 3–5 days

The lack of bowel contraction is supported by absent bowel sounds. The stomach usually has an ileus for 1 or 2 days after surgery. During this time the patient will feel bloated, have no appetite, and will burp. If too much fluid or gas builds up in the stomach or proximal small bowel, the patient may vomit. The nondiseased small intestine continues with peristalsis and produces bowel sounds unless a resection or injury to the bowel wall occurs (e.g. lysis of adhesions, division of the mesentery). Small bowel that has been distended secondary to obstruction or has had an ileus (secondary to infections or metabolic conditions) will take a variable amount of time to return to normal motility [5]. In the absence of these conditions, the small intestine can handle fluids. For this reason, intraluminal fluid or nutrition can be administered safely immediately after surgery. The colon usually has an ileus for 3–5 days after surgery. Because most of the gas in the colon comes from swallowed air, the passing of flatus is a good indicator of colonic function. If food is ingested before the colon resumes its normal activity, intestinal contents (succus and air) will back up in the small intestine, resulting in distention, nausea, and vomiting [4].

Postoperative nausea and vomiting (PONV) is a common early complication after gastrointestinal surgery. Approximately 25% of patients experience PONV within 24 hours. Among high-risk patients, the incidence may be as high as 70–80% [5]. PONV delays recovery of patients after in-patient surgery and accounts for a significant proportion of unanticipated hospitalizations following ambulatory surgery. PONV leads to patient discomfort and satisfaction, but is largely avoidable when properly addressed.

Risk factors and risk assessment for postoperative nausea have been well studied. Consensus guidelines for managing PONV highlight patient, anesthetic and surgical risk factors. Risk factors include female gender, previous PONV, duration of surgery, history of motion sickness and non-smoking status [5]. Prevention of PONV is centered on reducing anesthetic and surgical risks, while appropriately adding pharmacologic prophylaxis.

The management of an ileus depends on the cause and the symptoms. Patients with gastric distention or partial bowel obstruction associated with vomiting will receive relief with a functioning nasogastric tube. However, the routine use of nasogastric tubes in postoperative colorectal patients has been abandoned. Multiple retrospective and prospective controlled trials have confirmed the benefits of selective nasogastric decompression [6–9]. Overall, 90% of postoperative patients do well without a nasogastric tube and are spared the discomfort and morbidity associated with a nasogastric tube. Avoidance of nasogastric tubes reduces the length of postoperative hospital stays in most patients. Mild to moderate nausea is managed with antiemetics such as phenergan, zofran, reglan, or scopolamine patches. The few patients who develop significant distention or vomiting are managed with nasogastric decompression without additional sequelae.

Alvimopan (Entereg, Adolor and GlaxoSmithKline, Exton PA, USA) is a peripherally active μ opioid antagonist. Pooled data analysis of the three US trials showed that alvimopan speeded overall GI-2 (tolerance of solid food and first bowel movement) recovery by 12 hours and accelerated time to discharge order (hazard ratio = 1.35, $p < 0.01$) [10, 11]. A second meta-analysis of five studies demonstrated similar findings [12, 13]. In these studies, alvimopan has not been shown to have an increase in adverse event rates or complications. Alvimopan is currently approved for perioperative use only for hospitalized patients. The first dose of 12 mg should be given orally prior to surgery, and continued 12 mg BID for 7 days, or until discharge. Alvimopan is contraindicated for patients on chronic opioids, with bowel obstruction, or severe hepatic or renal disease [14].

A few patients in the postoperative period will develop a **small bowel obstruction**. The most common etiology is adhesions from previous abdominal surgery. Less frequent causes are neoplasms, hernias, and volvulus. Patients present with abdominal distention, nausea, and vomiting. Obstruction is differentiated from ileus by the clinical picture (presence of bowel sounds and history) and failure to resolve with conservative measures. A diagnostic study, such as an upper gastrointestinal contrast study (UGI) or CT scan, will often confirm the diagnosis. Initial treatment is intravenous hydration and bowel rest [15]. Patients who fail to resolve with conservative therapy or patients with signs or symptoms of bowel compromise (abdominal tenderness, fever, leukocytosis, or acidosis) should undergo abdominal exploration [15].

Oral Intake

When gastric function returns, the patient may be started on clear liquids. This stage is usually clinically apparent by the patient's feelings of hunger. When colonic function returns (passing flatus or formed bowel movements), a regular diet should be offered. If at any time the patient feels bloated or develops distention, oral feedings should be withheld. Several prospective trials support the safety and cost effectiveness of this management plan [16,17].

Diarrhea medications

Excessively loose or frequent stools may result from several conditions. Inflammatory and infectious conditions are covered in Chapters 14 and 20. An additional cause is the loss of bowel associated with many colorectal procedures. After resection, the remaining bowel can adapt to varying degrees. With small resections the patient may have a postoperative bowel pattern similar to his or her preoperative state. The more bowel removed, the more likely that stools will be looser and more frequent. The medications described below can be used to modify the consistency and frequency of stool.

Psyllium (e.g. Metamucil or Konsyl) is a hydrophilic, high-fiber grain product that acts to normalize stool (**Table 10.1**). In constipated patients, it adds bulk to the stool. For patients with diarrhea, it helps by absorbing the bowel fluid content, turning a liquid stool into a bulkier formed or semiformed stool. Psyllium is almost flavorless in its natural form and dissolves poorly in water. Several brands are available, and most vary in their additives. While these products are well tolerated, occasional problems with compliance can result from patients' dislike of the taste or because of mild bloating. Because these products are relatively inexpensive and have no long-term health risks, they should form the initial therapy.

Methylcellulose (Citrucel, Citrucel Fiber Tablets) and **calcium polycarbophil** (Fibercon or Konsyl Fiber Tablets) are synthetic fiber products that many patients find more palatable than psyllium. Taken in adequate amounts, they work well but are more expensive than other fiber products. The amount of fiber in available products is listed in **Table 10.1**.

Loperamide hydrochloride (Imodium) inhibits peristaltic activity by a direct effect on all muscles of the intestinal wall. This prolongs intestinal

Type of fiber	Trade name	Available fiber*
Bran	Whole bran	
Psyllium	Metamucil	3.4 g/teaspoon in 240 mL water
	Konsyl	6 g/teaspoon in 240 mL water
Methylcellulose	Citrucel	2 g in 240 mL water
	Citrucel fiber tablets	0.2 g/capsule
Calcium polycarbophil	Fibercon	0.5 g/capsule
	Konsyl fiber tablets	0.5 g/capsule

Table 10.1 Amounts of fiber in synthetic fiber products

* Initial dosage is increased as tolerated to relieve symptoms

transit time, resulting in increased fluid resorption. Loperamide is helpful for the management of diarrhea associated with chemotherapy and in patients with ileal anal pouches. This medication has few side effects, and physical dependence has not been observed. It is available by prescription and over the counter as 2 mg capsules and liquid 1 mg/5 mL. The recommended dosage is 2–4 mg PO four times per day, 30 minutes before meals and at bedtime.

Diphenoxylate hydrochloride with atropine sulfate (Lomotil) is available in either tablet or elixir form. It acts by direct effect on circular smooth muscle of the bowel, which results in prolongation of gastrointestinal transit time. The initial adult dose is one to two tablets or 5–10 mL of elixir four times per day, 30 minutes before meals and at night). This may be increased up to three tablets four times per day, if necessary. The elixir does not taste pleasant, but is preferable in short bowel situations. The quantity to prescribe is 300 mL. This is a Schedule V controlled substance.

Codeine sulfate is an analgesic with strong constipating side effects. It is available as either a tablet (30 mg) or a liquid (30 mg/5 mL). The recommended dose range is 30–60 mg, four times per day (one 30 minutes before meals and at night before retiring). Patients with a short small bowel will absorb tablets poorly, so they should be given elixir. The elixir tastes awful, but it is sometimes much more effective than tablets. Codeine is a Schedule II controlled substance, which requires a narcotic control number for prescriptions. Addiction can occur, and codeine will frequently cause drowsiness.

Tincture of opium is a suspension of crude opium powder. The usual starting dose is 10–15 drops PO, three times per day, one 30 minutes before meals and sometimes at night. It is a strong constipating agent but has a significant addiction potential. It is often difficult to obtain, since it is a Class A narcotic and not often used. The quantity to prescribe is 125 mL.

Tincture of morphine (Roxanol, Roxane Laboratories, Columbus, OH, USA) is available as a commercial preparation of 20 mg of morphine per mL. This is also a Schedule II drug that is supplied in 120 mL bottles and the dosage is similar to tincture of opium.

Bismuth subsalicylate (Pepto-Bismol, Procter & Gamble) is an over the counter medication that has several actions. It has a topical effect on stomach mucosa, an antimicrobial activity, binds bacterial toxins and normalizes fluid movement via an antisecretory mechanism. The usual dose is 2 tablespoons (30 mL) every 3–8 hours. This medication is helpful for gastrointestinal upset and as an antidiarrheal medication.

Belladonna and opium suppositories (B & O Supprettes #16) are suppositories made with a cocoa butter base containing 60 mg of crude opium and 15 mg of belladonna extract, which act by decreasing rectal motility. Patients should be instructed to insert a suppository after a bowel movement with the blunt end of the suppository going in first. If there is a painful anal condition, the suppository should be pushed up into the rectum with a swab stick. This is more comfortable for the patient and ensures that the suppository goes up above the anal sphincters rather than being caught at that level. The dosage is one half to one suppository when necessary, not to exceed four per day. Addiction can occur; this is a Schedule II controlled drug. The suppositories come in boxes of 12.

Octreotide acetate (Sandostatin and Sandostatin LAR Depot, Novartis Pharmaceuticals, East Hanover, NJ, USA) is a peptide that mimics the natural hormone somatostatin. In addition to inhibiting growth hormone, glucagon, and insulin, it decreases splanchnic blood flow and inhibits release of serotonin, gastrin, vasoactive intestinal peptide, secretin, motilin, and pancreatic polypeptide. The usual dose of Sandostatin is 100 μg SQ one to three per day. The Depot form is administered 10–20 μg IM each month. This is a potent medication with many potential adverse effects and it is very expensive. This medication has been used in refractory diarrhea secondary to chemotherapy [18], and in ileoanal pouch patients that fail to respond to other medication.

For patients with an intact gastrointestinal tract, Metamucil is usually tried first, followed by Imodium. For patients who have had colectomies, Metamucil may be less effective. In general, Imodium, Lomotil, and B & O suppositories are the first drugs used. Codeine and tincture of opium or morphine are used if simpler measures fail. Octreotide is a last resort.

Drains

A large body of literature exists to prove that the general abdominal cavity cannot be drained and that the use of closed suction drains is superior to use of Penrose drains. Therefore intra-abdominal drains are not used unless a well-formed abscess cavity is identified. When drainage is indicated, a closed suction drain (e.g. Blake, Ethicon, Inc, New Jersey, USA or Jackson-Pratt, Baxter, Chicago, IL, USA) is preferred because it has a lower potential as a source of contamination [19]. A sump drain (e.g. Axiom, Axiom Medical,

Inc., Rancho Dominguez, CA, USA) has an additional lumen to allow air or fluid to enter the drain, which assists in keeping surrounding tissue from collapsing around the drain.

Drainage of the presacral space deserves additional discussion. The bony nature of the pelvis results in a noncollapsible cavity after resection of the rectum. In the absence of tissue to fill this space (e.g. omentum or small bowel), blood and peritoneal fluid can accumulate. This fluid can serve as a culture medium. If it becomes contaminated (from bowel contents or skin flora) an abscess may form. To eliminate this fluid, many surgeons use closed suction or sump drains in the presacral space after a rectal resection [1]. When studied prospectively, infusion of saline solution into pelvic sump drains offered no advantage, and this practice has been abandoned by most surgeons [1, 20]. These drains are usually brought out through separate abdominal wall stab incisions and are removed when the postoperative drainage is less than 30 mL/day.

Nasogastric or orogastric tubes are used intraoperatively to decompress the stomach. As described above, their routine postoperative use has been abandoned. Postoperative nasogastric suction may be indicated in selected patients (e.g. those with preoperative small bowel obstruction or extensive adhesions). In these patients a large (18 Fr) nasogastric tube should be placed and correctly positioned intraoperatively. After surgery the tube should be checked frequently to ensure that it remains working. Allowing the patient to take small sips of water (20–30 mL/h) helps the tube remain patent. The tube can be removed when bowel function returns.

A **Foley catheter** is placed intraoperatively to decompress the bladder and allow urinary output monitoring. The length of time it is maintained after surgery depends on the surgical procedure and the comorbid conditions. In general, the Foley catheter is removed at the first to fifth postoperative day. The longer range is used in patients with extensive pelvic surgery (e.g. abdominoperineal resections, or restorative proctocolectomies) or preoperative voiding difficulty (e.g. benign prostatic hypertrophy). Urinary retention or incontinence after removal of the catheter is managed by another 1- to 4-day period of catheter drainage. Failure after this point requires urologic evaluation. The most frequent complication associated with urinary catheters is a urinary tract infection. This can be minimized by avoiding unnecessary catheterization, following meticulous aseptic technique during insertion, proper catheter care (adequate drainage, securing catheter to minimize movement), and removing the catheter as soon as possible.

Wound care

Wound care is an important part of postoperative care. A **surgical incision** can be managed in several ways. It may be primarily closed, packed open for delayed primary closure, or allowed to heal by secondary intention [21]. Selection of one of these options must be individualized, taking into account a multitude of operative and patient factors. These include the quality of bowel preparation, amount of operative contamination, patient status (e.g. nutrition, sepsis, medications), and experience of the surgeon.

A closed wound is easier to manage in healthy patients with minimal operative contamination. In healthy skin, the incision edges are sealed together within 24–48 hours. For this reason, the operative dressing is usually removed during the first postoperative visit. This allows the surgical team to inspect the patient's wound. The wounds of patients with significant risk factors for wound infections or with wound contamination at surgery should be packed open [22, 23].

An important part of postoperative care is monitoring wounds carefully and frequently for signs of infection. Skin erythema, warmth, edema, or increasing incisional pain may suggest infection and require that the wound be opened [21, 24].

Fistula tracts or drain tracts are managed to protect the surrounding skin. Options include dry gauze dressings or placing a stoma pouch around the site. The management of stomas is discussed in Chapter 7.

An additional option to aid healing in difficult wounds is the use of subatmospheric pressure dressings (SPD) [25,26]. In the United States, this type of dressing has been available since 1995 as the vacuum-assisted closure (VAC) device (Kinetic Concepts Inc., San Antonio, TX, USA). SPD requires placing a sponge directly onto the wound that is sealed by an adhesive airtight plastic drape [27]. An exiting tube connected to a special suction pump creates subatmospheric pressure over the wound, which increases local blood flow, decreases edema and bacterial count, and promotes the formation of granulation tissue [28].

The VAC device has been used in virtually every type of wound with empirically successful results [18]. At Ochsner, we have used this device in patients with difficult perineal wounds with good results. Portable suction devices are now available that allow outpatient management and increased mobility.

Intravenous fluids

Postoperative patients require maintenance fluid, as described in Chapter 8; deficits resulting from surgery must be corrected. Ongoing losses such as nasogastric or drain output should also be replaced. The best overall indicator of adequate hydration is a urine output of 0.5–1 mL/kg/h. Intravenous fluid should be maintained until the patient is taking adequate oral fluid.

Transfusions

Francis R. Rodwig, Jr., M.D., M.P.H.
Ochsner Clinic Foundation, New Orleans, Louisiana, U.S.A.

The objective of transfusion therapy is to provide the appropriate blood product to correct a deficiency of a particular component in the circulating blood. Red blood cells (RBC) are used to maintain or increase the oxygen delivery to the tissues. While the oxygen-carrying capacity of the blood depends almost entirely on the concentration and saturation of hemoglobin, actual oxygen delivery to the tissues is influenced by many other factors, including (but not limited to) cardiac output, blood viscosity, and the state of the peripheral microcirculation. The optimal hematocrit or hemoglobin concentration has not been determined; in the past it was generally thought to be 10–11 g of hemoglobin/L.

In 1988, a National Institutes of Health (NIH) consensus conference suggested that a hemoglobin concentration of 7 g/L might be a more reasonable transfusion threshold in an otherwise healthy person [29]. Since that time, a number of publications have provided similar insight on appropriate transfusion decisions in surgery and the critical care setting and the tolerance of mild anemia [30]. However, careful consideration should be given to elderly patients with significant coronary artery disease or acute myocardial infarction. A recent study indicates red blood cell transfusions may lower short-term mortality in these patients [31].

The decision to transfuse red blood cells should address the specific needs of each individual patient, and the clinician should cautiously consider the duration of the anemia, the probability of a large blood loss during an operative procedure, and coexisting medical conditions. One should differentiate between anemia and hypovolemia. In general, anemia is much better tolerated in a surgical patient than is hypovolemia. Blood volume is best maintained with colloid or crystalloid solutions, and red blood cells should not be given solely for repletion of the circulatory volume. For these reasons, most surgeons and anesthesiologists use preoperative transfusions in symptomatic patients, but defer transfusions in preoperative asymptomatic anemic patients. Transfusions are administered intraoperatively in response to physiologic changes or ongoing blood loss. The decision to transfuse should be based on comparing the risks to the benefits and should be individualized for each patient. One unit of packed red blood cells should increase the hemoglobin by 1 g/dL, or the hematocrit by 3–4%.

Platelets are minute fragments of megakaryocyte cytoplasm that are responsible for primary hemostasis. Like RBC transfusion decisions, there has been extensive debate about the decision to transfuse platelets and the appropriate dosage and expected benefit [32]. For most surgical procedures, the platelet count should be at least 50,000/mL. Platelets are commonly available in two preparations, an apheresis product (collected from a single donor) or a standardized pool (e.g. 6 units) of random platelets derived from a whole blood donation.

Fresh frozen plasma (FFP) contains all the components of the coagulation, fibrinolytic, and complement systems. The primary indication for the use of FFP is a history or clinical courses consistent with a congenital or acquired deficiency of coagulation factors, with active bleeding, or prior to an operative or other invasive procedure.

It is recommended that the coagulation defect by documented by the appropriate laboratory testing [25]. A typical unit of FFP has a volume of 200–250 mL. Cryoprecipitate is derivative of plasma, and provides a concentrated product of specific plasma proteins. The most common indication for cryoprecipitate is hypofibrinogenemia.

The risks of transfusion include hemolytic reactions, febrile reactions, allergic reactions, and transmission of infectious disease. Immediate hemolytic transfusion reactions are usually caused by transfusion of ABO incompatible blood resulting from clerical or laboratory error, usually from the misidentification of the patient, most often with the sample collection. Fever, chills, flushing, chest pain, hypertension or hypotension, bleeding, and hemoglobinuria (and not hematuria) are the presenting signs and symptoms. In the anesthetized patient, unusual bleeding or change in urine color may be the only signs. Treatment should include immediate cessation of transfusion, clerical check of the blood and patient identification, and efforts to increase the urine volume and alkaline content and maintain blood pressure. Dialysis or management of disseminated intravascular coagulation (DIC) may be needed. Delayed hemolytic reactions, usually due to weak or developing red blood cell antibodies, are often clinically mild and require no intervention other than transfusion of antigen negative blood. Non-immune hemolysis of transfused red blood cells can also occur from incompatible intravenous fluids, trauma from filters or bypass pumps, temperature extremes, and transfusion-associated sepsis.

Febrile, non-hemolytic reactions may be caused by transfused leukocytes or their released cytokines. While these reactions are not serious, they can be uncomfortable, and may require the discontinuation of the transfusion and an evaluation for incompatibility. Antipyretics may be useful, and leukocyte filtration can be used in patients with recurrent symptoms. Allergic (urticarial) reactions are triggered by exposure to soluble substances in plasma to sensitized individuals. This reaction responds favorably to antihistamines, which may be used prior to transfusion in susceptible patients. Anaphylactic reactions are extremely rare.

Although infectious diseases transmitted by the transfusion of blood and blood components are relatively uncommon, both recipients and physicians view this complication as the most important. The process of transfusion-transmitted disease prevention begins with the careful selection of donors, who must answer an extensive list of questions to identify those at risk for disease transmission. Each donation is extensively tested in the laboratory for hepatitis B and C, syphilis, and the human immunodeficiency virus (HIV), among others. While these two sections of the screening process have been improved continuously, the risk of disease transmission is not zero. Still, the blood supply is currently as safe as it has ever been.

In the mid-1970s, post-transfusion hepatitis was reported to occur in 7–12% of transfusion recipients [1, 33]. Greater than 85% of these cases were neither caused by hepatitis A nor hepatitis B viruses, and was called non-A, non-B hepatitis. The principal agent of this entity has been identified [34], and designated as the hepatitis C virus (HCV). A screening serologic assay has been in use since 1990, leading to a marked decrease in transfusion-transmitted hepatitis. However, 'window period' donations prior to seroconversion still led to occasional cases of post-transfusion hepatitis C. The use of nucleic acid amplification technology (polymerase chain reaction, PCR) to detect known sequences of hepatitis C RNA was added to the screening panel in 1999 [35]. The residual risk of transfusion-transmitted hepatitis C is now less than 1 in 12 million units [36, 37].

Transmission of HIV is the most feared complication of transfusion (see Chapter 20) Fortunately, HIV associated with blood transfusion has been virtually eliminated by donor screening for HIV, including the antibody for HIV, which started in 1985. Like hepatitis C, improvements in the antibody testing and the addition of nucleic acid testing for HIV RNA detection by PCR of donated blood has led to a significant reduction in the risk of transfusion-transmitted HIV, with the current residual risk approaching 1 in 8 million units [37].

When the West Nile virus (WNV) was identified as a risk of both transfusion and organ transplantation in 2002, the use of nucleic amplification testing was implemented, resulting in very few cases of transfusion-transmitted WNV infection [38].

Transfusion of cytomegalovirus (CMV)-infected blood rarely results in detectable disease in the recipient. When CMV does occur, the clinical course is usually mild and manifested as a heterophile negative mononucleosis. This usually benign infection can, however, be life threatening in immunocompromised hosts, such as bone marrow transplant recipients. These patient should receive serologically negative blood units if they are serologically negative [39]. Since the supply of CMV seronegative components is limited, leukocyte filtration of cellular components has been shown to reduce, if not eliminate, post-transfusion CMV transmission [40]. Other rare, but potentially transmissible infectious agents include *Treponema pallidum* (syphilis), Chagas' disease, new variant Creutzfeldt-Jakob disease (nvCJD), babesiosis, and malaria [1]. Testing for syphilis has been in place for many years, and an assay to detect antibody to *Trypanosoma cruzi* has recently been implemented. Potential donors are questioned about travel and other risks for CJD, babesiosis, and malaria to prevent donation by at-risk donors.

As the risks of transfusion-transmitted viral diseases have decreased, the risk of contamination of blood components with bacteria is receiving significant attention as an important cause of transfusion morbidity and mortality [41]. The usual sources of bacterial contamination are the skin and asymptomatic, afebrile but bacteremic donors. Currently, an additional screening test for the presence of bacteria in platelet products has decreased the incidence of transfusion associated sepsis.

Since pre-transplant transfusions were shown to prolong renal allograft survival, the immunosuppressive effect of transfusion has been studied both in the clinical and laboratory settings. Early retrospective studies implicated transfusions as causing an increased risk of bacterial infection and increased cancer recurrence rates after potentially curative resections of colorectal malignancies. Several analyses, including prospective, retrospective, and a meta-analysis, have failed to clarify the clinical significance of the immunomodulation associated with transfusion [42, 43]. Preventative strategies, including leukocyte reduction of transfused components, continue to be controversial [44].

Acute pulmonary edema associated with transfusion has been extensively studied in the past decade. It is well known that volume overload can occur in susceptible patients (e.g. compromised cardiac function) with transfusion therapy, which is now termed transfusion-associated circulatory overload (TACO). Affected patients can be treated with the traditional measures for pulmonary edema. Pulmonary edema without cardiac compromise can also be associated with transfusion, and is termed the transfusion-related acute lung injury (TRALI). The exact mechanism of lung injury in this TRALI has not been determined, but appears to be associated with the infusion of antibodies to leukocyte antigens and biologic response modifiers [45]. TRALI is now the leading cause of transfusion-related mortality in the United States [46].

Clearly, the safest blood is the patient's own. Plasma volume returns to normal by the third day after phlebotomy [1]. Thus, preoperative autologous donations can be given as frequently as every third day if anemia does not force lengthening of the interval. The last donation should be no sooner than 3 days before the planned surgery. An oral iron supplement ($FeSO_4$, 325 mg tid) or its equivalent should be prescribed if more than one unit is donated. The American Association of Blood Banks guideline recommends a threshold hemoglobin level of 11 g or a hematocrit of 33% for the harvesting of autologous blood. Intraoperative autologous transfusion using a cell-saver device is seldom, if ever, used in colorectal surgery, since the blood volume loss is usually not large and many procedures involve the open gastrointestinal tract. Normovolemic intraoperative hemodilution can be considered if significant blood loss is expected.

An additional option is the use of erythropoietin (epoetin alfa, Procrit, Ortho Biotech, Raritan, NJ, USA), although this indication is controversial, and should be used with caution. This glycoprotein stimulates red blood cell production. Prior to therapy the patient's iron stores, including transferrin saturation (serum iron and iron binding capacity) and serum ferritin, should be evaluated. For surgery patients the dose is Procrit 300 units/kg SQ daily for 10 days before surgery, on the day of surgery and for 4 days after surgery [48]. Alternate dose schedules include 600 units/kg SQ weekly (21, 14, and 7 days before surgery) or 100 mg SQ three times a week before surgery [49].

Although there will never be a zero-risk transfusion, the introduction of new serologic testing, increased educational efforts, the more discriminate use of blood products by physicians, and the use of autologous blood should allow us to approximate that goal. The development of artificial oxygen-carrying red blood cell substitutes holds promise, but has yet to be realized. Although several hemoglobin substitutes are in advanced clinical trials, there are currently no FDA approved substitutes for blood.

Antibiotics

The use of prophylactic antibiotics is discussed in Chapter 8. Most authors currently agree that these antibiotics should be used for 24 hours or less after surgery [49]. Longer usage results in development of resistant organisms, bacterial or fungal overgrowth, and no reduction in the incidence of wound infections [24]. Antibiotics are indicated in a therapeutic role for infectious conditions described in other chapters. Knowledge of the expected flora allows selection of an appropriate cost-effective antibiotic [50].

Rounds questions

1. Do patients need less medication with patient-controlled analgesia (PCA) or intramuscular injections?
2. What is adynamic ileus?
3. Do postoperative patients need routine placement of nasogastric tubes?
4. What is psyllium?
5. What is the mechanism of action of loperamide hydrochloride (Imodium)?
6. Can the general abdominal cavity be drained?
7. What are the options for managing a surgical wound?
8. What are the signs of a wound infection?
9. What is the best indication of adequate postoperative hydration?
10. Transfused blood is tested for what infectious agents?

References

1. Beck DE. Postoperative management. In: Beck DE, Welling DR. Patient Care in Colorectal Surgery. Boston: Little, Brown 1991;89–94.
2. Gordon PH, Nivatvongs S. Principles and Practice of Surgery for the Colon, Rectum, and Anus. St. Louis: Quality Medical Publishing, 1992;129–37.
3. Graber JW, Schulte WJ, Condon RE, et al. Duration of postoperative ileus related to extent and site of operative dissection. Surg Forum 1980;31:141–4.
4. Beck DE. Reoperative surgery for acute and chronic small bowel obstruction. In: Longo W, Northover J (eds). Reoperative Surgery of the Colon and Rectum. London: Taylor & Francis. 2003;53–75.
5. Stein SL, Delaney CP. Post Operative Management. In: Beck DE, Wexner SD, Roberts PL, Sacclarides TJ, Senagore A, Stamos M (eds). ASCRS Textbook of Colorectal Surgery, 2nd edition. New York: Springer-Verlag, 2007.
6. Arnell T, Stamos MJ. Small bowel obstruction. Clinics Colon Rectal Surgery 2001;14:69–80.
7. Wolff BG, Pemberton JH, Van Heerden JA, et al. Elective colon and rectal surgery without nasogastric decompression. Ann Surg 1989;209:670–5.
8. Colvin DB, Lee W, Eisenstat TE, et al. The role of nasogastric intubation in elective colonic surgery. Dis Colon Rectum 1986;29:295–9.
9. Bauer JL, Gelernt IM, Salky BA, et al. Is routine postoperative nasogastric decompression necessary? Ann Surg 1985;201:233–6.
10. Delaney CP, Wolff B, Viscusi E, et al. Alvimopan, for postoperative ileus following bowel resection: A pooled analysis of phase III studies. Ann Surg 2007;245:355–63.
11. Senagore A, Bauer J, Du W, et al. Alvimopan accelerates gastrointestinal recovery after bowel resection regardless of age, gender, race or concomitant medication use. Surg 2007;142:478–86.
12. Tan EK, Cornish J, Darzi AW, et al. Meta-analysis: Alvimopan vs. placebo in the treatment of postoperative ileus. Aliment Pharm & Ther 2006;25:47–57.
13. Herzog T, Coleman R, Guerrieri J, et al. A double blind randomized placebo-controlled phase III study of the safety of alvimopan in patients who undergo simple total abdominal hysterectomy. Am J Obstet Gynecol 2006;195:445–53.
14. Marderstein EL, Delaney CP. Management of postoperative ileus: Focus on alvimopan. Ther Clin Risk Management 2008;4:965–73.
15. Meltvedt R, Knecht B, Gibbons G, et al. Is nasogastric suction necessary after elective colon resection? Am J Surg 1985;140:620–2.
16. Binderow SR, Cohen SM, Wexner SD, Noyras JJ. Must early postoperative oral in-take be limited to laparoscopy? Dis Colon Rectum 1994;37:584–9.
17. Bufo AJ, Feldman S, Daniels GA, Lieberman RC. Early postoperative feeding. Dis Colon Rectum 1994;37:1260–65.
18. Zidan J, Haim N, Beny A, et al. Octreotide in the treatment of severe chemotherapy-induced diarrhea. Ann Oncol 2001;12:227–9.
19. Sarr MG, Parikh KJ, Minken SL, Zuidema GD, Cameron JL. Closed-suction versus Penrose drainage after cholecystectomy. A prospective, randomized evaluation. Am J Surg 1987;153:394–8.
20. Galandiak S, Fazio VW. Postoperative irrigation-suction drainage after pelvic colonic surgery: A prospective randomized trial. Dis Colon Rectum 1991;34:223–8.
21. Coit DG, Sclafani L. Care of the surgical wound. In: Wilmore OW, Brennan MF, Harken AH, et al (eds). Care of the Surgical Patient, vol 2. New York: Scientific American 1990;1–10.
22. Cruse PJE, Foord R. The epidemiology of wound infection: A 10-year prospective study of 62,939 wounds. Surg Clin North Am 1980;60:27–40.
23. Tobin GR. Closure of contaminated wounds-biological and technical considerations. Surg Clin North Am 1984;64:639–52.
24. Wexner SD, Beck DE. Sepsis prevention in colorectal surgery. In: Fielding LP, Goldberg SM (eds). Operative Surgery, 5th ed. London: Butterworth-Heinemann, 1993;41–6.
25. Greer SE, Duthie E, Cartolano B, et al. Techniques for applying subatmospheric pressure dressing to wounds in difficult regions of anatomy. J Wound Ostomy Continence Nurs N 1999;26:250–3.
26. Argenta LC, Morykwas MJ. Vacuum-assisted closure: a new method for wound control and treatment: clinical experience. Ann Plast Surg 1997;38:563–77.
27. Opelka FG. Unhealed perineal wound. Clinics Colon Rectal Surgery 2001;14:65–8.
28. Morykwas MJ, Argenta LC, Shelton-Brown EI, McGuirt W. Vacuum-assisted closure: a new method for wound control and treatment: animal studies and basic foundation. Ann Plast Surg 1997;38:553–62.

29. Consensus Conference. Perioperative red blood cell transfusion. JAMA 1988;260:2700–03.

30. Hebert PC, Yetisir E, Martin, C, et al. A multicenter, randomized, controlled clinical trial of transfusion requirements in critical care. Transfusion Requirements in Critical Care Investigators, Canadian Care Trials Group. N Engl J Med 1999;340:409–17.

31. Wu WC, Rathore SS, Wang Y, et al. Blood transfusion in elderly patients with acute myocardial infarction. N Engl J Med 2001;345:1230–36.

32. Development Task Force of the College of American Pathologists. Practice parameter for the use of fresh frozen plasma, cryoprecipitate, and platelets. JAMA 1994;271:777–81.

33. Alter HJ, Purcell RH, Feinstone SM, et al. Non-A, non-B hepatitis: A review and interim report of an ongoing prospective study. In Vyas GN, Cohen SR (eds). Viral Hepatitis. Philadelphia: Franklin Institute Press, 1978;359-69.

34. Choo QL, Kuo G, Weiner AJ, et al. Isolation of cDNA clone derived from a blood-borne non-A, non-B viral hepatitis genome. Science 1989;244:359–62.

35. Schreiber GB, Busch MP, Kleinman SH, Korelitz JJ. The risk of transfusion-transmitted viral infections. The Retrovirus Epidemiology Donor Study. N Engl J Med 1996;334:1685–90.

36. NAT implementation. Association Bulletin 99–3. Bethesda MD: American Association of Blood Banks.

37. O'Brien SF, Yi QL, Fan W, et al. Current incidence and estimated residual risk of transfusion-transmitted infections in donations made to Canadian Blood Services Transfusion. 2007;47:316–25.

38. Busch MP, Caglioti S, Robertson EF, et al. Screening the blood supply for West Nile virus RNA by nucleic acid amplification testing. N Engl J Med 2005;353:460–7.

39. Tegtmeier GE. Post-transfusion cytomegalovirus infections. Arch Pathol Lab Med 1989;113:236–44.

40. Bowden RA, Slichter SJ, Sayers M, et al. A comparison of filtered leukocyte-reduced and cytomegalovirus (CMV) seronegative blood products for the prevention of transfusion-associated CMV infection after marrow transplant. Blood 1995;86:3598–603.

41. Sazama K. Bacteria in blood for transfusion. A review. Arch Pathol Lab Med 1994;118:350–65.

42. Sibbering DM, Locker AP, Hardcastle JD, et al. Blood transfusion and survival in colorectal cancer. Dis Colon Rectum 1994;37:358–63.

43. Vamvakas EC. Perioperative blood transfusion and cancer recurrence: Meta-analysis for explanation. Transfusion 1995;35:760–8.

44. Blajchman MA. Allogeneic blood transfusions, immunomodulation, and postoperative bacterial infection: Do we have the answers yet? Transfusion 1997;37:121–5.

45. Siliman CC, Ambruso DR, Boshkov LK. Transfusion-related lung injury. Blood 2005;105:2266–73.

46. Kopko PM, Popovsky MA. Transfusion-related lung injury. In Popovsky MA (ed). Transfusion Reactions, 3rd ed. Bethesda: AABB Press 2007;207–28.

47. de Andrade JR, Jove M. Baseline hemoglobin as a predictor of risk of transfusion and response to Epoetin alfa in orthopedic surgery patients. Am J Orthroped 1996;25:533–42.

48. Goldberg MA, McCutchen JW, Jove M, et al. A safety and efficacy comparison study of two dosing regimen of epoetin alfa in patients undergoing major orthopedic surgery. Am J Orthrop 1996;25:544–52.

49. Vernava AM III, Dean P. Preoperative and postoperative management. In: Beck DE, Wexner SD, (eds). Fundamentals of Colon and Rectal Surgery. New York: McGraw-Hill, 1991;50–56.

50. Chapman S, Harford FJ. Perioperative antibiotics. Colon Rect Surg 2001;14:7–14.

Section 3

Disease Processes

Hirschsprung disease, colorectal anomalies, and pediatric colorectal conditions

Hirschsprung disease

Hirschsprung disease (HD) has been recognized since 1691, when Dutch anatomist Frederic Ruysch described a case of congenital megacolon at autopsy. Over the ensuing 300 years, the surgeons who struggle to treat this condition have slowly grown to understand it. Harald Hirschsprung [1a], the Danish pediatrician whose name the disorder bears, described two patients who died of chronic constipation and megacolon in 1887. Tittle noted an absence of ganglia in the distal bowel in 1901 [1b]. He was followed by Tiffin et al in 1940, who proposed that the aganglionic bowel lacked peristalsis which accounted for the symptoms [1c]. However, it was not until the pioneering work of Swenson and Bill [2], who performed the first surgical correction for the disorder in 1948, that effective treatment became available. Despite the amount of energy expended on HD by the medical community, its etiology has not yet been completely defined, and the dysfunction that it manifests still occasionally leads to 'cures' that are less than satisfying. It is to be hoped that the biochemical elucidation of the disorder during the last decade will allow a clearer understanding of the pathology.

Embryology and anatomy

During development, the neural crest cells begin to migrate into the gut at about the fifth week of gestation. This migration continues in a cranial to caudal direction until neuroblasts are present in the distal rectum around the twelfth week [3]. Maturation of the neuroblasts continues throughout the remainder of gestation and into the early part of infancy. The normal distal intestine contains two plexuses that innervate it and control peristalsis, the myenteric (Auerbach's plexus) and the submucosal (Meissner's plexus). Ganglia are found scattered among the nerve fibers in both plexuses. The normal distal colon will have ganglia in the submucosa distally to within 2 cm of the dentate line in newborns. In addition, the fibers form a characteristic meshwork that sends off branches to innervate the muscle in a predictable pattern. The fibers themselves have a standard caliber.

Histochemical techniques reveal a normal staining pattern for a variety of neurotransmitters that are found in the ganglia and throughout the fibers. Of primary importance are the presence and density of anticholinergic and nonadrenergic, noncholinergic (NANC) fibers.

Pathophysiology

Hirschsprung disease is a congenital disorder that occurs in 1 out of 5,000 births. It is characterized by an inability of the distal bowel and internal anal sphincter to relax, producing a state of tonic contraction. This is frequently manifested as a bowel obstruction in newborns or as a state of chronic constipation in older children. Grossly, the disease appears as a dilated colon proximally, which quickly tapers through a 'transition zone' to the constricted, diseased segment. Until recently the sine qua non of the disorder was a lack of neural ganglia in the myenteric and submucosal plexuses. In approximately 75-80% of infants with HD the migration of the neural crest cells is arrested in the sigmoid colon or rectum; in 10-15% the proximal colon is involved, and in less than 10% the migration is stopped in the small bowel.

Recently the focus of investigation into the pathology of the neural derangement in HD has shifted from an anatomic explanation to a biochemical one. The neurotransmitters of the distal gut have been more precisely delineated and their distribution in HD better defined. The primary deficiency is in the NANC neurons, which represent a heterogeneous group of nerve cells with a variety of neurotransmitters. NANC nerves mediate the relaxation phase of peristalsis and are essential for distal gut motility. In addition to a lack of ganglia in the 'diseased segment,' it has been shown that 80% of the more proximal ganglia lack nerve cell bodies reactive for normal neuronal peptides [4]. In addition, these specimens have abnormal nerve fiber architecture with disorganized muscle innervation.

Additional studies have looked at the distribution of nerve growth factor (NGF) and NGF receptors. NGF is thought to stimulate the ingrowth of certain nerve fibers. There are elevated levels of NGF in the submucosa of the aganglionic colon. By contrast, Kuroda et al [5] found none in the mucosa, which stains heavily for acetylcholinesterase and displays hypertrophied nerve fibers. NGF receptors are present in the myenteric plexus of ganglionic bowel but not in aganglionic bowel [6]. It is likely that the alteration of neurotrophic factors ultimately has some effect on distal bowel function in HD patients.

Although it is somewhat controversial, decreases in the number of c-kit positive interstitial cells of Cajal (intestinal pacemaker cells) in the aganglionic segment may also contribute to the pathophysiology of HD [7, 8]. Expression and distribution of interstitial cells of Cajal may also play a role in post-operative intestinal dysmotility [9-11].

Some evidence suggests that HD is related to genetic defects, both chromosomal abnormalities and point mutations. There is increased incidence in siblings of affected children and HD is associated with a 4 : 1 male to female ratio. Multiple susceptibility genes for HD have been identified [6]. The most common mutations observed include the RET gene family (most common), as well as in the glial cell neurotrophic factor gene, endothelin-B receptor gene (ENDRB) and endothelin-3 (END 3) genes. The genetics of HD are complex and do not follow simple Mendelian patterns of inheritance [12].

Total colon HD is a particularly difficult form of the disease in which all of the colon, as well as some length of the gastrointestinal tract proximal to it, lacks ganglia. Siblings of infants with total colonic involvement are at even higher risk of having HD than the siblings of patients with lesser involvement. The morbidity in this group is also higher, primarily as a result of excessive fluid loss, wound infections, stoma complications, and enterocolitis. Postoperatively these patients require more frequent anal dilations and rectal irrigations. In addition, enterocolitis is a major complicating factor in these children both before and after pull-through. In this group, the incidence of enterocolitis is 25% compared with 14% in standard HD patients.

A subset of HD patients with a very short-segment disease has been described; in these patients the abnormality of innervation extends only a short distance above the dentate line. The significance of this group is that the functional pathology resides primarily in the anal canal, which may require a different therapeutic approach. These patients are usually diagnosed at a later age, because the main symptom is mild to severe constipation. This allows diagnostic modalities not readily employed in the newborn to be used, particularly anal manometry.

Evaluation and treatment

Symptoms

Grossly, the bowel of a patient with HD is dilated and hypertrophied proximally and narrow distally, where there is a functional obstruction. The diseased area is unable to relax as in normal peristalsis. In the neonate this will most often manifest as a bowel obstruction in the first few days of life. Milder cases, or short-segment disease, in which only a small section of the distal rectum lacks ganglia, may present as constipation in infants. Failure to pass meconium in the first 24–48 hours is a strong clue that HD may exist and failure to pass meconium after 48 hours is an indication for rectal biospy

Enterocolitis is a common occurrence in HD, with an incidence of between 10% and 40% in patients before definitive operation. Symptoms may include fever, vomiting, abdominal distention, diarrhea, and manifestations of severe dehydration. Overt signs of sepsis and shock may be present and perforation may develop [13]. Undiagnosed patients may present initially with severe enterocolitis.

Constipation is the primary presenting symptom in older children. Constipation is a common problem in children and may be caused by a myriad of factors, including psychologic and developmental abnormalities. Constipation that develops after the first few years of life is most often caused by something other than HD [14]. By contrast, a child who has had difficulty with passing stool since infancy may, in fact, have HD.

Evaluation

Physical examination of an infant with HD may reveal a tight anal sphincter and a paucity of stool in the rectum. In the newborn, a digital rectal examination may precipitate explosive diarrhea after the examining finger is removed. In an older child, the abdomen may be distended, and stool may or may not be felt in the rectal vault. Overflow incontinence and encopresis is unusual in these patients. Long-standing and untreated HD can produce malnutrition and wasting in older children.

HD is frequently associated with other congenital disorders. These include cardiac, renal, and lower spinal anomalies, some of which may be life limiting. Down syndrome is found in 14% of patients with HD. If any of these congenital problems exist in an infant with even mild symptoms of constipation or enterocolitis, the diagnosis of HD should be strongly suspected.

Radiologic studies are commonly employed in the evaluation of patients for HD and may be helpful if there are positive findings. Plain abdominal films may show intestinal obstruction in the newborn or a large fecal collection in older patients. A contrast enema may demonstrate the classic transition zone where the caliber of the colon changes quickly from a dilated proximal segment to a normal caliber distal segment. Lateral views may be particularly helpful in demonstrating this finding (**Figure 11.1**). Unfortunately, the absence of this finding does not rule out HD and indeed, this may not be seen in the neonatal period.

Anorectal manometry has been used in the assessment of patients suspected of having HD. Manometry typically demonstrates elevated resting anal canal pressure and a lack of the normal recto-sphincteric reflex [15,16]. This reflex was first described by Gowers in 1878, and is characterized by relaxation of the anal canal produced by rectal distention. Its absence has been found to correlate strongly with HD. Unfortunately, anorectal manometry becomes more useful as the experience of the surgeon applying it increases, and the results of several series have not been reproducible at other centers. It may be most useful in older patients with short-segment disease as a screening tool before biopsy.

Definitive diagnosis of HD still depends on the absence of ganglia in the distal bowel. Full-thickness or submucosal suction biopsy is done to determine the level of involvement. The submucosal technique uses a modified small bowel suction biopsy kit. The specimens are taken

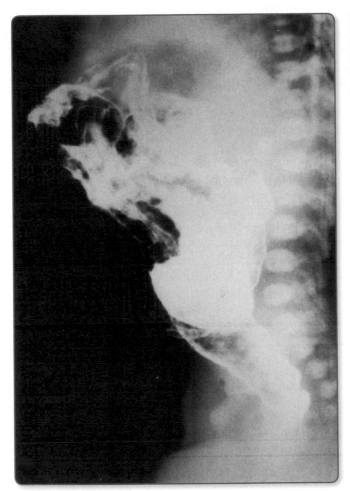

Figure 11.1 Lateral view of barium enema in patient with Hirschsprung disease. Note transition zone from the relatively normal diameter of the distal rectum to the dilated proximal bowel.

several centimeters proximal to the dentate line [17]. Interpretation of the biopsy specimens can be difficult and is most accurate in the hands of an experienced pathologist. The alternate method is to take full-thickness rectal biopsies or bowel wall biopsies if the patient requires an abdominal exploration. Despite the advantage of providing complete thickness of the bowel wall for interpretation, including both plexuses, open rectal biopsy requires an anesthetic and is more invasive. Suction biopsy is the most commonly employed method in infants and young children and can be performed at the bedside or in the clinic. Suction biopsy is not useful in older children because the bowel is thicker and it is difficult to obtain an adequate specimen. Full-thickness rectal biopsy is still advantageous if HD is suspected in older patients. Partial- or full-thickness bowel wall biopsy is used at the time of exploration for perforation or enterocolitis, or for long-segment disease, such as total colonic aganglionosis.

Identification of ganglion cells may be most difficult in the newborn, as immature cells may closely resemble endothelial or inflammatory cells [18]. Staining the biopsy specimen for acetyl-cholinesterase can be helpful in establishing the diagnosis [19]. The large longitudinal nerve fibers found in the submucosa at the level of aganglionosis stain heavily for this enzyme and suggest diseased bowel. A rapid acetylcholinesterase technique has been developed so that it may be used in conjunction with frozen section biopsy at the time of operation [20]. This allows a qualitative assessment of the 'transition zone', avoiding resection too distally. In addition, a rapid immunohistochemical staining technique has been developed using the fluorescent dye 4-Di-2-ASP on whole mounts so the architecture of the plexus can be observed, which may be particularly helpful in young infants in whom enteric nerve maturation is not complete [21]. Other stains, including those targeting neuron specific enolase, cathepsin D, tubulin, peripherin, MAP-2, and S-100 have been studied and demonstrated as helpful adjuncts in the diagnosis of HD, especially in newborns [18]. Staining for calretinin, a binding protein involved in calcium signaling, has been shown in small studies to be highly accurate in the diagnosis of HD [22–24]. Development of these methods reflects the need to more closely define the biochemical and structural abnormality of the diseased bowel in addition to simply determining if ganglia are present. No surgical treatment of HD should be undertaken without tissue diagnosis of the level of involvement. Impression of the extent of the disease at the time of operation by the surgeon is notoriously inaccurate and, if used to make operative decisions, risks a functionally poor result.

Initial therapy

If a neonate presents with a distal bowel obstruction or enterocolitis, and HD is suspected, the initial therapy should include intravenous hydration and nasogastric decompression. Rectal examination may provide temporary relief in the case of obstruction through decompression. Prolonged decompression can be achieved through repeated rectal irrigations or a colostomy. If a decision is made to create a decompressing colostomy, it should be placed proximal to the biopsy-proven transition zone; thus it should be located in an area that contains ganglia. The ideal location is just at the level of the normal bowel, creating a 'leveling' colostomy. This allows the colostomy site to act as the pull-through segment later. A loop colostomy or double barrel colostomy is preferred to allow decompression of the distal bowel if necessary. A right-sided transverse colostomy should be avoided if possible, because it can make a subsequent pull-through operation more difficult (see below).

Historically, most surgeons performed a leveling colostomy in neonates. Following colostomy, the infant was allowed to grow and mature until he was between 8 months and 2 years of age (8–10 kg) before a definitive pull-through repair was done. Definitive operation in the neonatal period to avoid a staged procedure is now the standard in most centers. The disease is initially controlled solely with rectal irrigation. Several series report very good success rates despite the technical demands of doing the operation at such a young age [25–27].

Surgical approach

The goal of the definitive operative correction of HD is to bring normally innervated bowel to the perineum, to allow bowel activity to approximate that of a normal child. The three commonly employed procedures are the Swenson, modified Duhamel, and Soave operations (i.e. the 'pull-through' procedures). Each has advantages, disadvantages, and its share of proponents. In addition, anal myectomy has been used as a first-line procedure in cases of short-segment disease or as a salvage operation after one of the pull-through procedures has had an unsatisfactory result.

Preparation of the older patient for a pull-through procedure who has a colostomy includes a gentle gastrointestinal lavage using room temperature electrolyte solution at a flow rate of 30 mL/kg/h via nasogastric tube for 2–4 hours. A cathartic bowel preparation can also be given although not all pediatric surgeons use a preoperative mechanical bowel preparation. If no diverting ostomy has been performed gentle rectal irrigation should be carried out. Antibiotics are administered either intraluminally or intravenously (see Chapter 8).

The **Swenson operation** was the first surgical procedure described to correct HD [2]. Dr Swenson's concept was to bring normal bowel to the perineum. The diseased rectum is dissected from the surrounding tissue down to the perineum. Care is taken to divide structures close to the rectal wall to avoid injury to the adjacent nerve plexuses, which could result in urinary or fecal incontinence, or impotence in the male. A two-layer anastomosis is performed immediately proximal to the dentate line (**Figure 11.2**).

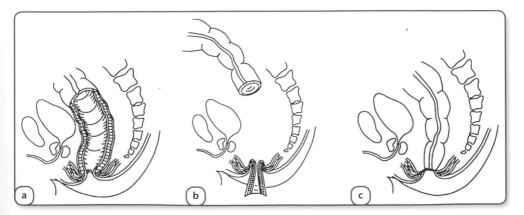

Figure 11.2 Swenson pull-through procedure. (a) The entire rectum is dissected. (b) The anastomosis is performed outside the anus, and (c) then returned to the pelvis.

The modified **Duhamel procedure**, using Martin's modification, requires dissection of the rectum from its posterior attachments distal to the levator muscles [28]. Normal bowel is drawn down posterior to the diseased rectum and anastomosed to its posterior aspect. Therefore, the anterior component of the rectal pouch is retained aganglionic rectum. A linear stapling device is used to divide the septum between the rectum and normal bowel more proximally, avoiding the small pouch that was left with the operation as originally described. The pouch had the tendency to collect fecal material, which eventually occluded the nondiseased segment as a 'fecaloma.' The Duhamel procedure requires the least dissection of the three and therefore is technically the easiest (**Figure 11.3**).

The **Soave operation** is accomplished by dissecting the mucosa of the distal rectum circumferentially from the deeper muscle layers, preserving a muscular sheath [29]. The normal bowel is drawn down through the sheath and anastomosed just proximal to the dentate line. Thus the normal bowel lies within the muscular sheath of the diseased rectum. This procedure avoids a perirectal dissection and has less propensity for nerve injury. The original procedure left a long muscular cuff, but recent modifications leave a very small cuff (**Figure 11.4**).

Although there is considerable argument among the proponents of each procedure as to which is best, each procedure has enjoyed success in the hands of those surgeons who perform them regularly. No adequate comparison can be made, because each series is made up of a majority of the favored procedure at that institution.

Recently the pull-through procedures have been accomplished using laparoscopy [26]. Exposure using laparoscopic techniques

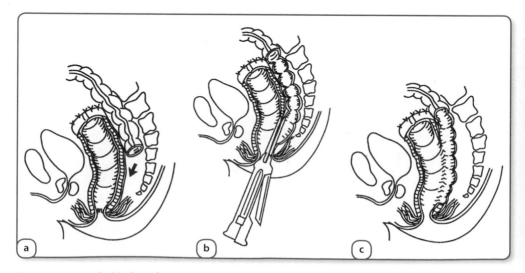

Figure 11.3 Modified Duhamel procedure. (a) The pull-through segment is brought to the perineum in the presacral space. (b) An anastomosis is performed, and (c) the septum separating the two segments is divided with the stapling device.

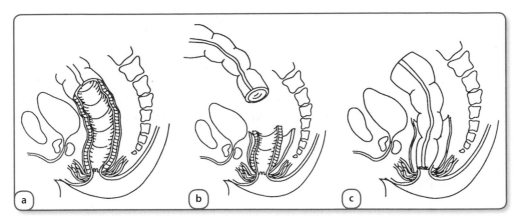

Figure 11.4 Modified Soave procedure. (a) The rectum before dissection. (b) The mucosa and submucosa are dissected, leaving a muscular cuff. (c) The pull-through segment is anastomosed just proximal to the dentate line.

is excellent, allowing less tissue retraction, dissection with more precision, and less manipulation of other structures. A review of the laparoscopic Swenson procedure found fewer complications when compared with the open version [30]. In addition, both the time to oral feeding and discharge were significantly less, which resulted in an overall reduction in cost for this small series. Besides the Swenson procedure, a laparoscopic technique has been developed that uses a transanal submucosal dissection similar to the open Soave procedure, as well as a laparoscopic version of the Duhamel technique [31, 32]. The application of laparoscopy (both pure and hybrid techniques) to the treatment of children with HD is expected to increase. Various groups have reported laparoscopic-assisted transanal pull-through at the time of intra-operative suction rectal biopsy with rapid acetylcholinesterase staining as one-stage initial management of children with HD [33]. and the use of laparoscopic-assisted suction colonic biopsy at time of transanal pull-through to identify the level of normoganglionosis [34]. In addition, single incision laparoscopic procedures for infants with HD have been reported [35].

As previously mentioned, several groups have recommended anorectal myectomy as the initial treatment of choice in patients with short-segment conditions or as a salvage operation after failed pull-through procedures [15, 36]. This operation involves removing a thin strip of the internal sphincter muscle in the posterior midline proximally, starting 1 cm above the dentate line. The strip is dissected as far proximally as allowed by the exposure, usually 3–15 cm. The approach may be made either through a transanal incision as described by Lynn and van Heerden [36], or a posterior sagittal incision as described by deVries and Peña [37]. Lynn and van Heerden treated 37 patients this way; in 28 it was the definitive procedure. Anal manometry has been applied in the postoperative assessment of rectoanal function. Evidence suggests that a resting pressure greater than 30 mmHg indicates an inadequate myectomy [15]. Re-do pull-through in selected patients after an initial failed operation (as manifested by recurrent obstructive symptoms and enterocolitis) has been associated with acceptable outcomes [38,39] Injection of botulinum toxin to address persistent non-relaxation off the internal sphincter has been shown to be beneficial for post-operative obstructive symptoms. Outcomes appear to be best if botulinum toxin is used after an initial workup to exclude mechanical obstruction, persistent aganglionosis, and other motility disorders [40–42].

Outcome

Although the assessment of the postoperative bowel function of HD patients is far from standardized, a number of large series report success in greater than 80% of cases [43–45] It is important to note that the incidence of adequate defecation improves as the length of follow-up increases. A series from Indianapolis is typical: of 103 patients, in those with follow-up of less than 5 years, 58% had bowel habits that were considered normal; for those followed for more than 15 years, it was normal in 88% [43]. A small minority of patients will require long-term anal dilation postoperatively. Even fewer may benefit from anal myectomy as a 'salvage' operation. In all, less than 5% continue to have debilitating symptoms such as frequent incontinence or impaction as adults. Longer term studies on quality of life in adulthood are generally similar. When patients who had reached the age of 18 or older were queried, over 80% reported satisfactory bowel function. Approximately 20% of patients still reported issues with incontinence and soiling [46]. Long-term quality of life may be related to length of the initial aganglionic segment [47].

As an operation to restore function to an area of the body that functions in such a complex manner, the surgical repair of HD must be viewed as a qualified success. Further understanding of the pathophysiology of the disease may yield even more improved results in the future.

Imperforate anus

Imperforate anus encompasses a wide spectrum of congenital defects. Some of these defects are minor and associated with an excellent functional prognosis, whereas others are significantly more complex and have a higher incidence of long-term problems. The incidence of imperforate anus is approximately 1 in every 4000–5000 live births. The frequency is slightly higher in boys than in girls. Associated anomalies are prevalent and play an important role in overall outcome. The two most crucial aspects in the surgical treatment of these children are an accurate preoperative identification of the rectal pouch location and meticulous operative technique.

Embryology and anatomy

The definitive embryologic explanation of anorectal malformations remains a subject of considerable debate [48]. The upper rectum and sigmoid colon develop from the hindgut, which joins the allantois (forerunner of the bladder) and the mesonephric ducts to form the cloaca, an endoderm-lined cavity [49]. The cloaca is separated from the amniotic cavity by the cloacal membrane, the location of the future perineum. The cloaca appears longitudinally as an inverted triangle, with the allantois, hindgut, and tailgut forming the apices. Classic teaching is that between the fifth and seventh week of gestation the urorectal septum, a transverse ridge of mesoderm between the allantois and hindgut, descends caudally to the cloacal membrane dividing the cloaca into a dorsal anorectal system and a ventral urogenital system. This descent is thought to be accompanied by a lateral infolding of cloacal mesoderm, which completes the separation process. Anorectal malformations were believed to occur secondary to defects in the proper descent of this septum. Recent investigations using scanning electron microscopy and three-dimensional reconstruction have challenged this theory and note no clear evidence of septation of the cloaca. They stress the importance of an absent dorsal cloacal membrane and dorsal cloaca as the fundamental components of this malformation [50–53].

Evaluation and treatment

Evaluation

The diagnosis of imperforate anus usually is readily apparent during the initial physical examination. Determining the level of the malpositioned rectal pouch is critical in planning the correct initial operative procedure. The Wingspread classification (**Table 11.1**), the most widely used classification for imperforate anus, established three anatomic categories based on the level of descent of the rectal pouch in relation to the puborectalis portion of the levator ani muscle [54]. High and intermediate anomalies are usually treated with

Table 11.1 The Wingspread classification of imperforate anus

	Female	Male
I.	*High*	
	Anorectal agenesis	Anorectal agenesis
	a. With rectovaginal fistula	a. With rectoprostatic urethral fistula
	b. Without fistula	b. Without fistula
	Rectal atresia	Rectal atresia
II.	*Intermediate*	
	Rectovestibular fistula	Rectobulbar urethral fistula
	Rectovaginal fistula	
	Anal agenesis without fistula	Anal agenesis without fistula
III.	*Low*	
	Anovestibular fistula	Anocutaneous fistula
	Anocutaneous fistula	Anal stenosis
	Anal stenosis	
IV.	*Cloacal malformations*	
V.	*Rare malformations*	

an initial diverting colostomy followed by a definitive repair; low lesions can normally be reconstructed primarily without a colostomy (**Figure 11.5**). Laparoscopic primary, one-stage repair in the neonate has been described and has gained popularity [55, 56]. Boys are twice as likely to have a high or intermediate anomaly compared with girls. In boys with a high or intermediate anomaly, over 85% have a rectourinary fistula.

Following diagnosis of an imperforate anus, all children should have intravenous lines established and be placed on NPO status. Conditions associated with imperforate anus that must be ruled out include esophageal atresia, congenital cardiac anomalies, and radial limb and vertebral anomalies. In all children with imperforate anus independent of the type, the presence or absence of neurologic symptoms or the coexistence of any bony sacral anomalies should be evaluated in early infancy to rule out a tethered spinal cord. Magnetic resonance imaging (MRI) is the current standard screening technique, but high-resolution ultrasound in the newborn is an equally effective, less expensive, and less invasive method [57–60]. Spinal ossification interferes with the use of ultrasound, however beyond 3–4 months of age. Early operative correction of a tethered spinal cord is essential to prevent the development of delayed neurologic sequelae. Evaluation of the urinary tract is also essential for all patients with imperforate anus. Genitourinary anomalies are found in 60–90% of children with high imperforate anus and 5–30% of those with a low anomaly [60, 61]. The most common lesions are renal agenesis and vesicoureteral reflux. A renal ultrasound and voiding cystourethrogram should be obtained in all children with an imperforate anus.

Evaluation in boys

In boys, perineal inspection and urinalysis are often enough to determine whether the patient needs a colostomy in 80–90% of cases. It may take nearly 24 hours for evidence of a perineal or urinary fistula to become apparent so it is important not to make any treatment

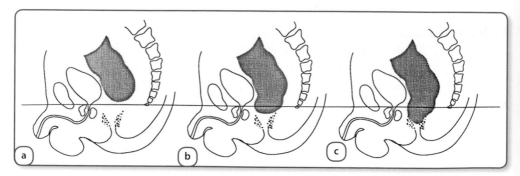

Figure 11.5 Variants of imperforate anus. (a) The 'high' lesion ends above the pubococcygeal line. (b) The 'intermediate' lesion ends between the pubococcygeal line and the ischium. (c) The low lesion ends below the ischium.

decisions immediately after delivery [62]. The most frequent fistula in boys is a rectourethral fistula. The presence of a 'flat bottom,' meconium in the urine, or air in the bladder is evidence of a high or intermediate anomaly and an indication for a diverting colostomy [63]. A perineal fistula is evidence of a low anomaly. In cases in which the level of the pouch is still unclear after 24 hours, additional diagnostic studies should be obtained. This invertogram, described by Wangensteen and Rice [64], is rarely used because of inaccuracy in some cases and the risk of desaturation in infants. Currrently, a cross-table lateral film with the child in a prone position, perineal ultrasound, CT scan, or MRI are the indicated studies [65–67]. Each of these tests can provide incorrect information if performed too early before air reaches the most distal aspect of the rectal pouch (16–24 hours of life). Measurements from lateral radiographs and ultrasound are frequently inaccurate [68,69]. Ultrasound, however, is of value in demonstrating abnormalities of the urogenital tract. MRI is the most accurate modality in determining level of termination of the rectal pouch, but only identifies a minority of rectourogenital fistulas [68].

If the measured rectal pouch to skin distance is less than 1 cm, indicating a low anomaly, no colostomy is needed and the child can be treated with a perineal procedure alone in the newborn period. Care must be taken using these criteria in infants with a relatively flat perineum. However, if the distance is greater than 1 cm, indicating a high or intermediate anomaly, a diverting proximal sigmoid colostomy is created initially followed by a definitive pull-through procedure when the patient is larger (1–6 months of age). There are proponents of immediate open or laparoscopic repair in the newborn period [55,56,70,71]. However, most recent reports of laparoscopic assisted pull-through operations describe the definite pull-through operation being performed several months after an initial diverting colostomy [72–74]. Perceived advantages of the laparoscopic-assisted approach include superior visualization and less extensive perineal dissection [74]. A colostomy should be performed in all cases where doubt exists regarding the level of the rectal pouch following completion of diagnostic studies.

Evaluation in girls

The decision making process in girls is usually easier than with boys. Diagnostic studies are rarely required and in nearly all patients, a thorough evaluation of the perineum is all that is needed. More than 90% will have a fistula connecting the rectum with the genitourinary tract [63]. A single orifice indicates the presence of a persistent cloaca, which constitutes a common opening for the urethra, vagina and rectum. If two orifices are seen including the urethra and vagina, and meconium is seen originating from within the hymen orifice, the diagnosis of rectovaginal fistula is made. The cloacal variant has been increasingly thought to be more common than a rectovaginal fistula [62]. A vestibular fistula, the most frequent defect in females, is located within the vestibule but immediately behind the hymen. Repair of a vestibular fistula can be performed with a cutback operation or, more often, an anal transposition with or without a protective colostomy. In some cases, the fistula will open in the middle of the perineum between the center of the external sphincter and the vestibule. This perineal or cutaneous fistula can also be treated with a cutback procedure or perineal anoplasty without a colostomy. As with boys, associated anomalies must be ruled out, the genitourinary tract must be evaluated, and in any case where the level of the rectal pouch is unclear, a colostomy should be performed.

Initial therapy

A completely diverting colostomy with separated stomas is the preferred type of colostomy construction for management of high and intermediate cases of imperforate anus [75]. Loop colostomies have a higher incidence of prolapse, are harder to adequately irrigate distally, and may increase the risk for urinary tract infections in children with a rectourinary fistula. The site chosen for the colostomy is also very important. The left descending colon and the upper portion of the sigmoid colon are the best sites. A colostomy opened too distal in the sigmoid colon will create a mechanical limitation for the subsequent pull through operation because of an insufficient length of bowel. Creation of a too-proximal colostomy will leave a long, defunctionalized segment that is difficult to empty. This can also lead to metabolic problems for the child with a large rectourinary fistula because of the absorption of an excessive amount of urinary chloride within the defunctionalized segment.

Surgical approach

Early experience with operations for high imperforate anus included either a combined abdominoperineal or a sacroabdominoperineal approach [76–78]. Currently the most widely practiced technique for the repair of intermediate and high anorectal malformations is the posterior sagittal anorectoplasty (PSARP) originally described by deVries and Peña in 1982 [37]. The child is placed in the prone position with the pelvis elevated. This approach is based on complete exposure of the anorectal region by means of a median sagittal incision that runs from the sacrum to the anal dimple and divides the entire muscle complex behind the rectum (**Figure 11.6**). All of the muscle structures are separated precisely in the midline to avoid nerve damage. It is important to adequately clean this blind-ending rectum before operation. Adequate lighting, optical magnification, and a muscle stimulator are essential to perform this procedure precisely. The rectal pouch is identified and opened and any urethral fistula is closed. The bowel is dissected free from the urinary tract or vagina so that enough length is gained to provide a tension-free repair. If necessary, the bowel should be tapered to permit reconstruction of the muscle complex around it. The rectum is then brought anterior to the levator ani and

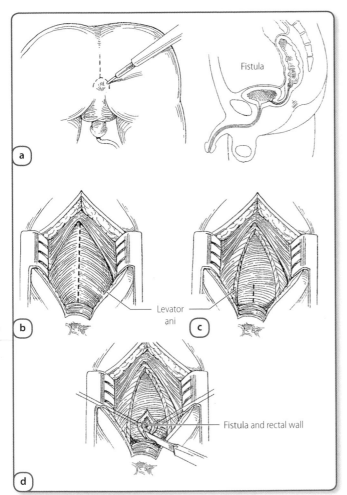

Figure 11.6 The deVries-Peña posterior sagittal anorectoplasty. (a) Electrical stimulation to identify the external sphincter location. (b) Midline incision through all posterior musculature. (c) Identification of the rectal pouch and incision into the posterior inferior wall of the rectum. (d) Identification and dissection of the rectourethral fistula from the rectum. (e) Closure of the rectourethral fistula and mobilization of the rectal pouch. (f) Closure of the striated muscle complex anteriorly. (g) Closure of the posterior musculature over the rectal pouch. (h) Skin closure and 'double diamond' method of anoplasty to promote sensation and to avoid stricture.

through the muscle complex to reach the skin where the anastomosis is performed. The colostomy is left in place and most children go home in 2–4 days. Anal dilations are normally begun approximately 2–3 weeks postoperatively, and parents are taught to perform these at home. Once or twice daily dilations are the key to good outcome. Dilator sizes are increased each week until the anus reaches the desired size. At that point the colostomy may be dosed. Dilations are continued for at least 6 months after operation.

Laparoscopic-assisted approaches for imperforate anus increasingly being utilized. Georgeson et al initially described the approach for high imperforate anus in 2000 and the majority of studies published since use the same general principles as that originally described [56]. General principles of the laparoscopic approach include laparoscopic rectal dissection, identification of the urinary/vaginal fistula with subsequent clip placement/division, and examination of the levators.

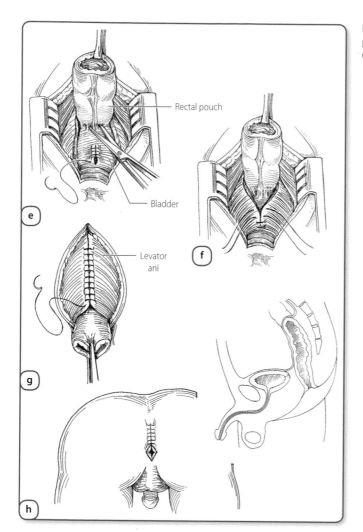

Figure 11.6 The deVries-Peña posterior sagittal anorectoplasty. *Continued.*

Perineal dissection commences after electrostimulation. An incision is made at the site of the proposed neo-anus after determination of the proposed boundaries and blunt dissection is performed using light from the laparoscope as a guide. A trocar that can be radially expanded is passed posterior to the urethra and advanced to a midline position between the bellies of the pubococcygeus. After radial dilation, the rectal pouch is brought through the tract and the anastomosis is completed (**Figure 11.7**) [56].

Outcome

Long-term outcome in terms of continence for these children is highly variable and is dependent on both the underlying anomaly and any associated abnormalities. The best outcome is in children with low anomalies. Those children with the worst prognosis for continence

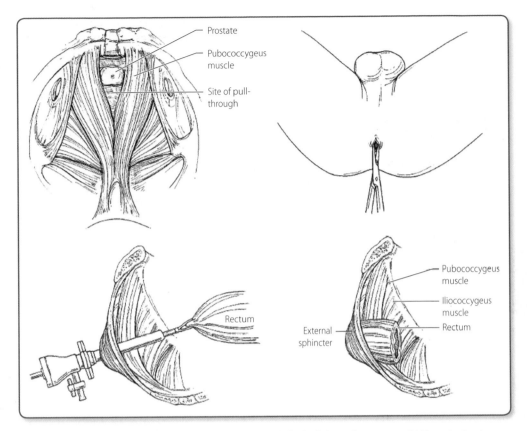

Figure 11.7 Laparoscopic assisted anorectal pull-through for high imperforate anus. (a) View obtained during laparoscopic dissection and identification of the pelvic floor. (b) Perineal blunt dissection is minimized and facilitated by illumination from the intra-abdominal laparoscopic light source. (c) Pull-through of rectum, and (d) completion anatomy.

are ones with high imperforate anus, sacral anomalies (more than two vertebrae missing), poor muscle structure, and a flat bottom (with little or no buttocks crease) [62]. Total continence is achieved in most patients with low lesions, but in patients with higher lesions may occur less than 50% of the time. Constipation is quite prevalent as well, and a structured bowel management program is important. Infertility may be a significant problem in patients as they reach maturity [79]. Secondary reconstructive procedures can be performed in children with incontinence following the original operation. However, these are usually reserved for children with a normal sacrum and evidence of a malpositioned rectum and anus clinically or by CT scan and/or MRI.

Duplications

A duplication of the alimentary tract is a rare entity and can occur at any location from the mouth to the anus. Only 4–18% of all cases are found in the colon and rectum [80]. Colonic duplications may be either cystic or tubular and are classified as either type I (partial duplication limited to the colon and/or rectum) or type II (complete duplication associated with duplication of other systems – i.e. lower urinary, reproductive, lumbosacral spine). Either type may or may not communicate with the true lumen of the bowel. The most frequent clinical picture includes intestinal obstruction, abdominal pain, abdominal mass and constipation. A rectal duplication can present as a presacral mass and may be confused for a pelvic tumor. Many patients, however, remain asymptomatic.

Barium enema is the procedure of choice for diagnosis. Because of the possibility of multiple malformations occurring with a colonic duplication, complete evaluation of the small intestine, lumbar spine, pelvis, and genitourinary tract is recommended [81]. Excision of the duplication is advised once the diagnosis is made. If there is a common blood supply, a concomitant intestinal resection might be required. For extensive duplications, it may be safer to simply create a common channel between the duplication and the true lumen [82]. This should only be performed in selected cases because of the risk of developing a malignancy in the duplication later in life [83].

Neonatal small left colon syndrome

Originally reported by Davis in 1974, neonatal small left colon (NSLC) syndrome is thought to represent a transient motility disorder of the distal colon [84]. Fifty-percent of infants with NSLC syndrome are born to diabetic mothers. It is hypothesized that an increase in glucagon production in response to neonatal hypoglycemia is responsible for the reduced bowel motility in these infants [85]. Within the first few days of life, these patients present with a clinical picture that is consistent with a distal intestinal obstruction (distention, bile-stained vomitus, and failure to pass meconium). Plain radiographs demonstrate dilated loops of bowel with air-fluid levels. A contrast enema should be performed early in the evaluation to rule out a mechanical obstruction. Characteristically, this will demonstrate a dilated colon proximal to a tapered transition zone, normally at the distal transverse colon or splenic flexure with a normal-sized rectum [86]. The colon should fill easily, and obstructing meconium plugs are usually not seen. This clinical and radiologic picture is similar to that of HD, except that a splenic flexure transition zone is rare with HD and there is no known association with maternal diabetes.

Normally, NSLC syndrome is a self-limiting condition and treatment is supportive, with intravenous fluids and gastric suction. The clinical obstruction should clear within 24–48 hours. In infants who fail to improve over a few days, dilute Gastrografin enemas are used to promote clearance of residual meconium. In some cases repeated enemas over several days may be required. In this group, a suction rectal biopsy is necessary to exclude the occasional Hirschsprung infant with a splenic flexure transition zone. Following resolution, feedings are instituted and advanced as tolerated. There do not appear to be any long-term complications from NSLC syndrome. Perforation has been reported, primarily in early case series describing this condition. It appears to be preventable by early contrast enema [87].

Necrotizing enterocolitis

Necrotizing enterocolitis (NEC) is an inflammatory disorder of the intestines found most commonly in the very low birth weight (VLBW, i.e. less than 1500 g) infant. NEC occurs in 2–10% of all VLBW infants and has an overall mortality ranging from 10–30% [88]. The etiology of the disease is unknown, but several factors, including intestinal immaturity, genetic susceptibilities, bacterial colonization, and ischemic injury are believed to contribute to the pathogenesis of NEC [89]. The large majority of infants with NEC are premature and the mean age at onset is around 34 weeks of gestation. Most infants with NEC have had enteral feedings instituted, although the timing and volume of feedings does not appear to be a factor. Breast fed infants do appear to have a lower incidence of NEC compared with formula fed infants. The disease may involve the small intestine alone, the colon alone or, frequently, both. Involvement of large sections of the small and large intestine is why NEC is the most common cause of short gut syndrome in children [90].

The diagnosis of NEC may be difficult unless the full-blown process is evident. Infants will manifest signs of sepsis including temperature instability, abdominal distention and feeding intolerance. Physical examination may also be nonspecific and include tenderness on examination, erythema or poor perfusion. Laboratory values do not offer any specific help since the white blood cell count may be high or low. The platelet count may also be decreased, but this is commonly seen in sepsis of any kind. Abdominal radiographs may show distended bowel loops or a fixed loop of bowel (secondary to ischemia) on repeat radiographs. Pneumatosis intestinalis is pathognomonic of NEC. Free air or portal vein air may also be seen on the plain radiograph. Ultrasound may also show portal vein air. Contrast studies are of no benefit in most patients.

Initial management of patients with NEC is supportive with volume resuscitation, broad-spectrum antibiotics and keeping the patient NPO. Over half of the infants with NEC will respond to medical management. The indications for operative intervention include free air, indicative of perforation, a fixed loop of bowel on repetitive radiographs, clinical deterioration, and portal vein air in most patients. Surgical options include primary drainage of the abdomen, either as a temporizing procedure or as definitive therapy and laparotomy with resection and creation of a diverting stoma. Overall survival for infants after surgical intervention is approximately 50–70% [91].

Colonic strictures can be seen commonly after NEC, both after medical or surgical intervention. Strictures should be carefully looked for prior to any stoma closure and can be dealt with by local stricturoplasty or resection. The long-term outlook for patients who survive the initial event is dependent on other problems such as intracranial hemorrhage, chronic lung disease and amount of remaining functional intestine.

Colonic atresia

Colonic atresia is rare, accounting for less than 15% of all gastrointestinal tract atresias [92]. It is most common in males and thought to be due to an in-utero vascular injury. Genetic factors may play a role as evidenced by reports of familial cases. Associated congenital abnormalities are generally rare. Associations with gastroschisis, HD, complex urological abnormalities, congenital varicella syndrome, and multiple small intestinal atresias have been reported [92,93]. Most commonly, colonic atresias are classified as described by Grosfeld et al and divides atresias into 4 major types [92,94]:
- Type 1 (atresia of mucosa only)
- Type 2 (fibrous cord connecting two atretic ends)
- Type 3a (mesenteric defect [V-shaped] separating two atretic ends)
- Type 3b (apple-peel atresia)
- Type 4 (multiple atretic segments)

Diagnosis may be suggested on prenatal ultrasound. Clinical symptoms may include emesis, failure to pass meconium, and abdominal distention. Plain abdominal radiographs may demonstrate distended loops of bowel with air fluid levels with a generously dilated proximal colon. Contrast enema demonstrates a small caliber distal colon with a sudden transition point at the level of obstruction. Prompt surgical management remains the mainstay of therapy and generally consists of an initial colostomy and mucus fistula. Intraoperatively, it is important to examine carefully for other proximal atresias as well as exclude the diagnosis of HD [95]. Outcomes are dependent on early diagnosis and surgery (mortality increased if surgery performed >72 hours after birth), presence or absence of associated abnormalities, and surgical procedure performed (one stage procedure with anastomosis may be associated with worsened outcomes) [92,93].

More recent studies report acceptable outcomes of one stage resection/primary anastomosis in uncomplicated cases of colonic atresia [96]. Although rare, the association of colonic atresia with HD necessitates its exclusion prior to restoration of intestinal continuity. Unfortunately, the diagnosis of HD or other intestinal neuronal dysplasias is frequently made by obstruction post-operatively. If a one stage procedure is to be performed, it is prudent to exclude the diagnosis of HD by intraoperative suction rectal biopsy [97].

Rounds questions

1. How does Hirschsprung disease present?
2. What establishes the diagnosis of Hirschsprung disease?
3. What is the most common anomaly associated with imperforate anus?
4. What is the appropriate initial treatment for high imperforate anus?
5. Neonatal small left colon syndrome is associated with what maternal condition?
6. Pneumatosis intestinalis in a newborn is pathognomonic for what disease?

References

1a. Hirschsprung H. Stuhltragheit neugeborener in folge von dilatation und hypertrophie des colons. Jahrb Kinderh 1887;27:1–7.

1b. Title K. Ubereine enageborene Missbildung des Dickdrmes. Wien Klin Wochenschr 1901;14:903.

1c. Tiffin ME, Chandler LR, Faber HK. Localized absence of ganglion cells of myenteric plexus in congenital mega colon. Am J Dis Child 1940;59:1071.

2. Swenson O, Bill AH. Resection of rectum and rectosigmoid with preservation of the sphincter for benign spastic lesions producing megacolon; an experimental study. Surgery 1948;24:212–20.

3. Heanue TA, Pachnis V. Enteric nervous system development and Hirschsprung's disease: advances in genetic and stem cell studies. Nat Rev Neurosci 2007;8:466–79.

4. Romanska HM, Bishop AE, Brereton RJ, et al. Immunocytochemistry for neuronal markers shows deficiencies in conventional histology in the treatment of Hirschsprung's disease. J Pediatr Surg 1993;28:1059–62.

5. Kuroda T, Ueda M, Nakano M, et al. Altered production of nerve growth factor in aganglionic intestines. J Pediatr Surg 1994;29:288–92; discussion 292–83.

6. Parisi MA, Kapur RP. Genetics of Hirschsprung disease. Curr Opin Pediatr 2000;12:610–7.

7. Wang H, Zhang Y, Liu W, et al. Interstitial cells of Cajal reduce in number in recto-sigmoid Hirschsprung's disease and total colonic aganglionosis. Neurosci Lett 2009;451:208–11.

8. Newman CJ, Laurini RN, Lesbros Y, et al. Interstitial cells of Cajal are normally distributed in both ganglionated and aganglionic bowel in Hirschsprung's disease. Pediatr Surg Int 2003;19:662–8.

9. Bettolli M, De Carli C, Jolin-Dahel K, et al. Colonic dysmotility in postsurgical patients with Hirschsprung's disease. Potential significance of abnormalities in the interstitial cells of Cajal and the enteric nervous system. J Pediatr Surg 2008;43:1433–8.

10. Rolle U, Piotrowska AP, Nemeth L, et al. Altered distribution of interstitial cells of Cajal in Hirschsprung disease. Arch Pathol Lab Med 2002; 126:928–33.

11. Taguchi T, Suita S, Masumoto K, et al. An abnormal distribution of C-kit positive cells in the normoganglionic segment can predict a poor clinical outcome in patients with Hirschsprung's disease. Eur J Pediatr Surg 2005;15:153–8.

12. Kusafuka T, Puri P. Genetic aspects of Hirschsprung's disease. Semin Pediatr Surg 1998;7:148–55.

13. Teitelbaum DH, Coran AG. Enterocolitis. Semin Pediatr Surg 1998;7:162–9.

14. Baker SS, Liptak GS, Colletti RB, et al. Constipation in infants and children: evaluation and treatment. A medical position statement of the North American Society for Pediatric Gastroenterology and Nutrition. J Pediatr Gastroenterol Nutr 1999;29:612–26.

15. Abbas Banani S, Forootan H. Role of anorectal myectomy after failed endorectal pull-through in Hirschsprung's disease. J Pediatr Surg 1994;29:1307–9.

16. Tamate S, Shiokawa C, Yamada C, et al. Manometric diagnosis of Hirschsprung's disease in the neonatal period. J Pediatr Surg 1984;19:285–8.

17. Andrassy RJ, Isaacs H, Weitzman JJ. Rectal suction biopsy for the diagnosis of Hirschsprung's disease. Ann Surg 1981;193:419–24.

18. Holland SK, Hessler RB, Reid-Nicholson MD, et al. Utilization of peripherin and S-100 immunohistochemistry in the diagnosis of Hirschsprung disease. Mod Pathol; 23:1173–9.

19. Nakao M, Suita S, Taguchi T, et al. Fourteen-year experience of acetylcholinesterase staining for rectal mucosal biopsy in neonatal Hirschsprung's disease. J Pediatr Surg 2001;36:1357–63.

20. Kobayashi H, Wang Y, Hirakawa H, et al. Intraoperative evaluation of extent of aganglionosis by a rapid acetylcholinesterase histochemical technique. J Pediatr Surg 1995;30:248–52.

21. Hanani M, Udassin R, Ariel I, et al. A simple and rapid method for staining the enteric ganglia: application for Hirschsprung's disease. J Pediatr Surg 1993;28:939–41.

22. Barshack I, Fridman E, Goldberg I, et al. The loss of calretinin expression indicates aganglionosis in Hirschsprung's disease. J Clin Pathol 2004;57:712–6.

23. Kapur RP, Reed RC, Finn LS, et al. Calretinin immunohistochemistry versus acetylcholinesterase histochemistry in the evaluation of suction rectal biopsies for Hirschsprung Disease. Pediatr Dev Pathol 2009;12:6–15.

24. Guinard-Samuel V, Bonnard A, De Lagausie P, et al. Calretinin immunohistochemistry: a simple and efficient tool to diagnose Hirschsprung disease. Mod Pathol 2009;22:1379–84.

25. Teitelbaum DH, Cilley RE, Sherman NJ, et al. A decade of experience with the primary pull-through for Hirschsprung disease in the newborn period: a multicenter analysis of outcomes. Ann Surg 2000;232:372–80.

26. Georgeson KE, Cohen RD, Hebra A, et al. Primary laparoscopic-assisted endorectal colon pull-through for Hirschsprung's disease: a new gold standard. Ann Surg 1999;229:678–682; discussion 682–73.

27. Santos MC, Giacomantonio JM, Lau HY. Primary Swenson pull-through compared with multiple-stage pull-through in the neonate. J Pediatr Surg 1999;34:1079–81.

28. Martin LW, Caudill DR. A method for elimination of the blind rectal pouch in the Duhamel operation for Hirschsprung's disease. Surgery 1967;62:951–3.

29. Soave F. A New Surgical Technique for Treatment of Hirschsprung's Disease. Surgery 1964;56:1007–14.

30. Curran TJ, Raffensperger JG. Laparoscopic Swenson pull-through: a comparison with the open procedure. J Pediatr Surg 1996;31:1155–6; discussion 1156–7.

31. Smith BM, Steiner RB, Lobe TE. Laparoscopic Duhamel pullthrough procedure for Hirschsprung's disease in childhood. J Laparoendosc Surg 1994;4:273–6.

32. Georgeson KE, Fuenfer MM, Hardin WD. Primary laparoscopic pull-through for Hirschsprung's disease in infants and children. J Pediatr Surg 1995;30:1017–21; discussion 1021–22.

33. Yamataka A, Kobayashi H, Hirai S, et al. Laparoscopy-assisted transanal pull-through at the time of suction rectal biopsy: a new approach to treating selected cases of Hirschsprung disease. J Pediatr Surg 2006;41:2052–5.

34. Yamataka A, Yoshida R, Kobayashi H, et al. Laparoscopy-assisted suction colonic biopsy and intraoperative rapid acetylcholinesterase staining during transanal pull-through for Hirschsprung's disease. J Pediatr Surg 2002;37:1661–3.

35. Muensterer OJ, Chong A, Hansen EN, et al. Single-incision laparoscopic endorectal pull-through (SILEP) for hirschsprung disease. J Gastrointest Surg; 2010;14:1950–4.

36. Lynn HB, van Heerden JA. Rectal myectomy in Hirschsprung disease: a decade of experience. Arch Surg 1975;110:991–4.

37. deVries PA, Peña A. Posterior sagittal anorectoplasty. J Pediatr Surg 1982;17:638–43.

38. Pini-Prato A, Mattioli G, Giunta C, et al. Redo surgery in Hirschsprung disease: what did we learn? Unicentric experience on 70 patients. J Pediatr Surg; 2010;45:747–54.

39. Lawal TA, Chatoorgoon K, Collins MH, et al. Redo pull-through in Hirschsprung's disease for obstructive symptoms due to residual aganglionosis and transition zone bowel. J Pediatr Surg; 2011;46:342–7.

40. Minkes RK, Langer JC. A prospective study of botulinum toxin for internal anal sphincter hypertonicity in children with Hirschsprung's disease. J Pediatr Surg 2000;35:1733–6.

41. Patrus B, Nasr A, Langer JC, et al. Intrasphincteric botulinum toxin decreases the rate of hospitalization for postoperative obstructive symptoms in children with Hirschsprung disease. J Pediatr Surg; 2011;46:184–7.

42. Langer JC. Persistent obstructive symptoms after surgery for Hirschsprung's disease: development of a diagnostic and therapeutic algorithm. J Pediatr Surg 2004;39:1458–62.

43. Rescorla FJ, Morrison AM, Engles D, et al. Hirschsprung's disease. Evaluation of mortality and long-term function in 260 cases. Arch Surg 1992;127:934–41; discussion 941–42.

44 Sherman JO, Snyder ME, Weitzman JJ, et al. A 40-year multinational retrospective study of 880 Swenson procedures. J Pediatr Surg 1989;24:833–8.

45. Yanchar NL, Soucy P. Long-term outcome after Hirschsprung's disease: patients' perspectives. J Pediatr Surg 1999;34:1152–60.

46. Ieiri S, Nakatsuji T, Akiyoshi J, et al. Long-term outcomes and the quality of life of Hirschsprung disease in adolescents who have reached 18 years or older-a 47-year single-institute experience. J Pediatr Surg 2010;45:2398–402.

47. Gunnarsdottir A, Sandblom G, Arnbjornsson E, et al. Quality of life in adults operated on for Hirschsprung disease in childhood. J Pediatr Gastroenterol Nutr 2010;51:160–6.

48. van der Putte SC. Normal and abnormal development of the anorectum. J Pediatr Surg 1986;21:434–40.

49 Skandalakis JE, Gray SW, Ricketts R. Colon and rectum. In: Skandalakis JE, Gray SW (eds). Embryology for Surgeons: The Embryological Basis for the Treatment of Congenital Anomalies. Baltimore: William & Wilkins 1994;242–81.

50. Kluth D. Embryology of anorectal malformations. Semin Pediatr Surg 19;201–8.

51. Ikebukuro KI, Ohkawa H. Three-dimensional analysis of anorectal embryology. Pediatric Surgery International 1994;9:2–7.

52. Kluth D, Hillen M, Lambrecht W. The principles of normal and abnormal hindgut development. J Pediatr Surg 1995;30:1143–7.

53. Paidas CN, Morreale RF, Holoski KM, et al. Septation and differentiation of the embryonic human cloaca. J Pediatr Surg 1999; 34:877–84.

54. Stephens FD, Smith ED. Classification, identification, and assessment of surgical treatment of anorectal anomalies. Pediatric Surgery International 1986;1:200–5.

55. Vick LR, Gosche JR, Boulanger SC, et al. Primary laparoscopic repair of high imperforate anus in neonatal males. J Pediatr Surg 2007;42:1877–81.

56. Georgeson KE, Inge TH, Albanese CT. Laparoscopically assisted anorectal pull-through for high imperforate anus-a new technique. J Pediatr Surg 2000; 35:927–930; discussion 930–1.

57. Long FR, Hunter JV, Mahboubi S, et al. Tethered cord and associated vertebral anomalies in children and infants with imperforate anus: evaluation with MR imaging and plain radiography. Radiology 1996;200:377–82.

58. Karrer FM, Flannery AM, Nelson MD, Jr., et al. Anorectal malformations: evaluation of associated spinal dysraphic syndromes. J Pediatr Surg 1988;23:45–8.

59. Tsakayannis DE, Shamberger RC. Association of imperforate anus with occult spinal dysraphism. J Pediatr Surg 1995;30:1010–2.

60. Rich MA, Brock WA, Peña A. Spectrum of genitourinary malformations in patients with imperforate anus. Pediatric Surgery International 1988;3:110–3.

61. Sheldon CA, Gilbert A, Lewis AG, et al. Surgical implications of genitourinary tract anomalies in patients with imperforate anus. J Urol 1994;152:196–9.

62. Peña A, Hong A. Advances in the management of anorectal malformations. Am J Surg 2000;180:370–6.

63. Peña A. Management of anorectal malformations during the newborn period. World J Surg 1993;17:385–92.

64. Wangensteen OH, Rice CO. Imperforate Anus: A Method of Determining the Surgical Approach. Ann Surg 1930;92:77–81.

65. Narasimharao KL, Prasad GR, Katariya S, et al. Prone cross-table lateral view: an alternative to the invertogram in imperforate anus. Am J Roentgenol 1983;140:227–9.

66. Donaldson JS, Black CT, Reynolds M, et al. Ultrasound of the distal pouch in infants with imperforate anus. J Pediatr Surg 1989;24:465–8.

67. Sachs TM, Applebaum H, Touran T, et al. Use of MRI in evaluation of anorectal anomalies. J Pediatr Surg 1990;25:817–21.

68. Rintala RJ. Congenital anorectal malformations: anything new? J Pediatr Gastroenterol Nutr 2009;48 Suppl 2:S79–82.

69. Pakarinen MP, Rintala RJ. Management and outcome of low anorectal malformations. Pediatr Surg Int 2010;26:1057–63.

70. Moore TC. Advantages of performing the sagittal anoplasty operation for imperforate anus at birth. J Pediatr Surg 1990;25:276–7.

71. Goon HK. Repair of anorectal anomalies in the neonatal period. Pediatric Surgery International 1990;5:246–9.

72. Lima M, Tursini S, Ruggeri G, et al. Laparoscopically assisted anorectal pull-through for high imperforate anus: three years' experience. J Laparoendosc Adv Surg Tech A 2006;16:63–6.

73. Podevin G, Petit T, Mure PY, et al. Minimally invasive surgery for anorectal malformation in boys: a multicenter study. J Laparoendosc Adv Surg Tech A 2009;19 Suppl 1:S233–5.

74. Al-Hozaim O, Al-Maary J, AlQahtani A, et al. Laparoscopic-assisted anorectal pull-through for anorectal malformations: a systematic review and the need for standardization of outcome reporting. J Pediatr Surg 2010;45:1500–4.

75. Wilkins S, Peña A. The role of colostomy in the management of anorectal malformations. Pediatric Surgery International 1988;3:105–9.
76. Santulli TV. The treatment of imperforate anus and associated fistulas. Surg Gynecol Obstet 1952;95:601–14.
77. Rhoads JE, Pipes RL, Randall JP. A simultaneous abdominal and perineal approach in operations for imperforate anus with atresia of the rectum and rectosigmoid. Ann Surg 1948;127:552–6.
78. Kiesewetter WB. Imperforate anus II. The rationale and technic of the sacro-abdomino-perineal operation. J Pediatr Surg 1967;2:106–10.
79. Holt B, Pryor JP, Hendry WF. Male infertility after surgery for imperforate anus. J Pediatr Surg 1995;30:1677–9.
80. Holcomb GW, Gheissari A, O'Neill JA, et al. Surgical management of alimentary tract duplications. Ann Surg 1989;209:167–74.
81. Yousefzadeh DK, Bickers GH, Jackson JH, et al. Tubular colonic duplication-review of 1876–1981 literature. Pediatr Radiol 1983;13:65–71.
82. Stern LE, Warner BW. Gastrointestinal duplications. Semin Pediatr Surg 2000;9:135–40.
83. Hickey WF, Corson JM. Squamous cell carcinoma arising in a duplication of the colon: case report and literature review of squamous cell carcinoma of the colon and of malignancy complicating colonic duplication. Cancer 1981;47:602–9.
84. Davis WS, Allen RP, Favara BE, et al. Neonatal small left colon syndrome. Am J Roentgenol Radium Ther Nucl Med 1974;120:322–9.
85. Philippart AI, Reed JO, Georgeson KE. Neonatal small left colon syndrome: intramural not intraluminal obstruction. J Pediatr Surg 1975;10:733–40.
86. Stewart DR, Nixon GW, Johnson DG, et al. Neonatal small left colon syndrome. Ann Surg 1977;186:741–5.
87. Ellis H, Kumar R, Kostyrka B. Neonatal small left colon syndrome in the offspring of diabetic mothers-an analysis of 105 children. J Pediatr Surg 2009;44:2343–6.
88. Caplan MS, Jilling T. New concepts in necrotizing enterocolitis. Curr Opin Pediatr 2001;13:111–5.
89. Neu J, Walker WA. Necrotizing enterocolitis. N Engl J Med; 364:255–64.
90. Sigalet DL. Short bowel syndrome in infants and children: an overview. Semin Pediatr Surg 2001;10:49–55.
91. Horwitz JR, Lally KP, Cheu HW, et al. Complications after surgical intervention for necrotizing enterocolitis: a multicenter review. J Pediatr Surg 1995;30:994–998; discussion 998–9.
92. Karnak I, Ciftci AO, Senocak ME, et al. Colonic atresia: surgical management and outcome. Pediatr Surg Int 2001;17:631–5.
93. Haxhija EQ, Schalamon J, Hollwarth ME. Management of isolated and associated colonic atresia. Pediatr Surg Int 2011;27:411–6.
94. Grosfeld JL, Ballantine TV, Shoemaker R. Operative mangement of intestinal atresia and stenosis based on pathologic findings. J Pediatr Surg 1979;14:368–75.
95. Seo T, Ando H, Watanabe Y, et al. Colonic atresia and Hirschsprung's disease: importance of histologic examination of the distal bowel. J Pediatr Surg 2002;37:E19
96. Dassinger M, Jackson R, Smith S. Management of colonic atresia with primary resection and anastomosis. Pediatr Surg Int 2009;25:579–82.
97. Cox SG, Numanoglu A, Millar AJ, et al. Colonic atresia: spectrum of presentation and pitfalls in management. A review of 14 cases. Pediatr Surg Int 2005;21:813–8.

12 Functional colorectal disorders

Even though functional disorders of the lower GI tract do not usually constitute an emergency on a par with trauma or bleeding, these problems will cause a physician in training to pause on many occasions The major categories of functional disorders are constipation and anal incontinence. A significant proportion of health care dollars is spent annually on the diagnosis and treatment of these problems. As the population ages, individuals will be seen in the emergency department with the extreme consequences of these problems. Therefore, it is helpful to have a basic plan readily available for evaluation and treatment of these problems [1].

Constipation

Definition

The definition of constipation has varied. Patients will report constipation based on a change in their pattern of bowel movements, the effort required to evacuate stool, or the consistency of their stool. Less than three bowel movements in a 7-day period, excessive straining (more than 25% of the time) at stool, and impacted hard stools all constitute symptoms of the severe form of constipation [2]. Constipation in itself is not a health problem until it changes the patient's quality of life or if it is caused by another more serious disease process. This chapter will deal only with the intrinsic non-life-threatening causes of constipation.

Causes

There are several major causes of functional constipation: inadequate fiber or water intake, the use of constipating medications, colonic inertia and megacolon, and pelvic floor outlet obstruction.

Inadequate fiber or water intake is a consequence of industrialization. The recommended daily fiber intake is 25–30 g of insoluble fiber; the usual daily intake of fiber by members of Western industrialized societies is 10–14 g [3]. Members of nonindustrialized countries may ingest as much as 80 g of fiber daily. These extremes have produced different problems in these populations that the medical profession must contend with. Recommended water intake is about 2–3 L per day. Inadequate fiber and water results in small, hardened stools and poor peristalsis leading to constipation.

Several ingested products result in constipation. The most common are narcotics, diuretics, calcium channel blockers, and antidepressants. The mechanism of each is different, but all have been shown to cause constipation. Fortunately, the effects of most are reversible, and the secondary constipation will be relieved by discontinuing the medication. Long-term use of laxatives has not been shown to damage the bowel, but their effectiveness may vary.

Colonic inertia is an uncommon cause of severe constipation. The exact cause of colonic inertia is unknown but theories include a hormonal component or neurotransmitter dysfunction which results in diminished peristalsis [4]. The resulting delay in colonic transit time can lead to secondary colonic dilatation and megacolon. An idiopathic version occurs in a young females who report a bowel movement every 2–3 weeks accompanied by distention, bloating, and a lack of urge to defecate [5]. Some of these patients also have delayed small bowel transit. One must differentiate between patients with true colonic inertia and those with short segment or adult Hirschsprung's disease with anal manometry or rectal biopsy [6]. Devroede and Girard have reported constipation and outlet obstruction in psychologically, physically, or sexually traumatized patients, which suggests a psychologic component in some of these patients [7].

A special type of colonic dysfunction is seen in a patient with pseudo-obstruction of the colon, often called **Ogilvie's syndrome.** Classic Ogilvie's syndrome occurs in patients with retroperitoneal infiltration of cancer at the sympathetic and parasympathetic nerve plexus along the aorta at the base of the bowel mesentery. More commonly, the syndrome occurs in elderly patients receiving narcotics after an orthopedic or cardiac procedure with an antecedent history of mild to moderate constipation. This form of colonic dysfunction can result in disaster if not recognized and treated appropriately. These elderly patients have a significant risk of cecal or transverse colon perforation and a lessened response to local peritonitis which often makes clinical assessment difficult.

Pelvic floor outlet obstruction is another source of constipation caused by nonrelaxation of the puborectalis muscle, rectal intussus-ception, or a rectocele. Nonrelaxation of the puborectalis muscle has been called anismus or paradoxical pelvic floor contraction [8]. The various names suggest a poorly understood entity. The puborectalis, pelvic floor muscles, and/or external sphincter fail to relax during defecation and patients typically relate prolonged periods (more than 1 hour in some cases) of straining or use digital maneuvers to empty the rectum. This condition is an acquired or learned phenomenon that eventually causes colonic retention that may be confused with colonic inertia. Since this condition may respond to nonoperative biofeedback techniques and can affect the outcome of an operation for colonic inertia if misdiagnosed, efforts should be made to identify a nonrelaxing puborectalis muscle in all patients suspected of having colonic inertia.

Anal manometry, balloon expulsion testing, or defecography are useful in diagnosing outlet obstruction. Outlet obstruction has also been related to underlying psychologic factors including a need to control, a previous history of sexual abuse or physical abuse, or an event that caused the patient to change or forget their normal defecatory pattern. These factors should be considered when evaluating constipated patients.

Intussusception of the rectum (discussed in Chapter 15) is the formation of a funnel-shaped infolding of the rectum into itself without the complete expulsion of the rectum seen with rectal prolapse. However, internal intussusception of the rectum can be seen on defecography in normal asymptomatic individuals. Therefore, the evaluating physician must be cautious in attributing symptoms to the intussusception. The cause of the intussusception is variable. A redundant, mobile rectosigmoid junction may fold into the distal rectum by no fault of the patient, or a patient may strain excessively when the rectum is essentially empty and cause the rectum to funnel into itself. Neither theory is proven. The funnel of bowel, when large enough, will plug the upper portion of the anal canal and obstruct the outlet despite all efforts to evacuate the rectum. This may be the precursor to full rectal prolapse. Patients complain of the feeling of incomplete evacuation and strain to empty what they perceive to be as a bowel movement from the rectal vault. Intussusception is potentially surgically correctable and must be differentiated from a nonrelaxing puborectalis muscle which is not. Large rectoceles can also hinder evacuation. The need to digitally stent the posterior vagina or perineal body to assist evacuation suggests their functional significance.

Evaluation

The first priority when faced with a patient complaining of constipation is to take a history and perform a physical examination and endoscopy to rule out other life-threatening or significant causes of constipation. The majority of these patients have a fear of cancer and may only need reassurance that theirs is a benign process. Patients at high risk for colon cancer should be screened appropriately, since constipation is a change in bowel habits.

A simple trial of fiber may be the next step in evaluation. Psyllium (3 g orally once or twice a day) is usually an adequate supplement to restore regularity or normalcy to most diets and bowel patterns [9]. The upper limit of fiber supplementation is unknown; however, one should hesitate before prescribing more than 36 g of psyllium per day. The majority of patients with complaints of constipation, inadequate rectal emptying, rectal pressure, straining, hard stools, and irregularity will respond to fiber supplementation with adequate water intake and need no further treatment. Thus a fiber trial is not only a test but a treatment and should be the initial step before embarking on an otherwise costly workup.

The workup for severe constipation not resulting from Hirschsprung's disease includes colonic transit times, and balloon expulsion or defecography. These tests help to differentiate among colonic inertia, internal intussusception, and a nonrelaxing puborectalis muscle as the cause of the problem.

Colonic transit times are evaluated by giving a gel capsule containing 24 radiopaque markers or a meal containing 24 slices of a nasogastric tube (1 mm thick) followed by anterior-posterior abdominal X-ray examinations 1, 3 and 5 days later (see Figure 4.29) [10]. It is helpful to have the patient on a known dose of fiber supplement (e.g. 1 tsp/3 g psyllium bid). The markers should progress to the rectum by day 3 and be expelled from the rectum by day 5. If more than 20% of the markers are scattered throughout the colon on day 3 and this pattern persists by day 5, this is consistent with colonic inertia. Movement of at least 80% of the markers to the rectum by day 3 and retention of the markers in the rectum to day 5 is consistent with outlet obstruction.

Balloon expulsion is a very simple maneuver, usually performed in conjunction with anal manometry but possible to perform as a specific test. A latex manometry or helium balloon is inflated with 60 mL of air, water or saline solution within the rectum. The patient is asked to expel the balloon in a private bathroom using any means other than pulling out or deflating the balloon [11]. Straining to expel the balloon for less than 8 minutes denotes normal expulsion time. While there is potential for variation and inaccuracy, this test has been shown to reliably predict the presence of a nonrelaxing puborectalis muscle or rectal dysmotility [12]. Other tests of rectal evacuation have been described including defecating scintigraphy and anal surface electrode electromyography (Chapters 2 and 4). Failure to empty the rectum and relax the puborectalis muscle may be artifactual or be the result of patient embarrassment as well as true paradoxical motion of the puborectalis muscle.

Defecography is performed using cinefluoroscopy to obtain video images of the rectum from the lateral view during the patient's attempts to evacuate barium thickened with methylcellulose from the rectal vault (see Figure 4.30). Contrast medium in the small bowel and vagina provide additional information about the anterior pelvis and cul-de-sac. A special commode seat is used to improve images at the air-anal interface. The defecogram will demonstrate internal intussusception, an impression on the posterior rectum made by the puborectalis muscle during paradoxical motion, anterior displacement of the posterior wall of the vagina (rectocele), downward impression of the small intestine on the vagina (enterocele), and incomplete emptying of the rectum. The defecogram is very sensitive and there is a documented incidence of intussusception, a nonrelaxing puborectalis muscle, rectocele, and enterocele in asymptomatic controls [13, 14]. The diagnosis of a nonrelaxing puborectalis muscle made by defecography should be confirmed by both balloon expulsion and colonic transit time evaluation.

Treatment

Inadequate fiber

Supplementation of fiber in the diet is simple. Insoluble fiber is found in the form of psyllium or other vegetable fiber. The highest fiber content in vegetable form is found in broccoli, green peas, and bran cereals. The addition of fiber is effective in more than 90% of patients with constipation [15]. As mentioned earlier, a maximum of 36 g of fiber in a 24-hour period should be adequate; this must be accompanied by appropriate amounts of water to avoid concretions of fiber.

Colonic inertia

The first line of treatment of colonic inertia is a high dose of fiber. Some patients may also require the addition of laxatives to stimulate motility. It is important to avoid irritant laxatives, since these can make the problem worse.

Several motility agents are available. Cisapride (Propulsid, Janssen, Pharmaceuticals, Titusville, NJ, USA) which stimulates peristolic activity in the small bowel and colon, is very effective. Unfortunately, due to an association with serious cardiac arrhythmias, this drug is currently available only as part of very restrictive protocols. Erythromycin has also been documented as a motility agent. Another option is a 17 g dose of a polyethylene glycol laxative (Miralax, Braintree Laboratory, Braintree, MA, USA) taken orally on a daily basis to propel colonic contents [16, 17]. A colonic chloride channel activator, lubiprostone (Amitiza, Takeda Pharmaceutical America) is also available for the treatment of chronic constipation.

Only when medical therapy has failed and the patient remains symptomatic should surgical treatment of constipation be considered [18]. A patient with colonic inertia who has been diagnosed by evaluation of colonic transit times and who has no evidence of pelvic floor outlet obstruction may be considered for a total colectomy and ileorectal anastomosis [18–20]. Lesser operations, such as a segmental resection, have resulted in a high rate of recurrence of constipation. Long-term results of total colectomy, in properly selected patients, have been good [20]. For patients older than 70 years of age and those with anal incontinence, special consideration should be given to their having a colectomy and ileostomy. Diarrhea can be as debilitating as constipation, and diarrhea in combination with anal incontinence is worse than a permanent ostomy. Therefore complete evaluation of the anal canal is helpful in any patient with colonic inertia for whom surgery is contemplated if there is a possibility of anal sphincter dysfunction.

Pseudo-obstruction of the colon

A patient in the hospital, recovering from a nonabdominal procedure, who develops massive abdominal distention from an acute dilatation of the colon poses a challenging management problem. The first therapeutic maneuver is to remove all constipating agents from the treatment plan if possible. This includes narcotics, calcium channel blockers, and psycholeptic agents. There is controversy over the order in which the subsequent evaluations or treatments should proceed. Colonoscopy, water soluble enemas, neostigmine, and epidural injection of anesthetic agents have all been used to treat colonic pseudo-obstruction.

Epidural anesthesia at the thoracic/lumbar area will result in a block of the sympathetic fibers at the base of the colonic mesentery, producing unhindered peristalsis of the colon and decompression of the colon through the rectum. This is especially helpful in a patient in the intensive care unit who cannot be moved to the radiology or endoscopy suites. Success is variable with this technique, but it should be considered before recommending operative decompression [21].

Neostigmine is parasympathomimetic drug that has shown impressive results in several studies [22, 23]. A dosage of 2.5 mg given intravenously over 1–3 minutes produces evacuation of the colon. Administration of this drug should be performed with close monitoring of cardiac rhythm and blood pressure. Atropine should be available to treat bradycardia; neostigmine is contraindicated in patients on beta blockers and those who are acidotic or have suffered recent myocardial infarctions.

The use of a water soluble (Hypaque or Gastrografin) enema has both diagnostic and therapeutic potential in the treatment of pseudo-obstruction. In most patients, the colon can be decompressed with fluoroscopic guidance of a water-soluble contrast medium through the entire colon. A subsequent mass peristalsis after controlled distention and further dilution of the usually semiliquid stool in the colon can empty the entire colon. The use of water soluble contrast avoids barium concretions within the colon if decompression is unsuccessful and barium peritonitis if perforation should occur. The diagnosis of obstructing cancer or volvulus is also easily made.

Colonoscopic decompression of a dilated colon is possible if the contents are gas or liquid [24]. However, this is not always predictable. The skill of the colonoscopist greatly influences the outcome and care must be taken to avoid overinflation of the colon during efforts to negotiate stool and anatomy. It is sometimes helpful to leave a colonic tube in the colon proximal to the sigmoid colon to facilitate decompression. The tube can be dragged to the level of the left colon or placed as an oversheath on the colonoscope. The tube can lead to erosion through the colonic wall if left in place too long.

The decision to intervene surgically depends on the clinical status of the patient and the presence of signs that suggest impending perforation of the colon. The colon is most likely to perforate from ischemia at the cecum. However, the transverse colon and sigmoid colon have also been known to be the site of perforation. The options for operative therapy include decompressing loop transverse colostomy, cecostomy, segmental colectomy and ileostomy, or total abdominal colectomy. Loop transverse colostomy or cecostomy are temporizing maneuvers that should only be used in a patient with no peritoneal signs in whom all conservative measures have failed. A cecostomy is used infrequently because it is not very effective and almost always results in a fecal fistula that requires operative closure. The transverse colostomy is a simple procedure that can be performed under local or epidural anesthesia. A helpful practice is to place a coin over the umbilicus and obtain an abdominal X-ray film before marking the site of the planned stoma over the most dilated portion of the transverse colon. A blowhole colostomy (see Figure 7.8) using only one side of the colon wall is all that is necessary [25]. The opening may close spontaneously when the patient returns to a normal state.

In the unlikely event that the colon looks ischemic at the time of exploration, the decision to perform a colonic resection is the only reasonable plan. The extent of resection may be the most difficult decision in that instance. Right colonic ischemia necessitates at least a right colectomy, but the patient may be better served by a total abdominal colectomy with ileostomy and rectal stump, ileorectal anastomosis, or ileorectal anastomosis and protecting loop ileostomy. When a right colectomy is performed, the small bowel may be reanastomosed to the transverse colon and protected with a loop ileostomy. This decision should be based on the state of the transverse colon-whether it is full of stool or dilated with air and essentially clean. If the transverse colon is filled with stool, a mucous fistula may be necessary. Once again, a total abdominal colectomy may be more appropriate in this circumstance.

Pelvic floor outlet obstruction

Nonrelaxation of the puborectalis muscle has been treated successfully with biofeedback techniques [26]. Patients with this condition respond to a form of operant conditioning using surface electromyography, balloon expulsion, and simulated rectal filling using a psyllium slurry. The principle behind the technique is to document the existence of the problem to the patient's satisfaction, restore the sensation of rectal filling and anal canal relaxation, and restore spontaneous rectal evacuation using only the abdominal muscles to raise the intra-abdominal pressure. Psychologic testing has shown that these patients score high in the areas of need to control and anxiety. Thus it is helpful to have them receive relaxation training before embarking on their operant conditioning therapy. The conditioning can be performed in an outpatient setting in the clinic or at home after instructional sessions. Success can be expected in 80% of patients treated in this way.

The pelvic floor outlet obstruction due to severe internal intussusception may respond to high doses of fiber (>18g/day). If this is unsuccessful, an operation to remove the internal prolapse or fix the mobile segment of the rectum to the sacrum should be contemplated (see Chapter 15).

Anal incontinence

Definition

Anal incontinence is the inability to control the release of rectal contents until a socially acceptable time and place. There are varying degrees of anal incontinence, depending on the type of material leaked (gas, liquid, or solid) and the frequency with which incontinence occurs [28]. However, the critical feature in determining the significance of anal incontinence is the patient's perception that the incontinence severely affects quality of life. Thus only one episode of incontinence of solid stool at a public event may be enough to cause a patient to consider the problem significant. Another patient may consider the problem significant only if the incontinence is recurrent on a frequent basis (weekly or monthly). The loss of gas may be significant to one patient and not to another. The problem of incontinence is becoming more prevalent or at least recognized more frequently, especially in nursing homes.

Causes

Anal incontinence may be primarily related to anal sphincter function or to altered rectal capacity and bowel function. Sphincter function may be altered as a result of mechanical or neurogenic causes. There is a small group of incontinent patients in whom no cause can be determined for their loss of control.

Mechanical injury

The most common cause of mechanical injury to the anal sphincter is obstetric trauma, especially from a midline episiotomy during vaginal delivery [27]. There is a higher likelihood of persistent sphincter dysfunction after a third- or fourth-degree episiotomy (third degree, into the rectal muscle; fourth degree, through rectal muscle and mucosa). An estimated 2% of all patients who undergo episiotomy at the time of vaginal delivery will develop anal incontinence. Mechanical injury to the sphincter is more likely to occur with midline than mediolateral episiotomy. An injury to the external sphincter in the anterior midline in a woman results in a weakening of the muscle at its weakest point. Disruption of the circular sphincter mechanism will result in varying degrees of incontinence of solid, liquid, or gas. The puborectalis sling at the posterior aspect of the anorectal ring is responsible for control of solid stool and may prevent loss of solid stool even when the entire anterior mechanism is disrupted. The external sphincter below the puborectalis is probably responsible for the control of liquid and gas. The complexity of factors involved in anal continence (sensation, rectal capacity, stool consistency, muscle integrity) prevent one from predicting an exact consequence in terms of function based on anatomic defect. However, injury to the anterior portion of the anal sphincter mechanism will often result in a functional problem.

Other causes of mechanical injury to the anal sphincter include anorectal trauma and fistulotomy for Crohn's fistula or cryptoglandular disease. Transecting the sphincter in the lateral and posterior quadrants of the anal canal usually does not result in major anal incontinence. Patients with mechanical injury to the anal sphincter may report leakage of liquid or mucus or gas. However, transection of the anterior sphincter mechanism (except the most superficial fibers) will result in significant dysfunction consistent with that seen with obstetric injury.

Neurogenic causes

Injury to the innervation of the anal canal usually occurs at the level of the pudendal nerves, which are terminal motor and sensory fibers of roots S2–4. The pudendal nerves travel through the ischiorectal fossa from Alcock's canal at the ischial spine to the posterolateral aspect of the external sphincter on either side of the anal canal. These nerves can be injured by stretch (during chronic straining, childbirth, or procidentia), systemic diseases (multiple sclerosis, diabetes), or local trauma (drainage of ischiorectal fosa abscess, rectal trauma) [28–31]. The injury of one pudendal nerve may not cause incontinence, but bilateral injury inevitably will result in significant incontinence.

Rectal prolapse is associated with anal incontinence in 60% of patients before repair and resolves in half of patients after repair. Persistent incontinence can be attributed to pure neurogenic incontinence in approximately half of these (i.e. 15%) of patients [30].

Irritable bowel syndrome (IBS)

It is not uncommon to see patients who complain of diarrhea alternating with constipation, abdominal cramps, bloating, food intolerance, and occasionally anal incontinence. This irritable bowel complex must be differentiated from inflammatory bowel disease, bacterial or other forms of colitis, and viral illness. It also is unusual for a patient with IBS to have incontinence without at least some mild defect in the anal sphincter. The volume and urgency of diarrhea required to overwhelm a normal sphincter is usually not produced by IBS.

Diminished rectal capacity

Radiation-induced or inflammatory bowel disease induced fibrosis of the rectum will reduce rectal capacity. The reduction in holding capacity can cause the sphincter mechanism to be overwhelmed by liquid or soft stool. The long-term consequences of pelvic radiation of greater than 50 Gy are fibrosis, vascular telangiectasias, and atrophy of the mucosa. Unfortunately, these are not reversible. The sphincter is unable to provide adequate pressure to resist transmitted sigmoid peristalsis, because the rectal vault can no longer accept the volume and pressure change. Pelvic radiation at the doses used for rectal and prostate cancer have little effect on the anal sphincter itself [32].

Idiopathic causes

Patients who cannot be fitted into the preceding diagnostic groups are considered to have idiopathic anal incontinence. This group is now small. In the past, those patients with neurogenic incontinence or unrecognized sphincter injury were considered to have idiopathic incontinence. Improved diagnostic methods have all but eliminated this group. Patients with occult prolapse and incontinence can be diagnosed with defecography. Nerve injury can be identified with electromyography. The complete workup for anal incontinence must be unrevealing before including a patient in this diagnostic group, because there is essentially no medical surgical or biofeedback therapy that has been shown to be effective.

Evaluation

Office evaluation of the patient complaining of incontinence begins with a detailed history that focuses on bowel habits, especially any recent change, and deals with the presence of urgency, frequency, and loss of stool. The nature of the incontinence should be quantitatively documented (i.e. type of incontinence, how often). A past history of obstetric injury, anal procedure, or rectal prolapse should be elicited. The details of abnormal straining patterns during defecation will also be pertinent.

Examination of the anal canal and perineum should include a digital rectal examination, which provides data regarding anal sphincter length, resting and squeezing tone, proper relaxation of the puborectalis during straining and contraction during squeeze, and an assessment of the thickness of the tissue in the rectovaginal septum and perineal body. The presence of a fistula between the rectum and vagina will usually be apparent on proctoscopy, as will inflammatory or fibrotic changes of the rectum that limit distensibility.

Anal physiology

The complete objective evaluation of the anal canal includes anal manometry, measurement of pudendal nerve terminal motor latency (PNTML) with electromyographic techniques, and endoluminal ultrasound of the anal sphincter [33]. Anal manometry can be performed in numerous ways, but the parameters measured should be the same. Anal canal resting and squeeze pressure in each quadrant throughout the length of the sphincter are the most important features [28]. Normal rest pressure is 40 mmHg and maximal squeeze pressure is at least 80 mmHg. Minimal sensory volume is measured by incremental inflation of a latex balloon within the rectum and normal is 20 mL of air. A mechanical sphincter defect will give a decreased rest and squeeze pressure in the quadrant of injury, but sensory volumes will be normal. Neurogenic incontinence will show normal rest pressure (the internal sphincter is normal and innervated by autonomic fibers) but diffusely low squeeze pressures and an increased sensory volume. Fibrotic changes of the rectum may or may not involve the sphincter. If not involved, the sphincter may be normal on testing. The only abnormality may be a very low sensory volume, indicating hypersensitivity and poor compliance of the distal rectum.

Measurement of PNTML using a stimulating and recording electrode on a disposable glove yields information about nerve conduction in the terminal fibers of the pudendal nerve [34]. Normal conduction time from Alcock's canal at the ischial spine to the external sphincter via the large, fast-conducting fibers is 2.0 +/− 0.2. A delay in conduction indicates damage to the larger fast-conducting fibers [35]. It is possible to have unilateral or bilateral nerve damage with corresponding unilateral or bilateral prolonged PNTML. Nerve stretch or systemic disease can cause a delay, whereas transection will result in an inability to identify any electrical activity. Spinal cord injury may cause pudendal nerve abnormality by virtue of antegrade degeneration after proximal nerve root injury.

Endoluminal ultrasound has become the method of choice for mapping or detecting anal sphincter defects (**Figure 12.1**) [36]. A probe with a 10 MHz rotating transducer gives a 360° cross-sectional image of the anal canal. The internal sphincter appears as a thick hypoechoic band surrounded by the thicker variable-echoic circular fibers of the external sphincter (see Figure 4.12). Hyperechoic lines within the external sphincter probably represent interfaces between fascicles. A mechanical defect will appear as a break in the symmetry of the circular patterns of the internal and external sphincter. Scar has a diffuse, more hyperechoic pattern than the internal sphincter but is less echogenic than the external sphincter and lacks the hyperechoic bands. Fistula tracts can also be identified as an absence of echogenicity in a traceable line through the sphincter.

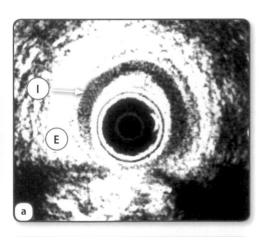

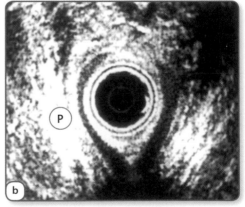

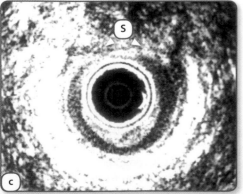

Figure 12.1 Ultrasounds of the anal sphincter.
(a) Transanal ultrasound demonstrating a normal hypoechoic internal sphincter (I) surrounded by the external sphincter (E). (b) Transanal ultrasound demonstrating a normal puborectalis muscle (P). (c) Transanal ultrasound demonstrating replacement by scar (S) of the normal sphincters in a patient with a sphincter defect.

Treatment
Medical

Minor incontinence, caused by either neurogenic or mechanical defects, usually responds to medical management that consists of added bulk-forming agents, constipating agents, such as loperamide, and a stimulated bowel routine with suppositories and/or enemas in the morning to empty the rectum as needed. As the severity of incontinence increases, medical management becomes less effective. It is at this point that surgical intervention may be considered to correct a mechanical cause of incontinence. Neurogenic incontinence has not responded to operations to reef sphincters, plicate the pelvic floor, or encircle the anal canal. Biofeedback and sacral nerve stimulation or an artificial sphincter have shown the best results. Biofeedback or operant conditioning are most successful in patients with minor degrees of mechanically induced incontinence in whom viable, functioning, innervated sphincter exists [36].

Operant conditioning uses manometry or surface anal electromyography to show the patient his or her own squeeze efforts. The objective is to both strengthen the muscles and make the squeeze efforts more timely and efficient. Anorectal sensation is also improved as the patient coordinates squeezes to a progressively smaller volume of air in a latex balloon. These patients are also the most likely to have an excellent outcome after an anal sphincter reconstruction.

Surgical

If medical therapy is inadequate and a defect in the sphincter mechanism is determined, a plan of treatment can be determined (**Figure 12.2**). **Sphincteroplasty** involves identifying the scarred, separated ends of the anal sphincter muscles in the lateral aspects of the perineal body and either reefing them in the midline or performing an overlapping repair. The procedure has been used extensively with good success in patients with obstetric injury and incontinence (**Figure 12.3**) [37]. If there is no associated nerve injury, there is a 75% chance of restoration of complete control of solid, liquid, and gas [38].

Patients with irretrievable neurogenic anal incontinence (e.g. patients who fail to recover control after repair of rectal prolapse) or those with severely injured sphincter muscles as a result of perineal and rectal trauma are now considered candidates for some of the newer techniques, such as the artificial sphincter (ABS) or sacral nerve stimulation [39,40]. Patients who can not be helped with these options or desires only one procedure with minimal risk may be best served by a standard **colostomy** after a very low Hartmann resection of the rectum.

The **artificial bowel sphincter** (ABS) is a device similar to that used for urinary incontinence. A urinary device was initially successfully placed around the anus in 1987 and has been subsequently modified for the use around the anus. The procedure involves creating a subcutaneous tunnel around the anus, typically through a transverse perineal

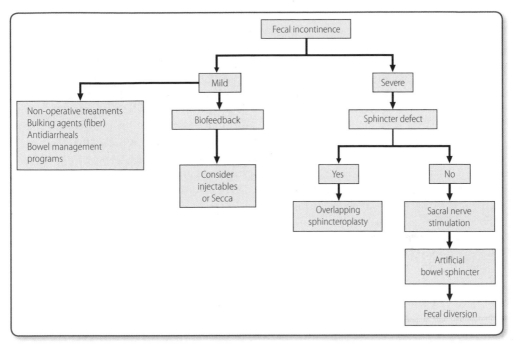

Figure 12.2 Algorithm for evaluation and management of anal incontinence.

incision. The cuff is situated around the anus. The pump is tunneled through a pfannensteil incision down to either the labia or scrotum, while the reservoir is placed in the space of retzius. (**Figure 12.3**). All of the tubing is tunneled subcutaneously. The device provides continence by keeping the perianal cuff full in the resting state. When the patient needs to evacuate, he/she needs to actively pump fluid from the cuff to the reservoir. The cuff will then passively refill. The device has a higher failure rate in patients who lack adequate soft tissue in the perineum to cover the devices and prevent erosion. It is also important that the patient has the manual dexterity to activate the device.

Infection has been the greatest challenge for patients and surgeons utilizing the artificial bowel sphincter. The results of a multi-center trial were published by Wong et al in 2002 [42]. Of the 112 patients implanted there were 384 device related adverse events in 99 patients. Seventy-three revisional operations were performed in 51(46%) patients and 25% of patients developed infection requiring surgical revision. Forty-one (37%) patients had devices completely explanted. While the intention to treat success rate was low at 53%, 85% of patients with a functional device had a successful outcome. Recent reports of the long-term outcome for patients with the artificial bowel sphincter have been published [43]. With a mean follow-up was 68 months (range: 3–133), all 17 patients had some complication and 65% required at least one re-operation. As with other published series, 53% of the patients had an implanted device at follow-up. Those patients enjoyed the benefit of

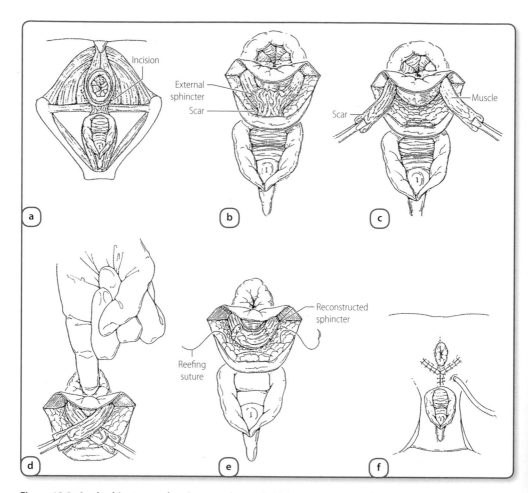

Figure 12.3 Anal sphincter overlapping muscle repair. (a) Anterior incision and perineal view of muscles. (b) Rectal flap is created and sphincter muscles are isolated. (c) Muscle flaps are fully mobilized. (d) Muscle flaps are overlapped around a 15 mm rubber dilator or fingertip. (e) Muscle flaps are sutured in place and the perineal body is repaired. (f) Drain is placed behind the vaginal wall and closed.

improved quality of life and significantly decreased fecal incontinence scores. Factors associated with failure include an early first post-operative bowel movement and a history of perineal sepsis. Early failure was more often related to infectious complications, while late failure was related to device associated mechanical complications [44]. The major challenge of this treatment for fecal incontinence is infection followed by device-related complications.

Sacral nerve stimulation (SNS) or neuromodulation was initially developed for the management of urinary incontinence. It was subsequently noted that in patients with fecal incontinence treated with SNS for urinary incontinence, the fecal incontinence also improved. This observation prompted use of SNS in patients with fecal incontinence [45]. Unlike other therapeutic modalities, SNS is a staged procedure. The first stage is the percutaneous nerve evaluation (PNE) which serves as a feasibility trial period lasting 2 weeks. Patients who experience an improvement of 50% or greater decrease in the number of incontinence episodes progress to the final stage and are offered placement of a permanent stimulator.

The electrode placement is performed under sterile conditions with fluoroscopic guidance. Stimulation of the S2, S3, and S4 nerve roots via their sacral foramina is tested. The goal is to elicit contraction of the levator ani and external anal sphincter with plantar flexion of the first two toes, seen with stimulation of S3. The purpose of direct stimulation of the sacral nerves is to recruit additional inactive motor units to improve muscle strength, resulting in an increase in resting anal pressure and to improve the rectal sensory threshold and balloon expulsion time [46,47].

Both the initial PNE and subsequent placement of the permanent stimulator are performed on an outpatient basis. Complications are rare and have all been minor with lead migration being most typical. Other complications include infection leading to explantation of the stimulator and pain attributed to either the leads or the stimulator [48].

An obvious benefit of sacral nerve stimulation is that it avoids creation of an incision around or near the anal canal. This avoids further anal scarring and decreases the risk of infection. Some authors have proposed SNS as the first line option due to the observed improved continence and decreased rate of outlet obstruction [49]. Promising short and long-term success has been reported with significant and sustained decreases in the Cleveland Clinic Florida Fecal Incontinence Score [50]. The device has obtained FDA approval for fecal incontinence in the United States and it has been used extensively in other countries [51].

Fecal diversion with a colostomy or ileostomy is typically the therapeutic option of last resort, when all other reasonable options have been exhausted. Most patients will be best served with an end sigmoid colostomy, but some patients with chronic constipation and slow transit may do better with an ileostomy. Acceptance of a stoma can be difficult even in the face of severe and debilitating incontinence. Patient education and a visit by an enterostomal therapist or a patient already with an ostomy can greatly ease anxiety.

Patients with irritable bowel syndrome or inflammatory bowel disease (IBD) have altered colorectal function. Management of these conditions is the subject of many books and cannot be covered in-depth here. The treatment of incontinence associated with these diseases works to normalize bowel function as much as possible using bulking agents and antidiarrheal and antispasmodic medications as needed. IBD will also require other disease-specific medications that are not necessarily related to bowel pattern but that will affect bowel function as the disease resolves. A rectum that is fibrotic as a result of radiation therapy or inflammatory changes poses a special problem that may respond to the medical management protocol suggested for minor sphincter problems. However, if the sphincter is normal, the rectum unusable, and the patient is a suitable candidate, a proctectomy with coloanal anastomosis may be considered [52]. The indications for this are rare and the procedure exceedingly difficult in patients with radiation injury to the pelvis. Once again, a colostomy may better serve these individuals.

In patients with idiopathic incontinence, the addition of bulking agents, long sessions of counseling, and reassurance are often all that is needed for these patients. It is occasionally worthwhile to restudy an individual with 'idiopathic' incontinence, since a definable, treatable cause may be found. Otherwise, the patient should be allowed to continue as before, since no procedure is appropriate. Biofeedback using operant conditioning techniques to help the patient strengthen unused muscles or relearn the signal for an impending bowel movement may be useful but will usually need to be repeated.

Rounds questions

1. Define constipation.
2. What are the major causes of constipation?
3. What is the first priority in evaluating a constipated patient?
4. What should the work-up include for non-Hirschsprung's severe constipation?
5. What is the appropriate therapy for a symptomatic constipated patient with documented colonic inertia, no evidence of pelvic floor outlet obstruction, and who has failed medical therapy?
6. What options are available to treat pseudo-obstruction of the colon?
7. Define anal incontinence.
8. What are the causes of anal incontinence?
9. What tests are used to objectively evaluate the anal canal?

References

1. Camilleri M, Thompson WG, Fleshman JW, et al. Clinical management of intractable constipation. Ann Intern Med 1994;121:520–8.
2. Thompson WG, Creed F, Drossman DA, et al. Functional bowel disease and functional abdominal pain. Gastroenterol Int 1992;5:75–91.
3. Burkitt DP, Walker AR, Painter NS. Effect of dietary fibre on stools and transit-times, and its role in the causation of disease. Lancet 1972;2:1408–12.
4. von der Ohe MR, Camilleri M, Carryer PW. A patient with localized megacolon and intractable constipation: Evidence for impairment of colonic muscle tone. Am J Gastroenterol 1994;89:1867–70.
5. Beck DE. Colectomy for colonic inertia. Seminars in Colon and Rectal Surgery 1992;3:115–9.
6. Pemberton JH. Anorectal and pelvic floor disorders: Putting physiology into practice. J Gastroenterol Hepatol 1990;5:127–43.
7. Devroede G, Girard G, Bouchoucha M, et al. Idiopathic constipation by colonic dysfunction: Relationship with personality and anxiety. Dig Dis Sci 1989;34:1428–33.
8. Kuijpers HC, Bleijenberg G. The spastic pelvic floor syndrome. A cause of constipation. Dis Colon Rectum 1985;28:669–72.
9. Cummings JH. Constipation, dietary fibre and the control of large bowel function. Postgrad Med J 1984;60:811–9.
10. Hinton JM, Lennard-Jones JE, Young AC. A new method for studying gut transit times using radioopaque markers. Gut 1969;10:842–7.

11. Beck DE. Simplified balloon expulsion test. Dis Colon Rectum 1992;35:597–8.
12. Fleshman JW, Dreznik Z, Cohen E, et al. Balloon expulsion test facilitates diagnosis of pelvic floor outlet obstruction due to nonrelaxing puborectalis muscle. Dis Colon Rectum 1992;35:1019–25.
13. Goei R, van Engelshoven J, Schouten H, et al. Anorectal function: Defecographic measurement in asymptomatic subjects. Radiology 1989;173:137–41.
14. Goei R. Anorectal function in patients with defecation disorders and asymptomatic subjects: evaluation with defecography. Radiology 1990;174:121–3.
15. Murtagh J. Constipation. Aust Fam Physician 1990;19:1693–7.
16. Andorsky RI, Goldner F. Colonic lavage solution (polyethylene glycol electrolyte lavage solution) as a treatment for chronic constipation: A double-blind, placebo-controlled study. Am J Gastroenterol 1990;85:261–5.
17. Dipalma JA, DeRidder PH, Orlando RC, et al. A randomized, placebo-controlled multicenter study of the safety and efficacy of a new polyethylene glycol laxative. Am J Gastroenterol 2000;95:446–50.
18. Pemberton JH, Rath DM, Ilstrup DM. Evaluation and surgical treatment of severe chronic constipation. Ann Surg 1991;214:403–11.
19. Beck DE, Fazio VW, Jagelman DG, Lavery IC. Surgical management of colonic inertia. South Med J 1989;82:305–9.
20. Pikarsky AJ, Singh JJ, Weiss EG, et al. Long-term follow-up of patients undergoing colectomy for colonic inertia. Dis Colon Rectum 2001;44:179–83.
21. Lee JT, Taylor BM, Singleton BC. Epidural anesthesia for acute pseudo-obstruction of the colon (Ogilvie's syndrome). Dis Colon Rectum 1988;31:686–91.
22. Stephenson BM, Morgan AR, Salaman JR, Wheeler MH. Ogilvie's syndrome: A new approach to an old problem. Dis Colon Rectum 1995;38:424–7.
23. Turegano-Fuentes F, Munoz-Jimenez F, Del Valle-Hernandez E, et al. Early resolution of Ogilvie's syndrome with intravenous neostigmine: a simple, effective treatment. Dis Colon Rectum 1997;40:1353–1357.
24. Geller A, Petersen BT, Gostout CJ. Endoscopic decompression for actue colonic pseudo-obstruction. Gastrointest Endosc 1996;44:144–50.
25. Turnbull RB, Hawk WA, Weakley FL. Surgical treatment of toxic megacolon. Ileostomy and colostomy to prepare patients for colectomy. Am J Surg 1971;122:325–31.
26. Kuijpers HC, Bleijenberg G. Assessment and treatment of obstructed defecation. Ann Med 1990;22:405–11.
27. Miller R, Bartolo DCC, Locke-Edmunds JC, et al. Prospective study of conservative and operative treatment for faecal incontinence. Br J Surg 1988;75:101.
28. Fleshman JW, Kodner IJ, Fry RD, et al. Anal incontinence. In: Zuimeda GD (ed). Shackelford's Surgery of the Alimentary Tract, vol 4. Philadelphia: WB Saunders, 1996.
29. Jones PN, Lubowski DZ, Swash M, et al. Relation between perineal descent and pudendal nerve damage in idiopathic fecal incontinence. Int J Colorectal Dis 1987;2:93–5.
30. Snooks SJ, Henry MM, Swash M. Anorectal incontinence and rectal prolapse: Differential assessment of the innervation to puborectalis and external anal sphincter muscles. Gut 1985;26:470–6.
31. Neill ME, Parks AG, Swash M. Physiological studies of the anal musculature in faecal incontinence and rectal prolapse. Br J Surg 1981;68:531–6.
32. Birnbaum EH, Dreznik Z, Myerson RJ, et al. Early effect of external beam radiation therapy on the anal sphincter: A study using anal monometry and transrectal ultrasound. Dis Colon Rectum 1992;35:757–61.
33. Smith LE. Practical Guide to Anorectal Testing. 2nd ed. New York: Igaku-Shoin, 1995.
34. Fleshman JW. Determination of pudendal nerve terminal motor latency. In: Smith LE. Practical Guide to Anorectal Testing, 2nd ed. New York: Igaku-Shoin 1995.
35. Kiff ES, Swash M. Slowed conduction in the pudendal nerves in idiopathic (neurogenic) faecal incontinence. Br J Surg 1984;71:614–6.
36. Tjandra JJ, Milsom JW, Stolfi VM, et al. Endoluminal ultrasound defines anatomy of the anal canal and pelvic floor. Dis Colon Rectum 1992;35:465–70.
37. Goldberg SM, Gordon PH, Nivatvongs S. Essentials of Anorectal Surgery. Philadephia: JB Lippincott, 1980:389.
38. Fleshman JW, Peters WR, Shemesh EI, et al. Anal sphincter reconstruction: Anterior overlapping muscle repair. Dis Colon Rectum 1991;34:739–43.
39. Hetzer FH, Hahnloser D, Clavien PA, Demartines N. Quality of life and morbidity after permanent sacral nerve stimulation for fecal incontinence. Arcg Surg 2007;142:8–13.
40. Madoff RD, Baeten CG, Christiansen J, et al. Standards for anal sphincter replacement. Dis Colon Rectum 2000;43:135–41.

41. Christiansen J, Lorentzen M. Implantation of artificial sphincter for anal incontinence. Lancet 1987;2(8553):244–5.

42. Wong WD, Congliosi SM, Spencer MP, et al. The safety and efficacy of the artificial bowel sphincter for fecal incontinence: results from a multicenter cohort study. Dis Colon Rectum. 2002;45(9):1139–53.

43. Ruiz Carmona MD, Alós Company R, Roig Vila JV, et al. Long-term results of artificial bowel sphincter for the treatment of severe faecal incontinence. Are they what we hoped for? Colorectal Dis. 2009;11:831–7.

44. Wexner SD, Jin HY, Weiss EG, et al. Factors associated with failure of the artificial bowel sphincter: a study of over 50 cases from Cleveland Clinic Florida. Dis Colon Rectum. 2009;52:1550–7.

45. Matzel KE, Bittorf B, Stadelmaier U, et al. Sacral nerve stimulation in the treatment of faecal incontinence. Chirurg. 2003;74:26–32.

46. Kenefick NJ, Emmanuel A, Nicholls RJ, et al. Effect of sacral nerve stimulation on autonomic nerve function. Br J Surg. 2003;90:1256–60.

47. Ganio E, Masin A, Ratto C, et al. Short-term sacral nerve stimulation for functional anorectal and urinary disturbances: results in 40 patients: evaluation of a new option for ano-rectal functional disorders. Dis Colon Rectum. 2001;44:1261–7.

48. Jarrett ME, Mowatt G, Glazener CM, et al. Systematic review of sacral nerve stimulation for faecal incontinence and constipation. Br J Surg. 2004;91:1559–69.

49. Meurette G, La Torre M, Regenet N, et al. Value of sacral nerve stimulation in the treatment of severe faecal incontinence: a comparison to the artificial bowel sphincter. Colorectal Dis. 2009;11:631–5.

50. Wexner SD, Coller JA, Devroede G, et al. Sacral nerve stimulation for fecal incontinence: results of a 120-patient prospective multicenter study. Ann Surg 2010;251:441–9.

51. Sands D, Madsen M. Fecal incontinence. In: Beck DE, Wexner SD, Roberts PL, Sacclarides TJ, Senagore A, Stamos M (eds). ASCRS Textbook of Colorectal Surgery 2nd ed. New York: Springer-Verlag, 2011; In press.

52. Goldstein SD. Radiation injury of the rectum. In: Zuimeda GD, (ed). Shackelford's Surgery of the Alimentary Tract, vol. 4. Philadelphia: WB Saunders, 1996:408–420.

Diverticular disease

Pathophysiology

Incidence

The prevalence of colonic diverticular disease and related complications has increased during this century [1]. Diverticulosis is common in Western industrialized societies and may be present in 50% of the elderly population. With the proportion of the elderly in the population growing, the complications of diverticulosis will likely represent a significant health problem in the 21st century.

Colonic diverticula are false diverticula of mucosal pouches that protrude through the colonic musculature alongside any of the three taeniae. Typically, diverticula are located along the mesenteric side of the two antimesenteric taeniae. The mucosal defect escapes through the colon musculature by traversing the tunnel created by the vasa recta, small arteries that supply blood to the mucosa (**Figure 13.1**). It is generally accepted that **diverticulosis** (the presence of colonic diverticula) is an acquired condition. In 95% of people with diverticulosis the sigmoid colon is involved, and in 65% of cases it may be the only segment involved. Cecal, or right-sided, diverticula are not as common, occurring in 6–7% of cases [2]. The right-sided diverticula were once thought to represent true diverticula, but recent evidence suggests that they are false diverticula.

The pathologic condition of diverticulosis was not well recognized until the mid-nineteenth century. Cruveilhier in 1849 [3] detailed the first pathologic description of diverticular disease. Over the next several years, isolated reports of colonic diverticula and related complications appeared in the literature. Subsequent autopsy studies and barium enema studies in the early 1900s reported a 5% incidence of diverticulosis in patients older than 40 years of age [5]. Since then, numerous studies conducted in industrialized nations have demonstrated an increasing prevalence of diverticulosis and its complications. The incidence of diverticulosis increases with age and reaches a peak in the sixth through eighth decades of life. It is now reported that at least 30% of the population older than 60 years of age and as many as 50% of those 80 years of age have diverticulosis [5–7].

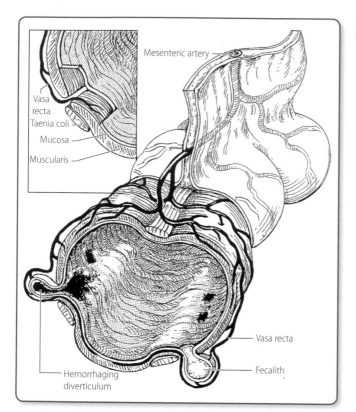

Figure 13.1 Anatomy of colonic diverticulosis.

Pathogenesis

Several theories have been postulated to explain the increasing prevalence of diverticulosis [8]. Many factors appear to predispose the colon to the development of diverticula, including decreased colonic wall strength, increased intraluminal pressure, decreased stool bulk, and lack of dietary fiber. No well controlled studies have determined whether one factor alone or a combination of several factors leads to the development of diverticular disease. Painter and Burkitt [9]. noted that industrialization correlates directly with an increase in diverticulosis. Industrialization leads to more refined foods, canned goods, and decreased cereal-fiber consumption. Changing from grist mills to roller mills at the turn of the century removed whole wheat from the Western diet and contributed significantly to the lowering of fiber content in the diet. Based on Laplace's law (pressure = tension/ radius) Painter and Burkitt postulated that decreased stool bulk causes a decrease in colonic diameter and subsequently increases the intraluminal pressure. They also believed that a narrow colon contains small bladders, or segments, caused by nonpropulsive colonic motility (segmentation). These areas are normally dilated by large bulky stools that do not allow significantly increased colonic pressure gradients.

A colon containing small stool is not distended, creating narrow segments with increased intraluminal pressure that causes the mucosa to herniate through defects in the colonic musculature. They suggested that increasing dietary fiber might prevent diverticulosis.

Others, reporting from industrialized nations, reviewed dietary fiber consumption and changes in stool weight for normal patients and those with diverticulosis and found wide variability, with no significant difference between the two groups [9–10]. Clearly, other factors may be involved. Arfwidsson [10] assessed colonic motility in people with diverticular disease by measuring intraluminal pressure in the sigmoid colon. He noted increased intraluminal pressure in diverticular colons when compared with pressure in colons in normal subjects during a resting state, after meals, and following cholinergic stimulation. Painter and Burkitt found no difference in pressure between normal subjects and patients with diverticular disease during the resting state. These investigators confirmed the differences noted postprandially and with cholinergic stimulation. Other reports show conflicting results [11]. Normal motility patterns are seen in patients with diverticulosis, and increased pressures are noted in patients with spastic colons but no evidence of diverticulosis. Eastwood [11] noted that abnormalities of colonic motility are more directly related to the symptoms of irritable bowel syndrome than to the presence of diverticulosis. Abnormalities of colonic motility alone do not appear to be the major cause of diverticulosis.

The shortened, thickened colon seen in diverticulosis suggests increased intraluminal pressure, altered motility, and increased colonic wall strength. However, several authors have shown that the colonic wall is weakened in patients with diverticulosis [12]. Colonic wall tensile strength is related to the age of the patient and to changes in the colonic connective tissue. Structural changes in tissue elastin increase with age. Whiteway and Morson [12] noted that these changes appear to correlate with the presence of diverticulosis, suggesting a cause-and-effect relationship. The exact pathogenesis of diverticulosis is unknown. However, perhaps for genetic reasons, certain people appear to have a predisposition to colonic wall weakness. Lack of dietary fiber results in increased intraluminal pressure and altered colonic motility. The result is mucosal protrusions through colonic wall defects, which creates diverticula. Many other factors may be involved in the development of colonic diverticula, but their exact contribution to the pathogenesis is not yet clear.

Diagnosis and treatment

The majority of patients with diverticulosis remain symptom free. However, as many as 10–20% of patients with diverticulosis develop symptoms such as infection (diverticulitis), fistula, obstruction, or hemorrhage. The inflammatory complications of diverticulitis involve a spectrum of infection (**Table 13.1**). Minimal involvement begins with

Table 13.1 Complications of diverticulitis

Acute	Chronic
Peridiverticular inflammation	Fistula Colovesical Colocutaneous Coloenteral Colovaginal
Peridiverticular abscess/phlegmon	Obstructions
Intra-abdominal or pelvic abscess	–
Generalized peritonitis	–

peridiverticular inflammation. The infectious process may progress to a peridiverticular abscess or phlegmon. Toxicity increases still further as intra-abdominal or pelvic abscess develops. Generalized peritonitis results from a free peritoneal perforation [13]. A classification system, proposed by Hinchey, Schaal, and Richards [14] for perforated diverticulitis is presented in **Table 13.2**.

Acute diverticulitis

Peridiverticular inflammation

Inspissated stool, a fecalith trapped within a diverticulum, produces thinning of the diverticular wall, resulting in localized infection or peridiverticular inflammation. The patient typically seeks treatment for acute left lower abdominal discomfort. An abdominal examination reveals minimal lower abdominal tenderness with no appreciable mass. No further diagnostic evaluation is needed for acute discomfort. The patient may have low-grade fever, is usually not tachycardic, and the white blood cell count is mildly elevated.

Treatment consists of broad-spectrum oral antibiotics (trimethoprim/sulfamethoxazole and metronidazole or ciprofloxin) and a fiberrestricted

Table 13.2 Hinchey classification and management of perforated diverticulitis

Stage	Description	Preferred initial management
I	Pericolic or mesenteric abscess	Antibiotics and bowel rest CT- or US-guided drainage
II	Walled-off pelvic abscess	Antibiotics and bowel rest CT- or US-guided drainage
III	Generalized purulent peritonitis	Fluid resuscitation and antibiotics Resect perforated segment Proximal colostomy Closure of distal segment (Hartmann's procedure)
IV	Generalized fecal peritonitis	Fluid resuscitation and antibiotics Resect perforated segment Proximal colostomy Closure of distal segment (Hartmann's procedure)

diet. Patients will usually respond in 24–48 hours of treatment. Failure to respond or progression of symptoms should prompt additional evaluation and intravenous antibiotics.

Follow-up clinical examination should include flexible sigmoidoscopy and a barium enema after the inflammation has resolved. These examinations are postponed for a month or more to ensure complete resolution of the inflammation and associated subclinical complications of diverticulitis.

Peridiverticular abscess/phlegmon

A patient may complain of moderate to severe left lower abdominal pain and anorexia. The abdominal examination reveals a tender mass (representing the inflamed colon) and voluntary guarding in the lower abdomen. Rebound tenderness or Rovsing's sign may also be present. The infection is localized by the adjacent structures, the abdominal wall, mesentery, omentum, small bowel, bladder, or retroperitoneal fat. Pyrexia, tachycardia, and leukocytosis are usually present. An upright chest radiograph and flat and upright abdominal radiographs exclude the pressure of free intraperitoneal air or intestinal obstruction. Urinalysis excludes urinary tract infection, fecaluria, and ureterolithiasis. The patient is best treated with hospitalization, intestinal rest, intravenous fluids, and intravenous antibiotics (e.g. ampicillin sodium/sulbactam sodium, ciprofloxacin, or gentamicin and clindamycin). Nasogastric decompression is generally unnecessary except for persistent emesis or obstruction. A water-soluble contrast enema or CT scan is useful to confirm the diagnosis in atypical presentations [15]. Experienced ultrasonographers have identified acute diverticulitis, but this examination is examiner dependent and the result is not as reproducible as with CT scans or contrast enemas.

Intra-abdominal or pelvic abscess

Occasionally a patient with a peridiverticular abscess will not improve and will develop a persistent fever, prolonged ileus, or sustained leukocytosis [1]. This clinical picture represents more than a small, contained infection. Usually an intra-abdominal or pelvic abscess has developed. A CT scan of the abdomen and pelvis with intraluminal contrast will define the walled-off cavity. The abscess appears as a fluid-filled, often loculated collection, which may contain gas. Ultrasonography may identify subphrenic or pelvic abscesses but is less useful for other intra-abdominal locations. Ultrasound offers a portable, inexpensive, real-time method to guide percutaneous drainage of these abscesses and is particularly useful for unstable patients in the intensive care unit. However, CT-directed drainage of the abscess is preferred. Under radiologic guidance a drainage catheter is placed and connected to closed suction drainage. Percutaneous drainage allows resolution of the inflammation and a delayed, one-stage surgical resection. If the abscess cannot be localized by CT scan or ultrasound or safely drained percutaneously, surgical exploration and drainage are necessary. A two-stage procedure is preferred, with resection of the involved colon, colostomy, closure of the distal bowel (rectum), and drainage of the abscess cavity.

Generalized peritonitis

Generalized peritonitis occurs when the inflamed colon or abscess freely perforates into the peritoneal cavity. Patients usually complain of severe diffuse abdominal pain with anorexia, and vomiting. The toxic patient is tachycardic, pyrexic, and dehydrated. Severe tachycardia and hypotension are signs of septic shock, which may accompany free perforation. On examination, the abdomen is diffusely tender, and involuntary guarding is present. Rebound and percussion tenderness are also usually present, and severe leukocytosis develops. An upright chest radiograph and an acute abdominal series may reveal free intraperitoneal air (see Figure 4.1). The first step in the management of peritonitis is volume replacement with intravenous fluids. Treatment also includes insertion of a nasogastric tube and Foley catheter and administration of intravenous antibiotics. Surgical exploration should follow immediately. Surgical treatment involves resection of the involved colon, colostomy, closure of the distal bowel, abdominal irrigation, and drainage of any abscesses.

A new alternative to resection and Hartman's pouch in selected patients with perforated diverticular disease is laparoscopic lavage. Myers et al described using laparoscopic peritoneal lavage to treat generalized peritonitis resulting from perforated diverticulitis in 100 patients [16]. They converted 8 patients using a Hartmann's procedure who had feculent peritonitis, the remaining 92 were followed with only a 4% morbidity and 3% mortality. Only 2 patients required additional procedures for pelvic abscesses and 2 patients had recurrent diverticulitis, one at 12 months and the other at 84 months post procedure. Additional studies are needed to determine what role this management option may play in acute diverticular disease.

Fecal peritonitis is the least common but most devastating form of perforation [5]. The morbidity and mortality are high. The patient presents with acute onset of abdominal pain and distention, peritoneal signs, and leukocytosis. An abdominal series will usually reveal free air. Patients with fecal peritonitis demand immediate fluid resuscitation, antibiotics, and exploration. Surgical treatment is similar to that described above.

Chronic diverticulitis

Diverticular fistulas

A peridiverticular abscess may erode into an adjacent viscus, causing a fistula [17]. The most common fistula involves the bladder (a colovesical fistula). Colovesical fistulas usually occur in men, because in women the uterus may be interposed between the colon and the bladder. Patients typically complain of urinary frequency, dysuria, pneumaturia, fecaluria, or hematuria. Intravenous antibiotics are administered, and a Foley catheter is used during the acute infectious period. After the acute infection has been treated, the suspected colovesical fistula is confirmed. Several procedures used to identify colovesical fistulas include cystoscopy, a barium enema, and a CT scan. Cystoscopy is the most sensitive examination to identify a colovesical fistula and demonstrates bullous edema at the site of the fistula. The CT scan may demonstrate contrast medium or air in the bladder. Sigmoidoscopy is necessary to exclude inflammatory bowel disease. Once the fistula is defined, patients may undergo an elective one-stage colonic resection with closure of the fistula. A section of bladder need not be removed if fibrosis involving the bladder wall is minimal. Many surgeons will place a closed suction drain adjacent to the involved bladder. The Foley catheter should remain in place for 5–10 days and its removal is often preceded by a cystogram to confirm the absence of a leak. If the clinical picture describes a colovesical fistula but it cannot be identified by any test, operative intervention remains indicated.

Other fistulas include colocutaneous, coloenteral, and colovaginal. Colocutaneous fistulas with minimal contamination can be managed conservatively; they will close, allowing for elective colonic resection. If the contamination from a colocutaneous fistula is difficult to control, a diverting colostomy or ileostomy is performed. Once the inflammation has subsided, the involved colonic segment is resected. Coloenteral fistulas are uncommon and usually present with persistent diarrhea after resolution of the diverticulitis. A barium upper gastrointestinal series with small bowel follow-through, barium enema, or flexible sigmoidoscopy may reveal the fistula site. Surgical treatment entails elective resection of the involved small and large bowel and primary anastomosis. Colovaginal fistulas, involving feculent drainage from the vagina, are rare and generally occur only in women who have previously undergone hysterectomy. Vaginal inspection reveals reactive granulation around the fistula. Elective surgical resection of the involved colonic segment with primary anastomosis resolves the condition.

Colonic obstruction

Colonic obstruction occurs as the result of chronic fibrosis and inflammation in the sigmoid colon. This may be difficult to differentiate from carcinoma, ischemic strictures, or inflammatory bowel disease. The obstruction may be partial or complete. Complete obstruction requires correction of electrolyte and fluid imbalances and operative intervention. A two-stage operation consisting of primary resection and end colostomy is preferred. Partial obstruction usually allows for careful preoperative bowel preparation with one-stage elective resection and primary anastomosis.

Surgical procedures for diverticulitis

Emergency operations

In 1907, Mayo et al [18] recommended the use of a **temporary diverting colostomy** and subsequent elective resection of the involved segment of colon for the treatment of acute diverticulitis. Since that time, a wide range of operations have been used to treat diverticulitis (**Figure 13.2**). Initial emphasis involved irrigation of the peritoneal cavity, drainage of infection, and diversion of the fecal stream. Smithwick [19] in 1942 was a proponent of a **three-stage procedure** designed to decrease the morbidity and mortality in surgical interventions for diverticulitis. Initially, the patient underwent diverting colostomy and drainage of intra-abdominal infection. The second stage involved resection of the diseased segment. The diverting transverse colostomy was not closed until final stage. Smithwick felt this would protect the anastomosis performed in proximity to the previously inflamed colon. However, three-stage procedures were associated with high mortality rates (29–32%).

Alternatively, an **exteriorization procedure** was used to create a colostomy and remove the inflamed segment from the peritoneal cavity. Unfortunately, the toxins present in the inflamed colon remain a source of sepsis with access to the bloodstream. The exteriorized

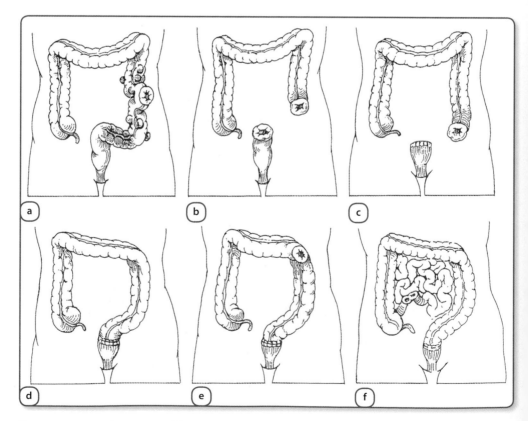

Figure 13.2 Surgical treatment of diverticulitis. (a) Exteriorization. (b) Resection, end colostomy, mucous fistula. (c) Resection, end colostomy, oversew rectum (Hartmann's procedure). (d) Resection, primary anastomosis. (e) Resection, primary anastomosis, diverting colostomy. (f) Resection, primary anastomosis, diverting loop ileostomy.

segment develops a malodorous serositis, produces dermatitis, and is difficult for even an experienced enterostomal therapist to control. Exteriorization requires enough mobilization of the colonic mesentery that resection of the diseased segment can be performed and is not generally recommended.

A two-stage procedure has several advantages. In the initial procedure the infected colon is removed and the fecal stream is diverted with a colostomy. Removing the septic focus during the initial surgery reduces the mortality rate to 10–12%. In the final stage, the colostomy is closed. To minimize the morbidity and mortality associated with additional surgery (i.e. the third stage) the two-stage procedure has become the preferred operative approach.

Several variations of resectional procedures have been described, including the Hartmann procedure; surgical excision, end-descending colostomy, and creation of a mucous fistula; the Paul-Mikulicz procedure (double-barrel colostomy); and surgical excision and primary closure with or without a protective colostomy [20].

The **Hartmann procedure** involves removal of the inflamed sigmoid colon, closure of the rectal stump, and a descending colostomy. This procedure removes the involved diverticular segment and facilitates the second stage of the procedure. During the second stage, closure of the colostomy usually requires no further resection of the distal segment. As described in Chapter 6, this colostomy takedown can often be accomplished with laparoscopic techniques. If a mucous fistula is used, the distal segment often contains residual diverticula that will be a source of recurrent symptoms. This retained segment of colon often proves difficult to resect during colostomy closure because of pericolic fibrosis remaining after resolution of the inflammation. The Paul-Mikulicz procedure involves a double-barreled colostomy. It is unlikely that after resecting the affected colon during the first stage there will be adequate length of distal colon for a double-barreled colostomy. Furthermore, a Paul-Mikulicz procedure often leaves sigmoid diverticulosis in the distal segment, with the potential for problems much like those with a separate mucous fistula. Removal of the remaining distal segment to close the colostomy often proves difficult.

One-stage procedures for acute diverticulitis have a limited role [21]. Exploration of the abdominal cavity may reveal a mesenteric abscess or limited inflammatory reaction in the left lower quadrant, which allows the infected colon and involved mesentery to be resected with minimal contamination. Intraoperative colonic washout of the remaining colon and rectum with saline solution may allow a primary anastomosis, which may be protected with a diverting colostomy or ileostomy.

Elective resection

Most patients with diverticulitis do not require surgical intervention. Elective resection is recommended for patients who have required hospitalization for repeated (more than three) attacks of moderate to severe diverticulitis. Treatment of acute attacks typically consists of administration of intravenous antibiotics and intestinal rest. Repeated attacks of diverticulitis increase the risk of future attacks of diverticulitis. Emergency surgery of complicated diverticular disease is associated with a higher morbidity and mortality than a one-stage elective colon resection. Thus elective resections are recommended for patients with recurrent attacks [22].

In 1983, Ouriel and Schwartz [23], recommended elective resection for young patients (less than 40 years of age) after their first significant attack of diverticulitis. They noted that younger patients more frequently required readmission during the follow-up period (55%). Twenty-three percent had a serious complication, and 45% of medically managed patients eventually required elective resection. Although the disease is less common among young patients, diverticulitis is associated with more complications, and early elective surgical intervention is recommended.

Elective resection is recommended in several less common situations, such as when radiographic or endoscopic studies cannot exclude carcinoma. Persistent urinary tract symptoms following attacks of diverticulitis also indicate possible fistula formation and suggest a need for elective resection. Immunosuppressed patients and transplant patients with mild diverticular symptoms have a high incidence of complicated diverticulitis and should be considered for elective sigmoid resection.

For an elective resection, the patient receives a mechanical and antibiotic bowel preparation and is positioned in a modified Lloyd-Davies (lithotomy) position. The abdomen is explored through a midline incision. Diseased, thickened bowel (sigmoid) is resected. The distal line of resection should be healthy rectum. This ensures uninvolved bowel (there are no diverticula in the rectum) with a good supply and a large diameter. The proximal limit of resection is soft, pliable, uninvolved colon. Proximal diverticula are not a problem if the bowel is soft and pliable and of adequate diameter. This point is usually in the left colon, but occasionally distal transverse colon may have to be used for the anastomosis.

Recent advances in laparoscopic surgery have extended the use of this technology into the area of colon surgery [24]. Laparoscopically assisted colon resection has become a standardized surgical technique. Initial learning curves have established criteria for good patient selection, better operative logistics, and awareness of the dangers and pitfalls of laparoscopic surgery. As described in Chapter 6, the left or sigmoid colon can be resected and delivered through a small incision. The anastomosis is performed intracorporeally or extracorporeally using a double-staple technique. Beart [24] claims laparoscopic colon resection results in quicker return of intestinal function, decreased postoperative narcotics and shorter hospital length of stay. Other reports demonstrate conflicting views, representing a need for a large, controlled clinical trial to assess the benefits and differences of open and laparoscopic-assisted colectomy. Controversial issues include the ability to establish adequate margins for resection of the colon involved with diverticular disease and to limit the recurrence of the disease. The postoperative patient management considerations of diets and narcotics after open colectomy may vary from other laparoscopic procedures. A randomized trial of comparable patients is needed to answer these questions.

Diverticular hemorrhage

Diverticular bleeding occurs in 5–15% of patients with diverticulosis; the average age of patients with diverticular hemorrhage is 65 years. Elderly patients with diverticular hemorrhage have associated cardiac, pulmonary, and renal dysfunction, which contributes to a reported mortality rate as high as 20%.

Diverticular hemorrhage is generally massive but self-limited [25]. Patients require many transfusions, with an average of 7.6 units of blood. Diverticular bleeding stops spontaneously with supportive management in 70–95% of cases. Recurrent episodes of hemorrhage requiring a second admission to the hospital occur in 25% of patients. After the second episode of diverticular hemorrhage, the chance of a third event increases to 50%.

Classic diverticular bleeding is painless. However, the cathartic effect of intracolonic blood may cause mild, crampy abdominal pain. Painless lower gastrointestinal bleeding may also arise from colonic angiodysplasia, carcinoma, and Meckel's diverticulum. Significant abdominal pain associated with bleeding suggests a cause such as ischemic colitis, whereas diarrhea suggests inflammatory bowel or infectious causes.

The precise mechanism of diverticular hemorrhage is unknown. In the late 1800s, Kebs outlined the vascular anatomy of the vasa recta and the mucosal blood supply and Drummond [26] in 1917 displayed the relationship between the vasa recta and the neck of the diverticulum. In 1976, Meyers et al [27] defined the bleeding sites as the ruptured vasa recta in the diverticulum, noted structural changes located eccentrically in the vasa recta at the site of rupture, intimal thickening with thinning of the media, the absence of any acute or chronic inflammation and stated that these vascular changes were typically the result of focal injury. It is generally accepted that thinning of the media in the vasa recta predisposes to intraluminal rupture: focal injury may occur from trauma related to a fecalith.

In the past, nearly 70% of patients were reported to have bleeding diverticula in the right colon [1]. However, within the last 20 years, the advent of selective mesenteric angiography and endoscopy revealed that angiodysplasia of the colon was a significant alternative cause of lower GI hemorrhage. Eighty percent of angiodysplasias are located in the right colon, and at least 50% of patients with angiodysplasia have diverticulosis [28]. The discovery of angiodysplasia as a source of lower

GI bleeding has created uncertainty in identifying the precise cause in individual patients. Data from several reports further complicate the incidence of diverticular hemorrhage by attributing bleeding to angiodysplasias seen on arteriography without actual contrast extravasation.

The history of lower GI bleeding includes the duration and amount of bleeding, the presence of melena or hematochezia, and whether the bleeding is associated with abdominal, rectal, or anal pain. The patient is also asked about previous episodes of rectal bleeding or the results of a previous barium enema or colonoscopy; use of aspirin, dipyridamole, or warfarin; and about alcohol abuse or renal or liver disease that may predispose the patient to rectal bleeding. The patient's vital signs and cardiopulmonary stability are evaluated. The abdominal examination in diverticular bleeding is typically unremarkable, but the digital anal examination reveals gross evidence of intestinal bleeding. Intravenous resuscitation is initiated immediately, and blood is drawn for type and crossmatch, complete blood cell count, coagulation profile, serum electrolytes, liver function tests, and a bleeding time. Anorectal causes are excluded by anoscopy and proctosigmoidoscopy. Flexible sigmoidoscopy may be necessary to exclude such diagnoses as ischemic colitis and carcinoma. If flexible sigmoidoscopy fails to identify a distal bleeding source, placement of a nasogastric tube helps exclude an upper GI source. If the nasogastric aspirate contains no bile, an upper GI source cannot be excluded but is unlikely. If the nasogastric aspirate contains evidence of bleeding, an urgent esophagogastroduodenoscopy is indicated.

In acute massive lower GI hemorrhage, the priority after resuscitation is to determine the site of bleeding in order to allow a limited surgical resection in patients with continued hemorrhage. Modern techniques to identify the site and etiology of lower GI bleeding include nuclear scintigraphy, colonoscopy, and selective mesenteric arteriography (**Figure 13.3**). The intermittent nature of lower GI hemorrhage typically requires the combined results from several of these tests. A barium enema study was once thought to be useful in identifying the potential source of lower GI hemorrhage and producing tamponade. However, barium has proven to be a deterrent to more valuable diagnostic techniques: barium precludes the use of scintigraphy, obscures angiography, and impairs colonoscopy. A barium enema will identify diverticulosis but not hemorrhage or angiodysplasia.

Despite recent advances in diagnostic imaging, the exact cause and site of bleeding often remain undetermined. **Nuclear scintigraphy** using the ^{99m}Tc-labeled RBC scanning technique can detect intermittent bleeding, and delayed scanning provides a cumulative bleeding image. To detect a site of hemorrhage, ^{99m}Tc-labeled RBC scanning requires a bleeding rate of only 0.1–0.5 mL/min. Nuclear scintigraphy has 90% sensitivity, 100% specificity, and 93.5% accuracy [29]. Nuclear scintigraphy can confirm active bleeding and identify patients who are likely to demonstrate bleeding arterio-graphically. Careful selection

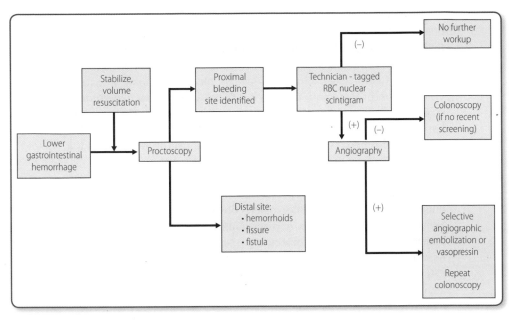

Figure 13.3 Algorithm for the management of lower gastrointestinal hemorrhage.

of patients for arteriography minimizes the number of negative arteriograms. Ng et al [30] demonstrated that a positive scintigraphic result within the first 2 minutes of imaging is highly predictive of a positive angiographic result. Scintigraphic localization permits selective arterial injection and reduces the amount of dye necessary during arteriography, thus limiting the risk of contrast nephrotoxicity in elderly, hypovolemic patients.

Mesenteric arteriography is accurate in identifyng the precise cause of lower GI bleeding if extravasated contrast medium is detected [31]. To demonstrate hemorrhage, arteriography requires an active bleeding rate of 0.5–2 mL/min. The angiographic catheter can be left in place for repeat arteriograms or therapeutic interventions to identify potential sources that are not actively bleeding at the time of injection. Continuous selective arterial infusion of vasopressin at a rate of 0.2–0.4 units/min for a period of 12–24 hours can be administered through the catheter [32]. After the bleeding stops, the vasopressin is tapered over 12–24 hours. Vasopressin has been successful in controlling hemorrhage in 82% of patients with lower GI bleeding identified by arteriography. However, rebleeding may occur in as many as 41% of patients once therapy has been stopped. Vasopressin infusion increases the risk of myocardial infarction or intestinal ischemia and infarction and can increase fluid retention. Continuous-infusion vasopressin therapy requires intensive care monitoring. More recently, angiographic embolization of the distal bowel vessel through angiographic micro catheters has replaced vasopressin infusion. Continued uncontrolled bleeding requires surgical resection.

Colonoscopy has long been used to identify the source of colonic bleeding. Reports of cases in which emergency colonoscopy successfully identifies the source of hemorrhage typically involve cancer or colitis and not the picture of massive lower GI bleeding [33]. In massive lower GI hemorrhage, clots and active bleeding impair adequate visualization of the colon, making it difficult even for an experienced colonoscopist to identify the source of hemorrhage [25]. If the patient appears to be stable and is not actively bleeding, colonic preparation can be performed. Colonoscopy may then be useful in identifying a potential source of hemorrhage.

Emergency resection for lower GI hemorrhage is controversial. Blind left colectomy without precise knowledge of the bleeding site was once encouraged. The selection of left colectomy was predicated on the knowledge that the majority of diverticula are located in the left colon. Patients treated with a left colectomy revealed a 63% rate of persistent hemorrhage and 12% postoperative mortality. McGuire and Haynes [34] and Drapanas et al [35] recommend subtotal colectomy as an alternative. They reported no rebleeding and a mortality of 9.4%. Others reported complications related to blind subtotal colectomy [34]. These include rebleeding from a small intestinal source and, in the elderly, fecal incontinence and intractable diarrhea associated with ileorectostomy. Segmental colectomy is the preferred operation for continued lower GI hemorrhage from an identified site. Subtotal colectomy is best reserved for treatment of massive lower GI bleeding when the clinical condition of the patient will not allow attempts to localize the bleeding site.

Conclusion

Diverticulosis is a growing health care problem. The incidence of diverticular disease continues to increase in industrialized nations. The elderly population, often afflicted with diverticular disease, continues to grow as well. Complications of the disease include diverticulitis, fistula, obstruction, and hemorrhage. Early diagnosis and treatment may decrease the risk of emergency resection. Identification of patients for elective colon resection before diverticular complications develop can limit surgical treatment to a one-stage procedure.

Rounds questions

1. What are colonic diverticula?
2. What section of the colon is most frequently involved with diverticulosis?
3. What factors predispose to the development of colonic diverticula?
4. What is Laplace's law?
5. What are the signs and symptoms of acute diverticulitis?
6. Ideally, how would a well-localized abscess cavity be managed?
7. What is the most common type of diverticular fistula?

8. What is the most sensitive test for confirming the presence of a colovesical fistula?
9. What previous operation has a woman with a colovaginal fistula previously undergone?
10. What are the five surgical options available to treat acute diverticulitis?
11. What are the generally accepted elected operative indications for diverticular disease?
12. When performing a resection for diverticular disease, what are the proximal and distal limits of resection?

References

1. Thorson AG, Goldberg SM. Benign colon: Diverticular disease. In: Wolff BG, Fleshman JW, Beck DE, Pemberton JH, Wexner SD, (eds). ASCRS Textbook of Colorectal Surgery. New York: Springer-Verlag, 2007;269–307.
2. Rankin FW, Brown PW. Diverticulitis of the colon. Surg Gynecol Obstet 1930;50:836–847.
3. Cruveilhier J. Traite Anat Pathol Paris: Bailliere 1849;1593–5.
4. Heller SN, Hackler LR. Changes in the crude fiber content of the American diet. Am J Clin Nutr 1978;31:1510–4.
5. Gordon PH. Diverticular disease of the colon. In: Gordon PH, Nivamongs S, (eds). Principles and Practice of Surgery for the Colon, Rectum, and Anus, 2nd ed. St. Louis: Quality Medical Publishing 1999;975–1043.
6. Parks TG. Natural history of diverticular disease of the colon. Clin Gastroenterol 1975;4:53–69.
7. Morson BC. Pathology of diverticular disease of the colon. Clin Gastroenterol 1975;4:37–52.
8. Ryan P. Changing concepts in diverticular disease. Dis Colon Rectum 1983;26:12–18.
9. Painter NS, Burkitt DP. Diverticular disease of the colon: A deficiency disease of Western civilization. Br Med J 1971;2:450–4.
10. Arfwidsson S. Pathogenesis of multiple diverticula of the sigmoid colon in diverticular disease. Acta Chir Scand 1964;342:5–68.
11. Eastwood MA. Colonic diverticulosis: Medical and dietary management. Clin Gastroenterol 1975;4:85–97.
12. Whiteway J, Morson BC. Pathology of the aging diverticular disease. Clin Gastroenterol 1985;14:829–46.
13. Chappuis CW, Cohn I. Acute colonic diverticulitis. Surg Clin North Am 1988;68:301–13.
14. Hinchey EJ, Schaal PGH, Richards GK. Treatment of perforated diverticular disease of the colon. Adv Surg 1978;12:85–109.
15. Hulnick DH, Megibow AJ, Balthazar EJ, et al. Computed tomography in the evaluation of diverticulitis. Radiology 1984;152:491–5.
16. Myers E, Hurley M, O'Sullivan GC et al. Laparoscopic peritoneal lavage for generalized peritonitis due to perforated diverticulits. Br J Surg 2008;95:97–101.
17. Corman ML (ed). Colon and Rectal Surgery. Philadelphia: Lippincott, 1984.
18. Mayo WJ, Wilson LB, Griffin HZ. Acquired diverticulitis of the large intestine. Surg Gynecol Obstet 1907;5:8–15.
19. Smithwick RH. Experiences with the surgical management of diverticulitis of the sigmoid. Ann Surg 1942;115:969–85.
20. Greif JM, Fried G, McSherry CK. Surgical treatment of perforated diverticulitis of the sigmoid colon. Dis Colon Rectum 1980;23:483–7.
21. Marshall SF. Earlier resection in one stage for diverticulitis of the colon. Am Surg 1963;29:337–46.
22. Thorson AG. Diverticular disease. In: Beck DE, Wexner SD, Roberts PL, Sacclarides TJ, Senagore A, Stamos M (eds). ASCRS Textbook of Colorectal Surgery, 2nd edition. New York: Springer-Verlag 2011; in press.
23. Ouriel K, Schwartz SI. Diverticular disease in the young patient. Surg Gynecol Obstet 1983;156:1–5.
24. Beart RW. Laparoscopic colectomy: Status of the art. Dis Colon Rectum 1994;37(Suppl):47–9.
25. Opelka FG, Timmcke AE. Management of bleeding diverticulosis. Semin Colon Rectal Surg 1990;1:109–15.

26. Drummond H. Sacculi of the large intestine. Br J Surg 1916;4:407–13.

27. Meyers MA, Alonso DR, Gray GF, Baer JW. Pathogenesis of bleeding colonic diverticulosis. Gastroenterology 1976;71:577–83.

28. Boley SJ, DiBiase A, Brandt LJ, Sammartano RJ. Lower intestinal bleeding in the elderly. Am J Surg 1979;137:57–64.

29. Nicholson ML, Neoptolemos JP, Sharp JF, et al. Localization of gastrointestinal bleeding using in vivo technetium-99m-labelled red blood cell scintigraphy. Br J Surg 1989;76:358–61.

30. Ng DA, Opelka FG, Beck DE, et al. Predictive value of Tc99m-labeled red blood cell scintigraphy for positive angiogram in massive lower gastrointestinal hemorrhage. Dis Colon Rectum 1977;40:471–7.

31. Browder W, Cerise EJ, Litwin MS. Impact of emergency angiography in massive lower gastro-intestinal bleeding. Ann Surg 1986;204:530–6.

32. Baum S, Rosch J, Dotter CT, et al. Selective mesenteric arterial infusions in the management of massive diverticular hemorrhage. N Engl J Med 1973;288:1269–72.

33. Rossinni FP, Ferrari A. Emergency colonoscopy. In: Hunt RH, Wayne DJ (eds). Colonoscopy, Techniques, Clinical Practice and Color Atlas. Chicago: Year Book Medical Publishing, 1981;289–99.

34. McGuire HH, Haynes BW. Massive hemorrhage from diverticulosis of the colon: Guidelines for therapy based on bleeding patterns observed in fifty cases. Ann Surg 1972;172:847–855.

35. Drapanas T, Pennington DG, Kappelman M, Lindsey ES. Emergency subtotal colectomy: Preferred approach to management of massively bleeding diverticular disease. Ann Surg 1973;177:519–26.

36. Gianfrancisco JA, Abcarian H. Pitfalls in the treatment of massive lower gastrointestinal bleeding with blind subtotal colectomy. Dis Colon Rectum 1982;25:441–5.

14 Inflammatory bowel disease: ulcerative colitis and Crohn's disease

Inflammatory bowel disease (IBD) encompasses the two enigmatic disease processes of ulcerative colitis and Crohn's disease. These diseases continue to challenge and frustrate the surgeon, gastroenterologist, and, most importantly, the patient. The term IBD links these two conditions, which are related by common clinical symptoms and overlapping histological features of recurrent inflammation with an unknown etiology.

The medical and surgical management of these two disease processes are different and will be discussed separately. However, the differences and similarities between the two diseases and how they affect management will be emphasized.

Ulcerative colitis

Ulcerative colitis (UC) is an inflammatory disease of unknown etiology of the mucosa of the large intestine and rectum. This chronic disorder is characterized by remissions and exacerbations of colitis associated with abdominal cramps, rectal bleeding, and diarrhea. The disease usually affects patients in their youth or early middle age and has devastating local and systemic short- and long-term effects, including side effects from medical therapy used to treat the condition. The disease is variable in its topographic distribution: some patients have limited proctitis, proctosigmoiditis, or left-sided colitis, some patients have a mild disease process that may become quiescent for variable periods, and in others the entire colon may be involved, with acute onset of fulminant colitis or toxic megacolon.

There is no specific medical cure, except for removal of the entire colon and rectum. Medical therapy may control 'flares'; however, it does not provide a definitive treatment for the disease. By contrast, total or restorative proctocolectomy provides a cure, although newer surgical alternatives have supplemented total proctocolectomy and ileostomy in most patients [1]. Continuing experience with the ileoanal reservoir has led to a positive alternative for patients with UC and has influenced patients and gastroenterologists to consider surgical cure earlier in the course of disease [2].

History

The distinction between UC and infectious colitis was not apparent until 1859, when Samuel Wilks [3] described the post mortem appearance of the intestine and coined the term 'ulcerative colitis.' He further characterized the disease in 1875 and reported distinguishable clinical and pathologic criteria from common infectious enteritides [4]. In 1932, Crohn et al [5] noted a transmural inflammation of the terminal ileum and affixed the appelation 'regional ileitis' thus distinguishing it from UC. The two diseases initially appeared to have distinct pathologic features. Moreover, during the past 50 years clinical, pathologic, endoscopic, radiologic, and anatomic overlap has been appreciated between the two conditions; in 10–15% of cases, a clear distinction cannot be made. This distinction is important because the surgical approaches for these conditions are quite different. The ileoanal reservoir has become paramount and relegated most other surgical options, especially the continent ileostomy, to a limited role.

Epidemiology

The incidence and classification of UC vary considerably throughout the world, limiting incidence data. The incidence is about 6 per 100,000 per year, and the prevalence is between 50 and 70 per 100,000 per year [6]. The incidence of UC is highest in developed regions of the world and lowest in developing regions, although there are clues that this trend may reverse. UC is reported with increasing frequency in Japan, India, Thailand, and other Asian countries. It appears to be more common in Jewish than in non-Jewish people and in whites than in non-whites; however, recently the incidence has been increasing in these other populations [7].

Most cases of UC are diagnosed in patients between 15–40 years of age, but the range extends from infants to the elderly; approximately 5% of cases of UC have their onset after 60 years of age. Males and females are equally affected. The disease has a familial pattern, but there is no conclusive evidence regarding the genetic or environmental determination of this pattern [6,7].

Etiologic factors

The cause of IBD remains elusive. Current theories include genetic factors, infectious agents, immunologic dysfunction and vasculitis. The lack of a true animal model further hinders the progress toward elucidation of a cause. Immunologic, genetic, and infectious etiologic factors continue to be actively investigated [8].

Infectious causes

Ulcerative colitis (UC) has been attributed to bacterial causes for many years. In 1928, Bargen [9] claimed that a transmittable diplococcus was the responsible agent. Subsequent studies failed to conclusively demonstrate an association with bacterial agents. Electron microscopy of affected tissue has also implicated viral particles [10]. Whether the infectious agents are the triggers or perpetuators of the disease is controversial.

Immunologic causes

An immunologic origin is supported by efficacious responses with immunosuppressants such as cyclosporine and azathioprine [11].

Perhaps corticosteroids help in a similar way. Increasing evidence points to a role for cytokines in IBD [11,12]. Cytokines are proteins secreted by activated immunocytes that influence the activity, differentiation, and rate of proliferation of other cells. They exert autocrine, paracrine, and endocrine responses; they mediate both inflammation and immunologic responses and initiate the inflammation characteristic of IBD. Specific cytokines have been implicated but the precise cascade of inflammatory events is unknown. **Interleukin-1β** (IL-1β) has been shown to be elevated in UC as well as in experimental models of colitis [13]. In animal models of experimentally induced colitis, the increased concentration of IL-1β in colonic mucosa correlates with the severity of histologic inflammation [12–14]. In addition, IL-1β stimulates the secretion of potent chemotactic cytokines that may promote fibrosis by stimulating fibroblasts [12,15]. Similar fibrosis may result in stricture formation that is much more characteristic of Crohn's disease than UC. The concentration of other cytokines has also been altered in IBD. Thus it appears that cytokines are integrally involved in the pathogenesis of IBD through both immunoregulatory and proinflammatory properties. The clinical effectiveness of biological therapies such as anti-tumor necrosis factor lends additional support to an immunologic cause of IBD.

Genetic causes

Genetic predisposition for the development of IBD exists: relatives of IBD patients are more likely to develop IBD than are people with relatives that are unaffected; the relative risk of a family member of a patient with UC developing it is 15. The high degree of disease concordance among relatives, and not spouses, suggests a genetic predisposition or environmental factors requiring exposure at an early age [6–8]. The majority of cases of UC have their onset in individuals who are 15–40 years of age, and only 5% occur in patients older than 60 years of age. Monozygous twins have a higher concordance for IBD than dizygous twins. In addition, the HLA phenotypes Aw24 and Bw35 are associated with UC, particularity in Israeli Jews of European origin. The Aw24 phenotype is increased in frequency in patients with early onset of chronic UC with severe disease. Nevertheless, there are no conclusive data regarding genetic versus environmental determination of familial patterns.

Several age-related exposures have been described that could influence the incidence of IBD. Smoking has been demonstrated to be an independent risk factor for recurrence of IBD [16–18]. The nicotine patch has been used successfully to treat patients with UC, relieving UC symptoms in 82% of cases [19].

Clinical Features

History

A diagnosis of IBD is not confirmed by any single laboratory test; rather the diagnosis is often one of exclusion. Diagnostic evaluation should assess the urgency of resuscitative intervention and expeditiously exclude other diagnoses. UC and Crohn's disease can usually be distinguished on the basis of the clinical course, the symptomatology, and the endoscopic and histologic findings. **Table 14.1** summarizes a number of characteristic features of each disease.

Rectal bleeding is virtually always present in UC but is relatively rare for patients with Crohn's disease; 25% of patients with Crohn's disease will never manifest rectal bleeding. However, UC is confined to the colon and rectum, whereas Crohn's disease can occur anywhere in the alimentary tract from the mouth to the anus. Perianal sepsis is virtually pathognomic for Crohn's disease. Similarly, the presence of fissures and stenosis increases the likelihood of Crohn's disease rather than UC.

Table 14.1 Features of inflammatory bowel disease		
	Ulcerative colitis	**Crohn's disease**
Course	Exacerbations and remissions	Continuous, progressive
Bleeding	Virtually always	Uncommon
Abdominal pain	Uncommon	Common
Perianal disease	Fissures or hemorrhoids only	Also fistulas and abscesses
Fistulas	No	Common
Abdominal mass	Never	Occasional
Carcinoma	Increased	Increased, but less than with ulcerative colitis
Radiographic and endoscopic features		
Distribution	Contiguous from rectum No skip areas Always rectal involvement Confined to colon	Segmental, skip lesions Eccentric Often rectal sparing Can be mouth to anus Creeping fat
Small bowel	Spared	Often involved
Stricture	Rare, virtually always malignant	Frequent, virtually always benign
Mucosa	Mucosa contact bleeding; granular Shallow and wide superficial ulcers Pseudopolyps	Fissuring Deep and narrow longitudinal ulcers Cobblestone appearance
Aphthous ulcers	Rare	Common
Microscopic features		
Extent	Mucosa and submucosa (difficult to interpret after toxicity)	Transmural
Granulomas	Never	Common
Dysplasia	Occasional	Rare
Lymph nodes	Reactive	With granulomas
Crypts and abscesses	Common	Present
Mucus production	Decreased	Increased

Modified from Corman MC. Ulcerative colitis. In: Corman MC, (ed). Colon and Rectal Surgery, 3rd ed. Philadelphia: JB Lippincott, 1993, 901.

Physical examination

Patients with distal disease are usually healthier than are individuals with pancolitis. The patient will often appear cushingoid, anemic, and osteopenic with cataracts and other complications of corticosteroid use, such as a history of peptic ulcer disease, mood swings, hypertension, diabetes, and fractures secondary to prolonged steroid use. However, there are usually fewer outward physical signs of disease compared with a patient with Crohn's disease. Most abdominal examinations are unremarkable, except in patients with toxic colitis. The perineum is usually disease free; however patients with UC can have an occasional fissure or rectovaginal fistula from obstetric trauma [7]. In UC, a digital examination is less likely to reveal induration of the anal canal and more likely to reveal bloody mucoid discharge or friability in the lower rectum.

Endoscopic findings

Proctosigmoidoscopic examination is of paramount importance, especially noting the appearance of the rectal mucosa. Although a finding of normal rectum almost always excludes UC, topical rectal preparations can also lead to the normalization of rectal mucosa.

Characteristic changes in the rectum include contact bleeding, granularity, and ulcerations and lack of compliance in the rectum. Although 40% of patients with Crohn's colitis will have a normal rectum [7]. It may be difficult to differentiate Crohn's disease from UC when the rectum is diseased. Stool specimens should be analyzed for ova and parasites and be cultured and analyzed for the presence of *Clostridium difficile.*

Radiologic studies

The importance of radiographic evaluation of patients with IBD should not be underestimated. In an acutely ill patient, an upright chest X-ray film should be obtained to search for free air. The plain abdominal film is useful to assess bowel distention, particularly in a patient with toxic colitis (**Figure 14.1**) [7]. When toxic dilatation is suspected a barium enema is contraindicated, but serial plain films are used to determine the progression or resolution of the critical state. This serial study is important, because the patient may be obtunded or signs and symptoms may be obscured by corticosteroid use. In acute toxic colitis, the colon is dilated to greater than 10 cm and the haustra are effaced. This condition is seen in less than 5% of cases and is declining in incidence [6,7].

A double-contrast barium enema (ACBE) has been the most useful radiographic technique for evaluation of patients with UC, more recently CT enterography is being used. Typical radiographic findings on ACBE include edema, ulceration, and changes in colonic motility. The ulcerations may have a collar button appearance (**Figure 14.2**), indicating severe colitis [20]. Alternatively, edema and ulceration may result in thumbprinting, as with ischemic colitis. In the early stages of UC, the haustra are less prominent as a result of reduced distensibility,

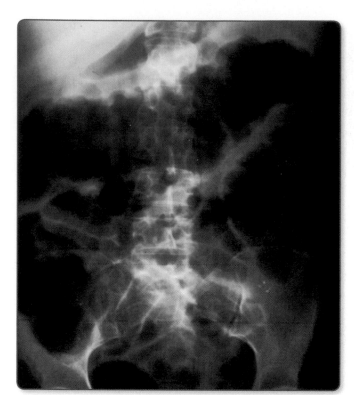

Figure 14.1 The plain abdominal X-ray film reveals marked dilatation of the transverse colon.

and the mucosa assumes a finely granular (spica) appearance. Eventually progression will result in complete loss of haustration with a 'lead pipe' appearance, including narrowing of the lumen, shortening of the longitudinal axis, and rigid, smooth contours with constriction and shrinkage of the entire colon and rectum. Chronic inflammation may lead to diffuse mucosal atrophy, leaving behind hypertrophic islands of inflamed mucosa and granulation tissue that assumes a polypoid shape called **pseudopolyps** [7]; pseudopolyps may be non-neoplastic or preneoplastic. CT findings of UC include colonic wall thickening with fat stranding of the colonic mesentery.

Other radiographic guidance can be derived from the pattern of distribution of the disease. Only about 25% of patients have pancolitis; however, the disease is always continuous, as opposed to Crohn's colitis, which can be segmental [6]. Colonic strictures in UC must be considered malignant until proven otherwise although endoscopy is superior to radiography for such evaluation [7]. Before elective surgery, it is advisable to perform either a small bowel series or CT enterography to help exclude Crohn's disease.

Histopathologic Findings

Macroscopic

Ulcerative colitis (UC) is an inflammatory condition confined to the mucosa and submucosa of the colonic and rectal walls. It is a continuous

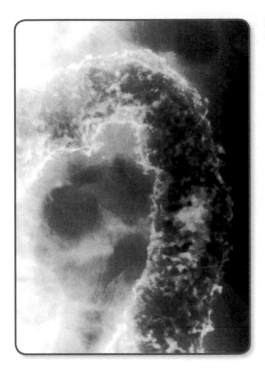

Figure 14.2 Acute ulcerative colitis. Note loss of haustra and collar button ulcers.

disease always involving the rectum and extending proximally for varying distances; usually the most severe involvement is distal. The disease should never involve the small bowel. However, occasionally the terminal ileum may show secondary mild inflammatory changes called 'backwash' ileitis [6]. Grossly, the colonic mucosa demonstrates healed granular superficial ulcers superimposed on a friable, thickened mucosa with increased vascularity. The result of the confluence of numerous ulcers leaving islands of hypertrophied heaped-up mucosa gives the pseudopolyp appearance [6,7].

Microscopic

Microscopic changes in UC include an intense inflammation in the mucosa and submucosa with multiple crypt abscesses. There is infiltration of round cells and polymorphonucleocytes into the crypts of Lieberkühn at the base of the mucosa [6]. Marked vascular engorgement accounts for the propensity for rectal bleeding. The number of crypt epithelial cells that produce mucin (goblet cells) are diminished and rendered dysfunctional by injurious toxins or cytokines, and hence the production of mucus is decreased [21–23]. Episodes of inflammation and healing lead to an irregular branching of the glands. The base of the glands does not reach the basement membrane. As the inflammation progress, there is a coalescence of crypt abscesses and desquamation of overlying cells to form an ulcer that should be limited to the mucosa and submucosa. In toxic megacolon, however, there is full-thickness involvement of the bowel, with necrosis and friability. In this situation, the colon may perforate, rendering definitive diagnosis more difficult.

Nonoperative treatment

Categories of drug treatment for UC include sulfasalazine, its analogs (aminosalicylates), corticosteroids, immunomodulators, and biologic agents [24]. Other medical therapies that have shown promise include topically absorbed steroids, soluble mediator blockade, immune mediator blockade, oxygen radical scavenger, and dietary modification [25–28]. Once a diagnosis of UC has been established, medical therapy depends on the severity of symptoms and the severity and extent of disease as indicated by clinical, radiographic, and endoscopic examinations.

Sulfasalazine and aminosalicylates (ASA)

Sulfasalazine, an inhibitor of mucosal prostaglandin synthesis, has been a mainstay of therapy for the past 50 years. Sulfasalazine consists of a 5-aminosalicylic acid (5-ASA) molecule linked by an azo bond to sulfapyridine; 5-ASA is thought to be the therapeutically active component with sulfapyridine acting as a transporter to the lower GI tract. Bacteria in the colon splits the azo bond to release the 5-ASA, which acts topically on the inflamed mucosa [25–28]. The typical dose is 4 g/day in divided doses. Twenty-five percent to 30% of patients experience side effects such as headaches, nausea, anorexia, and dyspepsia; other individuals may be allergic to the sulfa. Other more serious complications include Steven–Johnson syndrome and sterility. Sulfasalazine induces remission in up to 80% of patients with mild to moderate acute attacks of UC; 2 g/day may also be effective in preventing relapse [26, 27].

Table 14.2 Aminosalicylate products and uses					
Drug	Relative cost	Delivery method	Dose	Use in ulcerative colitis	Use in Crohn's disease
Sulfasalazine (Azulfidine)	1.0	Colonic bacterial azo reductases	2–4 g	Active colitis Maintenance	Active colonic disease
Olsalazine (Dipentum)	2.9	Colonic bacterial azo reductases	1 g	Active colitis Maintenance	Active colonic disease
Mesalamine (Asacol)	1.5	Eudragit-S Release at pH > 7	800–2400 mg	Active colitis Maintenance	Active colonic disease
Mesalamine (Pentasa)	1.4	Ethylcellulose microgranules (time-release)	1500–4000 mg	Active colitis Maintenance	Active colonic disease
Mesalamine (Lialda)		Multi-matrix system	2.4–4.8 g	Active colitis	Active colonic disease
Mesalamine enemas (Rowasa)	2.3	Directly available	4 g	Active left-sided disease	Distal colonic disease
Mesalamine suppositories (Rowasa)	5.6	Directly available	1000 mg	Active proctitis Maintenance	Crohn's proctitis

In an effort to eliminate the side effects associated with the sulfa carrier, newer formulations of 5-ASA have been developed; 5-ASA is rapidly absorbed in the small intestine, which has necessitated development of alternative delivery methods [25] (**Table 14.2**). For example, mesalamine (Asacol) is a coated tablet that dissolves only at an alkaline pH of 6 or 7, corresponding to the pH of the terminal ileum and colon. These compounds have been shown to be as efficacious as sulfasalazine in treating acute attacks of UC as well as preventing relapses [26]. A number of other medications with varied delivery mechanisms and dosing schedules are currently available.

Corticosteroids

The other common modality for the treatment of UC, corticosteroids, are potent inhibitors of the release of arachidonic acid from cell membranes and of the inflammatory response, which inhibit IL-1 and IL-2 and are lympholytic [21–28]. Whether they are administered in oral, intravenous, or rectal forms, they may control symptoms and induce remission. However, low-dose maintenance therapy in inactive disease does not prevent relapse.

Patients must be monitored for the long-term adverse sequelae of corticosteroids such as ulcer disease, cataracts, diabetes, renal failure, and osteoporosis. Morbidity from long-term steroid use is significantly greater than that of elective or urgent surgical therapy for patients with severe ulcerative colitis [29].

Newly developed steroid enemas are poorly absorbed and quickly metabolized, thus free of most adverse side effects. These new compounds include budesonide, beclomethasone dipropionate, and tixocortol pivalate, all of which undergo extensive first-pass metabolism in blood and liver and result in metabolites without significant toxicity [27]. The oral form of budesonide has also shown promise in IBD patients [28].

Approximately 10–20% of patients with UC have a severe enough course to require hospitalization. These patients need nutritional support: generally intravenous hyperalimentation and fluid resuscitation, bed rest, and correction of anemia and require parenteral steroids [8]. Besides 5-ASA and corticosteroids, a number of immunosuppressive agents have been used for the management of UC, including azathioprine, 6-mercaptopurine (6-MP), and cyclosporine. Azathioprine and its metabolite h-mercaptopurine are not helpful in acute attacks, although they may decrease steroid dependence. Cyclosporine inhibits cytokine production, which may be the basis for improvement in inflammation [12, 25–28]. Lichtiger et al [19] reported a response rate of 82% for patients with severe UC that was refractory to steroid therapy. However, the morbidity associated with this medication has been high, and no studies to date have shown that use of this drug has reduced the need for subsequent surgery.

A broad array of agents and strategies have been tried in the treatment of IBD. They include fish oils, zileuton (a specific 5-lipo-oxygenase inhibitor), sucralfate enemas, clonidine, plaquenil, methotrexate, superoxide dismutase, IL-1 receptor antagonist, and the nicotine patch for the treatment of UC [24, 25]. These agents or undiscovered ones will likely improve the medical management of patients with IBD; however, specific curative therapy awaits elucidation of the cause of IBD or surgical extirpation of the colon and rectum.

Operative treatment

The surgical indications for UC (**Table 14.3**) can be classified as elective, urgent, and emergent.

Elective indications

Intractability is the commonest indication for surgery in UC; however, it is also the hardest to define. Unfortunately, the surgeon usually does not see the patient until late in the course of the disease. As a result, patients referred for resection are often malnourished, critically ill, and receiving high doses of steroidal and immunosuppressant medications. These patients are predestined to do poorly, with higher morbidity [29], thus creating a self-fulfilling prophecy for the reluctant gastroenterologist. Today, with the success of the ileoanal reservoir (IAR), there is no justification for procrastination [1, 2, 6, 7]. The best results are obtained when the patient is referred early in the course of the disease. A colectomy can ameliorate the extraintestinal manifestations of UC and as such can be the primary indication. Arthritis, pyoderma gangrenosum, erythema nodosum, and eye lesions may regress following total proctocolectomy. Unfortunately, ankylosing spondylitis and sclerosing cholangitis usually do not improve. Colectomy can be of dramatic benefit in children with UC who previously demonstrated growth retardation. High-grade dysplasia or suspected malignancy is a clear indication for colectomy [21, 30], as is low-grade persistent dysplasia. Carcinoma is not a contraindication to restorative proctocolectomy with ileoanal anastomosis unless the tumor is located in the distal third of the rectum.

Table 14.3 Surgical indications in ulcerative colitis

Elective
Intractability and failure of medical therapy
Extraintestinal manifestations
Growth retardation
Dysplasia or malignancy
Complications from medical therapy: unable to wean from steroids
Urgent
Toxic colitis
Continued hemorrhage
Obstruction from stricture
Emergent
Perforation
Hemorrhage
Toxic megacolon

Urgent indications

UC may progress to a toxic state, relegating the patient to multiple hospital admissions with little or no benefit from steroidal therapy. In this situation or with continued hemorrhage or intermittent obstruction from stricture, urgent surgical therapy may be required.

Emergent indications

Uncontrollable hemorrhage and perforation are uncommon indications for emergent total colectomy ($\leq$1%) [6]; proctectomy should be assiduously avoided. Total abdominal colectomy with either Hartmann's closure of the rectal stump or mucous fistula for toxic megacolon is usually the best alternative in an acutely ill patient [31, 32]. Rarely, the Turnbull 'blowhole' procedure is indicated when the colon is too friable to be manipulated (see Chapter 7) [33]. This operation includes creation of an antimesenteric 'blowhole' transverse colostomy and a loop ileostomy; an optional antimesenteric blowhole sigmoid colostomy is another option. This temporary option avoids spillage by limiting bowel manipulation.

Procedure

The ideal surgical procedure for UC removes all potentially colitic or dysplastic mucosa while preserving anal sphincters and normal bowel function. Historically, a proctocolectomy with a permanent Brooke ileostomy was the procedure of choice. Despite the fact that all the mucosa is excised, this operation clearly falls short of the ideal goal to preserve the anal sphincters. An ileostomy alters body image and is fraught with appliance and stoma-related complications. Furthermore, the proctectomy may result in sexual dysfunction, delayed perineal wound healing, pelvic sepsis, and other postoperative surgical complications. Alternatives to proctocolectomy include ileoproctostomy, proctocolectomy with continent ileostomy (Kock pouch), subtotal colectomy with ileostomy and rectal retention, and restorative proctocolectomy (IPAA).

Proctocolectomy

Prior to the 1980s, total proctocolectomy with ileostomy was the procedure of choice. This large operation cures the patient since the entire colon and rectum are removed but leaves the patient with a permanent ileostomy. The external appliance for the ileostomy may need emptying four to eight times per day. The overall elective morbidity rate ranges from 20–40%, [33] and 10–25% of patients require stoma revision [34]. At least 20% of patients will present with small bowel obstruction in the postoperative period [34, 35], while perineal wound healing is a problem in 4–9%, and sexual dysfunction occurs in up to 12% [6, 7, 36]. (Table 14.4). These complications are minimized by performing the proctectomy in an intersphincteric plane (between the internal and external sphincter). This dissection minimizes blood loss, reduces the risk of nerve injury, and leaves a small perineal wound that is closed primarily.

Table 14.4 Major complications of proctocolectomy

	Unhealed perineal wound (%)	Sexual dysfunction (%)
Bacon et al, 1960 [38]	–	2.8
Waits et al, 1982 [39]	4	–
Metcalf et al, 1986 [40]	–	12
Bauer et al, 1986 [41]	–	2.3
McLeod et al, 1986 [42]	8	–
Phillips et al, 1989 [43]	9	–

Additionally, there are metabolic consequences to ileostomy formation. Despite the complications and disadvantages, a proctocolectomy and Brooke ileostomy is a simple, one-stage operation that rapidly restores health to many patients with UC. The experience at the Mayo Clinic with total proctocolectomy and Brooke ileostomy has been favorable: 76% of patients had few limitations in lifestyle, 95% reported no dietary restrictions, 98% were employed, and 72% would not change the type of ileostomy [43].

Ileorectostomy

Because of the complications associated with a proctectomy, some surgeons preferred abdominal colectomy with ileorectostomy (ileoproctostomy) (**Figure 14.3**). The anastomosis is usually performed at the sacral promontory with an end-to-end technique using an intraluminal stapler. The reported leak rate is less than 2% and the mortality rate is 1.4% [44]. Since the rectum is not mobilized and there is no pelvic dissection, the potential chances of sexual dysfunction, bladder dysfunction, and presacral hemorrhage are negligible [31–36]. Other advantages include acceptable transanal bowel evacuation frequency and low complication rates, avoiding an unhealed wound (**Table 14.5**) [49]. Finally, the option for a restorative ileoanal reservoir or total proctocolectomy still exists. This procedure is selected most often in very young patients (preteens) who have relatively healthy distensible rectums.

The disadvantages of ileorectostomy include the risks of proctitis and rectal carcinoma. The risk of cancer is related to the length of retained rectum and duration of disease. Cancer has not been reported at less than 10 years after the procedure, but the incidence is 2–6% at 10–19 years and 13–15% at 20–30 years [49, 50]. Approximately 50% of patients will require an additional operation to deal with their retained rectum [44].

Patients offered this procedure must be motivated and understand the necessity of lifelong rectal surveillance. Contraindications to ileorectostomy include a nondistensible diseased rectum, severe proctitis, perianal disease, fecal incontinence, colorectal neoplasia or dysplasia, or a patient who cannot reliably be seen for periodic rectal surveillance. Surveillance of the retained rectum should include a

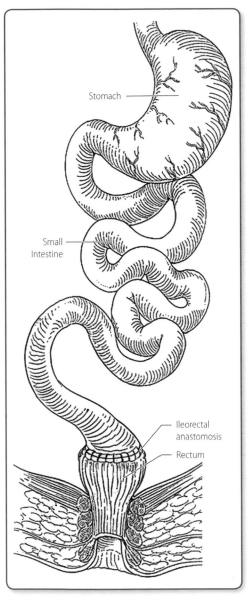

Figure 14.3 Colectomy with ileorectal anastomosis.

Stomach

Small Intestine

Ileorectal anastomosis

Rectum

	No. of patients	Mortality (%)	Anastomotic leak (%)	Failure rate (%)	Cancer rectal (%)	Mean no. of bowel movements
Table 14.5 Ileoproctostomy results						
Oakley et al, 1985 [46]	145	0	2	24	3.4	4.3
Parc et al, 1989 [47]	197	–	–	25	–	4.5
Khubchandani et al, 1989 [48]	110	0	2	10	–	1.4

proctoscopy with biopsy on a 6–12 month basis after the patient has had ulcerative colitis for more than 7 years.

Continent ileostomy (Kock pouch)

The continent ileostomy described by Professor Nils Kock of Goteborg, Sweden in 1969 consisted of an internal intestinal pouch that would serve as a reservoir for stool. The reservoir was coupled with an intestinal nipple valve (**Figure 14.4**) between the pouch and a flush cutaneous stoma situated lower on the abdominal wall than a Brooke ileostomy (see Figure 7.6) [51]. Patients empty the pouch by passing a soft plastic tube through the valve via the stoma 4–6 times a day. A continent eliminates the requirement for an external appliance, which simplifies social and recreational activities. Thus this procedure offers the patient a cosmetic option [52].

Nevertheless, the continent ileostomy has been associated with a high reoperation and complication rate, including slippage of the nipple

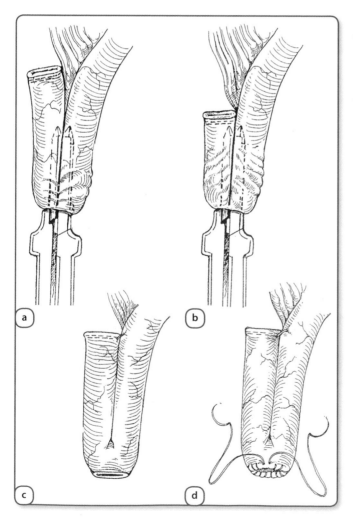

Figure 14.4 Creation of stapled J pouch. (a) Linear cutting stapler inserted through apex of pouch. (b) Second application of stapler. (c) Completed pouch. (d) Purse-string placed at apex in preparation for doubled-stapled ileoanal reservoir.

valve, obstruction, metabolic complications, and pouchitis (**Table 14.6**) [56]. Despite multiple technical modifications [57], valve slippage remains a significant problem and reported occurs in 5–15% of patients having long-term follow-up. If significant valve slippage occurs (usually manifested by pouch incontinence or difficulty with pouch intubation), surgical correction is required. A patient who develops difficulty in intubating the pouch must seek medical attention. A continent pouch that cannot be intubated results in a complete bowel obstruction. If the pouch cannot be intubated with a catheter, endoscopic intubation may be required. Pouchitis occurs in 5–43% of patients with a continent ileostomy [58].

Development of restorative proctocolectomies (discussed on pages 253–259) has significantly reduced the demand for continent ileostomies. However a small select group of patients are best served with this option. [56]. This includes patients who are not candidates for a restorative proctocolectomy (UC and rectal cancer or anal incontinence) and in whom a pelvic pouch or ileoanal reservoir has not been successful; usually because of septic complications. It is also a consideration for patients who are dissatisfied with their Brooke ileostomy.

Subtotal colectomy

A subtotal colectomy, with an end Brooke ileostomy and either a Hartmann closure of the rectum or a mucous fistula, is the procedure of choice in an emergent setting. If the diagnosis of UC cannot be clearly established, a preliminary subtotal colectomy with either ileoproctostomy or ileostomy may be indicated [59].

Restorative proctocolectomy (ileoanal reservoir)

The restorative proctocolectomy, IPAA or pouch procedure has become the most common definitive operation for UC [31–35, 44]. Parks and Nicholl [59], from St. Mark's hospital in London, first described this procedure in 1978; it has since been modified and has gained widespread acceptance. The original operation entailed a total abdominal colectomy with rectal mucosectomy, ileal reservoir, and ileoanal anastomosis. A temporary diverting loop ileostomy minimized the sequelae of pelvic sepsis. Currently, the pouch is created with two, three, or four loops of small intestine to act as a neorectum (**Figure 14.5**) [60]. The pouch is delivered through the rectal muscular cuff and anastomosed to the anus or anastomosed to the top of the anal canal (**Figure 14.6**).

Table 14.6 Results with continent ileostomy (Kock pouch)			
	Number of patients	Reoperation rate (%)	Excision rate (%)
Dozois et al, 1980 [54]	299	50.8	6.6
Kock and Myrvold, 1980 [55]	396	54.0	4.3
Fazio and Church, 1988 [56]	168	42.5	5.0

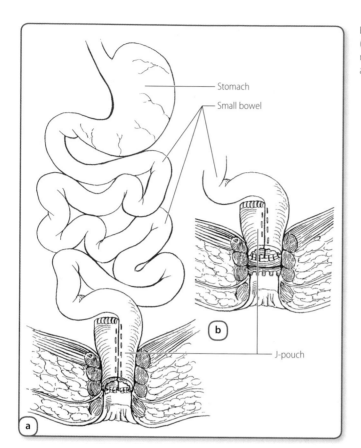

Figure 14.5 Ileoanal reservoir.
(a) Hand-sewn anastomosis after mucosectomy; (b) Double-stapled anastomosis.

Stomach

Small bowel

b

J-pouch

a

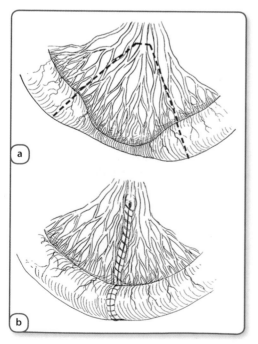

Figure 14.6 Small bowel resection. (a) Extent of small bowel resection. (b) Completed end-to-end anastomosis.

a

b

Table 14.7 Functional results of restorative proctocolectomy

	No. of patients	Frequency of evacuation	Leakage (%)	Incontinence (%)
Becker and Raymond, 1986 [62]	100	5.4 ± 0.2	25	?
Pemberton et al, 1987 [63]	389	6 ± 2	22–52	?
Fonkalsrud, 1987 [64]	138	4.8	?	?
Fleshman et al, 1988 [65]	102	6.2 ± 3.1	18–23	1–7
Wexner et al, 1989 [66]	114	5.4 ± 2.5	12–29	1–2
Kelly, 1992 [67]	1193	4.5	25	?
Reissman et al, 1995 [68]	140	5.4	0.4–3.2	0–0.8
Blumberg et al, 2001 [69]	145	4.5	10	0

Regardless of configuration, the IPAA has well-documented functional results (**Table 14.7**). The average number of daily bowel movements ranges from four to six. Nocturnal bowel movements generally occur one or two times per evening. Most series note continued improvement in function for at least 1–2 years. The majority of patients can resume normal work, social activities, and sexual intercourse. Impotence and retrograde ejaculation are rarely seen; infertility and dyspareunia have been less well studied [61–68].

Several controversies persist relative to technical aspects of the procedure. Most surgeons currently perform a double-stapled IPAA which obviates the need for rectal mucosectomy and may improve postoperative continence [34, 35, 67]. The rectal mucosectomy has the potential to adversely affect anal continence in two distinct ways: first, anal dilation for adequate exposure to the entire rectal circumference and dilation during fashioning of the anastomosis may damage or disrupt the sphincters [70]; second, the anal transition zone is permanently extirpated, ablating the rectoanal inhibitory reflex. The anal transition zone is rich in sensory nerves, which helps in discriminating among gas, liquid, and solid stool. This sensory mechanism plays a role in maintaining continence [70].

The problems with mucosectomy are not limited to incontinence and leakage. O'Connell et al [71] showed that after mucosectomy, small islands of residual mucosa remained between the rectal cuff and the IAR in 21% of patients. These findings are of concern, because extra reservoir inflammation, dysplasia, or even carcinoma may arise in an inaccessible area of tissue that cannot be easily subjected to surveillance [72,73].

Although technically easier to create, the double-stapled IPAA has disadvantages if improperly performed. The anal transition zone occasionally contains some columnar epithelium, and its retention can lead to subsequent inflammation. This is more likely the higher the anastomosis is placed. If the anastomosis is greater than 2–3 cm above the dentate line, some true rectal mucosa may be retained. Several reports have described development of inflammation (anitis) in the retained anal transition zone or anorectal mucosa [74,75]. Patients with significant symptoms resulting from an inappropriately cephalad anastomosis may require topical or systemic immunosuppressive medications or surgical removal of the anal transition zone and advancement of the pouch to the dentate line. This has been performed transanally or with an abdominoperineal approach [76]. As in patients after a mucosectomy [72,73], persistent or recurrent disease also raises the question of whether the patient has Crohn's disease.

The risk of cancer in this retained segment has yet to be determined. Most surgeons performing a double-stapled technique recommend periodic surveillance (often including biopsies), and to date no cancers have been reported after a double-stapled technique has been used. Conversely, with longer follow-up, at least three cancers have been reported after mucosectomy [72,73,77]. If the anastomosis is placed too low (at or within 1 cm of the dentate line), a significant portion of the internal sphincter may be removed and the patient will have reduced continence [78]. Proponents of performing a mucosectomy argue that the double-stapled technique does not 'cure' the patient of colitis, which for many is the goal of the operation.

Two small prospective randomized studies have compared a double-stapled IPAA to mucosectomy [79,80]. These studies produced similar functional results for each operation. Other larger retrospective reviews have confirmed these finding [81,82]. A final concern is that for technical reasons a double-staple technique may not be possible. These patients will then require a mucosectomy, and surgeons performing this type of surgery must be able to perform a mucosectomy if required.

An increasing number of surgeons perform restorative procto-colectomy using laparoscopic techniques [83,84]. A laparoscopic restorative proctocolectomy has cosmetic advantages, no increased rate of complications, but slightly longer operative time (1–2 hours). To reduce operative times some surgeons use a hand assisted laparoscopic technique [85].

Technical tips for the mucosectomy

A lighted Chelsea-Eaton retractor is inserted into the anus and a 1 : 100,000 solution of epinephrine solution is infiltrated using a spinal needle into the submucosa around the anus (circumferentially from the dentate line to the anal rectal ring). This reduces bleeding and delineates the correct dissection plane. The mucosa is incised at the dentate line with electrocautery, and with sharp scissor dissection, a mucosal flap is created. Dissection is continued proximally to a level above the pelvic dissection performed by the abdominal team. After an adequate mucosal dissection, the residual rectal wall is divided at the anorectal ring by either the perineal or abdominal surgeon using scissors or electrocautery. Eight or twelve sutures of 2-0 polyglycolic acid are placed at the dentate line, splayed in a radial fashion and held in place to the operative drapes with clamps. When placed correctly, these sutures incorporate anoderm (which is advanced slightly up into the anal canal) and a small portion of the internal sphincter.

The pelvis and anal canal are irrigated, and adequate hemostasis is confirmed. The end of the ileal pouch is carefully passed through the anal canal. The previously placed sutures are then sequentially placed through the open end of the pouch and tied (constructing an ileal pouch–anal anastomosis). After all sutures are tied, a small lighted Hill-Ferguson retractor is placed through the anastomosis to confirm complete mucosal approximation. Any gaps are closed with additional sutures.

Technical tips for the double-stapled ileoanal reservoir

The operation is performed in the lithotomy position with the patient's legs in Allen stirrups (Allen Medical, Cleveland, Ohio, USA). The tip of the coccyx should be at the back of the table with a small pad used as a sacral rest for easy access to the anal canal in case a mucosectomy is necessary. A total abdominal colectomy is performed, transecting the ileum flush with the cecum and maintaining the ileal blood supply. After ligation of the inferior mesenteric or superior rectal vessels, the presacral space is sharply entered with electrocautery. Dissection and mobilization of the rectum is continued with the electrocautery down to the level of the levator muscles until only a narrow sleeve of muscle remains at the anorectal junction. Great care must be taken to avoid injury to the vagina and presacral anatomic nerves. A 30 mm linear stapler should fit easily around the anorectal circumferential sleeve between the levators. No more than 1 cm of anal canal should remain cephalad to the dentate line; the result should not be a pouch–rectal but rather a pouch–anal anastomosis.

Reservoir construction

A number of configurations of the reservoir exist. However, functional outcome is not related to pouch configuration [6,7,60]. The J pouch is the simplest and most popular technique [60]. After mobilization of the entire small bowel to the origin of the SMA at the inferior aspect of the pancreas, the distal 20–40 cm of ileum is configured as the two limbs of the J reservoir. The apex should easily reach several centimeters below the pubis. Another advantage of the double-stapled technique is that a tension free anastomosis is seldom a problem. However, a variety of lengthening techniques can be employed [86]. A W or an S configuration may provide increased length and decrease tension in patients with a short mesentery [6,7,62]. A J pouch is constructed using two to three sequential firings of a long linear cutter through the apex of the pouch. The pouch length varies from 15–20 cm. (**Figure 14.5**) [35]. A circular 2-0 or 0-Prolene whipstitch is placed around the base of the enterotomy and the detachable anvil from a 29 mm circular stapler (Ethicon Endo-Surgery, Inc., Cincinnati, Ohio, USA) is secured with the previously placed Prolene suture. A circular stapler is inserted in the anus against the linear anal canal staple line and with the aid of a lipped retractor; the vagina is reflected anteriorly to prevent injury as the stapler is closed and fired. Anastomotic integrity is verified by air insufflation under water and by palpation. A closed suction drain may be placed in the presacral space for 2–4 days. Because many patients with UC are on large doses of steroids or immunosuppressants, are malnourished and often anemic, a temporary loop ileostomy has traditionally been constructed. The ileostomy should help protect patients from the consequences of anastomotic leaks and pelvic sepsis, the most devastating complications of IPAA which may ultimately compromise functional results [6,7]. In selected cases, surgeons who frequently perform the operation may elect to omit the stoma.

Complications

The most common complications after restorative proctocolectomy with an IPAA are small bowel obstruction and pouchitis. An obstruction rate of 9–27% is reported in most series; in half of these cases a laparotomy is required (**Table 14.8**). The long-term rate of laparotomy for small bowel obstruction rises to 17%. Recent use of Seprafilm, an adhesion prevention product, in pouch patients may help reduce adhesions, which can cause small bowel obstruction [87,88].

Pouchitis consists of an increase in the frequency of evacuation, often with bloody or mucoid watery stools, which can be accompanied by abdominal cramps, tenderness, fever, and dehydration. The incidence of pouchitis is 10–33% [63–66,89]. Endoscopically, friable edematous mucosa is seen. This condition is more common in patients with UC than in those with familial adenomatous polyposis (FAP) and more frequent in patients with UC who have had pre-existing extraintestinal manifestations of UC [32]. The cause of pouchitis is unclear, but it generally responds to a course of metronidazole or ciprofloxacin and rehydration administered on an outpatient basis.

Pelvic sepsis is the most devastating complication, but fortunately its incidence has decreased from 10–25% in the early 1980s to less than

Table 14.8 Complications of restorative proctocolectomy					
Author	No. of patients	Sepsis (%)	Small bowel obstruction/ laparotomy (%)	Pouchitis (%)	Stricture (%)
Fonkalsrud, 1987 [64]	138	4	?/9	29	–
Schoetz et al, 1987 [85]	86	8	27/12	10	–
Fleshman et al, 1988 [65]	102	17	?/19	23	8
Wexner et al, 1990 [3]	178	11	27/15	27	12
Kelly, 1992 [67]	1193	5	15/5	–	–
Blumberg et al, 2001 [69]	145	8	26/?	11	–

5% at present. The sequela of pelvic infection is fibrosis, which probably does not allow the pouch to distend and may yield poor functional results. If a laparotomy is required for pelvic sepsis, pouch failure and excision approach 50% [90].

A pouchogram is performed before ileostomy closure to exclude anastomotic leak [89]. If a leak is found, ileostomy closure should be delayed. Pelvic collections can be percutaneously drained or accessed through the pouch if a communication already exists. An advantage of a double-stapled IPAA is that elimination of mucosectomy also obviates the potential for a cuff abscess [34, 35]. Rates of pelvic sepsis after creation of a double-stapled IRA have been lower than 5% [6, 89–93].

The incidence of pouch vaginal fistula is 8–10% [92–96]. A pouch vaginal or cutaneous fistula should alert one to the possible presence of Crohn's disease. Despite a variety of both perineal and abdominal approaches to eradicate the pouch vaginal fistula, the need for ultimate pouch excision occurs in approximately 20% of cases [31, 92, 93]. Overall rates of IPAA failure range from 5–10%, necessitating pouch excision and permanent ileostomy [31]. Failure is generally attributable to pelvic sepsis and IPAA complications that occur within the first 2 years after ileostomy closure.

Eventually a significant proportion of patients with UC require an operation, with the realization that colectomy does not reflect a therapeutic failure but rather a permanent cure. A colectomy with an IPAA is currently the operation of choice. Several studies have demonstrated that patients have an extremely high level of satisfaction and performance after IPAA, particularly when compared with proctocolectomy, continent ileostomy, and permanent Brooke ileostomy [31, 64–68].

Crohn's disease

Crohn's disease is a chronic transmural inflammatory disorder that can involve the entire alimentary tract from the mouth to the anus. Crohn's disease predominantly affects a young, economically productive patient population. The disease is a lifelong condition that can be either chronically debilitating or intermittently exacerbated. Its course is unpredictable, medical therapy is limited, and surgery temporizes rather than cures. Not surprisingly, the disease has a significant adverse impact on the patient's quality of life.

Crohn's disease is usually segmental; the terminal ileum and proximal colon are the most commonly affected. The disease appears to be systemic; it can involve both the entire alimentary tract and extraintestinal tissues.

History

Crohn, Ginzberg, and Oppenheimer described a transmural inflammatory condition of the terminal ileum in 1932 [5]. The authors allegedly listed their names in alphabetical order for the publication and hence an everlasting eponym was established. The latter caused the well-known controversy between these physicians, since the majority of cases were that of surgeon A. Borg at Mount Sinai Hospital in New York, where Crohn was Chairman of the Department of Gastroenterology [7,97].

In actuality, in 1903 Dalziel reported an obscure tuberculosis-like condition that he called 'chronic interstitial enteritis,' which may have been Crohn's disease [98]. In 1923, Moschowitz and Wilensky [99] also described a granulomatosis condition of the intestine. In 1959, Morson and Lockhart-Mummery [100] described Crohn's colitis, which was accepted as a clinical entity distinct from UC.

Epidemiology

Since the historic description of Crohn's disease in 1932, its incidence appears to have markedly increased. The worldwide prevalence is estimated to be 10–70 cases per 100,000 population, with an incidence in 1 year of one to six cases per 100,000 population [97]. The disease is almost exclusively encountered in industrialized nations of Western Europe and the United States, which suggests that environmental factors are important. The disease is more common among Jewish people and urban residents and is associated with patients with higher levels of education [5–7].

Aggregation in families occurs mostly among first-degree relatives, suggesting a role for genetic factors. Crohn's disease occurs in men and women with equal frequency and occurs most often between 15 and 30 years of age, with a second peak at 55–60 years [97].

Etiologic factors

Many advances have been made since Crohn et al described the clinical entity more than 70 years ago, yet the cause of this disease remains speculative. The efficacy of corticosteroids and immunosuppressive agents such as 6-MP and cyclosporine suggests an immunologic origin [10,11]. Epidemiologic data suggest genetic, dietary, environmental, and infectious causes. Two major hypotheses have evolved: the infectious theory contends that an unidentified agent causes the disease and the subsequent immune response; the immunologic theory suggests that the immune system reacts inappropriately to antigenic challenge (i.e. cytokines and antibiotics). In both theories, the immune system plays a major role in the cause [8].

Clinical Features

History

Abdominal pain is a frequent complaint of patients with Crohn's disease. The pain is intermittent, colicky in nature, and tends to be localized to the right lower quadrant. Patients usually have anorexia, nausea, vomiting, and diarrhea and are generally malnourished, with weight loss and general fatigue; peritoneal irritation causes more severe constant pain.

Clinical consequences of impaired absorption and the resultant malnutrition cause detrimental alteration in many systems:

- Diarrhea with dehydration and electrolyte imbalance
- Steatorrhea
- Gallstones
- Protein-losing enteropathy
- Growth retardation
- Anemia
- Hypoproteinemia with edema
- Demineralization of bone
- Hypovitaminosis
- Renal oxalate stones

The consequences are particularly serious in children, resulting in growth retardation and delayed maturation in 10–40% of children with Crohn's disease [8, 101, 102].

Physical examination

Because patients with Crohn's disease typically present with pain, often accompanied by a tender mass in the right lower quadrant with febrile episodes, the differential diagnosis must include appendicitis. Perianal disease is common and includes eccentrically placed, deep, indolent fissures, multiple fistulas-in-ano, abscesses, ulcers, and skin tags [31,103]. The prevalence of perianal disease is about 25% for patients with ileitis, 50% with ileocolitis, and 40% for individuals with isolated colonic involvement [31,103,104]. Crohn's disease is frequently associated with extraintestinal manifestations: the skin, eyes, and joints are the most common sites. The prevalence is higher in patients with colonic disease than those with small bowel disease (**Table 14.9**) [97].

Endoscopic findings

Endoscopic examination is the most important tool for evaluating the bowel and confirming the presence or absence of Crohn's disease. Proctosigmoidoscopic examination is particularly important in differentiating Crohn's disease from other colitides. The cancer risk

Table 14.9 Extraintestinal manifestations of irritable bowel disease	
Skin	**Joints**
Pyoderma gangrenosum	Arthritis
Erythema nodosum multiform	Ankylosing spondylitis
Vasculitis	Hypertrophy, osteoarthropathy
Aphthous stomatitis	
Eyes	**Liver**
Conjunctivitis	Sclerosing cholangitis
Iritis	Pericholangitis (rare)
Iridocyclitis, episcleritis	Granulomatous hepatitis (rare)
Uveitis	
Vasculitis	

From Schraut WH, Medick D. Crohn's disease. In: Greenfield LT, Mulholland MW, Oldham K, et al. (eds). Surgery: Scientific Principles and Practice. Philadelphia: JB Lippincott, 1993; 741.

for patients with Crohn's disease is increased over that of the general population, and thus periodic surveillance is indicated. This will be discussed in more detail later in this chapter. Upper endoscopy is also important, since Crohn's disease may involve the esophagus, stomach, and duodenum in up to 3% of all patients. Endoscopic examination may reveal ulceration, stricture, or fistula. Colonoscopy is a useful tool to confirm disease, evaluate strictures, grade disease activity and response to treatment, and for surveillance of dysplasia and cancer. Random biopsies should be taken at random sites throughout the entire colon in both involved and uninvolved segments. Granuloma is the most useful lesion found on colonoscopic biopsy.

The rectum is often spared in Crohn's disease. Diseased segments of mucosa appear as deep, indolent, linear ulcers or there may be cobblestoning, friability, strictures, aphthoid ulcers, and most important, segmental involvement with skip lesions; toxic dilatation is rare; colonoscopy can precipitate toxic dilatation, so its presence is a contraindication to colonoscopy.

Radiologic findings

Contrast radiographs are useful for the differential diagnosis and delineation of the extent and severity of disease. Barium studies may show fistula, strictures, and segmental involvement, but these studies are being supplanted by CT or MR enterography. A CT scan delineates masses and abscesses amenable to percutaneous drainage before resection. Correlation between the extent of disease seen radiographically and the clinical picture is often absent [103]. Recurrent disease after surgical resection is often radiographically apparent (mucosal irregularity proximal to the anastomosis) before the development of clinical signs and symptoms [97]. Another technique for assessing the small bowel is enteroclysis. Intravenous pyelography may be helpful before resection to exclude ureteral obstruction.

Histopathologic findings

The acute active phase is marked by aphthous mucosal ulcers, lymphoid aggregates, granulomas, and transmural chronic inflammation with fissures and fistulas [7]. The quiescent or healing phase is characterized by fibrosis, stricture formation, and chronic ulcers.

The bowel appears rigid, thickened from fibrosis, and inflamed, resulting in a narrowing of the lumen. The mesenteric fat creeps over the antimesenteric border and the mesentery is foreshortened, thickened, and edematous, containing enlarged, inflamed nodes. The inflammatory process is transmural and extends to adjacent tissues, sometimes causing fistulas and abscesses.

Noncaseating granulomas are pathognomonic; they are localized, well-formed aggregates of epithelioid histocytes surrounded by lymphocytes and giant cells. Although two thirds of patients exhibit granulomas, they are rarely identified by colonoscopic biopsy specimen. Fistulas that develop from confluent crypt abscesses and transmural inflammation are also found in Crohn's disease but not in UC (**Table 14.1**) [7, 22, 97]. Narrow, deeply penetrating fissures and ulcers are also characteristic, as is increased mucous secretion.

When a diagnosis of either Crohn's disease or UC cannot be determined, the condition is called 'indeterminate colitis.' In the 10% of cases that are indeterminate, the clinical course of the disease determines the eventual diagnosis [97].

Nonoperative treatment

Medical therapy for Crohn's disease includes supportive care with treatment of acute exacerbations [24]. Surgery is reserved for complications of chronic disease or complications of or refractoriness to medical therapy. There is no disease-specific therapy; thus emphasis is placed on nutritional support, alleviation of symptoms, and suppression of the inflammatory process.

Nutrition

Dietary modifications include supplementation with bulk-forming agents, reduction of fresh fruit and milk products, and addition of medications to slow the transit time. Total parenteral nutrition (TPN) may be helpful to induce short-term remission [106]. Nutritional support of malnourished patients with Crohn's disease increases body weight, visceral protein status, and nitrogen balance. Bowel rest and TPN may be used to treat acute disease and for preoperative therapy. In patients with short gut syndrome or patients who are extremely malnourished, TPN may be beneficial for fluid and electrolye repletion and fistula healing. It may also be used for treatment in the presence of chronic small bowel obstruction or growth retardation in these debilitated patients with Crohn's disease [107].

Corticosteroid therapy

Systemic corticosteroids have been used to treat Crohn's disease since its original description. Although the immunosuppressive effects of steroidal medications are useful in acute exacerbation of the disease, long-term treatment is not beneficial and is associated with many deleterious systemic side effects [26–28]. Topical steroidal agents with less systemic absorption and metabolism are currently available.

Aminosalicylates (ASA)

Sulfasalazine and its metabolite 5-ASA are more effective than placebo in achieving remission of acute disease and are more effective in patients with Crohn's colitis. Newer preparations of oral 5-ASA with varied absorptive patterns are being used clinically [21,26,27,29].

Antibiotics

Metronidazole is most often used to treat perianal disease, although it may also be effective in the treatment of acute disease [108]. Long-term use causes irreversible peripheral neuropathy, a metallic taste, and nausea. Ciprofloxacin has also been used as a single agent and in combination with metronidazole to treat Crohn's disease [24].

Immunosuppressive agents

Azathioprine and its metabolite 6-MP are used in patients with Crohn's disease to reduce steroid requirements, encourage the healing of fistulas, and, theoretically, to reduce recurrence rates. They require at least 3 months of treatment to be effective; side effects during this prolonged course include bone marrow suppression (2%), pancreatitis (2–4%), and nausea and vomiting [24,26–29].

Methotrexate and cyclosporine have been used as part of the immunologic pharmacopeia against Crohn's disease. Both interfere with cytokine production involved in the pathogenesis of IBD [29]. Brynskov et al [109] concluded that cyclosporine had a beneficial effect on 59% of patients who were refractory to steroid treatment. However, major concerns with this drug are its side effect of renal damage and the fact that remission cannot be maintained after its use is discontinued.

Biologicals

Progress in biotechnology has fostered the development of new agents that target pivotal processes in disease pathogenesis. An anti-tumor necrosis factor-α (TNF-α) monoclonal antibody (infliximab [Remicade], Centocor Ortho Biotech) produces rapid improvement in symptoms and clinical remissions in IBD patients [110,111]. The drug has been used in single dose therapy and multiple dose regimens. Experience is increasing with these agents. With infliximab, 20–30% of patients experience minor adverse effects and 26% of patients experience serious adverse events, which include infections in 3.8%. Tuberculosis is an increasing concern, and patients should have skin testing prior to starting therapy. An additional disadvantage is the cost of the drug and the potential for a HAMA (human antimularian antibody) reaction. This can be reduced by concurrent treatment with other immunosuppressant medications (including azathioprine and methotrexate), by maintaining a regular infusion schedule, and by giving patients a pre-treatment dose of steroid medication [112].

Etanercept (Enbrel, Amgen) is an engineered protein that blocks TNF receptor 2 [113]. Adalimumab (Humira, Abbott) is a humanized recombinant antibody to TNF. Both of these agents have shown effectiveness in patients with moderate-to-severe Crohn's disease [114]. Adalimumab has an advantage in that it is given by subcutaneous injection as opposed to infliximab, which is given by intravenous infusion.

In 2005, two other recombinant medications were reported to have benefit in moderate to severe Crohn's disease. Certolizumab pegol (Cimzia, Union chimique belge, Belgium) is a Fab fragment of a humanized anti-TNF-α monoclonal antibody that is attached to polyethylene glycol to increase its half-life in circulation. It was found to have efficacy over placebo medications for 10 weeks in the treatment of moderate to severe Crohn's disease in one large trial [115]. Natalizumab (Tysabri, Elan) is a humanized monoclonal antibody against the cellular adhesion molecule of α-4 integrin. The drug is thought to work by reducing the ability of inflammatory immune cells to pass through cell layers [116]. Unfortunately, this drug has been associated with progressive multifocal leukoencephalopathy, a usually fatal viral infection of the brain, that may limit its use [117].

Operative treatment

Surgical therapy is palliative and is therefore reserved for treatment of complications of the disease, including fistula, obstruction, perforation, abscess, malignancy, toxic megacolon, hemorrhage, growth retardation, and failure of medical management. Failure of or complications from medical management can result from the chronic debilitation associated with the disease, from intractability of symptoms, impairment of well-being or lifestyle, or from the debilitating side effects of medical therapy [28,118,119]. Basic perioperative principles are outlined in **Table 14.10**.

Specific situations

Anorectal

Fistulas Fistulas secondary to Crohn's disease almost never close permanently [26]. However, enteroenteric fistulas do not require surgery unless they are associated with sepsis, obstruction, intractability, or electrolyte abnormalities. Conversely, enterocutaneous fistulas almost always require surgery because of dehydration, malnutrition, and sequelae of loss of intestinal fluid. A patient with enterocutaneous fistulas may benefit from bowel rest and TPN while the fistula clears of fecal material and the skin and tract heal as much as possible.

Fistulous communication to the sigmoid colon, the bladder, the retroperitoneum, or any other intra-abdominal organ is handled in a similar manner. The opening in the nondiseased organ is cleared and

Table 14.10 Basic perioperative principles
1. Full preoperative evaluation
2. Colonoscopy +/– air contrast barium enema
3. Upper gastrointestinal series/small bowel follow through series
4. Computerized tomography scan, if clinically indicated
5. Intravenous pyelography, if clinically indicated
6. Stoma site marking
7. Mechanical bowel preparation
8. Oral antibiotic preparation
9. Intravenous antibiotic preparation
10. Perioperative steroids
11. Consider ureteric catheters
12. Midline incision
13. Meticulous search for skip lesions
14. Assess length of uninvolved intestine
15. Limit resection to gross disease without large normal margins
16. Careful handling of mesentery with suture-ligation of vessels
17. Strictureplasty, when indicated
18. Bypass only for duodenal Crohn's disease
19. Avoid appendectomy if base of appendix and cecum are involved

Nogueras JJ, Werner SD. Surgical management of primary and recurrent Crohn's disease. Probl Gen Surg 1993;10:123.

closed in layers. An ileosigmoid fistula is treated by resection of the diseased small bowel and either resection of the sigmoid or by simple closure of the colonic defect.

Stricture Patients with recurrent Crohn's disease may develop multiple strictures of the small bowel and large bowel. In selected patients strictures may be resected (**Figure 14.6**). Extensive or multiple small bowel resections could result in short bowel syndrome. To avoid this problem, a strictureplasty is an excellent alternative for short strictures [119, 120]. The basic principles of strictureplasty are shown in **Figure 14.7**. Resection and strictureplasty are complementary; resection or Finney strictureplasty should be performed for long segment strictures or for multiple short segment strictures confined to a small area of small bowel. Strictureplasty results are summarized in **Table 14.11**.

Ileocolic disease is usually managed with an ileocolic resection (**Figure 14.8**). Colonic strictures are usually resected as described below. Due to a significant association of malignancy with colonic strictures in inflammatory bowel disease patients, strictureplasties are rarely indicated.

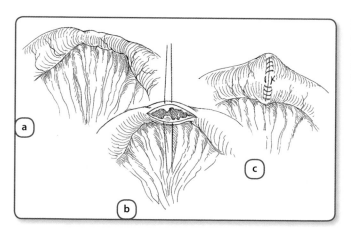

Figure 14.7 Heineke–Mikulicz strictureplasty (a). Longitudinal incision is made on the antimesenteric border (b). The incision is closed in a transverse fashion (c).

Table 14.11 Results of strictureplasty				
	No. of patients	No. of strictureplasties	Complications (%)	New strictures (%)	Recurrences (%)
Alexander-Williams, 1986 [122]	57	146	7	10	3
Fazio et al, 1989 [123]	50	225	16	8	4
Dehn et al, 1989 [124]	24	86	4	13	4
Spencer et al, 1994 [125]	35	–	–	–	0
Stebbing et al, 1995 [126]	52	241	–	–	3.7
Serra et al, 1995 [127]	28	–	–	–	–
Ozuner et al, 1996 [128]	162	798	5	17	5
Yamamoto and Keighley, 1999 [129]	43	–	–	–	–

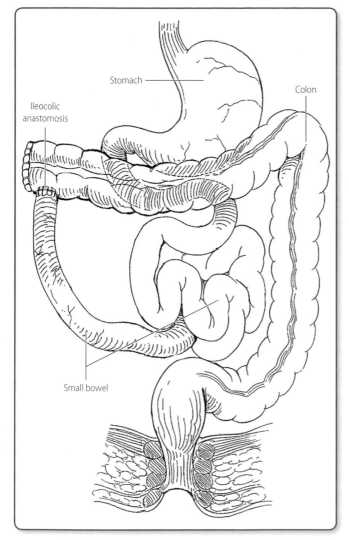

Figure 14.8 Ileocolic resection.

Colonic disease   Crohn's colitis is notorious for high recurrence rates if a partial colectomy is performed; therefore either a subtotal colectomy or a total proctocolectomy with ileostomy is a preferable alternative. If there is rectal sparing, an ileorectal anastomosis (**Figure 14.3**) can be fashioned. If the rectum is diseased, an intersphincteric proctectomy diminishes perineal wound problems [97, 129]. On rare occasions a subtotal colectomy with creation of a Hartmann's rectal pouch or even a near-total proctocolectomy with preservation of the anus and anal sphincters may be appropriate.

Perianal disease   The traditional approach to perianal Crohn's disease was to avoid surgery because of increased risk of poor wound healing and incontinence; recently, however, this approach has been challenged.

Many surgeons now advocate aggressive treatment for fissures and fistula [130,131]. Exceptions to aggressive surgical management include high complex and rectovaginal fistulas in which fistulotomy would entail division of a substantial percentage of the external anal sphincter muscle [31,103,118]. However, if one uses prompt abscess drainage, conservative fistulotomy for intersphincteric and low trans-sphincteric fistulas, and drainage by seton or mushroom catheter for high trans-sphincteric, multiple, and complex fistulas or rectovaginal fistulas, proctectomy can usually be avoided [132–135]. Rectal flaps tend not to fare well if the rectum is severely diseased, and a transvaginal approach may be used [136–137]. On occasion, a concomitant loop ileostomy may afford the opportunity for sufficient perianal and perineal healing to avoid a total proctocolectomy and permanent ileostomy [135–137]. However, routine stoma construction is unnecessary. More complex procedures such as sphincteroplasty and muscle transposition occasionally have a role after a failed advancement flap [11,138].

Surgery should be avoided for 'asymptomatic' hemorrhoids, fistulas, fissures, and skin tags. Patients with severe rectal disease with associated perianal disease may benefit from diversion and future treatment of the perianal condition. On occasion, metronidazole may be beneficial.

Ultimately, proctectomy is indicated in up to 25% of patients with severe anorectal or perianal Crohn's disease [139]. A perineal intersphincteric approach should be used to minimize wound healing problems [129]. A low Hartmann procedure or a near total proctocolectomy may serve as an alternative to proctectomy for severe anorectal disease, particularly if fistulous tracts exit a significant distance from the anal verge and if perianal sepsis predominates. Sher et al [140] reported an 88% healing rate within 12 months of proctectomy with this approach.

Pregnancy and inflammatory bowel disease

In most cases, pregnancy does not affect IBD, and inactive IBD does not affect the course of a pregnancy or result in premature birth. Active IBD will decrease the probability of conception, complicate the pregnancy by increasing the spontaneous abortion rate and fetal complication rate, and increase the likelihood of premature delivery. Pregnancy should not be postponed because of the fear of activating a quiescent case of IBD, and also pregnancy should not be terminated because of IBD, whether active or quiescent. If surgery is necessary during pregnancy, it is best to proceed rather than deleteriously waiting until after delivery. A subtotal colectomy is preferrable to a proctectomy because of the enlarged uterus and its blood supply. Medical therapy with prednisone, sulfasalazine, and TPN is usually safe during pregnancy. Laparoscopy and the use of anti-adhesion agents are suggested in women who require surgical therapy and desire to preserve their fertility. Patients with an IPAA are occasionally able to successfully deliver vaginally without permanent incontinence [141].

Surveillance

The risk of developing colon cancer in patients with IBD is undoubtedly increased both in patients with UC and in those with Crohn's disease. Since onset of the disease is often at an early age, it is logical that screening programs to detect dysplasia and prevent neoplasia would be beneficial.

Surveillance in ulcerative colitis

The duration and extent of disease are the best established risk factors. There is an increase of approximately 1% per year for an individual to develop colon cancer after 10 years of UC [142]. While two studies have indicated a decrease in colon cancer mortality with surveillance, others have failed to confirm this finding possibly due to issues of compliance [143,144].

Periodic surveillance colonoscopy is recommended after 8–10 years of pancolitis, because synchronous dysplasia is noted in 75% of patients with carcinoma of the colon. Colon cancer develops 10–20 years earlier in these patients than in the general population, and patients with UC are found to have synchronous cancers at twice the rate (11%) of individuals without colitis. In fact, the risk may rise by 50–60 times over the general population by the fourth decade of disease. Carcinomas tend to develop in areas of diseased bowel, and the presence of a stricture may increase the likelihood of harboring an underlying carcinoma [21].

Mucinous signet ring histologic features are seen in 25% of these tumors. There is an increased number of flat and infiltrating types of carcinoma with ill-defined edges, making colonoscopic detection in active disease difficult. The 5-year survival rate is similar to that seen in patients with sporadic cancers and is dependent on stage. Despite the equivalence of 'stage-matched' survival, detection at a later stage is more common with ulcerative colitis [22].

Dysplasia

The precancerous marker dysplasia is defined as unequivocal preneoplastic transformation of the epithelium. Dysplasia is classified as negative, indefinite or positive; the latter is further subdivided into low grade and high grade. In low-grade dysplasia, all nuclear changes are confined to the basal portion of the epithelial crypt. In high-grade dysplasia, the nuclear changes are more extreme, with pronounced nuclear polymorphism and hyperchromasia and extend beyond the basal epithelium [22,144]. The presence of dysplasia suggests a high likelihood of concomitant presence or eventual development of carcinoma. High-grade dysplasia associated with a mass has up to a 43% risk of malignancy, whereas low-grade dysplasia carries up to an 18% risk, and indefinite or negative dysplasia carries a low likelihood of cancer [22]. Unfortunately, it can be very difficult for a pathologist to differentiate between inflammation and dysplasia. Therefore, represen-tative biopsies from both abnormal and normal areas should be taken during colonoscopy. Furthermore, such sampling will enable better differentiation between Crohn's disease and UC.

Inflammation damages the epithelium, and the repair process leads to the appearance of immature cells that may be confused with cytologic changes of dysplasia. Therefore, high-grade dysplasia should be confirmed by a second opinion from a pathologist experienced in this area.

Impact of surveillance

The rationale for colonoscopic surveillance in patients with UC is focused on the premise that the cancer risk is increased, dysplasia is a predictive marker, and surgical resection provides the only effective cure. A single finding of high-grade dysplasia or persistent low-grade dysplasia warrants colectomy. A 22-year cancer study demonstrated that such surveillance methods increased the likelihood of detecting the cancer earlier [144].

Method of surveillance

A surveillance program comprises clinical and colonoscopic evaluation. Changes in symptoms such as bleeding, abdominal pain, anorexia, nausea, vomiting, and weight loss warrant further investigation and possibly colonoscopy. Periodic colonoscopy should otherwise begin after 8–10 years of disease. Screening should be performed during periods of remission at 1- to 2-year intervals. Two biopsies should be taken every 10–20 cm throughout the colon; in addition, biopsies should be taken of any mass lesions or strictures. Biopsy specimens from each segment should be labeled separately [144, 145].

In the absence of dysplasia, quiescent or active colitis should be followed through repeated colonoscopic biopsies every 1–2 years, possibly with an interval flexible sigmoidoscopic examination. Indefinite dysplasia mandates repeat colonoscopy plus biopsies in 1–6 months. Low-grade dysplasia warrants at least a repeat colonoscopy plus biopsies in 1–3 months if a colectomy is not elected. High-grade dysplasia or dysplasia associated with mass lesions warrants an immediate colectomy. Since the advent and success of the IAR, there has been more enthusiasm for surgery [22, 144, 146].

Cancer surveillance has been shown to decrease mortality from colon cancer in patients with UC. Whether it will decrease the risk of the development of cancer or be cost effective enough for our society remains to be determined.

Surveillance in Crohn's disease

Carcinoma is much less common in Crohn's disease than in UC. These tumors are more difficult to diagnose and tend to be aggressive, multicentric, and of advanced stage at the time of diagnosis. A high percentage of cases occur in bowel that has been bypassed and is therefore not readily accessible to screening methods. Dysplasia is also present in Crohn's disease and is associated with strictures; thus periodic surveillance colonoscopy with biopsies is recommended.

Future directions

With further advances in our understanding of the pathogenesis of IBD, it is to be hoped that we can improve on the medical and surgical approaches to these enigmatic diseases. The overall ledger shows that prompt surgical cure of UC has a lower rate of adverse sequelae and a superior functional result to prolonged medical management. Similarly, the efficacy of surgery to treat primary and recurrent Crohn's disease should prompt such intervention prior to rendering the patient malnourished, anemic, immunocompromised, and experiencing the ravages of inappropriately prolonged medical management.

Rounds questions

1. Which extraintestinal manifestations usually do not improve following colectomy for ulcerative colitis?
2. What procedures would you recommend for a patient with ulcerative colitis and highgrade dysplasia in the distal third of the rectum?
3. What is the best emergency operative procedure for acute fulminating ulcerative colitis that has not been responsive to medical therapy?
4. A patient presents after having had an ileoanal reservoir created surgically and now has abdominal pains, increased stool frequency, watery diarrhea, and fever. What is the most likely diagnosis, how is it confirmed, and what is the therapy?
5. Who was Crohn?
6. What is the best drug for treating perianal Crohn's disease and what are its potential side effects?
7. What surgery would you perform to treat patients with Crohn's disease and an enterovesical fistula?
8. What is the best therapy for rectovaginal fistula for Crohn's disease?
9. What are the risk factors for carcinoma in ulcerative colitis?

References

1. Jagelman DG. Surgical alternatives for ulcerative colitis. Med Clin North Am 1990;74:155–67.
2. Wexner SD, Wong WD, Rothenberger DA, et al. The ileoanal reservoir. Am J Surg 1990;159:178.
3. Wilks S. The morbid appearances in the intestines of Miss Bankes. Med Times Gaz 1859;2:264.
4. Wilks S, Moxon W (eds). Lectures on Pathological Anatomy, 2nd ed. London: J & A Churchill, 1875;408.
5. Crohn BB, Ginzberg L, Oppenheimer GD. Regional ileitis: A pathologic and clinical entity. JAMA 1932;99:1323.
6. Becker J. Ulcerative colitis. In: Greenfield LJ, Mulholland MW, Oldham K, et al (eds). Surgery: Scientific Principles and Practice. Philadelphia: JB Lippincott 1993;988.
7. Corman ML. Ulcerative colitis. In Corman ML, (ed). Colon and Rectal Surgery, 3rd ed. Philadelphia: JB Lippincott 1993;901.

8. Sartor RB. Current concepts of the etiology and pathogenesis of ulcerative colitis and Crohn's disease. Gastroenterol Clin North Am 1995;24:475–507.

9. Bargen JA. Chronic ulcerative colitis associated with malignant disease. Arch Surg 1928;17:561.

10. Donnelly BJ, Delaney PV, Healy TM. Evidence of a transmissible factor in Crohn's disease. Gut 1977;18:360–3.

11. Sartor RB. Pathogenetic and clinical relevance of cytokines in inflammatory bowel disease. Immunol Res 1991;10:465–71.

12. Sher ME, D'Angelo AJ, Stein TA, et al. Cytokines in Crohn's colitis. Am J Surg 1995;169:133–6.

13. Brynskov J, Tvede N, Andersen CB, et al. Increased concentrations of interleukin 1-beta, interluken OC and soluble interluken OC receptors in endoscopical mucosal biopsy specimens with active inflammatory bowel disease. Gut 1992;33:55–8.

14. Cominelli F, Nast CC, Clark BD, et al. Interleukin 1 (IL-1) gene expression synthesis and effect of specific IL-1 receptor blockade in rabbit immune complex colitis. J Clin Invest 1990;86:972–80.

15. Stevens C, Walz G, Singaram C, et al. Tumor necrosis factor-alpha, interleukin 1-beta, and interleukin-6 expression in inflammatory bowel disease. Dig Dis Sci 1992;37:818–26.

16. Lashner B. Epidemiology of inflammatory bowel disease. Gastroenterol Clin North Am 1995;24:467–74.

17. Cottone M, Rosselli M, Orlando A, et al. Smoking habits and recurrence in Crohn's disease. Gastroenterology 1994;106:643–8.

18. Boyko EJ, Koepsell TD, Perera DR, et al. Risk of ulcerative colitis among former and current cigarette smokers. N Engl J Med 1987;316:707–10.

19. Lichtiger S, Present DH, Kornbluth A, et al. Cyclosporine in severe ulcerative colitis refractory to steroid therapy. N Engl J Med 1994;330:1841–5.

20. Altaras J. Ulcerative colitis imaging techniques. In: Serio GG, Delaini GG, Hulten L, et al (eds). Inflammatory Bowel Disease. Edinburgh: Graffham Press 1994:13.

21. Choi PM, Kim WH. Colon cancer surveillance. Gastroenterol Clin North Am 1995;24:671–87.

22. Kirsner JB, Shorter RG. Recent developments in 'nonspecific' inflammatory bowel disease inflammatory bowel disease, Part 1. N Engl J Med 1982;306:775.

23. Seldenrijk CA, Morson BC, Meuwissen SGM, et al. Histopathologic evaluation of colonic mucosal biopsy specimens in chronic inflammatory bowel disease: Diagnostic implications. Gut 1991;32:1514–20.

24. Brzezinski A. Medical treatment of Crohn's disease. Clin Colon Rect Surg 2001;14:167–73.

25. Friedman LS. New medical therapies. Semin Colon Rectal Surg 1993;4:14.

26. Griffin MG, Miner PB. Conventional drug therapy in inflammatory bowel disease. Gastroenterol Clin North Am 1995;24:509–21.

27. Hanouer SB, Scholman MI. New therapeutic approaches. Gastroenterol Clin North Am 1995;24:523–40.

28. Peppercorn MA. Advances in drug therapy for inflammatory bowel disease. Ann Intern Med 1990;112:50–60.

29. Sher ME, Weiss EG, Nogueras JJ, Wexner SD. Morbidity of medical therapy for ulcerative colitis: what are we really saving? Int J Colorectal Dis 1966;11:287–93.

30. Collins RH, Jr, Feldman M, Fordtran JS. Colon cancer, dysplasia and surveillance in patients with ulcerative colitis: A critical review. N Engl J Med 1987;316:1654.

31. Wexner SD. General principles of surgery in ulcerative colitis and Crohn's disease. Semin Gastroenterol Dis 290, 1995.

32. Binderow SR, Wexner SD. Current surgical therapy for mucosal ulcerative colitis. Dis Colon Rectum 1994;37:610–24.

33. Turnbull RB, Jr, Hank WA, Weakley FL. Surgical treatment of toxic megacolon. Ileostomy and colostomy to prepare patients for colectomy. Am J Surg 1971;122:325–31.

34. Wexner SD, Jagelman DG. The double-stapled ileal reservoir and ileoanal anastomosis. Perspect Colon Rectal Surg 1990;3:132–56.

35. Wexner SD, James K, Jagelman DG. The double-stapled ileal reservoir and ileoanal anastomosis. A prosective review of sphincter function and clinical outcome. Dis Colon Rectum 1991;34:487–94.

36. Corman ML, Veidenheimer MC, Collen JA. Impotence after proctectomy for inflammatory bowel disease of the bowel. Dis Colon Rectum 1978;21:418–9.

37. Bacon ME, Barlow SP, Berkley JL. Rehabilitation and long term survival after colectomy for ulcerative colitis. JAMA 1960;172:324–38.

38. Waits JO, Dozois RR, Kelly KA. Primary closure and continuous irrigation of the perineal wound after proctectomy. Mayo Clin Proc 1982;57:185–8.

39. Metcalf AM, Dozois RR, Kelly KA. Sexual function in women after proctocolectomy. Ann Surg 1986;204:624–7.

40. Bauer JJ, Gelernt IM, Salk BA, et al. Proctectomy for inflammatory bowel disease. Am J Surg 1986;151:157–62.

41. McLeod RS, Lavery IC, Letherman JR, et al. Factors affecting quality of life with a conventional ileostomy. World J Surg 1986;10:474–80.

42. Phillips RK, Ritchie JK, Hawley PR. Proctocolectomy and ileostomy for ulcerative colitis: The longer term story. J R Soc Med 1989;82:386–7.

43. Beart RW. Surgical management of chronic ulcerative colitis. Semin Colon Rectal Surg 1990;1:186–94.

44. Beck DE, Gathright JB Jr. Ulcerative colitis: Surgical indications and alternatives. South Med J 1994;87:773–9.

45. Oakley JR, Jagelman DG, Fazio VW, et al. Complications and quality of life after ileorectal anastomosis for ulcerative colitis. Am J Surg 1985;149:23–30.

46. Parc R, Legrand M, Frileux P, et al. Comparative clinical results of ileal-pouch anal anastomosis and ileorectal anastomosis in ulcerative colitis. Hepatogastroenterology 1989;36:235–9.

47. Khubchandani IT, Sanfort MR, Rosen L, et al. Current status of ileorectal anastomosis for inflammatory bowel disease. Dis Colon Rectum 1989;32:400–3.

48. Jagelman DG, Lewis CB, Rowe-Jones DC. Ileorectal anastomosis: appreciation by patients. Br Med J 1969;1:756–7.

49. Baker WNW, Glass RE, Ritchie JK, et al. Cancer of the rectum following colectomy and ileorectal anastomosis for ulcerative colitis. Br J Surg 1978;65:862–8.

50. Grundfest SF, Fazio V, Weiss RA, et al. The risk of cancer following colectomy and ileorectal anastomosis for extensive mucosal ulcerative colitis. Ann Surg 1981;193:9–14.

51. Kock NG. Intra-abdominal 'reservoir' in patients with permanent ileostomy: Preliminary observations in a procedure resulting in fecal 'continence' in five ileostomy patients. Arch Surg 1969;99:223–31.

52. Whitlow CB, Beck DE. Continent ileostomies. Ostomy Quarterly 1997;35:42–6.

53. Dozois RR, Kelly KA, Beart RW, Beahrs OH. Improved results with continent ileostomy. Ann Surg 1980;192:319–24.

54. Kock NG, Myrvold HE, Nilsson LO. Progress report on the continent ileostomy. World J Surg 1980;4:143–8.

55. Fazio VW, Church JM. Complications and function of the continent ileostomy at the Cleveland Clinic. World J Surg 1988;12:148–54.

56. Vernava AM, Goldberg SM. Is the Kock pouch still a viable option? Int J Colorectal Dis 1988;3:135–8.

57. Fazio VW, Tjandra JJ. Technique for nipple valve fixation to prevent valve slippage in continent ileostomy. Dis Colon Rectum 1992;35:1177–9.

58. Gorfine SR, Bauer JJ, Gelernt IM. Continent stomas. In: MacKeigan J, Cataldo PA (eds). Intestinal Stomas. Principles, techniques and management. St Louis: Quality Medical Publishing, 1993;154–79.

59. Parks AG, Nicholls RJ. Proctocolectomy without ileostomy for ulcerative colitis. Br Med J 1978;2:85–8.

60. Beck DE. Effect of pouch design. Semin Colon Rectal Surg 1996;7:109–13.

61. Becker JM, Raymond JL. Ileal pouch-anal anastomosis. A single surgeon's experience with 100 consecutive cases. Ann Surg 1986;204:375–83.

62. Pemberton JH, Kelly KA, Beart RW, et al. Ileal pouch anal anastomosis for chronic ulcerative colitis. Long-term results. Ann Surg 1987;206:504–73.

63. Fonkalsrud EW. Update on clinical experience with different surgical techniques of the endorectal pull-through operation for colitis and polyposis. Surg Gynecol Obstet 1987;165:309–16.

64. Fleshman JW, Cohen Z, McLeod RS, et al. The ileal reservoir and ileoanal anastomosis procedure: Factors affecting technical and functional outcome. Dis Colon Rectum 1988;31:10–6.

65. Wexner SD, Jensen L, Rothenberger DA, et al. Long-term functional analysis of the ileoanal reservoir. Dis Colon Rectum 1989;32:275–81.

66. Kelly KA. Anal sphincter-saving operations for chronic ulcerative colitis. Am J Surg 1992;163:5–16.

67. Reissman P, Piccirillo M, Ulrich A, et al. Functional results of the double-stapled ileoanal reservoir. J Am Coll Surg 1995;181:444–50.

68. Blumberg D, Opelka FG, Hicks TC, et al. Restorative proctocolectomy: Ochsner Clinic experience. South Med J 2001;94:467–71.

69. Liljeqvist L, Lindquist K, Ljungdahl I. Alterations in ileoanal pouch technique 1980 to 1987: Complications and functional outcome. Dis Colon Rectum 1988;31:929–38.

70. Miller R, Bartolo DC, Orrom WT, et al. Improvement of anal sensation with preservation of the anal transition zone after ileoanal anastomosis for ulcerative colitis. Dis Colon Rectum 1990;33:414–8.

71. O'Connell PR, Pemberton JH, Weiland LH, et al. Does rectal mucosa regenerate after ileoanal anastomosis? Dis Colon Rectum 1987;30:1–5.

72. Puthu D, Rajan N, Rao R, et al. Carcinoma of the rectal pouch following restorative proctocolectomy: Report of a case. Dis Colon Rectum 1992;35:257–60.

73. Stein H, Walfisch S, Mullen B, et al. Cancer in an ileoanal reservoir: A new late complication? Gut 1990;31:473–5.

74. Lavery IC, Sirimarco MT, Ziv Y, et al. Anal canal inflammation after ileal pouch-anal anastomosis: The need for treatment. Dis Colon Rectum 1995;38:803–6.

75. Curran FT, Sutton TD, Jass JR, Hill GL. Ulcerative colitis in the anal canal of patients undergoing restorative proctocolectomy. Aust N Z J Surg 1991;61:821–4.

76. Delaurier GA, Nelson H. Ileal pouch-anal anastomosis. In: Hicks TC, Beck DE, Opelka FG, Timmcke AE (eds). Complications of Colon & Rectal Surgery. Baltimore: Williams & Wilkins, 1996:339.

77. Ziv Y, Fazio VW, Sirimarco MT, et al. Incidence, risk factors, and treatment of dysplasia in the anal transitional zone after ileal pouch-anal anastomosis. Dis Colon Rectum 1994;37:1281–5.

78. Deen KI, Williams JG, Grant EA, et al. Randomized trial to determine the optimum level of pouch-anal anastomosis in stapled restorative proctocolectomy. Dis Colon Rectum 1995;38:133–8.

79. Seow-Choen AT, Tsunoda A, Nicholls RJ. Prospective randomized trial comparing anal function after hand sewn ileoanal anastomosis with mucosectomy versus stapled ileoanal anastomosis without mucosectomy in restorative proctocolectomy. Br J Surg 1991;78:430–4.

80. Luukkonen P, Javinen H. Stapled vs hand-sutured ileoanal anastomosis in restorative proctocolectomy: A prospective, randomized study. Arch Surg 1993;128:437–40.

81. McIntyre PB, Pemberton JH, Beart RW, et al. Double-stapled vs. handsewn ileal pouch-anal anastomosis in patients with chronic ulcerative colitis. Dis Colon Rectum 1994;37:430–3.

82. Wettergren A, Gyrtrup HJ, Grosmann E, et al. Complications after J-pouch ileoanal anastomosis: Stapled compared with handsewn anastomosis. Eur J Surg 1993;159:121–4.

83. Roberts PL. Operative techniques for ileoanal pouches. Clin Colon Rect Surg 2001;14:42–7.

84. Zuri Murrel Z, Fleshner P. Ulcerative colitis : Surgical management. In: Beck DE, Wexner SD, Roberts PL, Sacclarides TJ, Senagore A, Stamos M (eds). ASCRS Textbook of Colorectal Surgery, 2nd ed. New York: Springer-Verlag; in press.

85. Rivadeneira DE, Marcello PW, Roberts PL, et al. Benefits of hand-assisted laparoscopic restorative proctocolectomy: a comparative study. Dis Colon Rectum 2004;47:1371–6.

86. Burnstein MJ, Schoetz D, Coller JA, et al. Technique of mesenteric lengthening in ileal reservoir-anal anastomosis. Dis Colon Rectum 1987;30:863–6.

87. Becker JM, Dayton MT, Fazio VW, et al. Prevention of postoperative abdominal adhesions by a sodium hyaluronate-based bioresorbable membrane: A prospective, randomized, double-blind multicenter study. J Am Coll Surg 1996;183:297–306.

88. Beck DE, Cohen Z, Fleshman JW, et al. A prospective, randomized, multicenter, controlled study of the safety of Seprafilm adhesion barrier in abdominopelvic surgery of the intestine. Dis Colon Rectum 2003;46:1310–19.

89. Schoetz DJ, Coller JA, Veidenheimer MC. Can the pouch be saved? Dis Colon Rectum 1988;31:671–5.

90. Scott NA, Dozois RR, Beart RW, et al. Postoperative intra-abdominal and pelvic sepsis complicating ileal pouch-anal anastomosis. Int J Colorectal Dis 1988;3:149–53.

91. Tsao JI, Galandiuk S, Pemberton JH. Pouchogram: Predictor of clinical outcome following ileal pouch-anal anastomosis. Dis Colon Rectum 1992;35:547–51.

92. Wexner SD, Rothenberger DA, Jensen L, et al. Ileal pouch vaginal fistulas: Incidence, etiology, and management. Dis Colon Rectum 1989;32:460–5.

93. Schmitt SL, Wexner SD, James K, et al. Sepsis is not a problem after stapled ileoanal anastomosis. J South Med 1992;85:14.

94. Nicholls RJ, Moskowitz RL, Shepherd NA. Restorative proctocolectomy with ileal reservoir. Br J Surg 1985;72:576–9.

95. Hleald RJ, Allen DR. Stapled ileo-anal anastomosis: A technique to avoid mucosal proctectomy in the ileal pouch operation. Br J Surg 1986;73:571–2.

96. Keighley MRB. Abdominal mucosectomy reduces the incidence of soiling and sphincter damage after restorative proctocolectomy and J-pouch. Dis Colon Rectum 1987;30:386–90.

97. Schraut WH, Medick D. Crohn's disease. In: Greenfield LT, Mulholland MW, Oldham K, et al. (eds). Surgery: Scientific Principles and Practice. Philadelphia: JB Lippincott, 1993:741.

98. Dalziel TK. Chronic intestinal enteritis. Br Med J 1913;2:1068–1070.

99. Moschowitz E, Wilensky AO. Non-specific granulomata of the intestine. Am J Med Sci 1923;166:48–66

100. Morson BC, Lockhart-Mummery HE. Crohn's disease of the colon. Gastroenterologia 1959;92:168.

101. Rosenthal SR, Snyder JD, Hendricks KM, et al. Growth factor and IBD: Approach to treatment of a complicated adolescent problem. Pediatrics 1983;72:481–91.

102. Motol KJ, Grand RJ, David-Kraft E. The epidemiology of growth failure in children and adolescents with IBD. Gastroenterology 1983;84:1254.

103. Wexner SD. Anal and perianal Crohn's disease. Inf Surg 1989;8:185.

104. Nogueras JJ, Rothenberger DA. Surgical management of anorectal Crohn's disease. Probl Gen Surg 1993;10:169.

105. Goldberg HI, Caruthers GB Jr, Nelson JA, et al. Radiologic findings of the National Cooperative Crohn's Disease Study. Gastroenterology 1979;77:925–37.

106. Teahon K. Bjorenson I, Pearson M, et al. Ten year's experience with an elemental diet in the management of Crohn's disease. Gut 1990;31:1133–7.

107. Fazio VW, Kodner I, Jagelman DG, et al. Inflammatory disease of the bowel: Parenteral nutrition for primary or adjunctive treatment (symposium). Dis Colon Rectum 1976;19:574–6.

108. Brandt LJ, Bernstein LH, Boley SJ, et al. Metronidazole therapy for perineal Crohn's disease: A follow-up study. Gastroenterology 1982;83:383–7.

109. Brynskov J, Freund L, Rasmussen SN, et al. A placebo-controlled, double-blind, randomized trial of cyclosporine therapy in active chronic Crohn's disease. N Engl J Med 1989;321:845–50.

110. Feagan B, Sandborn WJ, Baker JP, et al. A randomized, double-blind, placebo-controlled, multicenter trial of the engineered human antibody to TNF (CDP571) for steroid sparing and maintenance of remission in patients with steroid-dependent Crohn's disease. Gastroenterology 118:A655, 2000.

111. Sandborn WJ, Feagan BG, Hanauer SB, et al. An engineered human antibody to TNF (CDP571) for active Crohn's disease: a randomized double-blind placebo-controlled trial. Gastroenterology 2001;120:1330–8.

112. Sandborn WJ. 'Optimizing anti-tumor necrosis factor strategies in inflammatory bowel disease.' Curr Gastroenterol Rep 2003;5: 501–5.

113. Sandborn WJ, Hanauer S, Katz S, et al. Etanercept for active Crohn's disease: a randomized, double-blind, placebo-controlled trial. Gastroenterology 2001;121:1088–94.

114. Hanauer S, Sandborn W, Rutgeerts P, et al. Human anti-tumor necrosis factor monoclonal antibody (adalimumab) in Crohn's disease: the CLASSIC-I trial. Gastroenterology 2005;130:323–33; quiz 591.

115. Schreiber S, Rutgeerts P, Fedorak R, et al. A randomized, placebo-controlled trial of certolizumab pegol (CDP870) for treatment of Crohn's disease. Gastroenterology 2005;129:807–18.

116. Sandborn W, Colombel J, Enns R, et al. Natalizumab induction and maintenance therapy for Crohn's disease. N Engl J Med 2005;353:1912–25.

117. Van Assche G, Van Ranst M, Sciot R, et al. Progressive multifocal leukoencephalopathy after natalizumab therapy for Crohn's disease. N Engl J Med 2006;353:362–8.

118. Nogueras JJ, Wexner SD. Surgical management of primary and recurrent Crohn's disease. Probl Gen Surg 1993;10:123–35.

119. Fazio VW. Crohn's disease. In: Moody FG, Corey LC, Jones RS, et al (eds). Surgical Treatment of Digestive Disease, 2nd ed. Chicago: Year Book Medical Publishers 1990;655.

120. Hull TL. Strictureplasty for Crohn's disease. Clinics Colon Rect Surg 2001;14:135–43.

121. Alexander-Williams J. The technique of intestinal strictureplasty. Int J Colorectal Dis 1986;154–7.

122. Fazio VW, Galandiuk S, Jagelman DG, et al. Strictureplasty in Crohn's disease. Ann Surg 1989;210:621–5.

123. Dehn TCB, Kettlewell MG, Mortensen NJM, et al. Ten-year experience of strictureplasty for obstructive Crohn's disease. Br J Surg 1989;76:339–41.

124. Spencer MP, Nelson H, Wolff BG, Dozois RR. Strictureplasty for obstructive Crohn's disease: the Mayo experience. Mayo Clin Proc 1994;69:33–6.

125. Stebbing JF, Jewell DP, Kettlewell GW, et al. Recurrence and reoperation after strictureplasty for obstructive Crohn's disease: Long-term results. Br J Surg 1995;82:1471–4.

126. Serra J, Cohen Z, McLeod RS. Natural history of strictureplasty in Crohn's disease: 9-year experience. Can J Surg 1995;38:481–5.

127. Ozuner G, Fazio VW, Lavery IC, et al. How safe is strictureplasty in the management of Crohn's disease? Am J Surg 1996;171:57–61.

128. Yamamoto T, Keighley MRB. Long-term results of strictureplasty without synchronous resection for jejunoileal Crohn's disease. Scand J Gastroenterol 1999;2:180–4.

129. Marcello PW. Large bowel Crohn's disease. Clinics Colon Rect Surg 2001;14:159–66.

130. Fleshner PR, Schoetz DJ, Roberts PL, et al. Anal fissure in Crohn's disease: A plea for aggressive management. Dis Colon Rectum 1995;38:1137–43.

131. Beck DE. Management of anorectal Crohn's fistulas. Clinics Colon Rect Surg 2001;14:117–28.

132. Harper PH, Kettlewell MG, Lee ECG. The effect of split ileostomy in perianal Crohn's disease. Br J Surg 1982;69:608–10.

133. Fry RD, Shemesh EI, Kodner IJ, et al. Techniques and results in the management of anal and perianal Crohn's disease. Surg Gynecol Obstet 1989;168:42–8.

134. Radcliffe AG, Ritchie JK, Hawley PR, et al. Anovaginal and rectovaginal fistulas in Crohn's disease. Dis Colon Rectum 1988;31:94–9.

135. MacRae HM, McLeod RS, Cohen Z, et al. Treatment of rectovaginal fistulas that have failed previous repair attempts. Dis Colon Rectum 1995;38:921–5.

136. Bauer JJ, Sher ME, Jaffin H, et al. Transvaginal approach for repair of rectovaginal fistula complicating Crohn's disease. Ann Surg 1991;213:151–8.

137. Sher ME, Bauer JJ, Gelernt I. Surgical repair of rectovaginal fistulas in patients with Crohn's disease: Transvaginal approach. Dis Colon Rectum 1991;34:641–8.

138. Wexner SD, Gonzalez-Padron A, Teoh TA, et al. Stimulated gracilis neosphincter operation: Initial experience, pitfalls, and complications. Dis Colon Rectum 1996;39:957–64.

139. Keighley MR, Allan RN. Current status and influence of operation on perianal Crohn's disease. Int J Colorectal Dis 1986;1:104–7.

140. Sher ME, Bauer JJ, Gorphine S, et al. Low Hartmann's procedure for severe anorectal Crohn's disease. Dis Colon Rectum 1992;35:975–80.

141. Burakoff R, Opper F. Pregnancy and nursing. Gastroenterol Clin North Am 1995;24:689–98.

142. Greenstein AJ, Sachar DB, Smith H, et al. A comparison of cancer risk in Crohn's disease and ulcerative colitis. Cancer 1981;48:2742–5.

143. Bozdech JM, Oakley JR, Fanner RG. Cancer surveillance in ulcerative colitis. Evidence for improved survival. Gastroenterology 1991;100:199.

144. Choi PM, Nugent FW, Schoetz DJ, et al. Colonoscopic surveillance reduces mortality from colorectal cancer in ulcerative colitis. Gastroenterology 1993;105:418–24.

145. Lennard-Jones JE, Melville DM, Morson BC, et al. Precancer and cancer in extensive ulcerative colitis: Findings among 401 patients over 22 years. Gut 1990;31:800–6.

146. Schmitt SL, Wexner SD, Lucas FV, et al. Retained mucosa after double-stapled ileal reservoir and ileoanal anastomosis. Dis Colon Rectum 1992;35:1051–6.

Rectal prolapse and intussusception

Prolapse has been recorded as early as the ancient Egyptians (Ebers Papyrus, c. 1500 BC) [1]. In full-thickness rectal prolapse (procidentia), the rectum protrudes through the anal opening, whereas in internal prolapse (preprolapse or sigmoidorectal intussusception) the rectum does not protrude beyond the anal opening. Although the exact incidence of prolapse is not known, it is relatively uncommon. Despite its infrequency, a plethora of surgical options exist to treat rectal prolapse. This chapter outlines the current understanding of the causes of prolapse, the evaluation of the patient with prolapse, and the more commonly used surgical alternatives.

Pathophysiology

At least two classification systems exist for rectal prolapse. The first was described by Altemeier et al [2]. Type I rectal prolapse is a protrusion of redundant mucosa of the rectum and has been referred to as mucosal prolapse or false prolapse. Type II prolapse is internal prolapse and is thought to occur from rectosigmoid intussusception without a coexisting hernia of the cul-de-sac. Other patients have complete prolapse (type III), which Altemeier et al believed was caused by a sliding hernia through a defect in the pelvic diaphragm.

Beahrs et al [3] believed that rectal prolapse is an intussusception and proposed a classification based on the clinical spectrum of the disease. Type I prolapse is partial or mucosal prolapse. Type II prolapse involves all layers (complete prolapse) and is further divided into first-degree, second-degree, and third-degree prolapse. First-degree prolapse is high or concealed prolapse. Second-degree prolapse is externally visible with straining and a sulcus is evident between the rectal wall and anal canal. Third-degree prolapse is externally visible but no sulcus is present.

As demonstrated by the differences in the two classification systems and the many different surgical approaches to treatment, the etiologic factors in prolapse are incompletely understood. Two general theories exist to explain the cause of prolapse: one describes prolapse as a sliding hernia through a weakness in the pelvic floor [2,4] in the other theory, prolapse starts as an intussusception of the sigmoid into the rectum, which eventually progresses to prolapse through the anus [5].

Several anatomic features have been noted in patients with prolapse including redundant sigmoid colon [6], a deep rectovesical pouch (pouch of Douglas) [4], a patulous anal sphincter [7], diastasis of the levator ani [6], and loss of the normal attachments of the rectum to the sacrum and pelvic sidewalks [8]. Theories of development of prolapse disagree on whether these findings are causes of prolapse or the result of prolapse.

Evaluation

In adults, rectal prolapse is much more common in women than in men. The peak incidence in women is in their seventh decade, whereas in men the incidence drops after the fifth decade [9]. In children, prolapse is distributed equally between the sexes and most often presents by 3 years of age [10].

Clinical factors associated with prolapse include straining at bowel movements [11], neurologic diseases (such as cauda equina lesions, multiple sclerosis), and mental illness [12]. The role of parity is unclear.

In children, prolapse is most frequently of the mucosal type which begins at the mucocutaneous junction [10,13]. Factors related to development of prolapse in this age group include cystic fibrosis [14,15], coughing [16], diarrhea (frequently from parasitic infection) [17,18], constipation, malnutrition, spina bifida, and myelomeningocele [10]. An anatomic explanation for prolapse in children involves a lack of fixation of the rectum and the sacrum is shallow which causes the rectum to be more vertical than in adults. This may allow intra-abdominal pressure to be transmitted directly downward through the rectum toward the anus [19].

Patients with prolapse most frequently complain of protrusion of the rectum during defecation. This may reduce spontaneously or require manual reduction. As the condition progresses, the protrusion may occur with any event that results in increased intra-abdominal pressure. Patients frequently complain of constipation and tenesmus. Incontinence is a major complaint of more than half of patients [20]. Less frequent presenting symptoms include bleeding, pain, mucous discharge, and pruritus.

Physical examination

Spontaneous prolapse is obvious on inspection (**Figure 15.1**). Some patients may require straining to produce the prolapse, and the straining patient is best examined in the squatting or sitting position. The patient can be examined while he or she is on the toilet by having the patient lean forward or using a long rod to which a mirror is attached placed between the patient's legs to view the prolapse. Another option is to place a flexible endoscope into the toilet with the viewing end pointed toward the perineum.

Full-thickness prolapse is distinguished by its concentric rings and grooves as opposed to the radially oriented grooves associated

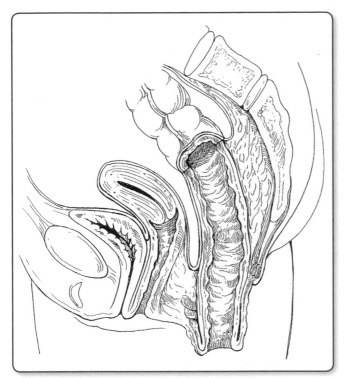

Figure 15.1 Sagittal view of full-thickness rectal prolapse.

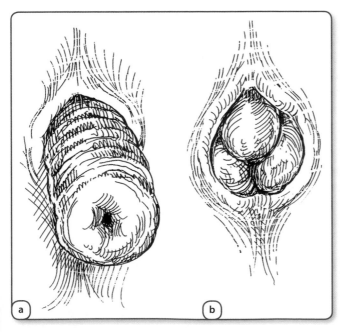

Figure 15.2 Physical examination. (a) Concentric folds of prolapsed rectum. (b) Radial folds of hemorrhoids (mucosal prolapse).

with mucosal prolapse (**Figure 15.2**). Inspection should also include examining the perianal skin for any maceration or excoriations. A thorough digital rectal examination is important to detect concomitant anal pathology and to determine adequacy of resting tone and squeeze pressure of the anal sphincters and function of the puborectalis muscle.

Endoscopic studies

All patients with rectal prolapse should have endoscopic examination of the colon and rectum. The entire colon should be evaluated prior to any surgery on that organ by colonoscopy or the combination of sigmoidoscopy and an air contrast barium enema. A biopsy should be performed for any abnormalities. Proctitis, colitis cystica profunda, and solitary rectal ulceration are conditions found in patients with prolapse that may require biopsy to differentiate them from rectal neoplasms or inflammatory bowel disease [21].

Radiologic studies

In patients who present with significant constipation in addition to prolapse, a colonic transit marker study is indicated (see Chapters 4 and 12). After the patient ingests a capsule containing 24 radiopaque rings, a plain abdominal radiograph is obtained within 24 hours of ingestion and again at 1, 3 and 5 days later. Normal patients should have no more than four rings remaining at 5 days [10]. At 7 days, no rings should remain. Abnormal results fall into one of two patterns: patients with pancolonic slow transit (colonic inertia) will have rings distributed throughout the colon, whereas those with pelvic outlet obstruction will demonstrate clustering of the remaining rings in the rectosigmoid. Either pattern may be seen in patients with prolapse [22].

In patients with symptoms of tenesmus, incomplete evacuation, fecal impaction, or unexplained constipation, or those found to have the solitary rectal ulcer syndrome, occult rectal prolapse should be suspected. Defecography should be performed to confirm this diagnosis [23]. Sigmoidorectal intussusception, puborectalis function, and perineal descent may be evaluated using this technique. A standard caulking gun is used to instill 200 mL of barium paste into the rectum. The patient sits on a radiolucent commode, and defecation is recorded with cineradiography or fluoroscopy with video recording (see Chapter 4).

Physiologic studies

There are several techniques for performing anorectal manometry. Typically a water-perfused or solid state catheter with four or eight radially oriented side ports is connected through transducers to a computer or polygraph. Data obtained include resting pressure, squeeze pressure, anal canal length, and presence of the rectoanal inhibitory reflex. Variable amounts of sphincter dysfunction have been found in patients with rectal prolapse. In two studies, resting and squeeze pressures were shown to be lower in prolapse patients than in control subjects [24,25]. In addition, Metcalf and Loenig-Baucke [24] found that patients with prolapse had decreased rectal capacity, as measured by decreased critical volume (mean rectal volume producing a lasting urge to defecate), decreased volume to produce constant relaxation, and decreased volume on the saline incontinence test. These findings, along with the decreased sphincter pressures, may explain why many prolapse patients experience incontinence before the sensation of the urge to defecate. Two studies have failed to show a return to normal of resting or squeeze pressures following repair of prolapse by rectopexy [26,27].

Electromyographic (EMG) measurements assess motor unit integrity by a concentric needle technique or by a single-fiber technique. These techniques have been used to document reduced amplitude of action potential in the external anal sphincter and puborectalis muscles and increased single fiber density in patients with incontinence. Farouk et al [27] reported that these changes were not noted in patients with prolapse who had normal continence, nor do they return to normal after repair of prolapse. Pudendal nerve terminal motor latency is also lengthened in patients with rectal prolapse, suggesting that nerve stretch contributes to sphincter dysfunction [28].

The studies described play an important role in our understanding of the causes of prolapse and incontinence associated with prolapse. Few studies have thoroughly evaluated treatment options based on the results of preoperative and postoperative physiologic testing. However, Yoshioka et al [26]. found that four parameters were significant in predicting continence following rectopexy: delayed leakage during a saline infusion test, a narrow anorectal angle, minimal pelvic floor descent, and long anal canal length. They suggested adding a pelvic floor repair for any patient who is likely to remain incontinent based on these criteria.

Treatment

Nonoperative treatment

Mucosal prolapse can be treated successfully by starting the patient on bulk-forming laxatives, avoidance of straining, and rubber band ligation [30]. In more severe cases, hemorrhoidectomy may be required.

Prolapse in children can usually be managed nonoperatively [10]. Underlying conditions should be treated; this may include treatment of parasitic infections, stool softeners for constipation, or nutritional support. Medical management also involves reduction of the prolapse and in some instances taping the buttocks together. In cases in which medical management is unsuccessful, one of the following procedures is recommended: injection of a sclerosing agent into the perirectal tissue [31], packing Gelfoam into the presacral space [10] or linear cauterization of the anorectal mucosa [32]. If these less invasive procedures fail, rectopexy, mucosal sleeve resection, or anal encirclement have also been successful [10, 33–36].

Operative treatment

The choice of surgical treatment for rectal prolapse depends on the condition of the patient, preoperative anatomic and physiologic testing, presence of incontinence or constipation, prior prolapse repairs, and the surgeon's preference. Repairs can be divided into perineal and abdominal approaches. Perineal approaches have less morbidity associated with them but in general have high recurrence rates and have therefore been typically reserved for high-risk elderly patients.

Comparison of results from various series in patients with prolapse can be confusing. Recurrence is recorded only in patients with full-thickness prolapse in some series, whereas others include full-thickness and mucosal prolapse. Discussion of recurrence rates in this chapter will include only full thickness prolapse unless otherwise stated. Length of follow-up differs from one report to another; those with longer follow-up report recurrences as late as 16 years postoperatively [29]. Incontinence and constipation may be improved or worsened by most procedures. When comparing the effects of a procedure on bowel or sphincter function it is important to note the preoperative status of patients. This is often omitted or recorded with different endpoints, making comparison between series impossible.

Preoperative preparation for most operations for repair of prolapse is the same. Patients are given a mechanical and antibiotic bowel preparation the day before surgery, as described in Chapter 6. Perioperative broad-spectrum intravenous antibiotics are also given. Patients undergoing an abdominal procedure are placed in the supine modified lithotomy position. Perineal procedures can be performed in the prone jackknife, lithotomy, or left lateral positions. A Foley catheter should be placed in all patients before the operation begins. Operative

Table 15.1 Treatment options

Treatment	Advantages	Disadvantages
Abdominal		
Anterior resection	Low recurrence	Resection required
Ripstein mesh sling	No resection	Impaction, constipation, foreign body
Well's Ivalon sponge	No resection	Constipation persists foreign body
Orr-Loygue	No resection	Constipation persists
Sigmoid colectomy with suture rectopexy	Low recurrence	Resection required
Perineal		
Altemeier (perineal rectosigmoidectomy)	Low morbidity/mortality, low recurrence	General/regional anesthesia, continued incontinence, anastomosis
Altemeier with levatorplasty	Low morbidity/mortality, low recurrence, incontinence improved	General/regional anesthesia, anastomosis
Delorme procedure	Low morbidity/mortality, local anesthesia	High recurrence rates, continued incontinence
Thiersch anal encirclement	Low morbidity/mortality, local anesthesia	Fecal impaction, infection, wire breakage, erosion

treatment options along with respective advantages and disadvantages are summarized in **Table 15.1**.

Abdominal procedures

Anterior resection of the rectosigmoid is a procedure familiar to most surgeons. In the treatment of prolapse, it is important to mobilize the rectum posteriorly down to the coccyx. Postoperative presacral adhesions that form in this area are felt to play a positive role in preventing recurrence. The main disadvantage of this approach is that it involves an anastomosis. Cirocco and Brown [37] reported on 41 patients who underwent anterior resection and had a recurrence rate of 7% at an average follow-up of 6 years. These surgeons reported no mortality and 15% morbidity (no anastomotic complications); 90% of patients had improvement or no change in their level of continence; and 10% of patients reported incontinence postoperatively. Of 150 patients who underwent anterior resection alone for prolapse, Wolff and Dietzen [29] reported an 8.9% recurrence rate at a mean of 7 years, a complication rate of 28% (9.3% anastomotic or wound), and a 0.7% mortality rate. The incontinence rate dropped 15.5% after surgery; however, 16 patients (10.7%) experienced new onset incontinence postoperatively.

Reporting on the same data several years earlier, Schlinkert et al. [38] noted a significant difference in morbidity based on the level of the coloproctostomy. Patients who underwent anastomosis to the peritonealized portion of the rectum had a complication rate of 19%, whereas those who had a lower anastomosis had a 52% complication rate. Several larger series are summarized in **Table 15.2**.

Most abdominal procedures for prolapse involve complete mobilization of the rectum down to the levator muscles, followed by fixation of the rectum to the sacrum (rectopexy). Various techniques for rectopexy have been described. The **Ripstein procedure** involves placing a 2 inch wide T-shaped sling of Teflon around the mobilized rectum (**Figure 15.3**). The sling is fixed to the sacrum, 2 inches caudal

Table 15.2 Rectosigmoid resection and rectopexy				
	No. of patients	Morbidity (%)	Mortality (%)	Recurrence (%)
Watts et al, 1985 [9]	102	4	0	1.9
Husa et al, 1988 [39]	48	0	2.1	9
Sayfan et al, 1990 [40]	13	2.3	0	0
Cirocco and Brown, 1993 [37]	41	15	0	7
McKee et al, 1992 [41]	9	0	0	0
Wolff and Dietzen, 1991 [29]	–	28	0.7	5.9
Luukonen et al, 1992 [42]	15	20	6.7	0
Canfrere et al, 1994 [43]	17	–	0	0
Huber et al, 1995 [44]	39	7.1	0	0

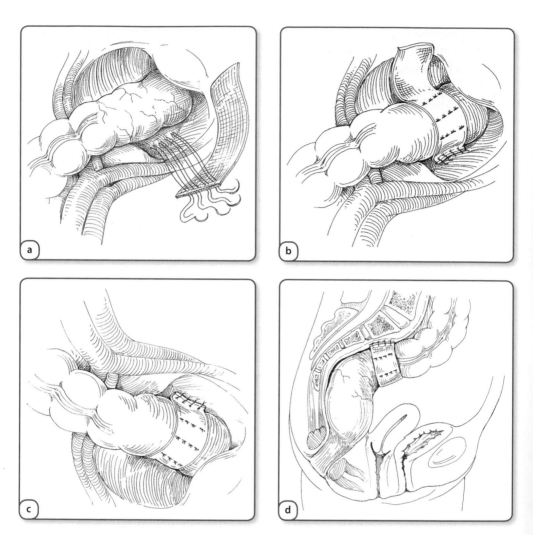

Figure 15.3 Mesh rectopexy (Ripstein procedure). (a) Posterior fixation of sling on one side. (b) Sling brought anteriorly around the mobilized rectum. (c) Sling fixed posteriorly on the opposite side. (d) Sagittal view of the completed rectopexy.

to the sacral promontory, passed around the rectum, and fixed back onto the sacrum. The edges of the sling are fixed to the circumference of the bowel [7]. More recently Marlex or Proline mesh has been used, and it has been recommended that the mesh be attached only for the posterior three fourths of the bowel circumference to decrease postoperative obstructive symptoms [45]. Several large series reported on results of the Ripstein procedure (**Table 15.3**). The mortality rate was low (0–2.8%), as was the recurrence rate (0–12.2%). Morbidity ranged from 3.7–52%. Although continence tends to be improved after this operation, difficulties with defecation including impaction, sling obstruction, and stricture are not infrequent. Presacral hemorrhage accounted for 8% of complications in one series and was the second

Table 15.3 Ripstein procedure							
	No. of patients	Morbidity (%)	Mortality (%)	Improved (%)	Constipation worsened (%)	ilmproved (%)	Incontinence worsened (%)	improved (%)
Launer et al, 1982 [46]	57	26	0	NA	18	41	10*	12
Roberts et al, 1988 [47]	135	52	0.7	69	31	78	22*	10
Holmstrom et al, 1986 [48]	108	3.7	2.8	**	NA	***	NA	4
Leeneen and Kuijpers, 1989 [49]	64	28	0	NA	NA	NA	NA	0
Keighley et al, 1983 [50]	100	NA	0	NA	NA	64	36	0

* Includes patients whose condition had not improved or worsened after surgery.
** Number of patients with poor defecation changed from 25 preoperatively to 40 postoperatively (P < 0.05)
*** Number of patients with normal continence changed from 32 preoperatively to 66 postoperatively (P < 0.0001)

most frequent complication reported in a survey of colon and rectal surgeons [51]. Infrequent complications include colocutaneous fistula, erosion of mesh into the rectum, pelvic abscess, and impotence.

In 1959, Wells [52] described a procedure similar to that described by Ripstein; it has been used widely in the United Kingdom and Canada. The rectum is mobilized posteriorly to the tip of the coccyx. An **Ivalon sponge** (polyvinyl alcohol) is sutured to the sacrum and the posterolateral aspect of the rectum (**Figure 15.4**). Others have modified the procedure by not suturing to the sacrum [53]. Morgan et al [54] reported on the largest series of patients treated by the Wells procedure: the rate of pelvic sepsis was 2.6%, as was the mortality rate. All four patients with septic complications eventually required removal of the sponge. The recurrence rate was 3.2% at 5.5 years. Incontinence was present in 80.6% preoperatively and only 38.8% postoperatively. Twenty-seven percent of patients reported constipation after surgery, compared with 65% before operation. Results of this procedure are summarized in **Table 15.4**.

Other materials have been used for rectopexy. Orr described the use of 1–2 cm wide strips of fascia lata sutured to the lateral aspects of the rectum and posteriorly to the fascia just proximal to the sacral promontory [59]. Loygue et al [60] reporting on 257 cases over a 29-year period, modified the procedure by replacing the fascia lata with nylon strips. Mortality was 0.8% and morbidity (sepsis, presacral hemorrhage, and intervertebral disk infection) was 2%. Recurrence of prolapse was 5.6%, and 84% of patients had normal anal continence postperatively [61].

Suture rectopexy has been used alone or, more commonly, in combination with sigmoid resection (Frykman-Goldberg procedure) [62]. After complete mobilization of the rectum, the lateral stalks of

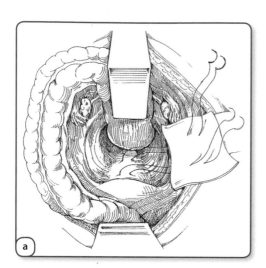

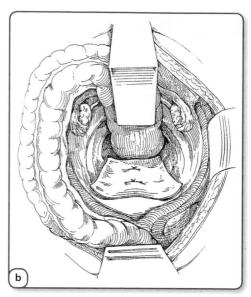

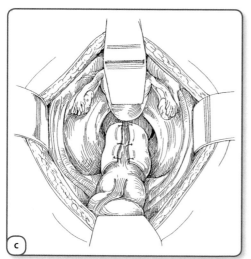

Figure 15.4 Ivalon sponge rectopexy (Wells). (a) Ivalon sponge being fixed to the sacrum. (b) Sponge in place before fixation to the rectum. (c) Incomplete encirclement of the rectum anteriorly with the sponge sutured in place.

the rectum are sutured posteriorly to the presacral fascia. The use of suture eliminates the 2% over all risk of infection related to the use of the previously mentioned foreign materials and is effective at repairing prolapse [63]. The benefit of adding colon resection is not completely resolved. Those who support it believe the functional results are improved over suture rectopexy alone. Recurrence rates for resection rectopexy are 1.9–9% [9,39,64]. Mortality rates have been low. Morbidity includes anastomotic leak, small bowel and colonic obstruction, and presacral hemorrhage. Constipation improved in 50–75% of patients, and rates of incontinence improved in 38–94%.

Table 15.4 Wells posterior rectopexy (Ivalon sponge)						
	No. of Patients	Morbidity (%)	Mortality (%)	Constipation (%)	Incontinence (%)	Recurrence (%)
Morgan et al, 1972 [54]	150	3	2.6	Preoperatively, 65 Postoperatively, 27	Preoperatively, 81 Postoperatively, 39	3.2
Penfold and Hawley, 1972 [55]	101	6	0	Postoperatively, 29	Preoperatively, 72 Postoperatively, 41	3
Boutsis and Ellis, 1974 [1]	26	8	4	Preoperatively, 44 Postoperatively, 32	Preoperatively, 69 Postoperatively, 36	12
Atkinson and Taylor, 1984 [56]	40	0	0	NA	Preoperatively, 35 Postoperatively, 25	10
Mann and Hoffman, 1988 [57]	59	51*	0	Preoperatively, 29 Postoperatively, 47	Preoperatively, 44 Postoperatively, 15	0
Yoshioka et al, 1989 [26]	165	19	0			
Novell et al, 1994 [58]	31	19	0	Postoperatively, 48	Preoperatively, 32 Postoperatively, 29	3

* 39% of patients developed urinary retention.

In a randomized prospective trial, McKee et al [41] reported no recurrence at 20 months for patients undergoing suture rectopexy with or without sigmoidectomy. Constipation was reduced in patients who underwent sigmoidectomy in addition to suture rectopexy.

In a randomized prospective trial comparing Ivalon sponge posterior rectopexy with sutured rectopexy, Novell et al [58] found similar recurrence rates. Patients undergoing suture rectopexy had better preservation of continence and a lower incidence of postoperative constipation. On the basis of these results, they recommended that Ivalon sponge rectopexy be abandoned.

Another prospective randomized trial compared posterior rectopexy with absorbable mesh (polyglycolic acid) versus rectopexy with sigmoid resection [42]. No recurrence was seen in either group at a mean follow-up of 2.1 years. The number of incontinent patients decreased a similar amount in both groups. Constipation improved in some patients in both groups. In the mesh rectopexy group, five patients became severely constipated postoperatively, and one of these eventually required colectomy [42].

Suture rectopexy, mesh rectopexy and rectosigmoid resection are being increasingly performed with **laparoscopic assistance** [65–68]. Recent reports have documented that resectional and fixation procedures can be performed with the same efficacy as traditional open approaches with short term follow-up. Cosmetic results are superior short term morbidity has been better or equal to open procedures. Additional randomized studies with long term follow-up will be needed to substantiate recurrence rates and morbidity.

Perineal procedures

In the late 19th and early 20th centuries several perineal procedures for the treatment of prolapse were described. Their use declined as abdominal surgery under general anesthesia became safe and it became clear that recurrence rates were lower with abdominal repairs. Preference for abdominal procedures has continued with the adoption of laparoscopy. However, perineal procedures still have a role for elderly patients with significant medical problems, for whom a major abdominal procedure carries a prohibitive risk. In addition, modern trends toward minimizing invasiveness and outpatient management have led to these procedures being offered to young and low risk patients.

Altemeier

Perineal rectosigmoidectomy was first described by Mikulicz in 1889 and then reintroduced by Miles in 1933 [69]. However, it is Altemeier's name that is attached to the operation that he and his colleagues originally reported on in 1952 [70]. The operation can be performed with the patient under general or regional anesthesia in either the lithotomy, left lateral, or prone jackknife position (**Figure 15.5**). After the rectum is prolapsed, the outer cylinder is circumferentially incised through its full thickness 1–2 cm proximal to the dentate line. Stay sutures are then placed at the distal edge of the rectum, and traction is placed on the inner cylinder. As the inner cylinder is delivered, the mesentery is serially divided and ligated until the bowel cannot be pulled out any farther. If the pouch of Douglas is encountered anteriorly, the hernia sac is opened and a high ligation may be performed. A levator repair can be performed anterior and/or posterior to the rectum. The inner cylinder is then transected about 2 cm distal to the outer rectal stump, and stay sutures are placed in each quadrant. Anastomosis is then performed, suturing a full thickness of bowel to the remaining rectal stump [71]. The anastomosis can also be performed with a circular stapler [72]. The length of bowel excised is from 5–30 cm. Patients are allowed to eat a regular diet on postoperative day 1, and the Foley catheter is generally removed by postoperative day 1 or 2.

Mortality in several series has been extremely low, and morbidity ranged from 0–25% (**Table 15.5**). Complications are mostly medical but have included anastomotic dehiscence and bleeding. Recurrence rates have been reported between 0% and 10%. Incontinence has improved in a large percentage of patients in series in which levatorplasty has been used. Of 114 patients, Williams reported 67 suffered from incontinence preoperatively [71]. Only 15 of 56 patients who did not have a levatorplasty were continent following operation. Of 11 patients who underwent levatorplasty, seven were continent postoperatively. Prasad et al [74] advocate levator repair and posterior suture rectopexy in addition to the perineal proctectomy. They reported on 25 patients with incontinence and rectal prolapse who underwent this repair. Twenty-two (88%) were completely continent by 4 weeks after surgery, and 100% were continent by 3 months.

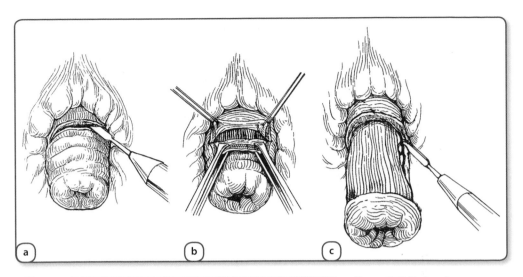

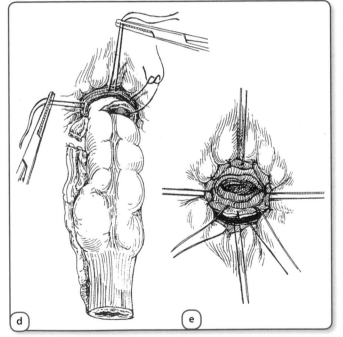

Figure 15.5 Perineal rectosigmoidectomy (Altemeier procedure). (a–c), Full-thickness excision of the outer cylinder of the prolapse. (d) Mesenteric vessels ligated; stay sutures placed in distal edge of inner cylinder. (e) Anastomosis of the distal aspect of the remaining colon to the rectal stump.

A randomized trial by Deen et al [80] compared abdominal resection and rectopexy with perineal rectosigmoidectomy with pelvic floor repair in patients older than 50 years of age. There were no deaths or anastomotic leaks. One patient developed an anastomotic stricture following perineal rectosigmoidectomy. There was one recurrence in the perineal group and none in the abdominal group at a median follow-up of 17 months. More patients who underwent perineal rectosigmoidectomy experienced fecal soiling (6 versus 2 in the

Table 15.5 Perineal rectosigmoidectomy					
	No. of patients	Morbidity (%)	Mortality (%)	Recurrence (%)	Incontinence (%)
Altemeier et al, 1971 [2]	106	25	0	3	NA
Gopal et al, 1984 [73]	18	17	6	6	NA
Prasad et al, 1986 [74]	25	0	0	0	Preoperatively, 100 Postoperatively, 0
Ramanujam and Venkatesh, 1988 [75]	41	15	0	5	Preoperatively, 100 Postoperatively, 22
Williams et al, 1992 [71]	114	12		10	Preoperatively, 36 Levatorplasty, 36 No levatorplasty, 80 Overall postoperatively, 73
Ramanujam et al, 1994 [76]	72			6	
Kim et al, 1999 [77]	183			16	
Agachan et al, 1997 [78]	53			10	
Whitlow et al, 1997 [79]	8	10	0	10	

abdominal resection group). Maximal resting and maximal squeeze pressure decreased postoperatively in patients undergoing perineal repair. These pressures increase in patients undergoing abdominal repair. The advantage of perineal rectosigmoidectomy was a shorter hospital stay (mean 5 days versus 11 days, $P < 0.05$).

Delorme

The French surgeon Delorme described a mucosal stripping procedure for procidentia in 1899 [81], and several authors have since modified the procedure. Unlike other perineal procedures, the Delorme procedure has also been used for internal prolapse. This procedure is most commonly performed with the patient under local anesthesia, supplemented by intravenous sedation. The patient is placed in the prone jackknife or left lateral position. The rectum may be prolapsed or reduced. Local anesthesia with 1 : 200,000 epinephrine is used to establish a perianal block and infiltrate the submucosal plane just proximal to the dentate line (**Figure 15.6a**). A circumferential incision is made through the mucosa 1 cm proximal to the dentate line. The mucosa and submucosa are dissected into the apex of the prolapse in a circumferential manner. This dissection is more difficult in patients with a history of diverticulitis or extensive diverticulosis. Presence of these conditions may warrant consideration of an alternative approach. Hemostasis is maintained during the dissection with electrocautery. The proximal mucosal sleeve is then amputated and the remaining edge is reapproximated to the distal mucosal edge. The muscular wall of rectum between the two mucosal edges is plicated with the same stitch used to perform the mucosal closure. Typically

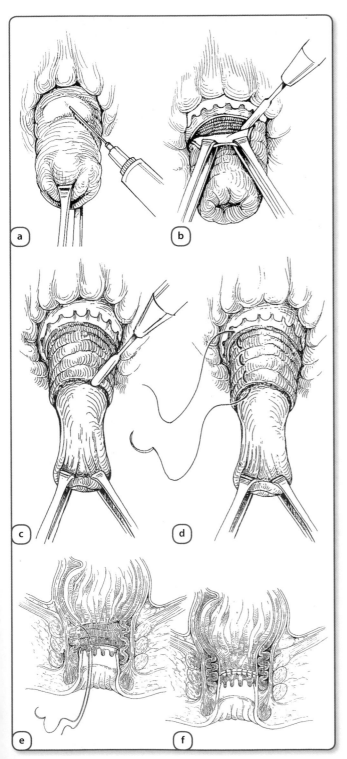

Figure 15.6 Mucosal proctectomy (Delorme). (a) Submucosal infiltration with lidocaine with epinephrine. (b) Circumferential mucosal incision. (c) Dissection of mucosa away from muscular layer. (d) and (e) Plicating stitch including cut edge of mucosa and muscular wall. (f) Completed anastomosis.

four quadrant sutures are placed, followed by four bisecting sutures. Tying the sutures is deferred until all eight are in place (**Figure 15.6**).

Recent series have shown a mortality for the Delorme procedure of 0–2.5% (**Table 15.6**) when it is performed on elderly patients who have significant medical problems. Morbidity (4–33%) has included bleeding, anastomotic dehiscence, stricture, diarrhea, and urinary retention. Recurrence rates have ranged from 7–22%, and recurrences have frequently been treated with a repeat Delorme procedure. Incontinence improved in 40–50% of patients who were incontinent preoperatively, and generally incontinence was not worsened by the procedure. Constipation was not a problem in most series.

Thiersch

Anal encirclement was first described by Thiersch in 1891 [90]. He placed a silver wire subcutaneously around the anus with the patient under local anesthesia. The mechanism of this procedure was to mechanically supplement or replace the anal sphincter and stimulate a foreign body reaction in the perianal area. There were several reports of the use of this procedure in the early part of this century, especially in Europe [90].

William Gabriel is credited with reviving interest in Thiersch's operation in the 1950s [91]. He reported on 25 cases of incontinence or minor rectal prolapse. He did not recommend this operation for major degrees of prolapse.

For this operation the patient is placed in the prone jackknife, lithotomy, or left lateral position (**Figure 15.7**). A local anesthetic is administered and a radial incision made on both sides of the anus about 2 cm from the anal verge. A curved hemostat or special circular needle is used to tunnel from one incision to the other above the anoperineal ligament anterior to the anus and keeping external to the external anal sphincter. The material for encirclement is brought through the tunnel.

Table 15.6 Delorme's procedure					
	No. of patients	Morbidity (%)	Mortality (%)	Recurrence (%)	Incontinence (%)
Nay and Blair, 1972 [82]	30	7	0	10	NA
Uhlig and Sullivan, 1979 [83]	44	32	0	7	Postoperatively, 41
Christiansen and Kirkegaard, 1981 [84]	12	0	0	17	Preoperatively, 50 Postoperatively, 33
Graf et al, 1992 [85]	14	0	0	21	Preoperatively, 79 Postoperatively, 50
Tobin and Scott, 1994 [86]	49	8	0	22	Preoperatively, 82 Postoperatively, 41
Oliver et al, 1994 [87]	40	75	2	22	Preoperatively, 45 Postoperatively, 39
Senapati et al, 1994 [88]	32	6	0	13	Preoperatively, 88 Postoperatively, 41
Plusa et al, 1995 [89]	104			17	

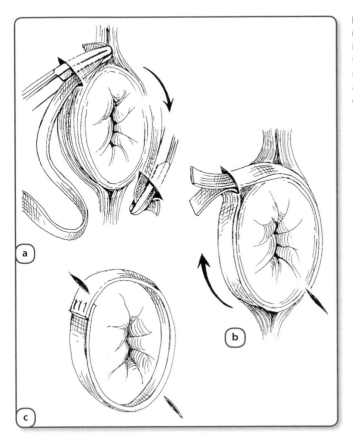

Figure 15.7 Anal encirclement (Thiersch procedure). (a) Lateral incisions with prosthetic mesh tunneled around the anus. (b) Mesh completely encircling the anal opening. (c) Completed anal encirclement procedure.

Tunneling is continued posterior to the anus above the anococcygeal ligament and the encircling material brought through so that the two ends meet [92]. The encircling material is then secured by tying snuggly over an index finger in the anus. A variety of materials used for encirclement include nylon, silk, Silastic rods, silicone, Marlex mesh, Mersilene mesh, fascia, tendon, and Dacron [71]. Complications of this procedure include breakage of the suture or wire, fecal impaction, sepsis, and erosion into the skin or anal canal. The Thiersch operation does not correct the prolapse but narrows the anus enough that the prolapse is confined to the rectum, accomplishing this goal in 54–100% of cases [69]. Because of its failure to correct prolapse and the morbidity of this procedure, it is reserved for the most seriously ill patients who are unable to undergo one of the previously described perineal procedures.

Conclusion

Rectal prolapse and intussusception are infrequently encountered problems. The causes as well as the ideal treatment for prolapse remain uncertain. Selection of the best procedure for a given patient depends on the patient's medical condition, the presence of incontinence or constipation, and prior surgery for prolapse. The surgeon weighs these factors, along with a knowledge of the available surgical options to arrive at a treatment decision.

Rounds questions

1. What pelvic anatomic abnormalities are associated with rectal prolapse?
2. What are the presenting symptoms of patients with rectal prolapse?
3. What surgical options are available for repair of prolapse through an abdominal approach?
4. What is the Altemeier procedure for rectal prolapse? How does it differ from the Delorme procedure?
5. What is the Thiersch procedure for the treatment of rectal prolapse?

References

1. Boutsis C, Ellis H. The Ivalon-sponge wrap operation for rectal prolapse: An experience with 26 patients. Dis Colon Rectum 1974;17:21–37.
2. Altemeier WA, Culbertson WR, Schowengerdt C, Hunt J. Nineteen years' experience with the one-stage perineal repair of rectal prolapse. Ann Surg 1971;173:993–1006.
3. Beahrs OH, Theuerkauf FJ Jr, Hill JR. Procidentia: Surgical treatment. Dis Colon Rectum 1972;15:337–46.
4. Moschowitz AV. The pathogenesis, anatomy, and cure of prolapse of the rectum. Surg Gynecol Obstet 1912;15:7–21.
5. Broden B, Snellman B. Procidentia of the rectum studied with cineradiography: A contribution to the discussion of causative mechanism. Dis Colon Rectum 1968;11:330–34.
6. Swinton NW, Palmer TE. The management of rectal prolapse and procidentia. Am J Surg 1960;99:144–51.
7. Ripstein CB. Surgical care of massive rectal prolapse. Dis Colon Rectum 1965;8:34–8.
8. Ripstein CB, Lanter B. Etiology and surgical therapy of massive prolapse of the rectum. Ann Surg 1963;157:259–64.
9. Watts JD, Rothenherger DA, Buls JG, et al. The management of procidentia: 30 years' experience. Dis Colon Rectum 1985;28:96–102.
10. Corman ML. Rectal prolapse in children. Dis Col Rectum 1985;28:535–9.
11. Keighley MRB, Shouler PJ. Abnormalities of colonic function in patients with rectal prolapse and faecal incontinence. Br J Surg 1984;71:892–5.
12. Corman ML. Rectal prolapse. In: Corman ML, (ed). Colon and Rectal Surgery, 3rd ed. Philadelphia: JB Lippincott, 1993:293–336.
13. Qvist N, Rasmussen L, Klaaborg KJ, et al. Rectal prolapse in infancy: Conservative versus operative treatment. J Pediatr Surg 1986;21:887–8.
14. Zempsky WT, Rosenstein BJ. The cause of rectal prolapse in children. Am J Dis Child 1988;142:338–9.
15. Kulczycki LL, Shwachman H. Studies in cystic fibrosis of the pancreas: Occurrence of rectal prolapse. N Engl J Med 1958;259:409–12.
16. Freeman NV. Rectal prolapse in children. J R Soc Med 1984;77:9–12.
17. Bhandari B, Ameta DK. Etiology of prolapse rectum in children with special reference to amoebiais. Indian Pediatr 1977;14:635–7.

18. Soriano LR, del Mundo F, Naguit-Sim L. Rectal prolapse in children with trichuriasis. J Philipp Med Assoc 1966;42:843–8.
19. Carter HG. Treatment of procidentia of the rectum. South Med J 1971;64:1238–47.
20. Marcello PW, Roberts PL. Surgery for rectal prolapse. In Hicks TC, Beck DE, Opelka FG, Timmcke AE, (eds). Complications of Colon & Rectal Surgery. Baltimore: Williams & Wilkins, 1996;237–62.
21. Tjandra JJ, Fazio VW, Church JM, et al. Clinical condundrum of solitary rectal ulcer. Dis Colon Rectum 1992;35:227–34.
22. Hinton JM, Lennard-Jones JE, Young AC. A new method for studying gut transit times using radioopaque markers. Gut 1969;10:842–7.
23. Berman IR, Manning DH, Dudley-Wright K. Anatomic specificity in the diagnosis and treatment of internal rectal prolapse. Dis Colon Rectum 1985;28:816–26.
24. Metcalf AM, Loenig-Baucke V. Anorectal function and defecation dynamics in patients with rectal prolapse. Am J Surg 1988;155:206–10.
25. Sun WM, Read NW, Donnelly TC, et al. A common pathophysiology for full thickness rectal prolapse, anterior mucosal prolapse and solitary rectal ulcer. Br J Surg 1989;76:290–5.
26. Yoshioka K, Hyland G, Keighley MRB. Anorectal function after abdominal rectopexy: Parameters of predictive value in identifying return of continence. Br J Surg 1989;76:64–8.
27. Farouk R, Duthie GS, Bartolo DCC, MacGregor AB. Restoration of continence following rectopexy for rectal prolapse and recovery of the internal anal sphincter electromyogram. Br J Surg 1992;79:439–40.
28. Snooks SJ, Nicholls RJ, Henry MM, Swash M. Electrophysiological and manometric assessment of the pelvic floor in the solitary rectal ulcer syndrome. Br J Surg 1985;72:131–3.
29. Wolff BG, Dietzen CD. Abdominal resectional procedures for rectal prolapse. Semin Colon Rectal Surg 1991;2:184–6.
30. Mathai V, Seow-Choen F. Anterior rectal mucosal prolapse: An easily treated cause of anorectal symptoms. Br J Surg 1995;82:753–4.
31. Kay NRM, Zachary RB. The treatment of rectal prolapse in children with injections of 30 per cent saline solutions. J Pediatr Surg 1970;5:334–7.
32. Hight DW, Hertzler JH, Philipappart AI, Benson CD. Linear cauterization for the treatment of rectal prolapse in infants and children. Surg Gynecol Obstet 1982;154:400–2.
33. Heald CL. A simple, bloodless operation for anorectal prolapse in children. Surg Obstet Gynecol 1926;42:840–1.
34. Chwals WJ, Brennan LP, Weitzman JJ, Woolley MM. Transanal mucosal sleeve resection for the treatment of rectal prolapse in children. J Pediatr Surg 1990;25:715–8.
35. Momoh JT. Quadrant mucosal stripping and muscle pleating in the management of childhood rectal prolapse. J Pediatr Surg 1986;21:36–8.
36. Ashcraft KW, Amoury RA, Holder TM. Levator repair and posterior suspension for rectal prolapse. J Pediatr Surg 1977;12:241–5.
37. Cirocco WC, Brown AC. Anterior resection for the treatment of rectal prolapse: A 20-year experience. Am Surg 1993;59:265–9.
38. Schlinkert RT, Beart RW, Wolff BG, Pemberton JH. Anterior resection for complete rectal prolapse. Dis Colon Rectum 1985;28:409–12.
39. Husa A, Sainio P, Smitten K. Abdominal rectopexy and sigmoid resection (Frykman-Goldberg operation) for rectal prolapse. Acta Chir 1988;154:221–4.
40. Sayfan J, Pinho M, Alexander-Williams J, Keighley MRB. Sutured posterior abdominal rectopexy with sigmoidectomy compared with Marlex rectopexy for rectal prolapse. Br J Surg 1990;77:143–5.
41. McKee RF, Lauder JC, Poon FW, et al. A prospective randomized study of abdominal rectopexy with and without sigmoidectomy. Surg Gynecol Obstet 1992;174:145–8.
42. Luukkonen P, Mikkonen U, Jarvinen H. Abdominal rectopexy with sigmoidectomy vs. rectopexy alone for rectal prolapse: A prospective, randomized study. Int J Colorect Dis 1992;7:219–22.
43. Canfrere VG, des Varannos SB, Mayon J, Lehar PA. Adding sigmoidectomy to rectopexy to treat rectal prolapse: A valid option? Br J Surg 1994;81:2–4.
44. Huber FT, Stein H, Siewert JR. Functional results after treatment of rectal prolapse with rectopexy and sigmoid resection. World J Surg 1995;19:138–43.
45. McMahan J, Ripstein CB. Rectal prolapse. An update on the rectal sling procedure. Am Surg 1987;53:37–40.
46. Launer DP, Fazio VW, Weakley FL, et al. The Ripstein procedure: A 16-year experience. Dis Colon Rectum 1982;25:41–5.
47. Roberts PL, Schoetz DJ Jr, Coller JA, Veidenheimer MC. Ripstein procedure: Lahey Clinic experience: 1963–1985. Arch Surg 1988;123:554–7.
48. Holmstrom B, Broden G, Dolk A. Results of the Ripstein operation in the treatment of rectal prolapse and internal rectal procidentia. Dis Colon Rectum 1986;29:845–8.

49. Leenen LPH, Kuijpers JHC. Treatment of complete rectal prolapse with foreign material. Neth J Surg 1989;41:129–31.

50. Keighley MRB, Fielding JWL, Alexander-Williams J. Results of Marlex mesh abdominal rectopexy for rectal prolapse in 100 consecutive patients. Br J Surg 1983;70:229–32.

51. Gordon PH, Hoexter B. Complications of the Ripstein procedure. Dis Colon Rectum 1978;21:277–80.

52. Wells C. New operation for rectal prolapse. Proc R Soc Med 1959;52:602–3.

53. Wedell J, zu Eissen PM, Fiedler R. A new concept for the management of rectal prolapse. Am J Surg 1980;139:723–5.

54. Morgan CN, Porter NH, Klugman DJ. Ivalon (polyvinyl alcohol) sponge in the repair of complete rectal prolapse. Br J Surg 1972;59:841–6.

55. Penfold JCB, Hawley PR. Experiences of Ivalon-sponge implant for complete rectal prolapse at St. Mark's hospital, 1960–70. Br J Surg 1972;59:846–8.

56. Atkinson KG, Taylor DC. Wells procedure for complete rectal prolapse: A ten-year experience. Dis Colon Rectum 1984;27:96–8.

57. Mann CV, Hoffman C. Complete rectal prolapse: The anatomical and functional results of treatment by an extended abdominal rectopexy. Br J Surg 1988;75:34–7.

58. Novel JR, Osborne MJ, Winslet MC, Lewis AA. Prospective randomized trial of Ivalon sponge versus sutured rectopexy for full-thickness rectal prolapse. Br J Surg 1994;81:904–6.

59. Orr TG. A suspension operation for prolapse of the rectum. Ann Surg 1947;126:833–40.

60. Loygue J, Huguier M, Malafosse M, Biotois H. Complete prolapse of the rectum: A report on 140 cases treated by rectopexy. Br J Surg 1971;58:847–8.

61. Loygue J, Nordlinger B, Cunci O, et al. Rectopexy to the promontory for the treatment of rectal prolapse: Report of 257 cases. Dis Colon Rectum 1984;27:356–9.

62. Frykman HM, Goldberg SM. The surgical treatment of rectal procidentia. Surg Gynecol Obstet 1969;129:1225–30.

63. Ejerblad S, Krause U. Repair of rectal prolapse by rectosacral suture fixation. Acta Chir Scand 154:103–5.

64. Madoff RD, Williams JG, Wong WD, et al. Long-term functional results of colon resection and rectopexy for overt rectal prolapse. Am J Gastroenterol 1992;87:101–4.

65. Xynos E, Chrysos E, Tsiaoussis J, et al. Resection rectopexy for rectal prolapse. The laparoscopic approach. Surg Endosc 1999;13:862–4.

66. Bruch HP, Herold A, Schiedeck T, Schwandner O. Lapsroscopic surgery for rectal prolapse and outlet obstruction. Dis Colon Rectum 1999;42:1189–95.

67. Kellokumpu IH, Vironen J, Scheinin T. Laparoscopic repair of rectal prolapse: a prospective study evaluating surgical outcome and changes in symptoms and bowel function. Surg Endosc 2000;14:634–40.

68. Zittel TT, Nanncke K, Haug S, et al. Functional results after laparoscopic rectopexy for rectal prolapse. J Gastrointest Surg 2000;4:632–41.

69. Williams JG. Perineal approaches to repair of rectal prolapse. Semin Colon Rectal Surg 1991;2:198–204.

70. Altemeier WA, Giuseffi I, Hoxworth PI. Treatment of extensive prolapse of rectum in aged and debilitated patients. Arch Surg 1952;65:72.

71. Williams JG, Rothenherger DA, Madoff RD, Goldberg SM. Treatment of rectal prolapse in the elderly by perineal rectosigmoidectomy. Dis Colon Rectum 1992;35:830–4.

72. Bennett BH, Geelhoed GW. A stapler modification of the Altemeier procedure for rectal prolapse: Experimental and clinical evaluation. Am Surg 1985;51:116–20.

73. Gopal KA, Amshel AL, Shonberg IL, Eftaiha M. Rectal procidentia in elderly and debilitated patients: Experience with the Altemeier procedure. Dis Colon Rectum 1984;27:376–81.

74. Prasad ML, Pearl RK, Abcarian H, Orsay CP, Nelson RL. Perineal proctectomy, posterior rectopexy, and postanal levator repair for the treatment of rectal prolapse. Dis Colon Rectum 1986;29:547–52.

75. Ramanujam PS, Venkatesh KS. Perineal excision of rectal prolapse with posterior levator ani repair in elderly high-risk patients. Dis Colon Rectum 1988;31:704–6.

76. Ramanujam PS, Venkatesh KS, Fietz MJ. Perineal excision of rectal procidentia in elderly high-risk patients. A ten-year experience. Dis Colon Rectum 1994;37:1027–30.

77. Kim DS, Tsang CBS, Wong WD, et al. Complete rectal prolapse - evolution of management and results. Dis Colon Rectum 1999;42:460–9.

78. Agachan F, Pfeifer J, Joo JS, et al. Results of perineal procedures for the treatment of rectal prolapse. Am Surg 1997;63:9–12.

79. Whitlow CB, Beck DE, Opelka FG, et al. Perineal procedures for prolapse. J La State Med Soc. 1997;149:22–6.

80. Deen KI, Grant E, Billingham C, Keighley MRB. Abdominal resection rectopexy with pelvic floor repair versus perineal rectosigmoidectomy and pelvic floor repair for full-thickness rectal prolapse. Br J Surg 1994;81:302–4.

81. Classic articles in colonic and rectal surgery. Edmond Delorme. On the treatment of total prolapse of the rectum by excision of the rectal mucous membranes or recto-colic. Dis Colon Rectum 1985;28:544–53.

82. Nay HR, Blair CR. Perineal surgical repair of rectal prolapse. Am J Surg 1972;123:577–9.

83. Uhlig BE, Sullivan ES. The modified Delorme operation: Its place in surgical treatment for massive rectal prolapse. Dis Colon Rect um 1979;22:513–21.

84. Christiansen J, Kirkegaard P. Delorme's operation for complete rectal prolapse. Br J Surg 1981;68:537–8.

85. Graf W, Ejerblad S, Krog M, et al. Delorme's operation for rectal prolapse in elderly or unfit patients. Eur J Surg 1992;158:555–7.

86. Tobin SA, Scott IHK. Delorme operation for rectal prolapse. Br J Surg 1994;81:1681–4.

87. Oliver GC, Vachon D, Eisenstat TE, et al. Delorme's procedure for complete rectal prolapse in severely debilitated patients: An analysis of 41 cases. Dis Colon Rectum 1994;37: 461–7.

88. Senapati A, Nicholls RJ, Thomson JPS, Phillips RKS. Results of Delorme's procedure for rectal prolapse. Dis Colon Rectum 1994;37:456–60.

89. Plusa SM, Charig JA, Balaji V, et al. Physiological changes after Delorme's procedure for full-thickness rectal prolapse. Br J Surg 1995;82:1475–8.

90. Goldman J. Concerning prolapse of the rectum with special emphasis on the operation by Thiersch. Dis Colon Rectum 1988;31:154–5.

91. Gabriel WB. Thiersch's operation for anal incontinence and minor degrees of rectal prolapse. Am J Surg 1953;86:583–90.

92. Khanduja KS, Hardy TG, Aguilar PS, et al. A new silicone prosthesis in the modified Thiersch operation. Dis Colon Rectum 1988;31:380–3.

Hemorrhoids and the symptoms they produce have plagued mankind throughout recorded history [1, 2]. Large sums of money are spent on products to control these symptoms, and the amount of work lost because of hemorrhoids is economically important. Our understanding of etiology and symptoms helps us to make recommendations for therapy. This chapter discusses the anatomy, pathophysiology, and methods of treatment of symptomatic hemorrhoids.

Anatomy

Hemorrhoids are cushions of vascular tissue found in the anal canal [2]. Hemorrhoidal tissue is normal and present at birth. Microscopically, this tissue contains vascular structures whose walls do not contain muscle. Thus hemorrhoids are not veins (which have muscular walls) but are sinusoids (**Figure 16.1**) [3]. Recent studies have also demonstrated that hemorrhoidal bleeding is arterial and not venous. When these sinusoids are injured (disrupted), hemorrhage occurs from presinusoidal arterioles. The arterial nature of the bleeding explains why hemorrhoidal hemorrhage is bright red and has an arterial pH [4].

In humans, hemorrhoidal tissue is thought to contribute to anal continence by forming a spongy bolster which cushions the anal canal and prevents damage to the sphincter mechanism during defecation [2]. This tissue also acts as a compressible lining that allows the anus to close completely. The three main cushions (or bundles) lie at the left lateral, right anterolateral, and right posterolateral portion of the anal canal. Smaller secondary cushions may occasionally lie between these main cushions. Each bundle starts superiorly in the anal canal and extends inferiorly to the anal margin. The superior portion of the hemorrhoidal tissue (above the dentate line) is covered by anal mucosa and the inferior portion (below the dentate line) is covered by anoderm or skin.

Pathophysiology

Etiologic factors

Enlargement of or a pathologic change in hemorrhoidal tissue results in symptoms of the 'hemorrhoidal syndrome'. Proposed etiologic factors for these changes include constipation, prolonged straining, pregnancy, and derangement of the internal sphincter [2]. All of these conditions work toward stretching and slippage of the hemorrhoidal tissue.

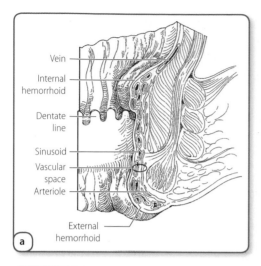

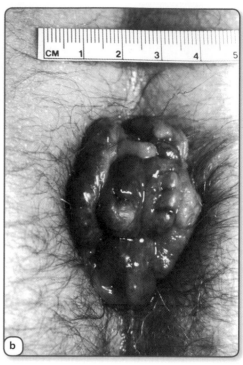

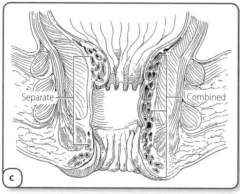

Figure 16.1 Hemorrhoidal anatomy. (a) Arteriovenous anastomosis (AV shunts) forming hemorrhoidal plexus. (b) Fourth degree hemorrhoids. (c) Usual position of the hemorrhoids. Separate external and internal hemorrhoids are seen on the left and a combined internal-external hemorrhoidal complex is seen on the right.

The overlying skin or mucosa is stretched and additional fibrous and sinusoidal tissue develops. The extra tissue tends to move toward the anal verge, making it susceptible to injury. Symptoms may then develop.

Hemorrhoids are not related to portal hypertention [4]. With increased portal venous pressure, the body develops portosystemic communications in several locations. In the pelvis, communications enlarge between the superior and middle hemorrhoidal veins; this results in the development of rectal varices. These varices are located in the lower rectum, not the anus. Because of the rectum's large capacity, they rarely bleed. Older literature suggested a relationship between portal hypertension and hemorrhoids partly as a result of the fact that hemorrhoids are common and therefore many portal hypertensive patients will have hemorrhoids. If portal hypertension were an etiologic factor, hemorrhoidal bleeding would be venous blood rather than arterial bleeding as described above. Hemorrhoidal symptoms may be difficult to manage in patients with portal hypertension as their liver disease frequently is associated with coagulation and platelet problems.

Classification

For anatomic and clinical reasons hemorrhoidal tissue has been divided into two types: external and internal. **External hemorrhoids** are located in the distal third of the anal canal (distal to the dentate line) and are covered by anoderm or skin. This overlying tissue is innervated by somatic nerves and thus is sensitive to touch, temperature, stretch, and pain. Symptoms from external hemorrhoids usually result from thrombosis of the hemorrhoidal plexus. The rapid tissue expansion produced by the clots and edema causes pain. Physical effort is felt to be an etiologic factor in thrombosis of external hemorrhoids. Physical examination in these patients reveals a tender blue mass at the anus. Additional symptoms are discussed next.

Internal hemorrhoids are located proximal to the dentate line and covered by mucosa. Based on size and clinical symptoms, internal hemorrhoids can be further subdivided by grades [5]: **Grade 1** hemorrhoids protrude into but do not prolapse out of the anal canal; **Grade 2** hemorrhoids prolapse out of the anal canal with bowel movements or straining, but spontaneously reduce; **Grade 3** hemorrhoids prolapse during the maneuvers just described and must be manually reduced by the patient; **Grade 4** hemorrhoids are prolapsed out of the anus and cannot be reduced. Hemorrhoids that remain prolapsed develop ischemia, thrombosis, or gangrene.

Evaluation and treatment

Symptoms

Patients with any anal complaints commonly present to physicians complaining of 'hemorrhoids.' Careful exploration of the symptoms will lead to the correct diagnosis. Symptoms associated with hemorrhoidal disease include mucosal protrusion, pain, bleeding, a sensation of incomplete evacuation, mucous discharge, difficulties with perianal hygiene, and cosmetic deformity.

Except when thrombosis or edema occurs, hemorrhoids are painless. Painless bleeding occurs from internal hemorrhoids, is usually bright red, and is associated with bowel movements. The blood will occasionally drip into the commode and stain the toilet water bright red. After trauma by firm stools or forceful bowel movements, bleeding may continue to occur with bowel movements for several days. The bleeding will often then resolve for a variable period of time.

Prolapse may be perceived by the patient as an anal mass, a feeling of incomplete evacuation, or a mucous discharge. It should be ascertained whether the patient must manually reduce prolapsed hemorrhoids. If thrombosis or gangrene occurs, it will be apparent on physical examination and may be associated with systemic symptoms.

Physical examination

An adequate evaluation for a patient with hemorrhoidal symptoms includes anoscopy and proctoscopy. If the patient is less than 40 years of age and hemorrhoidal disease compatible with symptoms is seen on physical examination, most authors feel that no additional workup is required. If the patient is older than 40 years of age and hemorrhoidal disease is not observed or additional symptoms are present, a barium enema or colonoscopy is obtained to identify other causes for bleeding that were not observed by proctoscopy.

Nonoperative treatment

Diet and stool-bulking agents

Most patients benefit from alterations in diet and the addition of bulk stool normalizers (e.g. psyllium) [6]. The goal is to produce a soft stool that is easy to pass. This type of stool reduces the requirement to strain with bowel movements and lessens the chance of damage to the hemorrhoids. It is important to counsel the patient to ingest an appropriate amount of water with the fiber.

If diet and bulking agents fail to relieve symptoms, other procedures are indicated. The goals of the various techniques described next are to remove excess anal tissue and mucosa and fixate the adjacent tissue, reducing prolapse.

Rubber band ligation

The most common office procedure for the treatment of symptomatic internal hemorrhoids is rubber band ligation [2]. Informed consent is obtained and an anoscope is inserted into the anus (I prefer a slotted lighted anoscope; **Figure 16.2**). A hemorrhoid bundle is identified and through the anoscope a band is placed using one of two types of ligators. A suction ligator (McGown) draws the hemorrhoid bundle into the ligator and closing the handle places the band around the hemorrhoidal tissue. With a Barron or McGivney ligator, an atraumatic clamp (**Figure 16.3**) is used to retract mucosa and redundant

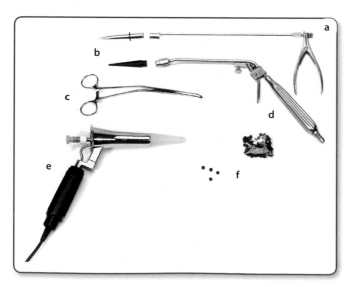

Figure 16.2 Hemorrhoidal banders. (a) Band ligator. (b) Baud loader. (c) Avascular clamp. (d) Suction ligator. (e) Fiberoptic anoscope. (f) Rubber bands.

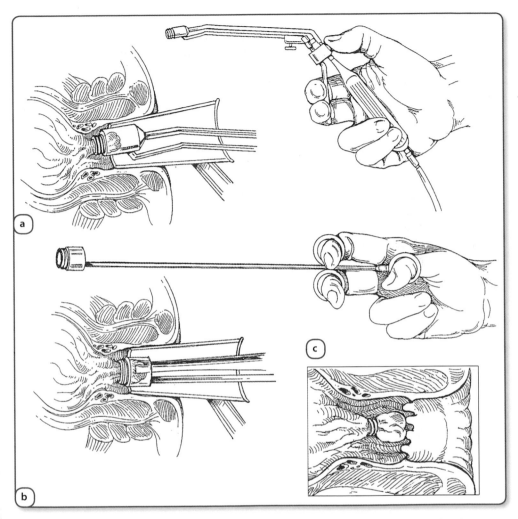

Figure 16.3 Banding an internal hemorrhoid. The internal hemorrhoid is teased into the barrel of the ligating gun with, (a) a suction (McGown) ligator or (b) a McGivney ligator. (c) The apex of the banded hemorrhoid is well above the dentate line to minimize pain.

hemorrhoidal tissue at the apex of the bundle into the applicator and a small rubber band is placed. This tight band causes ischemia of the enclosed tissue. After it necroses, the tissue sloughs, forming a small ulcer. Excess tissue is eliminated and as healing occurs, the remaining lining becomes fixed in the anal canal. Rubber band ligation works best for Grade 2 or 3 internal hemorrhoids.

Several points require additional elaboration. First, it is crucial that the bands be placed on tissue covered by anal mucosa. If bands are placed too distal and include somatically innervated skin, the patient will develop excruciating pain. The pain is usually so severe that the patient will demand removal of the band. To prevent this from occurring, it is recommended that the band be placed at the apex of the hemorrhoid bundle or just cranial to it. As an additional check, the proposed site of banding is tested by placing a clamp on the mucosa. If the patient feels the pain, the procedure should be abandoned. It is important that the clamp not be pulled after being applied. As the anal and rectal mucosa is sensitive to stretch, traction on the mucosa will produce inappropriate pain.

A second consideration is to resist too forceful retraction of the hemorrhoidal tissue. If pulled too hard, the hemorrhoidal tissue may be torn, resulting in hemorrhage that is sometimes difficult to control. Finally, this type of bander requires two hands and an assistant to stabilize the anoscope during the procedure. The McGowan ligator can be used with one hand, but it is more difficult to control the amount of tissue drawn into the bander.

Controversy exists about the appropriate number of bands that may be applied at one session. The author prefers to place one or two bands at a time. Banding this number will eliminate symptoms in most patients and does not produce too large an amount of banded tissue in the anal canal or cause excessive discomfort.

The patient is instructed that he or she may have a feeling of incomplete evacuation. If the urge to defecate or urinate is noted, patients are instructed to sit and try to pass the stool. If no stool is produced, they should refrain from prolonged straining. Normal activities should be continued. The sensation of fullness is from the bunched tissue in the anal canal. At 5–7 days the bands and necrotic tissue will slough. This may be associated with a small amount of bleeding. If the symptoms have not resolved at reexamination 2–3 weeks later, additional bands are placed.

Millions of bands have been applied with minimal morbidity. However, a few cases of postbanding sepsis have been described [7–9]. Difficulty urinating, fever, and pelvic pain are symptoms of postbanding sepsis. In a few patients, delayed diagnosis and treatment led to fatal results. More recent reports describe complete resolution with early hospitalization, adequate diagnostic examinations, and intravenous antibiotics [9]. Additional potential complications include failure to relieve symptoms and bleeding. Some patients with very sensitive anal mucosa do not tolerate rubber band ligation. They are better managed with an infrared coagulator (IRC).

Infrared photocoagulation

A newer technique to treat internal hemorrhoids is photocoagu-lation [10]. An IRC delivers a controlled amount of infrared energy (**Figure 16.4**). An anoscope is used to identify the hemorrhoidal tissue. Several applications of energy are delivered at the superior portion of the hemorrhoid bundle (**Figure 16.5**). The physics of the energy are such that the majority of energy is deposited into the submucosa. This results in a small mucosal ulcer, which causes fixation after healing [11]. The IRC works best on patients with small bleeding hemorrhoids. Two to three bundles are treated at each session.

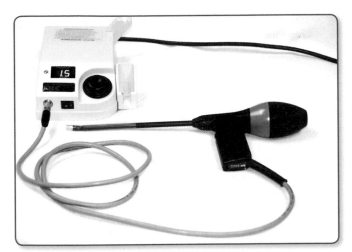

Figure 16.4 Infrared photocoagulator.

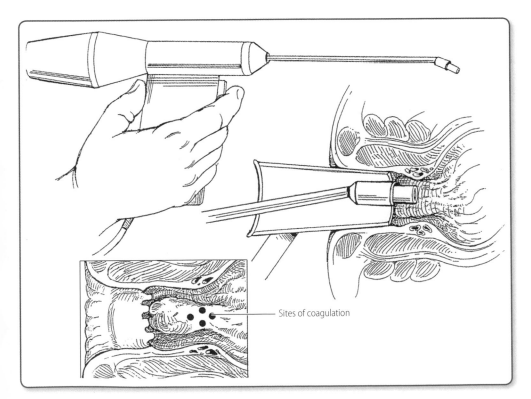

Sites of coagulation

Figure 16.5 The infrared photocoagulator creates a small thermal injury. Thus several applications are required for each hemorrhoidal column.

An advantage of this technique is that maximal discomfort occurs at the time of IRC treatment and not at a later time, as is seen with incorrectly placed bands. Disadvantages of this technique are that the cost of the instrument is significantly higher than a bander and that this method is less effective in eliminating bulky hemorrhoids [9].

Sclerotherapy

Sclerotherapy (injection therapy) is an older method that causes submucosal necrosis and subsequent fixation. Although the results produced by this method are similar to those of IRC, sclerotherapy is being used less frequently. Similar to IRC, sclerotherapy works best for Grade 1 or 2 hemorrhoids.

After the hemorrhoidal bundle is identified with an anoscope, a submucosal injection of 1–2 mL of a sclerosing agent (sodium morrhuate, 5% quinine urea, or 5% phenol in almond oil) is accomplished with a long needle (25-gauge spinal or Gabriel needle). The proper site of injection is just proximal to the hemorrhoidal plexus and the injection should be sufficiently deep to not blanch the mucosa, but not so deep as to injure the underlying muscle.

Cryotherapy

Cryotherapy is discussed here for completeness, but it is an infrequently used method. Through a cryoprobe inserted into the anus, cold is delivered to freeze a hemorrhoidal bundle. One disadvantage is the inability to control the amount of destruction that occurs. A prolonged necrotic tissue slough results, causing increased pain and an unpleasant anal discharge [9].

Electrocautery

Bipolar and direct current devices are currently available for electrocautery. Direct current therapy uses a special probe (Ultroid; Microinvasive, Watertown, MA, USA) to deliver an electrical current for up to 10 minutes to the internal hemorrhoid bundle. Bipolar diathermy (Circon ACMI, Stamford, CN, USA) uses an electrical current to generate a coagulum of tissue at the end of a cautery tipped applicator. The equipment for both methods is expensive, and neither method offers any advantage over the methods described previously [9].

Operative treatment

Thrombosed external hemorrhoids

The management of thrombosed hemorrhoids depends on when in the course of the disease the patient is seen. The natural course of this condition starts with thrombosis of an external hemorrhoid. The tissue around these clots swells, causing moderate to severe pain. If not treated in 2–4 weeks, the clot in the thrombosed vessels will either spontaneously drain through the thinned overlying skin or be gradually resorbed, and the discomfort will gradually diminish. After resolution, redundant anal skin will remain.

If symptoms have stabilized or are improving, nonoperative care including stool-bulking agents and pain medication is indicated. The patient should be reassured that the symptoms will resolve in 1–2 weeks. If the patient presents early, the procedure of choice is excision (**Figure 16.6**). The remaining wound may be left open or closed. The goal with excision is to remove the clots and leave a cosmetically pleasing wound. The procedure can be performed with local anesthesia. Incision and drainage is avoided as it removes only a portion of the clot and when healing occurs excess skin may remain.

Operative hemorrhoidectomy

For symptomatic combined external and internal hemorrhoids, a hemorrhoidectomy is indicated [12–15]. Various types of hemorrhoidectomies have developed throughout the years. These include a closed (Ferguson) technique, an open (Milligan–Morgan) technique, a circumferential (Whitehead), stappled rectopexy and transanal deartertalization with rectopexy. All of these procedures adhere to several basic principles which include decreasing blood flow to the anorectal ring, removing redundant hemorrhoidal tissue, and fixation of redundant mucosa and anoderm.

Each of these procedures can be performed with general, spinal, or local anesthesia. The choice must be individualized for each patient, but the national trend is toward the use of local anesthesia. With a general anesthetic, the author prefers the Sims' position (left lateral decubitus; see Figure 3.1b). With all other anesthetics, the prone jackknife position is used (see Figure 3.1a).

The **Ferguson** or **closed hemorrhoidectomy** is the most popular procedure performed in the United States. With this technique the anus is prepared with a povidone-iodine solution. If a local anesthetic (a 50/50 mixture 1% xylocaine with 1:100,000 epinephrine and 0.5% bapivocaine) is not being used, the anal submucosa is infiltrated with 0.5 % bapicocaine with 1:100,000 epinephrine solution. The perineum is reprepared and draped. An examination confirms the preoperative findings and determines the number of hemorrhoidal bundles to be excised. A medium or large Hill–Ferguson retractor placed in the anus

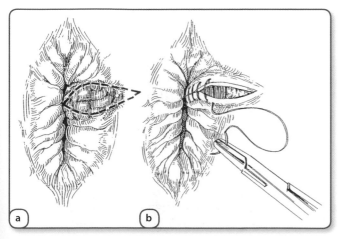

Figure 16.6 Thrombosed external hemorrhoid. (a) Site of incision. (b) A running stitch is used for wound closure.

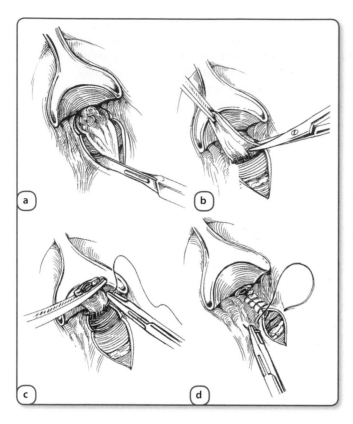

Figure 16.7 Modified Ferguson excisional hemorrhoidectomy. (a) Double ellipitical incision made in mucosa and anoderm around hemorrhoidal bundle with a scalpel. (b) The hemorrhoid dissection is carefully continued cephalad by dissecting the sphincter away from the hemorrhoid. (c) After dissection of the hemorrhoid to its pedicle, it is either clamped, secured, or excised. The pedicle is suture ligated. (d) The wound is closed with a running stitch. Excessive traction on the suture is avoided to prevent forming dog ears or displacing the anoderm caudally.

exposes a hemorrhoidal bundle. A double elliptical incision is made in the mucosa (**Figure 16.7**). For a pleasing cosmetic result, the incision should be at least three times as long as it is wide. The distal edge is grasped with a fine-toothed pick-up and the dissection is performed with scissors. Dissection in the proper plane results in elevation of all the varicosities with the specimen, while the muscles remain in their normal anatomic position. With the previously scored mucosa as a guide, the dissection is continued into the top of the anal canal.

At the superior edge of the hemorrhoidal bundle, the remaining vascular pedicle is clamped and the hemorrhoid is detached. The hemorrhoid specimen may be labeled by quadrant (e.g. left lateral, right posterior) and sent for pathologic evaluation. Location labeling is important if the hemorrhoids look unusual or clinically suspicious. Any bleeding vessels are cauterized with the electrocautery. An absorbable suture (e.g. 4-0 Vicryl or chromic) is used to suture-ligate the pedicle beneath the clamp. This suture is then used to reapproximate the mucosal edges. It is important to take small bites at the edge of the mucosa and a small bite of the sphincter with each bite. This running suture is continued to close the wound and eliminate dead space. As sutures are placed, the mucosa is advanced in a cranial direction to reestablish the normal anal anatomy and result in a 'plastic' closure.

At the outer edge the suture is loosely tied to itself to provide an escape for any hematoma developing after surgery. The other hemorrhoidal bundles are handled in a similar manner. One, two or three hemorrhoidal bundles may be excised in this fashion and the number of bundles that are excised will depend on the amount of excess tissue. Modifications of the technique include the use of electrocautery to incise the hemorrhoidal tissue, the type of suture used, and the extent of wound closure. Alternate energy sources have been tried, but they offer little advantages and add significant cost. It is essential with this type of hemorrhoidectomy that only minimal amounts of anoderm are excised. If large amounts of anoderm are excised, closing the anal wounds or secondary healing can result in significant postoperative pain and anal stenosis.

In the United Kingdom, the **Milligan–Morgan hemorrhoidectomy** is most commonly used [15]. This technique involves ligation and excision of the hemorrhoids while leaving the wounds open. In this technique, the anus is gently dilated and the hemorrhoidal tissue and perianal skin are everted just outside the anorectal ring. The triangular shaped hemorrhoid is excised down to the underlying sphincter muscle. The pedicle is then ligated with suture. The wound is left open and a light dressing applied. One, two or three hemorrhoids may be treated in this manner (**Figure 16.8**).

Laser hemorrhoidectomy (using a laser rather than a scalpel or scissors to remove the hemorrhoidal tissue) has received a lot of attention. Proponents have claimed that this technique involves less pain and has a better cosmetic result. Unfortunately, several well-controlled prospective studies have demonstrated no advantage of a laser over traditional techniques [9]. The additional cost and safety requirements of the laser equipment militate against its routine use.

The **Whitehead hemorrhoidectomy** was first described in 1882 [16]. This technique involves circumferential excision of hemorrhoidal veins and mucosa beginning at the dentate line and proceeding proximally (**Figure 16.9**). It is still used commonly in the United Kingdom but rarely employed in the United States due to technical difficulties and the potential for ectropion. Ectropia results from starting the incision distal to the dentate line and resuturing the edges of the mucosal flaps too distally in the anal canal. This technique is somewhat similar to the Delorme, used for rectal prolapse, and to the newly developed stapled anoplasty described in the following paragraphs.

Over the past few years, the **stapled rectopexy** has been developed as an alternative to standard Ferguson or Milligan–Morgan hemorrhoidectomy [15]. Several names have been applied to this procedure including 'stapled hemorrhoidectomy', 'stapled hemorrhoidopexy' and procedure for prolapsing hemorrhoids (PPH), and it is hoped that this procedure will avoid the pain associated with traditional hemorrhoid surgery. It was first described by Pescatori et al [17] and refined by Longo [18]. Since then, it has been written about by many authors and subjected to three randomized controlled trials [19–21].

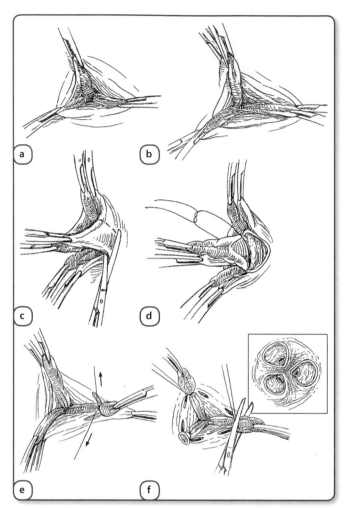

Figure 16.8 Open (Milligan–Morgan) hemorrhoidectomy.
(a) External hemorrhoids grasped with forceps and retracted outward.
(b) Internal hemorrhoids grasped with forceps and retracted outward with external hemorrhoids.
(c) External skin and hemorrhoid excised with scissors. (d) Suture placed through proximal internal hemorrhoid and vascular bundle.
(e) Ligature tied. (f) Tissue distal to ligature is excised. Insert depicts completed three bundle hemorrhoidectomy.

Stapled rectopexy involves transanal, circular stapling of redundant anorectal mucosa with a modified circular stapling instrument (Proximate HCS 33 mm PPH, Ethicon Endosurgery, Cincinnati, OH, USA). There is continued debate about the mechanisms by which it relieves symptoms. As hemorrhoids are thought to be redundant fibrovascular cushions, most treatments reduce blood flow and remove redundant tissue. Stapled rectopexy is thought to work by similar mechanisms. Redundant mucosa is drawn into the instruction and excised within the 'stapled doughnut.' Additionally, mucosal and submucosal blood flow is interrupted by the circular staple line. No incisions are made in the somatically innervated, highly sensitive anoderm which significantly reduces postoperative pain.

Patients are prepared as for a standard hemorrhoidectomy with partial or complete mechanical bowel preparation. General, spinal, and local anesthesias have all been described. Patients may be positioned in prone, lithotomy, or Sim's position depending upon the surgeon's preference.

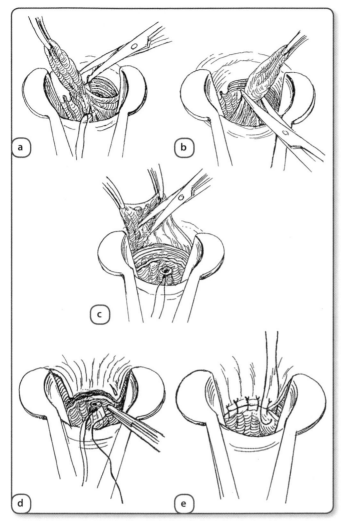

Figure 16.9 Whitehead hemorrhoidectomy. (a) Suture placed through proximal internal hemorrhoid for orientation. Excision started at dentate line and continued to proximal bundle. (b) Internal hemorrhoidal tissue excised above ligated bundle. (c) Vascular tissue excised from underside of elevated anoderm. (d) End of anoderm reaproximated with sutures to original location of dentate line. (e) Completed procedure.

After thorough examination of the anal canal and perianal tissues, a specially designed anoscope in inserted and a pursestring suture is placed. The purse-string should be 2–4 cm proximal to the dentate line and include only mucosa and submucosa. Suture 'bites' should be close together as large gaps will allow redundant mucosa to evade the stapler resulting in persistent hemorrhoids. Most surgeons place eight bites of the purse-string suture. The circular stapling instrument is then introduced (usually a 33 mm), fully opened, into the anal canal, and the suture tightened between the anvil and shaft of the instrument. Ends of the suture are drawn through slots of the stapler drawing distal redundant mucosal proximally into the jaws of the stapler. After tightening the stapler, a finger is placed transvaginally in females to assure that the anovaginal septum has not been included within the stapler. The stapler is then fired and removed (**Figure 16.10**).

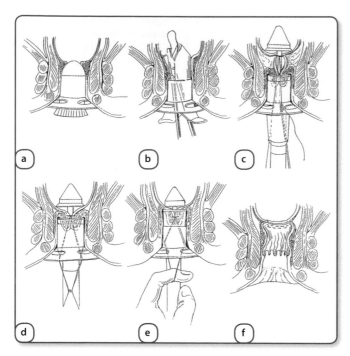

Figure 16.10 Stapled anoplasty (procedure for prolapse and hemorrhoids, PPH). (a) Retracting anoscope and dilator inserted. (b) Monofilament purse-string suture (eight bites) placed using operating anoscope approximately 3–4 cm above anal verge. (c) Stapler inserted through purse-string. Purse-string suture tied and ends of suture manipulated through stapler. (d) Retracting on suture pulls anorectal mucosa into stapler. (e) Stapler closed and fired. (f) Completed procedure.

Following this, the staple line is inspected for gaps and particularly for bleeding points, which can then be cauterized or oversewn. Some authors routinely place three figure of eight sutures at the location of the primary hemorrhoidal bundles to minimize the chances of postoperative bleeding.

Three randomized, prospective trials have compared stapled rectopexy to traditional surgery. Mehigan, Monson, and Hartley at the University of Hull randomized 40 patients with third or fourth degree hemorrhoids to stapled rectopexy or Milligan–Morgan hemorrhoidectomy [19]. All procedures were performed under general anesthesia. Complications were minor and rare in both groups. Hospital stay and return of bowel function were similar in both groups. The stapled group, however, experienced significantly less pain (average 2.1 vs. 6.5 on a pain scale of 1–10) and returned to normal activity sooner (17 vs. 34 days).

Rowsell, Bello, and Hemingway at the Leicester Royal Infirmary, UK included 22 patients in a prospective randomized trial comparing conventional (excision with partial closure) hemorrhoidectomy to stapled rectopexy [20]. Again both groups were without major complications. These authors found stapled rectopexy to be associated with a shorter postoperative hospital stay (1.09 vs. 2.82 nights), less postoperative pain (total pain score 20 vs. 44) and quicker return to normal function (8.1–16.9 days).

Finally, Ho et al. at Singapore General Hospital randomized 119 patients to stapled rectopexy vs. Milligan–Morgan hemorrhoidectomy

[21]. All their patients were described as having Grade 4 or irreducibly prolapsed hemorrhoids. In addition, they followed all patients with endoanal ultrasound and anal manometry for three months postoperatively. Manometric and ultrasound results were similar in both groups. Open hemorrhoidectomy was associated with a higher likelihood of slowly healing perineal wounds, postoperative bleeding and pruritus. Hospital stay was similar for both groups, but traditional hemorrhoidectomy was associated with more pain on defecation and total analgesic requirements at 6 weeks [21]. A multicenter prospective controlled trial with long term follow-up compared stapled rectopexy to a modified Ferguson technique [22]. The authors demonstrated that stapled rectopexy offered less postoperative pain, less requirement for analgesics, and less pain at first bowel movement, while providing similar control of symptoms and need for additional hemorrhoid treatment at one-year follow-up from surgery.

In summary, stapled rectopexy is a technique available to patients otherwise requiring surgical hemorrhoidectomy. In limited studies, stapled rectopexy it is associated with significantly less pain and similar complication rates when compared to conventional treatment. Considering the technique, however, the potential for disastrous complications may be higher (rectovaginal or rectourethral fistula due to including too much tissue within the pursestring). Bleeding also remains a problem and cases of perforation and leaks have been reported. It is also important to note that stapled rectopexy has not been compared to office treatments for Grade 1 and 2 hemorrhoids and should not replace these techniques for minimally symptomatic hemorrhoid disease.

A new addition to surgical armamentarium is **Doppler-guided arterial ligation with hemorrhoidopexy** [23]. The technique has evolved and currently uses a Doppler-guided ligation of hemorrhoidal arterial inflow with a suture rectopexy. There are currently two commercial products available in the United States [24]: transanal hemorrhoidal dearterialization (THD; American Ankeny, IA, USA) and hemorrhoidal artery ligation and rectoanal repair (HAL-RAR; AMI, Inc., Natick, MA, USA). These non excisional techniques rely on detection and ligation of the branches of the superior hermorhoidal artery in the insate mucosa well above the dentate line. The associated suture rectopexy reduces the redundant prolapsing mucosa and internal hemorrhoids.

The procedure is performed in the operating room and requires anesthesia similar to a traditional hemorrhoidectomy. A specially designed anoscope with a removable Doppler ultrasound probe and a slot for suture placement is used. After insertion, the anoscope is rotated until one of the arterial branches is located. Through the anoscope slot the vessel is suture ligated. Loss of the Doppler signal confirms accurate placement of the ligating suture. After ligating the vessel, the suture is used to oversew the internal hemorrhoid with a running technique from proximal to distal direction. The suture is completed proximal to the dentate line to minimize pain. Usually four to six arteries are ligated depending on the patient's anatomy and two to four hemorrhoids are fixated.

The operation has a short operating time and purports to accomplish the same goals as a stapled hemorrhoidopexy [24]. It is an operative procedure which includes anesthesia risks, operating room expense, and surgical risks of bleeding, infection, urinary retention, and postoperative pain. The specialized anoscope and Doppler probe are disposable and add cost to the procedure which is somewhat less that a stapled hemorrhoidopexy. A variety of publications have documented safety, reduced pain and short recovery with the technique [25]. It appears effective for Grades 2 and 3 hemorrhoids, but long-term results and cost-benefit analysis need additional study.

Complications

Hemorrhoid surgery is very safe and the incidence of complications is low [9,15, 26]. Potential complications that may occur include bleeding, urinary retention, and infection. Long-term complications include stenosis and mucosal ectropion [9].

Summary

The majority of patients with anal complaints visiting a colon and rectal surgeon will ascribe all their problems to hemorrhoids. A thorough history and physical examination will often determine that these complaints are secondary to other common anorectal problems such as fissures, fistulae, condylomata or pruritus ani. For the majority of patients who do truly have symptomatic hemorrhoids, treatment can often be performed in the office with minimum morbidity and discomfort. A summary of current treatment options is provided in **Table 16.1**. In patients with family histories of colorectal cancer, change in bowel habits or other systemic symptoms, proximal evaluation of the GI tract to rule out neoplasia is mandatory. In the majority of individuals, reassurance, treatment of underlying constipation and change in defecatory habits will resolve hemorrhoidal symptoms.

Table 16.1 Treatment alternatives for hemorrhoids

	Internal (grade)				External
Treatment	1	2	3	4	
Diet modification	X				
Sclerotherapy	X	X			
Infrared coagulation	X	X	(X)		
Rubber band ligation	(X)	X	X		
Stapled hemorrhoidectomy (PPH)		X	X		
Excisional hemorrhoidectomy		(X)	X	X	X
(X) selected					

In other individuals, office treatment such as banding, sclerotherapy or photocoagulation may be necessary.

In the rare individuals not responding or not appropriate for office treatments surgical hemorrhoidectomy will be necessary. Traditional Ferguson or Milligan–Morgan hemorrhoidectomy is associated with significant postoperative discomfort but relieves symptoms with low recurrence in over 90% of individuals.

Rounds questions

1. When hemorrhoids bleed acutely, is the hemorrhage arterial, venous, or portal blood?
2. Are hemorrhoids associated with portal hypertension?
3. What is the difference between internal and external hemorrhoids?
4. Describe the grades of internal hemorrhoids.
5. After rubber band ligation of internal hemorrhoids, a patient develops anal pain, fever, and inability to urinate. What evaluation and treatment should be considered?
6. What additional serious complications are associated with a stapled rectopexy?

References

1. Beck DE. Hemorrhoids. In: Beck DE, Welling DR, (eds). Patient Care in Colorectal Surgery. Boston: Little, Brown 1991;213–24.
2. Milsom JW. Hemorrhoidal disease. In: Beck DE, Wexner SD, (eds). Fundamentals of Anorectal Surgery. New York: McGraw-Hill 1992;192–214.
3. Thompson WHE. The nature of hemorrhoids. Br J Surg 1975;62:542–52.
4. Thulesius O, Gjores JE. Arterio-venous anastomoses in the anal region with reference to the pathogenesis and treatment of haemorrhoids. Acta Chir Scand 1973;139:476–8.
5. Corman ML. Colon and Rectal Surgery, 2nd ed. Philadelphia: JB Lippincott, 1989;49–105.
6. Moesgaard F, Nielsen ML, Hansen JB, Knudsen JT. High fiber diet reduces bleeding and pain in patients with hemorrhoids: A double-blind trial of Vi-Siblin. Dis Colon Rectum 1982;25:454–6.
7. O'Hara VS. Fatal clostridial infection following hemorrhoidal banding. Dis Colon Rectum 1980;23:570–1.
8. Scarpa FJ, Hillis W, Sabetta JR. Pelvic cellulitis: a life-threatening complication of hemorrhoidal banding. Surgery 1988;103:383–5.
9. Larach SW, Cataldo PA, Beck DE. Nonoperative treatment of hemorrhoidal disease. In: Hicks TC, Beck DE, Opelka FG, Timmcke AE (eds). Complications of Colon & Rectal Surgery. Baltimore: Williams & Wilkins, 1996:173–80.
10. Neiger S. Hemorrhoids in everyday practice. Proctology 1979;2:22–8.
11. O'Connor JJ. Infrared coagulation of hemorrhoids. Pract Gastroenterol 1979;10:8–14.
12. Ferguson JA, Mazier WP, Ganchrow MI, Friend WG. The closed technique of hemorrhoidectomy. Surgery 1971;70:480–4.
13. Mazier WP, Halleran DR. Excisional hemorrhoidectomy. In: Kodner IJ, Fry RD, Roe JP (eds). Colon, Rectal, and Anal Surgery: Current Techniques and Contraversies. St. Louis: Mosby, 1985:3–14.
14. Buls JG, Goldberg SM. Modern management of hemorrhoids. Surg Clin North Am 1978;58:469–78.
15. Cataldo PA. Hemorrhoids. Clinics Colon Rect Surg 2001;14:203–14.
16. Whitehead W. The surgical treatment of hemorrhoids. Br Med J I 1882;148–50.
17. Pescatori M, Favetta U, Dedola S, Orsini S. Trans anal stapled excision of rectal mucosal prolapse. Tech Coloproct 1997;1:96–8.

18. Longo A. Treatment of haemorrhoidal disease by reduction of mucosa and haemorrhoidal prolapse with a circular stapling device: a new procedure—6th World Congress of Endoscopic Surgery. Mundozzi Editore 1998; 777–84.

19. Mehigan BJ, Monson JR, Hartley JE. Stapling procedure for haemorrhoids versus Milligan-Morgan haemorrhoidectomy: randomised controlled trial. Lancet 2000;355:782–5.

20. Rowsell M, Bello M, Hemingway DM. Circumferential mucosectomy (stapled haemorrhoidectomy) versus conventional haemorrhoidectomy: randomised controlled trial. Lancet 2000;355:779–81.

21. Ho YH, Cheong WK, Tsang C, et al. Stapled hemorrhoidectomy—cost and effectiveness. Randomized, controlled trial including incontinence scoring, anorectal manometry, and endoanal ultrasound assessments at up to three months. Dis Colon Rectum 2000;43:1666–75.

22. Sennagore AJ, Singer M, Abcarian H, et al. A prospective, randomized, controlled, multicenter trial comparing stapled hemorrhoidopexy and Ferguson hemorrhoidectomy: perioperative and one year result. Dis Colon Rectum 2004;47:824–36.

23. Morianga K, Hasuda K, Ikeda T. A novel therapy for internal hemorrhoids: ligation of the hemorrhoidal artery with a newly devised instrument (Moricorn) in conjunction with a Doppler flowmeter. Am J Gastroenterol 1995;90:610–3.

24. Singer M. Hemorrhoids. In: Beck DE, Wexner SD, Roberts PL, Sacclarides TJ, Senagore A, Stamos, M (eds). ASCRS Textbook of Colorectal Surgery. 2nd ed. New York, Springer-Verlag 2007; in: press.

25. Giordano P, Overton J, Madeddu F, Zaman S, Gravante G. Transanal hemorrhoidal dearterialization: A systemic review. Dis Colon rectum 2009;52:16665–71.

26. Smith LE. Current therapy on colon and rectal surgery. In: Fazio VW (ed). Current Therapy in Colon and Rectal Surgery. Philadelphia: BC Decker 1990;9–14.

Anorectal abscess and fistula-in-ano

Fistula-in-ano and anorectal abscesses share a common cause and differ only with respect to proportion. The abscess represents the acute phase, whereas the fistula represents the chronic phase.

Anorectal abscess

Anatomy

Successful treatment of fistula-in-ano and abscesses requires an in-depth understanding of anorectal anatomy. Essential is an understanding of the existence of potential anorectal spaces (**Figure 17.1**) [1]. The perianal space is in the area of the anal verge. It becomes continuous with the ischiorectal fat laterally while it extends into the lower portion of the anal canal medially. It is continuous with the intersphincteric space. The ischiorectal space extends from the levator ani to the perineum. Anteriorly, it is bounded by the transverse perineal muscles; the lower border of the gluteus maximus and the sacrotuberous ligament form its posterior border. The medial border is formed by the levator ani and external sphincter muscles; the obturator internus muscle forms the lateral border. The intersphincteric space lies between the internal and external sphincters and is continuous inferiorly with the perianal space and superiorly with the rectal wall. The supralevator space is bounded superiorly by peritoneum, laterally by the pelvic wall, medially by the rectal wall, and inferiorly by the levator ani muscle.

At the level of the dentate line, the ducts of the anal glands empty into the anal crypts. The glands enter the submucosa, two-thirds enter the internal sphincter, and half of these cross in the intersphincteric space [2]. They do not penetrate the external sphincter and number from four to ten in a normal individual.

Pathophysiology

Etiologic factors

Ninety percent of abscesses result from nonspecific cryptoglandular infection; the remainder result from specific causes (**Table 17.1**). The cryptoglandular theory as proposed by Parks [3] suggests that abscesses result from obstruction of the anal glands and ducts. Persistence of anal gland epithelium in part of the tract between the crypt and the blocked part of the duct leads to formation of a fistula.

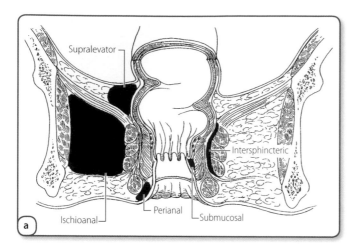

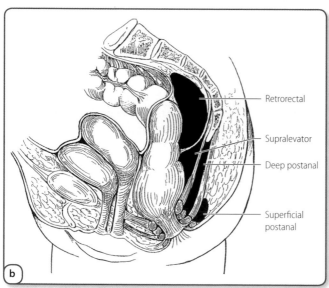

Figure 17.1 Anorectal spaces.
(a) Coronal section. (b) Sagittal section.

Table 17.1 Etiologic factors in anorectal abscesses
Nonspecific
Cryptoglandular origin
Specific
Inflammatory bowel disease
Infection (tuberculosis, actinomycosis, lymphogranuloma venereum)
Trauma (impalement, foreign body, surgery: episiotomy, hemorrhoidectomy, prostatectomy)
Malignancy (carcinoma, leukemia, lymphoma)
Radiation

Classification

Abscesses are classified by their location in the aforementioned potential anorectal spaces: perianal, ischiorectal, intersphincteric, and supralevator (**Figure 17.2**). Perianal abscesses are the commonest

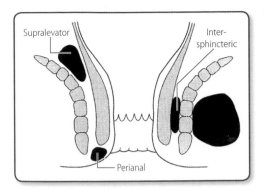

Figure 17.2 Classification of anorectal abscesses.

Supralevator

Inter-sphincteric

Perianal

type while supralevator abscesses are the rarest. Pus can also pass circumferentially through the intersphincteric, supralevator, and ischiorectal spaces, the latter via the deep postanal space, resulting in a horseshoe abscess.

Evaluation and Treatment

Symptoms

Pain, swelling, and fever are the hallmarks of an abscess. The patient with a supralevator abscess may complain of gluteal pain [4]. Rectal bleeding has been reported. Severe rectal pain accompanied by urinary symptoms such as dysuria, inability to void, and urinary retention may suggest an intersphincteric or supralevator abscess.

Assessment

Inspection will reveal erythema, swelling, and possible fluctulance with perianal or ischiorectal abscesses. It is crucial to recognize that with either intersphincteric or supralevator abscesses, no visible external manifestations are present despite the patient's complaint of excruciating pain [5]. With a supralevator abscess, a tender mass may be palpated on rectal or vaginal examination [4]. The presence of a black spot may be indicative of a widespread necrotizing infection [6].

Operative Therapy

Incision and drainage The primary treatment of acute anorectal suppuration is incision and drainage. Antibiotics are usually not necessary, except in patients with valvular or rheumatic heart disease, diabetes, immunosuppression, extensive cellulitis, or prosthetic devices. Fluctuance should not be allowed to develop under the guise of antibiotic treatment, because the inflammatory process will subsequently spread along tissue planes and result in possible damage to the anal sphincters. Rarely, delay in diagnosis and management of anorectal abscesses may result in life-threatening necrotizing infection and death [7].

Perianal abscesses can be drained with the patient under local anesthesia [4, 8], with the patient in the prone jackknife position. After determination of the tenderest point, the area around it may be infiltrated with 0.5% lidocaine with 1:200,000 epinephrine. A small elliptical or cruciate incision is made and the skin edges are excised to prevent coaptation, which may result in either poor drainage or recurrence (**Figure 17.3**). No packing is required.

Most ischiorectal abscesses can be incised and drained in a similar fashion. However, horseshoe abscesses should be drained with the patient under either regional or general anesthesia. An opening is made in the posterior midline and the lower half of the internal sphincter is divided to drain the postanal space, since this is believed to be the source of infection [4]. Counterincisions are made over each ischiorectal fossa to allow drainage of the anterior extensions of the abscess (**Figure 17.4**) [7].

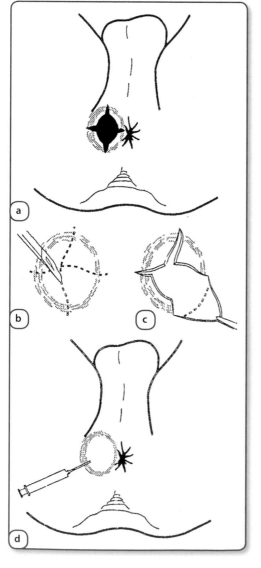

Figure 17.3 Drainage of abscess. (a) Injection of local anesthetic. (b) Cruciate incision. (c) Excision of skin. (d) Drainage cavity.

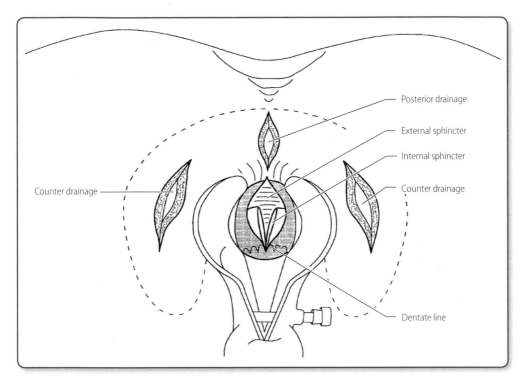

Figure 17.4 **Drainage of a horseshoe abscess.**

Since a diagnosis of an intersphincteric abscess is considered when the patient presents with pain out of proportion to the physical findings, an examination with the patient under anesthesia is mandatory to thoroughly assess the cause of pain. Once the diagnosis is made, the internal sphincter is divided along the length of the abscess cavity.

Before a supralevator abscess is drained its origin should be determined, because it may arise from an upward extension of an intersphincteric abscess, an ischiorectal abscess, or downward extension of a pelvic abscess [1,4]. If its origin is an intersphincteric abscess, it should be drained through the rectum and not through the ischiorectal fossa, since this will result in a suprasphincteric fistula. However, if it arises from an ischiorectal abscess, it should be drained as such and not through the rectum, since this will result in the creation of an extrasphincteric fistula (**Figure 17.5**). If the abscess is of pelvic origin, it can be drained through the rectum, ischiorectal fossa, or abdominal wall, depending on the direction to which it is pointing.

Following drainage, patients are advised to continue a regular diet, take a bulk-forming agent, a noncodeine analgesic, and sitz baths several times a day. They are seen in follow-up in 1 month, or in 2 weeks for intersphincteric and supralevator abscesses.

Catheter drainage An alternative method of treatment for selected patients is catheter drainage. Patients suitable for this technique should

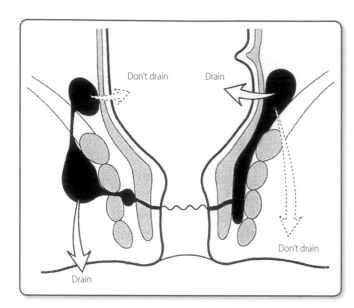

Figure 17.5 Drainage of a supralevator abscess.

not have severe sepsis or any serious systemic illness [9]. The patient is placed in either the prone jackknife or left lateral (Sims') position. The skin is prepared with a povidone-iodine solution and the fluctuant point of the abscess is determined. A local anesthetic of 0.5% lidocaine and 1:200,000 epinephrine is injected into the surrounding area, and a stab incision is made to drain the pus (**Figure 17.6a**). A 10–16 Fr soft latex mushroom catheter is inserted over a probe into the abscess cavity. When it is released, the shape of the catheter tip holds the catheter in place, thus obviating the need for sutures. The external portion of the catheter is shortened to leave 2–3 cm outside the skin when the tip is in the depth of the abscess cavity (**Figure 17.6b**). This reduces the chances of the catheter's falling out of or into the cavity. A small bandage is placed over the catheter. Antibiotics are unnecessary, and analgesics are prescribed.

The patient is instructed to keep the area clean and to return within 7–10 days. If at this visit the cavity has closed around the catheter and the drainage has ceased, the catheter may be removed. Sigmoidoscopy and anoscopy should be performed to exclude an associated fistula. Patients found to have fistulas should be scheduled for elective fistulotomy. If the abscess cavity has not healed, the catheter should be left in place or it should be replaced with a smaller catheter. The patient should be followed until healing has occurred.

Several portions of this technique deserve further comment. First, the stab incision should be placed as close as possible to the anus, minimizing the amount of tissue that must be opened if a fistula is found once the inflammation subsides (**Figure 17.6a**). Second, the size and length of the catheter should correspond to the size of the abscess cavity (**Figure 17.7a**). A catheter that is too small or too short

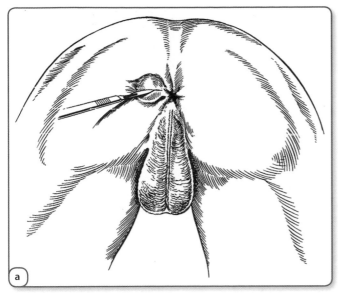

Figure 17.6 Catheter drainage of an abscess. (a) Stab incision. (b) Catheter in place.

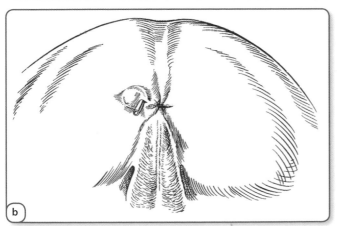

may fall into the wound (**Figure 17.7b**). If the patient waits too long for a follow-up visit, the skin may seal and a second incision will be required to retrieve the catheter, or the abscess may recur. Third, the length of time that the catheter should be left in place requires clinical judgment; factors involved in the decision include the size of the original abscess cavity, the amount of granulation tissue around the catheter, and the character and amount of drainage. If there is doubt, it is better to leave the catheter in place for an additional period of time. Alternatively, a contrast study through the catheter may be obtained. The catheter should remain in place until the cavity has closed down around the catheter. Finally, follow-up care is very important. An adequate physical examination, including sigmoidoscopy, is essential once the inflammation has resolved to rule out an associated fistula or other disease process.

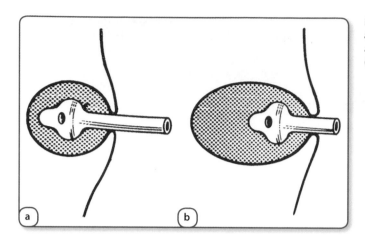

Figure 17.7 Catheter in an abscess cavity. (a) Correct size and length of catheter. (b) Catheter cut too short.

Primary fistulotomy and abscess drainage The incidence of a missed fistula during abscess drainage ranges from 18–95% [10–18]. Abscess drainage alone will suffice in 34–60% of patients [8,12,13]. Of those abscesses that are drained, 11% of patients may develop a fistula-in-ano, and 37% may develop a recurrent abscess [8]. This situation is more commonly seen with ischiorectal abscesses. The incidence of recurrent abscess or fistula following incision and drainage may be decreased substantially to 1.8% following primary fistulotomy [16].

Fistula-in-ano

Pathophysiology

An anorectal fistula is defined as a tract or cavity communicating with the rectum or anal canal by an identifiable internal opening. Our current understanding suggests that fistulas result from partial healing of an abscess.

Classification

The most helpful yet complicated classification of fistula-in-ano is that described by Parks et al (**Table 17.2**) [19].

Intersphincteric fistula-in-ano This fistula results from a perianal abscess. The tract passes within the intersphincteric plane (**Figure 17.8a**). This is the most common type and accounts for approximately 70% of fistula [19].

Trans-sphincteric fistula-in-ano This results from ano ischiorectal abscess and constitutes approximately 23% of fistulas seen [19]. The tract passes from the internal opening through the internal and external sphincters to the ischiorectal fossa (**Figure 17.8b**). A rectovaginal fistula is a form of trans-sphincteric fistula.

Suprasphincteric fistula-in-ano This fistula is the result of a supralevator abscess and accounts for approximately 5% in some series [19]. The tract passes above the puborectalis after arising as an inter-

Table 17.2 Classification of fistula-in-ano

Intersphincteric	Suprasphincteric
Simple low tract	Uncomplicated
High blind tract	High blind tract
High blind tract with rectal opening	
Rectal opening without perineal opening	
Extrarectal extension	
Secondary to pelvic disease	
Trans-sphincteric	**Extrasphincteric**
Uncomplicated	Secondary to:
High blind tract	Anal fistula
	Trauma
	Anorectal disease
	Pelvic inflammation

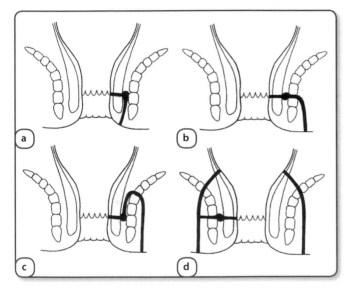

Figure 17.8 Classification of fistula-in-ano. (a) Intersphincteric fistula. (b) Trans-sphincteric fistula. (c) Suprasphincteric fistula. (d) Extrasphincteric fistula.

sphincteric abscess. The tract curves downward lateral to the external sphincter in the ischiorectal space to the perianal skin (**Figure 17.8c**).

Extrasphincteric fistula-in-ano This constitutes the rarest type and accounts for approximately 2% of fistulas as [19]. It passes from the rectum above the levators, through them to the perianal skin via the ischiorectal space (**Figure 17.8d**). This fistula may result from foreign body penetration of the rectum, with drainage through the levators; from penetrating injury of the perineum; or from Crohn's disease or carcinoma or its treatment. However, the most common cause is iatrogenic, resulting from vigorous probing during fistula surgery [7].

Evaluation and treatment

Symptoms

A patient with a fistula-in-ano will often give a history of an abscess that was drained either surgically or spontaneously. Drainage of bloody or purulent secretions, bleeding, pain with defecation, and a decrease in pain with drainage are common complaints.

Assessment

An external or secondary opening may be seen discharging pus. This may be expressed on digital rectal examination. The internal or primary opening in most cases is not apparent. However, the number of external openings and their location may be helpful in locating the primary opening. According to Goodsall's rule (**Figure 17.9**), an opening seen posterior to a line drawn transversely across the perineum will originate from an internal opening in the posterior midline. An anterior external opening will originate in the nearest crypt. Generally, the greater the distance from the anal margin, the greater the probability of a complicated upward extension.

Digital rectal examination may reveal a cordlike structure. It is necessary to determine sphincter tone because of the possible risk of incontinence following repair of the fistula. Anoscopy and sigmoidoscopy should always be done to identify the primary opening and to determine whether there is underlying proctitis. A barium enema or colonoscopy and an upper GI series with small bowel follow-through are indicated in patients who have symptoms of inflammatory bowel disease and in patients with multiple or recurrent fistulas. Although anal manometry is not generally required, it may be used as an adjunct

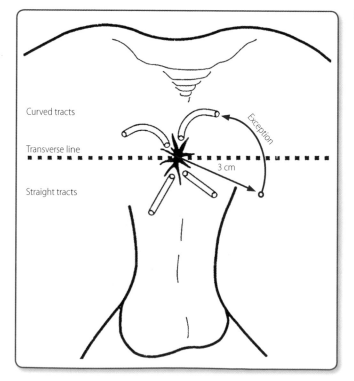

Figure 17.9 Goodsall's rule.

Curved tracts

Transverse line

Straight tracts

Exception

3 cm

to planning the operative approach in an elderly patient, a patient with Crohn's disease or AIDS, or in a patient with a recurrent fistula.

Fistulography involves injecting contrast material through a small catheter placed into the secondary fistula opening. Anterior-posterior and lateral radiographs are obtained. Contrast in the fistula tract may serve as a road map. Practically, however, due to the lack of radiologic identified landmarks and the differences in the patient's body position during the fistulogram and operative exploration, fistolography is often unreliable and may provide false positive results [20]. Its use is thought to be confined to the management of recurrent fistulas or in Crohn's disease, where previous surgery or disease may have altered anorectal anatomy [21].

Anal endosonography is a safe, accurate modality used to evaluate defects in the external sphincter and is the only method available to assess the internal sphincter [22, 23]. As described in Chapter 4, an anal probe may help to identify complex fistulas [24]. Hygrogen peroxide injected into the fistula tract serves as strong sonographic contrast and assists in identifying the fistula.

In the last decade, increasing attention has been given to magnetic resonance imaging (MRI) in the preoperative assessment of fistulas. This study has the ability to not only identify the tract but also to establish its relationship to the anal sphincter mechanism. In a comparative study of ultrasound and MRI, the endoluminal MRI was more accurate 61 vs 89% in classifying anorectal fistulas preoperatively [25]. No comparative studies have been done with hydrogen peroxide endosonography. Most studies have found good concordance rates between MRI and surgical findings both for the presence and course of the primary tract as well as the presence and site of secondary extensions or abscesses [26]. MRI can identify tracts in areas not explored at surgery. A recent study reported that tracts detected at MRI and not identified at surgery proved to be present at follow-up surgery. MRI was a better predictor of outcome than surgery with the positive predictive values and negative predictive values of 73 vs 57% and 87 vs 64%, respectively [25].

Decisions about what to do for the recurrent fistula ultimately depend on the findings of the above deliberations. If there is no suspicion for inflammatory bowel disease or other unusual cause for recurrence, the patient may simply require further surgery at which time the course of the tract must be delineated from primary to secondary opening, laying open all side or proximal tracts.

Operative treatment

The goals of treatment are to eliminate the fistula, prevent recurrence, and preserve sphincter function. Success is usually determined by identifying the primary opening and dividing the least amount of muscle possible.

Several methods have been proposed to identify the primary opening in the operating room [1, 4, 27, 28].

1. Passage of a probe or probes from the external to the internal opening or vice-versa
2. Injection of a dye, such as a dilute solution of methylene blue, milk, or hydrogen peroxide
3. Following the granulation tissue present in the fistula tract
4. Noting puckering of an anal crypt when traction is placed on the tract

Lay-open technique Although fistulectomy (excising the fistula tract) was once thought to be a satisfactory method of treating anal fistulas, fistulotomy or the lay-open technique is thought to be superior, since a much smaller wound is created, thus minimizing injury of the sphincter muscle [27].

For the treatment of a simple intersphincteric or trans-sphincteric fistula, the patient is placed in the prone jackknife position following induction of a regional anesthetic. Alternatively, a local anesthetic of 0.5% lidocaine or 0.25% bupivacaine with 1:200,000 epinephrine is injected along the fistula tract following placement of an anal speculum. A probe is inserted from the external opening to the internal opening at the dentate line. The tissue overlying the probe is incised and the granulation tissue extracted with a curette and sent to the pathology laboratory for analysis. A gentle probe is used to identify any high blind tracts or extensions, which are unroofed if found. The wound can subsequently be marsupialized on either edge by sewing the edges of the incision to the tract with a running locked absorbable suture (**Figure 17.10**).

If the tract is seen to cross the sphincter muscle at a high level, the use of the lay-open technique accompanied by insertion of a seton is safer: the lower portion of the internal sphincter is divided along with the skin to reach the external opening, and a nonabsorbable suture or elastic suture (the seton) is inserted into the fistulous tract. The ends of the suture or elastic are tied with multiple knots to create a handle for manipulation (**Figure 17.11**). The seton may act to stimulate fibrosis

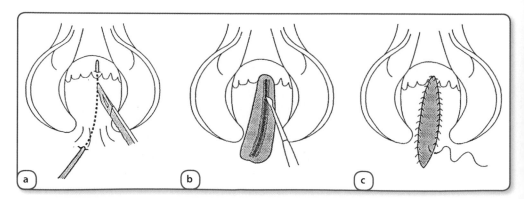

Figure 17.10 Lay-open technique. (a) Insertion of probe and incision of tissue overlying probe. (b) Curettage of granulation tissue. (c) Marsupialization of wound edges (optional).

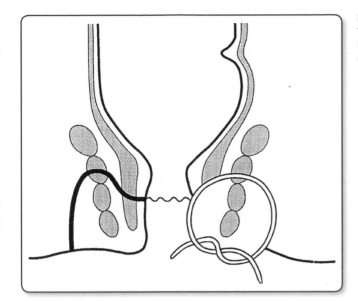

Figure 17.11 Insertion of a seton.
The anoderm and skin overlying the looped muscle have been incised (right side of drawing).

adjacent to the sphincter muscle to prevent gaping of the sphincter at a secondary stage repair. It allows delineation of the amount of remaining muscle and acts as a drain. Its use should be considered in high-level fistulas, in anterior fistulas in women, in patients with inflammatory bowel disease, in elderly patients with weakened sphincter muscles, and in patients with recurrent or complicated simultaneous fistulas. Although some surgeons sequentially tighten the seton (cutting seton), I avoid using this technique because of the resultant patient discomfort.

A horseshoe fistula results from circumferential spread of infection, resulting in multiple external openings. The key to treatment lies with the identification of the primary opening at the posterior midline and division of the lower part of the internal sphincter. The external openings are enlarged and the granulation tissue is removed with a curette or coarse gauze pulled through the tract.

Treatment for an extrasphincteric fistula depends on its cause. If the fistula arises as a result of an anal fistula, a secondary opening above the puborectalis is thought to be iatrogenic from extensive probing of a trans-sphincteric fistula. The lower portion of the sphincter is divided and the rectal opening is closed with a nonabsorbable suture. Although a temporary colostomy may be necessary, a medical colostomy consisting of preoperative mechanical and antibiotic bowel preparation followed by enteral feeding may suffice. If the fistula is the result of entrance of a foreign body, it must be removed, drainage must be established, the internal opening is closed, and a temporary colostomy performed to decrease rectal pressure. The fistula may be a manifestation of Crohn's disease. Treatment will depend on the nature of the anorectal mucosa and may be assisted by seton drainage. Finally, the fistula may be the result of downward tracking of a pelvic abscess that must be drained for the fistula to heal.

Although healing is a concern with Crohn's disease, simple fistulas can be treated with fistulotomy. The best results are seen in those patients with classic internal openings and in the absence of rectal involvement [29].

Following the lay-open technique or seton insertion, a regular diet is encouraged and bulk-forming agents and a non-codeine-containing analgesic are prescribed. Patients are instructed on perianal hygiene and the frequent use of sitz baths. They are evaluated every 2–3 weeks to ensure that healing has occurred from the depths of the wound. Excess granulation tissue is removed with silver nitrate sticks.

Continence disorders have been reported following use of the lay-open technique in up to 52% of patients [30]. Determining the patient's preoperative degree of fecal control is very important, since if it is marginal, the patient may be at greater risk. Although a seton is used primarily to preserve continence, minor control problems have been reported in 58%, whereas major fecal incontinence has been reported in 6.7% [10,31].

Recurrence after fistulotomy may result from failure to identify a primary opening or recognize lateral or upward extensions of a fistula [31–33]. Premature closure of the fistulotomy wound may result in fistula recurrence that can be obviated by diligent postoperative care to avoid the development of pocketing in the wound [32]. Epithelialization of the fistula tract may also be a factor [34]. Extra-anal pathologic conditions such as hidradenitis suppurativa, downward extension of a pilonidal abscess, or Crohn's disease should be considered when the previously mentioned reasons for recurrence have been ruled out [1,7,14].

Mucosal advancement flap The use of a rectal mucosal advancement flap has been proposed for rectovaginal fistulas, for patients with high trans-sphincteric or suprasphincteric fistulas, or for patients with inflammatory bowel disease with complicated fistula (**Figure 17.12**) [27,35]. A full mechanical and antibiotic bowel preparation is performed and the patient is placed in the prone jackknife position. The fistula tract is identified with a probe; the internal opening is identified, excised, and closed with an absorbable suture. The tract is either curetted or excised and an advancement flap consisting of rectal mucosa, submucosa, and part of the internal sphincter is dissected and advanced beyond the original internal opening and sutured to the anal canal distal to the opening. It is important to ensure that the base of the flap is twice the width of the apex to ensure good blood supply and prevent ischemic necrosis of the flap. Several advantages of this technique are that no muscle is divided, there is no resulting deformity of the anal canal, there is less discomfort, and there may be a reduction in healing time [35]. This repair is effective for a rectovaginal fistula, since it allows the interposition of healthy tissue to the high-pressure zone of the rectum [36].

Postoperatively, patients are maintained on intravenous therapy or clear liquids for 1–5 days to ensure adequate healing of the flap. Once

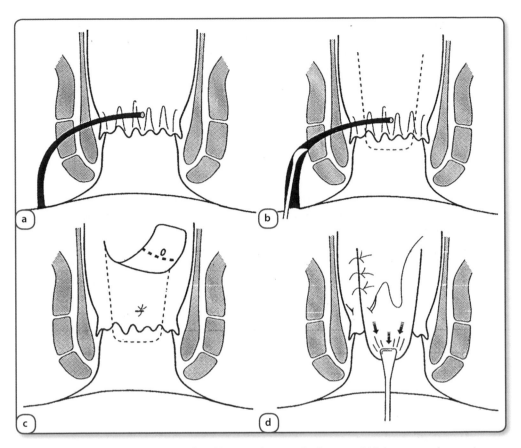

Figure 17.12 Anorectal advancement flap. (a) Trans-sphincteric fistula-in-ano. (b) Enlargement of external opening, curettage of tract, and outline of rectal flap. (c) Suture of internal opening, reflected anorectal flap. (d) Advancement of flap beyond internal opening and suturing to the anal canal.

this time has elapsed, the patient is progressed to regular diets and routine management is followed.

The use of fibrin sealant as a treatment for fistula has been described as a unique method to manage fistulas that is not surgically invasive and avoids the risk of fecal incontinence associated with fistulotomy. The initial preparations employed autologous tissues to prepare the fibrin sealant, but these products are now commercially available [37]. The technique for the instillation of fibrin sealant is simple. The fistula tract along with its internal and external openings is identified and thoroughly curetted. The fibrin and thrombin are then injected into the fistula tract through a Y-shaped connector so that the entire tract is filled and the fibrin sealant can be seen coming out of the internal opening. The injecting catheter is then slowly withdrawn so that the entire fistula tract is filled. Petroleum jelly gauze is applied over the secondary opening. The appeal of this technique is its simplicity and the minimal manipulation of the sphincter mechanism. Initial reports indicate a success rate approaching 70%, but longer follow-up and further research have been recommended since recurrences up to 1 year postoperatively have been reported [37–39]. It has not been found to be effective in fistulas with short tracts [37].

Anal fistula plug Recently, the use of a bioprosthetic plug made from lyophilized porcine intestinal submucosal has been described for the treatment of anal fistulas [40]. The Surgisis anal fistula plug (AFP), after implanted is colonized by host tissue cells and blood vessels and thus provides a scaffold to allow infiltration of the patient's connective tissue [40]. A consensus conference [41] defined the indications for the use of the plug in fistulous disease to include: 1) trans-sphincteric fistua 2) interspincteric fistula, if conventional fistulotomy posed a risk of incontinence such as in patients with inflammatory bowel disease, and 3) extrasphincteric fistula. Contraindications for the use of the plug included: 1) fistula with persistent abscess cavity 2) fistula with infection 3) allergy to porcine products, and 4) inability to identify both the external and internal openings. The latter constitutes an absolute contraindication for use of the plug. Following full mechanical bowel preparation or the use of a small volume enema along with a single preoperative dose of antibiotics, the patient is placed in the prone jackknife position. The internal and external openings must be clearly delineated. This can be accomplished by irrigation with saline or peroxide. Gentle passage of a probe is essential to confirm the position of the tract and facilitate insertion of the plug. Debridement or curettage of the tract is avoided. A seton should be used temporarily if there is acute inflammation or drainage. The anal plug should be immersed in sterile saline for 2 minutes for rehydration. An anal fistula probe is placed through the tract and a 2-0 suture is placed through the tapered end of the plug and the ends of this suture are attached to the fistula probe at the primary opening. The suture is pulled from the primary opening, through the fistula tract to exit at the secondary opening. For patients with a 'horseshoe' fistula, an incision is made over the fistula tract distal to the anal verge to create a secondary opening that the ends of the suture are brought through. With gentle traction on the suture, the porcine plug is pulled into the primary opening of the fistula until 'wrinkling' of the superficial layer of the plug is first seen. The plug is not forced tightly. Excess plug is removed by transecting the plug at the level of the primary opening. The plug is secured in the primary opening using a 2-0 absorbable suture placed in a figure of eight fashion with the suture crossing through the center of the plug and incorporating a generous portion of the sphincter mechanism on both sides. Any plug protruding through the secondary opening is also excised. The distal end of the plug is not sutured to the fistula tract and the distal opening is left open for drainage. Patients are advised to avoid vigorous physical activity for two weeks after plug placement to minimize the chance of plug dislodgement. No dietary restrictions are necessary nor are topical antibiotics indicated.

The first prospective study comparing the plug to fibrin glue in 25 patients with high trans-sphincteric or deeper fistulas found greater success rates with the plug (87% vs 40%) at 3 months [40]. The authors concluded that closure of the primary opening of a fistula tract using a suturable biologic anal fistula plug is an effective method of treating anorectal fistulas. Although the technique has appeal for its simplicity and avoidance of sphincter injury, more recent reports, however, have tempered enthusiasm with success rates ranging from 13.9–71%. Dislodgement occurred in 4–29% while sepsis requiring abscess drainage has been reported in 4–29% of patients [42].

Ligation of intersphincteric fistula tract Recently another sphincter-sparing technique has been introduced called the LIFT procedure (ligation of the intersphincteric fistula tract) [43]. This technique is based on the secure closure of the internal opening and removal of the infected cryptoglandular tissue in the intersphincteric space. The only patients not suitable are those with early fistulous abscess in which the intersphincteric tract is not well formed. Patients undergo mechanical bowel preparation or enemas and are placed in the prone jackknife position or left lateral position. A Fansler anoscope is inserted into the anal canal and the internal opening is identified. A fistula probe is inserted into the tract which assists tract identification during the procedure. A 1.5–2.0 cm curvilinear incision is made at the intersphincteric groove overlying the fistula tract. Cautery is used to dissect into the intersphincteric plane staying close to the external sphincter avoiding cutting through the internal sphincter and breaching anal mucosa. The internal and external sphincters are retracted. The intersphincteric tract is dissected and ligated next to the internal opening with a 3-0 absorbable suture. The tract next to the suture is also ligated. Tract excision is confirmed by injection or probing of the external opening. Granulation tissue may be curetted. The external opening is sutured through the intersphincteric wound and the incision is closed with 3-0 absorbable suture. Postoperatively wounds are cleansed with tap water twice a day and following bowel movements. Some patients are given 2 weeks of ciprofloxacillin and metronidazole.

A limitation of this technique is the intersphincteric approach for high tracts especially with horseshoe tracts. Also exposure of the intersphincteric space may damage the internal sphincter. Although there are only a few reports in the literature, success rates of 58–94% have been reported [43, 44]. Time to failure has ranged from 4–64 weeks with a median of 19 weeks [43, 44].

Rounds questions

1. What is thought to be the cause of anorectal infections?
2. What is the cryptoglandular theory?
3. How are anorectal abscesses classified?
4. How does an intersphincteric abscess present?
5. How are anorectal abscesses treated?

6. How are fistulas classified?
7. What is Goodsall's rule?
8. What is the most important technical aspect of fistulotomy to diminish the chances of recurrence?
9. What is a seton and when is its use indicated?
10. What is the ideal method of repair of a rectovaginal fistula?

References

1. Gordon PH. Anorectal abscesses and fistula-in-ano. In: Gordon PH, Nivatvongs S. Principles and Practice of Surgery for the Colon, Rectum, and Anus. St. Louis: Quality Medical Publishing, 1992;221–65.
2. Morson BC, Dawson IMP, Spriggs AI. Gastrointestinal Pathology. London: Blackwell Scientific Publications, 1979;715–8.
3. Parks AG. Pathogenesis and treatment of fistula-in-ano. Br Med J 1961;1:463–9.
4. Goldberg SM, Gordon PH, Nivatvongs S. Essentials of Anorectal Surgery. Philadelphia: JB Lippincott, 1980;100–27.
5. Parks AG, Thomson JPS. Intersphincteric abscess. Br Med J 1973;2537–9.
6. Bubrick MP, Hitchcock CR. Necrotizing anorectal and perineal infections. Surgery 1979;86:655–62.
7. Abcarian H. Surgical management of recurrent anorectal abscess. Contemp Surg 1982;21:85–91.
8. Vasilevsky CA, Gordon PH. The incidence of recurrent abscess or fistula-in-ano following anorectal suppuration. Dis Colon Rectum 1984;27:126–30.
9. Beck DE, Fazio VW, Lavery IC, Jagelman DG, Weakley FL. Catheter drainage of ischiorectal abscesses. South Med J 1988;81:444–6.
10. Pearl RK, Andrews JR, Orsay CP, et al. Role of the seton in management of anorectal fistulas. Dis Colon Rectum 1993;36:573–9.
11. Fucini C. One stage treatment of anal abscesses and fistulas: A clinical appraisal on the basis of two different classifications. Int J Colorectal Dis 1991;6:12–16.
12. Schouten WR, van Vroonhoven TJM. Treatment of anorectal abscess with or without primary fistulectomy: Results of a prospective randomized trial. Dis Colon Rectum 1991;34:60–3.
13. Scoma JA, Salvati EP, Rubin RJ. Incidence of fistulas subsequent to anal abscesses. Dis Colon Rectum 1974;17:357–9.
14. Chrabot CM, Prasad ML, Abcarian H. Recurrent anorectal abscesses. Dis Colon Rectum 1983;26:105–8.
15. McElwain JW, Maclean MD, Alexander RM, Hoexter B, Guthrie JF. Anorectal problems: Experience with primary fistuletomy for anorectal abscess, a report of 1000 cases. Dis Colon Rectum 1975;18:646–9.
16. Ramanujam PS, Prasad ML, Abcarian H, Tan AB. Perianal abscesses and fistulas. A study of 11023 patients. Dis Colon Rectum 1984;27:593–7.
17. Lockhart-Mummery HE. Anorectal problems. Treatment of abscesses. Dis Colon Rectum 1975;18:650–1.
18. Read DR, Abcarian H. A prospective survey of 474 patients with anorectal abscess. Dis Colon Rectum 1979;22:566–8.
19. Parks AG, Gordon PH, Hardcastle JD. A classification of fistula-in-ano. Br J Surg 1976;63:1–12.
20. Kuijpers HC, Schulpen T. Fistulography for fistula-in-ano: Is it useful? Dis Colon Rectum 1985;28:103–4.
21. Weisman RI, Orsay CP, Pearl RK, Abcarian H. The role of fistulography in fistula-in-ano: Report of five cases. Dis Colon Rectum 1991;34:181–4.
22. Law PJ, Kamm MA, Bartram CI. A comparison between electromyelography and anal endosonography in mapping external anal sphincter defects. Dis Colon Rectum 1990;33:370–3.
23. Law PJ, Kamm MA, Bartram CI. Anal endosonography in the investigation of faecal incontinence. Br J Surg 1991;78:312–4.
24. Law PJ, Talbot RW, Bartram CI, Northover JMA. Anal endosonography in the evaluation of perianal sepsis and fistula in ano. Br J Surg 1989;76:752–5.
25. Hussain SM, Stoker J, Schouten WR, et al. Fistula in ano: endoanal sonography versus endoanal MR imaging in classification. Radiology 1996;200:475–81.
26. Luchtefeld MA. Anorectal abscess and fistula-in-ano. Clin Colon Rectum Surg 2001;14:221–31.

27. Fazio VW. Complex anal fistulae. Gastroenterol Clin North Am 1987;16:93–114.

28. McLeod RS. Management of fistula-in-ano: 1990 Roussel Lecture. Can J Surg 1991;34:581–5.

29. Levien DH, Surrell J, Mazier WP. Surgical treatment of anorectal fistula in patients with Crohn's disease. Surg Gynecol Obstet 1989;169:133–6.

30. Van Tets WF, Kuijpers HC. Continence disorders after anal fistulotomy. Dis Colon Rectum 1994;37:1194–7.

31. MacLeod CAH, Balcos EG, Buls JG, Goldberg SM. Seton management of anorectal fistulas: A study of incontinence. Dis Colon Rectum 1990;33:P10.

32. Vasilevsky CA, Gordon PH. Results of treatment of fistula-in-ano. Dis Colon Rectum 1985;28:225–31.

33. Rosen L. Anorectal abscess-fistulae. Surg Clin North Am 1994;74:1293–308.

34. Lunniss PJ, Sheffield JP, Talbot IC, Thomson JPS, Phillips RKS. Persistence of idiopathic anal fistula may be related to epithelialization. Br J Surg 1995;82:32–3.

35. Lewis P, Bartolo DCC. Treatment of trans-sphincteric fistulae by full thickness anorectal advancement flap. Br J Surg 1990;77:1187–9.

36. Greenwald JC, Hoexter B. Repair of rectovaginal fistulas. Surg Gynecol Obstet 1978;146:443–5.

37. Park JJ, Cintron JR, Orsay CP, Pearl RK, et al. Repair of chronic anorectal fistulae using commercial fibrin sealant. Arch Surg 2000;135:166–9.

38. Gordon PH, Wiens TE, Orsay CP et al. What's new in the treatment of complicated fistula-in-ano. In: Schrock TR, ed. Perspectives in Colon and Rectal Surgery. New York, NY: Thieme Medical Publishers, Inc 1999;1:47–61.

39. Beck DE. Management of anorectal Crohn's fistulas. Clinics in Colon Rectal Surg 2001;14:117–28.

40. Johnson EK, Gaw JU, Armstrong DN. Efficacy of anal fistula plug vs fibrin glue in closure of anorectal fistulas. Dis Colon Rectum 2006;49:371–6.

41. The surgisis AFP anal fistula plug:report of a consensus conference. Colorectal Dis 2007;10;17–20.

42. Garg P, Song J, Stat AB et al. The efficacy of anal fistula plug in fistula-in-ano: A systematic review. Colorectal Dis: 2010; 12:965–70.

43. Rojanasakul A. LIFT procedure: a simplified technique for fistula-in-ano. Tech Coloproctol 2009;131:237–40.

44. Moloo H, Goldberg SM. Novel correction of intersphincteric perianal fistulas preserves anal sphincter. Presented at the American College of Surgeons, October 2008, San Francisco.

Pruritus ani

Anatomy

The anal and perianal skin, which is extremely sensitive, is richly supplied with sensory nerve endings in a pattern similar to that of the lips, fingers, and genitalia. The cutaneous sensation experienced in the perianal region and lining of the anal canal below the dentate line is conducted through afferent fibers contained in the inferior rectal nerves, branches of the pudendal nerves bilaterally. The pudendal nerves arise from dorsal sacral nerve roots of S2–4. As the pudendal nerves leave the pelvis bilaterally, they cross the ischial spine and continue in the ischioanal fossa through Alcock's canal. Other important branches include the perineal nerves to the urinary sphincter and the dorsal nerves to the penis or clitoris.

Pathophysiology

Etiologic factors

Factors predisposing the anal area to irritation are poor perianal hygiene, moisture, skin hypersensitivity, decreased resistance to infection, and injury to the perianal skin. Poor perianal hygiene can be the result of minor degrees of incontinence such as fecal seepage and soiling or excessively irregular or hairy perianal skin. Irregularities of the skin occur secondary to anal skin tags, condylomata accuminata, or previous surgery. Hairy perianal skin is one explanation for the fact that men develop pruritus four times as often as women [1]. Moisture from either sweat or perianal discharge can produce pruritus, especially when accompanied by poor ventilation because of obesity or tight-fitting, nonabsorbent garments. Perianal discharge can be associated with anal fistulas, fissures, perianal hidradenitis suppurativa, condyloma accuminata, or ulceration of the perianal skin caused by trauma such as that from excessive scratching or wiping [2]. Skin hypersensitivity is seen in the atopic individual or can occur as a result of ingested foods (e.g. tomatoes, pepper, coffee, chocolate, colas, beer, alcoholic beverages, citrus fruits and juices, nuts, and popcorn) [3] or medications (e.g. colchicine, quinidine), use of '-caine' type local anesthetic creams (eg. dibucaine, xylocaine, benzocaine), types of soaps, toilet tissues, lotions, or deodorants. Decreased resistance to infection can be the result of systemic disease (e.g. diabetes, leukemia, AIDS) or the use of broad-spectrum systemic antibiotics and systemic or topical application of antibiotic creams or lotions, or chemicals contained in various steroids. Perianal skin injury can result from excessive wiping, scrubbing, or scratching. Excessive wiping may occur when stools are soft and pasty or loose and watery. Also, stool frequency, as in diarrheal states, can increase the need for wiping. Often multiple potentially predisposing factors exist simultaneously. These multiple possible etiologic factors are what can make pruritus ani refractory to treatment. Some patients improve only after the offending agent or agents are identified and specific therapy is instituted. Fortunately, many patients' symptoms improve by the application of nonspecific treatments [1–4].

Classification

A useful classification is that employed by Dailey [5], which assigns symptoms to one of four categories: leakage, sensitivities, dermatoses, and infections. Frequently no causative factors can be identified and the pruritus is termed idiopathic.

Symptoms

Pruritus ani consists of intense perianal itching or burning that may be chronic or intermittent. Frequently symptoms are most vexatious at night, causing the patient to be awakened or sleepless. The perianal skin becomes erythematous or thickened. The thickening results in a pale whitish appearance with accentuation of the radial anal skin creases (**Figure 18.1**). In addition the skin may be excoriated or ulcerated, which when combined with thickening is referred to as lichenification. Occasionally, the skin may be so excoriated as to present as a large, coalescing, weeping ulcer.

Evaluation

A thorough history and physical examination are necessary to suggest possible causes of pruritus. Pruritus associated with chronic diarrhea should be investigated for the possible association of intestinal parasites (e.g. amebiasis, giardiasis, pinworms) or inflammatory

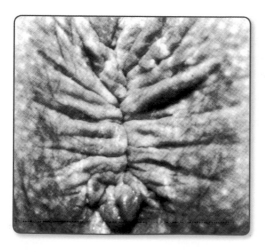

Figure 18.1 Idiopathic pruritis ani.

bowel disease. Systemic diseases such as diabetes mellitus, leukemia, and hyperbilirubinemia associated with biliary obstruction can be associated with pruritus. Dermatologic conditions that mimic pruritus such as psoriasis, intertrigo, and nonspecific neurodermatitis usually are not confined to the perianal area (**Figure 18.2**). Allergies to foods, drinks, and topical agents may result in periodicity of symptoms, suggesting the offending agent. Anorectal disorders such as fissure, fistula, and hemorrhoids may be associated with pruritus secondary to perianal discharge or difficult perianal hygiene. Prior anorectal surgery may result in anatomic deformity or minor degrees of incontinence that adversely affect perianal hygiene, resulting in pruritus.

Examination of the anorectum should be performed with the patient in the prone jackknife or left lateral position. Initial inspection of the perianal skin should be conducted with bright lighting and gentle retraction of the buttocks. No enemas or perianal cleansing should be performed before initial inspection to allow assessment of the usual condition of the perianal skin. The presence of stool, mucus, pus, or emollient cream should be noted. Examination of the patient's undergarments might suggest problems with perianal discharge or seepage and soiling of stool [6]. Digital rectal examination should be performed to assess anal sphincter competence both at rest and during maximal squeeze. Anoscopy and proctosigmoidoscopy can be performed following the administration of an enema; this will occasionally disclose proctitis or rectal lesions requiring additional investigations such as biopsies, cultures, inspection of stool for ova or parasites, and occasionally, colonoscopy. Physiologic studies may occasionally be useful [7–9]. Anal manometric studies have shown that patients with pruritus ani experience a greater fall in anal pressure

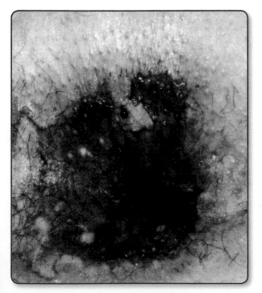

Figure 18.2 **Pruritis ani secondary to herpes simplex.**

when smaller volumes are instilled in the rectum [7,8], and patients with fecal seepage and soiling experience sphincter relaxation at low volumes of rectal inflation but require much higher volumes before the sensation of rectal filling is apparent [9]. Saline solution infusion testing showed pruritus patients leak at smaller volumes than asymptomatic patients [8].

Treatment

The principles of treating pruritus ani are simple. If an inciting cause can be identified, it should be eliminated or corrected. As stated earlier, frequently the cause of pruritus is elusive. Despite the inability to precisely identify the exact etiologic factors in pruritus ani, most patients can be managed using several simple principles.

Patients should **keep the perianal area dry.** This can be accomplished by placing a ball of cotton of fluffed cotton gauze at the anal orifice or dusting the perianal area lightly with a powder. I prefer an antifungal product such as miconazole nitrate 2%. Corn starch can be used, but it may promote the growth of *Candida*. Proprietary perfumed or deodorant powders should be avoided.

In addition, patients should avoid further trauma to the perianal area. Soap should be avoided. The area can be cleansed using a cleansing lotion specifically formulated for the perianal area (e.g. Balneol). The perianal area should be gently washed, never scrubbed. After showering the area should be patted dry or dried using a hair dryer on a low heat setting. Following bowel movements the anus should be cleaned using moistened toilet paper, medicated wipes (e.g. tucks or baby wipes). Wipes containing alcohol should be avoided. Excessive rubbing or wiping should be discouraged. Scratching or rubbing the anal area damages the perianal skin making it more susceptible to irritation.

Patients should be instructed to **avoid irritating foods and drinks** (described on p. 337) or any other foodstuffs found to be associated with increased gas, indigestion, or diarrhea. After 2 weeks, eliminated food items can be reintroduced one at a time in an attempt to identify the offending agent more specifically.

A **regular bowel habit should be maintained** using a fiber supplement (psyllium or methylcellulose preparation [Metamucil, Konsyl, Citrucel] and a healthy high-fiber diet. Regular bowel movements result in less trauma to the anal canal as can occur with either diarrhea or constipation. Bran and fiber supplements produce a well-formed stool that requires less wiping and potentially less soiling and trauma to the perianal skin. As they enlarge the stool, they may also dilute any irritating substances in the stool.

Patients should be instructed to **avoid all proprietary creams, lotions, or emollients**. If prescribed and supervised by a physician, a hydrocortisone cream may be applied sparingly to the affected area for a period of a week or less to initiate control of symptoms. It should be kept in mind that long-term application of steroid creams can result in thinning of the perianal skin, making it more susceptible to trauma and irritation. In particular, the fluorinated corticosteroid-containing creams and those containing '-caine' type local anesthetics should be avoided. Occasionally in refractory cases, a candidal yeast infection exists and a trial of antifungal lotion, solution, or powder is worthwhile.

Various treatments such as irradiation, undercutting the perianal skin, alcohol skin injections, have been advocated for refractory pruritus [10, 11]. These are associated with poor results and high complication rates and are mentioned here only to be condemned. Some authors have had limited success with tattooing the perianal skin with mythelene blue [12].

In general the principles of treating pruritus ani are to establish and maintain an intact, healthy, clean, and dry perianal skin. Frequently patients experience recurrent symptoms requiring reinstitution of the treatment routine that has been outlined. In cases that fail to improve, fungal and viral cultures and even biopsy may be necessary to exclude an infectious or neoplastic cause.

Fissure-in-ano

Anatomy

Fissure-in-ano is a painful longitudinal defect in the lining of the anal canal. This lining, called anoderm, begins proximally at the dentate line and extends to a level just distal to the intersphincteric groove. The anoderm is devoid of hair follicles and sebaceous or sweat glands and consists of a squamous epithelial mucous membrane. The mucosa proximal to the dentate line is an extension of the rectal mucosa and is insensitive, being supplied by autonomic nerves, whereas the anoderm distal to the dentate line is extremely sensitive to touch and pain, possessing somatic type innervation. Immediately deep to (or surrounding) the anoderm is the internal anal sphincter, which is a thickened extension of the circular smooth muscle layer of the rectum. The internal anal sphincter is responsible for 80–85% of the resting tone of the anal canal.

Deep to (or surrounding) the internal anal sphincter lies the external anal sphincter, which consists of a cylindrical extension of the funnel-shaped striated or voluntary muscles of the pelvic floor. The external anal sphincter is primarily responsible for deferring defecation to a socially acceptable time and place. It takes on a somewhat slit like shape due to its attachment to the anococcygeal ligament posteriorly and the transverse perineal muscles of the perineal body anteriorly. The external anal sphincter extends slightly distal to the internal anal sphincter creating a palpable intersphincteric groove. The distal (or caudal) most aspect of the external anal sphincter is referred to as the subcutaneous external anal sphincter or corrugator cutis ani muscle and is responsible for the radially directed skinfolds surrounding the anal opening.

Pathophysiology

The exact cause of fissure-in-ano has not been proved, but multiple factors have been suggested. It has been postulated that trauma, the anatomic configuration of the anal canal, internal anal sphincter dysfunction, and ischemia may contribute to the formation and perpetuation of anal fissures [13–15].

The majority of patients presenting with an anal fissure relate a history of having a large, hard, or otherwise traumatic bowel movement just before the onset of symptoms. Occasionally, frequent bowel movements associated with diarrhea are the initiating event. Insertion of a rectal thermometer, enema tip, or even a scope used to examine the rectum or anus can result in sufficient trauma to produce an anal fissure. Infrequently, a fissure can be the result of perineal trauma occurring during labor and a vaginal delivery.

The anatomic configuration of the anal canal probably predisposes fissures to occur predominantly in the posterior and occasionally the anterior locations. Anal fissures are consistently located in the posterior midline in 99% of men and 90% of women. The remaining 1% and 10%, respectively, are located anteriorly. The external anal sphincter muscle fibers run in an anterior to posterior direction decussating anteriorly at the perineal body and attaching posteriorly to the anococcygeal ligament. The internal anal sphincter is arranged in an elliptical configuration creating the aforementioned anteroposterior slit of the anal canal at rest. It is postulated that greater shearing forces occur posteriorly and anteriorly at these angled and fixed points, resulting in a greater tendency for the anoderm to tear (**Figure 18.3**) [16].

Nothmann and Schuster [17] demonstrated that although patients with an anal fissure exhibited a normal internal anal sphincter relaxation in response to rectal distention, the baseline pressure returned transiently to a higher level. This phenomenon they called the 'overshoot' and postulated that it was the result of a spastic or hyperreactive internal sphincter muscle and that it played a role in the cause of anal fissures. This 'overshoot' phenomenon can be demonstrated in some normal subjects without anal fissure, and even Nothmann and Schuster demonstrated overshoot in 26% of their control group compared with 90% of their fissure group [17]. They did state that in a very small number of patients (three) who were studied after treatment resolved their anal fissure, the 'overshoot' disappeared.

Initially Nothmann and Schuster [17] and later Hancock [18] and Arabi et [19] demonstrated that patients with anal fissures had elevated resting anal sphincter pressures when compared with normal controls. They were unable to state whether the abnormally high resting pressure was the result of an anal fissure or predisposed to its development. More recently, using anal manometry and Doppler laser flowmetry, Schouten et al [14] demonstrated less blood flow to the anoderm of the

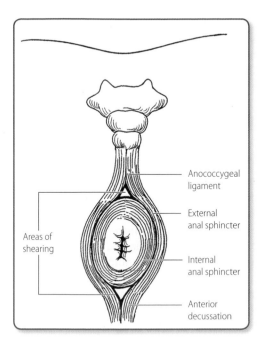

Figure 18.3 Anal sphincter muscle. Configuration predisposing to anterior and posterior fissure locations.

Anococcygeal ligament

External anal sphincter

Areas of shearing

Internal anal sphincter

Anterior decussation

posterior midline than is found in other areas of the anal canal. They also demonstrated a direct correlation between increasing resting anal canal pressure and decreasing posterior midline anodermal blood flow. These findings led them to postulate that ischemia may be responsible for the severe pain associated with anal fissures and may contribute to their failure to heal.

Symptoms

Patients with an anal fissure most commonly present with anal pain and particularly painful defecation. The pain is usually described as tearing, cutting, or burning in nature and occurs with the passage of stool. Anal fissure is the most common cause of painful rectal bleeding, and the pain is usually far more severe than would be expected from the size of the defect in the anal canal. The duration of the pain can be brief with resolution shortly after defecating or can be constant and made severe by the act of defecation. Indeed, the pain can be so severe as to prevent a patient from initiating defecation resulting in constipation and even fecal impaction. The passage of large hard constipated stools only further perpetuates the fissure.

In addition, anal fissures may produce bleeding, pruritus, and a malodorous discharge. Pruritus is thought to be secondary to the anal discharge produced by the anal ulceration and is said to occur in as many as 50% of cases. The bleeding associated with an anal fissure is bright red and usually seen on the toilet tissue. Occasionally, the bleeding can be more profuse, dripping into the toilet bowl or staining the undergarments. The bleeding is usually a small amount and virtually never, in the absence of a coagulopathy, results in hemorrhage or anemia. The pain from an anal fissure can occasionally be so severe as to result in urinary symptoms such as dysuria, frequency, and even retention [20]. Fissures can occur in all age groups but most frequently occur in the third and fourth decades of life. Both men and women are affected equally [21]. Fissure is the most common cause of rectal bleeding in infants and children [22].

Evaluation

In the majority of patients, a careful history and gentle inspection of the anus, retracting the buttocks and everting the anal orifice, is all the evaluation that is necessary to confirm the diagnosis (**Figure 18.4**). Even a digital rectal examination may evoke such severe pain that the patient will be unable to cooperate and indeed may never return to the office. If gentle eversion of the lower anal lining fails to disclose a fissure, digital examination, anoscopy, and proctosigmoidoscopy may be necessary. Occasionally, the use of xylocaine ointment 5% as a lubricant is necessary to facilitate the examination.

Rarely, it is necessary to perform these examinations under anesthesia. Acute fissures (**Figure 18.5a**) appear as simple tears, while chronic fissures (**Figure 18.5b**) are associated with a proximal hypertrophied anal papilla, a distal sentinel skin tag, and appearance of the internal sphincter muscle at the fissure base.

During the process of evaluation, anal fissure must be differentiated from other causes of anal ulceration, such as inflammatory bowel disease, infections, or malignancy (**Figure 18.6**). Anal manifestations are indeed well-known accompaniments of Crohn's disease and to a lesser extent ulcerative colitis. As many as 4% of patients with Crohn's disease present with anal disease as the initial manifestation. It has also been reported that nearly 50% of patients with Crohn's disease will experience an anal ulceration some time during the course of their disease. The distinguishing features of these ulcers are they are atypically located (not in the posterior or anterior midline), often multiple, broad based, and with shaggy or irregular margins. These lesions usually are attributed to inflammatory bowel disease only after

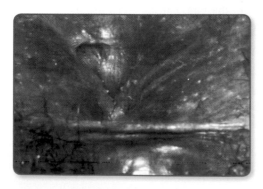

Figure 18.4 Identification of anal fissure by buttocks retraction.

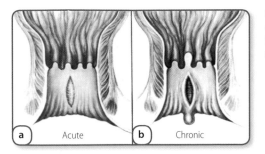

Figure 18.5 Anal fissures. (a) Acute fissure with exposed internal sphincter muscle fibers. (b) Chronic fissure with sentinel skin tag, hypertrophied anal papilla, and rolled, thickened margins.

| a | Acute |
| b | Chronic |

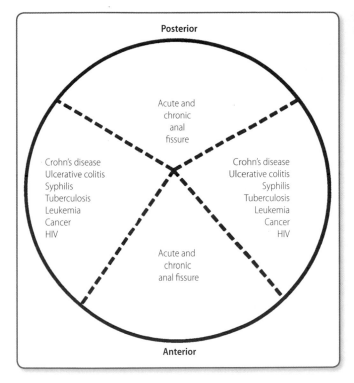

Figure 18.6 The location of anal fissures suggests their cause.

they fail to respond appropriately to medical or more often surgical management. A biopsy of the lesion is seldom helpful, and complete evaluation of the gastrointestinal tract may be necessary.

Anal infections can masquerade as an anal fissure. These include but are not limited to herpes, syphilis, chancroid, and tuberculosis. Herpes produces small superficial ulcerations often of the perianal skin which tend to coalesce and produce pain out of proportion to the apparent severity of the lesion. Viral culture of the lesions can confirm the diagnosis generally within 48–72 hours. The ulcerations associated with syphilis are deep, shaggy, moist, and often associated with mirror image lesions (**Figure 18.7** and see Figure 20.2). The diagnosis can be confirmed by rapid plasma reagin study. Dark-field examination of anal lesions is

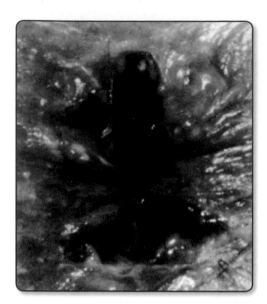

Figure 18.7 Anal fissure secondary to syphilis.

often difficult because of anatomic constraints in obtaining the requisite touch preparation. In the presence of prominent inguinal adenopathy, chancroid should be considered. Anal tuberculosis, although rare, is almost always associated with concomitant pulmonary disease.

Although they may mimic anal fissure, lesions of early carcinoma of the anus or rectum are usually so atypical in appearance as to be easily recognized and biopsied (see Figure 22.10). Ulceration of the anal and perianal region occurs in the setting of acute leukemia. These lesions can be extremely painful, represent leukemic infiltrates, require adequate surgical drainage and antibiotics, and often represent a preterminal event. Anal ulceration seen in the setting of AIDS can be caused by infections (e.g. herpes, cytomegalovirus) or AIDS-associated malignancies (e.g. Kaposi's sarcoma, B-cell lymphoma, or squamous cell carcinoma). These lesions are generally very atypical in location and appearance and are differentiated on the basis of cultures and biopsies (see Chapter 20).

Nonoperative treatment

A trial of conservative nonoperative therapy should represent the initial management in all patients with anal fissure. Such therapy consists of bulk stool softeners (e.g. psyllium or methylcellulose preparations), a diet high in fiber including unprocessed wheat or oat bran, increased hydration, polyethylene glycol preparations (Miralax, Schering-Plough Health Care Products, Inc.) and the liberal use of warm sitz baths or heating pads, particularly after defecation, to relax anal sphincter spasm and decrease the need for wiping, which may exacerbate both the pain and bleeding. The bulk agents consisting of the stool softeners and bran produce a large, soft, well-lubricated stool, increasing the ease of defecation and potentially dilating the spastic internal anal sphincter. Increased hydration is necessary to maintain soft well-lubricated stools. Even if symptoms resolve on this conservative regimen, patients should be encouraged to maintain soft, formed, regular stools for many weeks lest a single, large, hard stool result in recurrence.

The use of ointments, creams, and emollients containing various anti-inflammatory agents (e.g. hydrocortisone) or local anesthetics (e.g. dibucaine) has been advocated [23]. No well-controlled clinical trials have confirmed their efficacy. The little beneficial effect these agents may have could be attributed to the placebo effect of applying medication to the site of pain, their lubricating effect, or the natural history of spontaneous resolution that the majority of anal fissures exhibit. The use of anal suppositories is to be discouraged. Insertion is generally painful, and the suppositories tend to migrate to the upper rectum, where they can have little therapeutic benefit. It has been reported that as many as 50% of anal fissures will heal at least temporarily or at least symptoms resolve using nonoperative therapy.

Smooth muscle relaxants and antispasmodics (e.g. dicyclomine and oxybutynin) have been advocated under the assumption that the primary process is the result of smooth muscle spasm, but no clinical trials have been reported demonstrating their efficacy [24]. In a small uncontrolled study, Schouten and colleagues have reported the use of isosorbide dinitrate 1% ointment applied locally every 3–4 hours while awake results in healing of 82% of anal fissures [25]. Their rationale is that decreased anal smooth muscle spasm and increased blood flow are responsible for the healing of anal fissures.

The theory that a fissure is actually an ischemic ulcer of the anoderm has resulted in the use of topical nitroglycerin. Over the last decade topical nitroglycerin (NTG) ointment has been used with success rates varying from 48–78% [26–30]. NTG is metabolized and releases nitric oxide, which is believed to be an inhibitory neurotransmitter of smooth muscle. Nitric oxide binds to the iron moiety of guanylate cyclase in the smooth muscle, increasing levels of guanosine 3'5'-cyclic monophosphate (cGMP) [31]. Potassium channels are activated by the cGMP, which serves as a second messenger and results in hyperpolarization of the smooth muscle. As a result of neurogenic relaxation of the internal sphincter, a reduction in anal canal pressure is achieved, diminishing pain and spasm [32]. Typically 0.2% NTG is used three to five times a day but concentrations as high as 0.5% have been recommended [27–29]. The actual dosing is limited by its side effects, which may occur in up to 88% of patients [27–29,33]. Headaches are the predominant complaint but dizziness, lightheadedness, and hypotension may also occur. Caution must be exercised with this therapy in patients on cardiac medications and those with sensitivities to nitrates. A meta-analysis comparing topical nitroglycerin to sphincterotomy demonstrated that sphincterotomy is superior to topical NTG in the healing of chronic fissures [33].

The use of botulinum toxin has recently been reported to facilitate the healing of fissures in 78–90% of patients with an 8% recurrence rate in 6 months [34–36]. The toxin, produced by the bacterium *Clostridium botulinum*, acts by inhibiting the release of acetylcholine at the presynaptic membrane. As a result of blocked neurotransmission, spasms and contractions of the sphincter mechanism are diminished or eliminated.

Injections of 2.5–50 units are administered in 2–4 sites [34–36]. Although it still takes several days for the fissure to heal, pain relief is generally noted within 24 hours and there have been few complaints of incontinence with this form of therapy. The amount administered is small (compared to other applications) and is cautiously placed into the internal sphincter while avoiding the external sphincter. The effect, however, is transitory in nature, which may explain the 8% recurrence rate. The major drawback with use of this agent is cost, which can be up to $400 per 100-unit vial. Since the toxin is reconstituted and the manufacturer does not recommend storage after reconstitution, much of the toxin may be wasted.

Nifedipene ointment has also been used with varying degrees of success. Compounded from nifedipene, a dihydropyridine, it is mixed into a gel or ointment and acts as a calcium antagonist preventing the flow of calcium into the sarcoplasm of smooth muscle [37]. Reducing this active transport system decreases the local demand for oxygen and mechanical contraction of the muscle. Experimental studies suggest nifedipine may have locally effective anti-inflammatory properties [38]. 0.2% nifedipine ointment is applied topically similar to applying NTG ointment but seems to have fewer side effects. Caution using this agent should be exercised when used in cardiac patients or those patients who have demonstrated previous sensitivities. One multicenter study reported a 95% complete healing rate after 21 days of treatment [39]. Topical 2% diltiazem has also been used in patients with chronic fissures resulting in a 67% healing rate [40]. Experience with topical nifidipine suggests that it may be more beneficial in the treatment of the acute fissure rather than the chronic one.

The decision to persist with nonoperative management should be based upon the patient's response to treatment. The decision to use operative therapy ultimately depends on the lack of a symptomatic response that is acceptable to the patient. Frequently the patient decides that for reasons of unrelenting or intolerable pain or persistent bleeding, nonoperative therapy has been unsuccessful and immediate surgery is desirable.

Operative treatment

Operative therapy for chronic anal fissure involves dividing the distal aspect of the internal anal sphincter. Various approaches have been used to accomplish internal anal sphincter division including anal sphincter stretch, fissurectomy, internal anal sphincterotomy, and subcutaneous lateral internal anal sphincterotomy.

Recamier [41] in 1838 is credited with providing the first description of the use of **anal sphincter stretch** for the treatment of anal fissure. Goligher [42] in 1965 advocated anal sphincter stretch as an alternative to internal anal sphincterotomy. Lord in 1973 adapted the procedure for the treatment of hemorrhoids and his name has been attached to the procedure ever since [43]. Though often successful in alleviating the pain and promoting the healing of anal fissures, anal sphincter stretch has been shown ultrasonographically to produce a traumatic and uncontrolled disruption of the internal sphincter. The technique requires general anesthesia and involves inserting from four to eight fingers in the anal canal and stretching the sphincter in either an anterior to posterior or lateral direction. Various reports indicate only a 72% rate of fissure healing and also a 20% rate of 'minor' fecal incontinence [43, 44]. Because of the requirement of general anesthesia, uncontrolled sphincter disruption, and unacceptable complication rate, anal sphincter stretch has all but been abandoned for the surgical management of anal fissure.

Fissurectomy was described by Gabriel in 1948 for the treatment of chronic anal fissure [45]. He failed to recognize that the 'pecten band' that he was dividing during the procedure was actually the internal anal sphincter and was probably the reason for the procedure's success. The posterior midline wound created when performing fissurectomy is notoriously slow to heal and generally results in a 'keyhole deformity.' Such a deformity has been implicated as the cause of minor fecal incontinence. Fissurectomy is seldom employed and generally only when it is necessary to open an associated superficial fistula, remove a prolapsing hypertrophied anal papilla, or to excise a large, redundant anal skin tag which is interfering with perianal hygiene.

Internal anal sphincterotomy was first advocated by Eisenhammer of South Africa in 1951 [46–48]. He recognized that division of the distal aspect of the internal anal sphincter resulted in relief of pain and the subsequent healing of the anal fissure. Initially, he performed sphincterotomy in the base of the fissure, generally in the posterior midline. The poorly healing midline wound and resulting 'keyhole deformity' was reported by Bennett and Goligher [21] to cause fecal soiling in 22% of patients and incontinence of gas and stool in 19% and 9%, respectively. These poor results led Eisenhammer in 1959 [48] to modify the site of sphincterotomy to a lateral location. Initially, lateral internal anal sphincterotomy was performed through a longitudinal (radial) skin incision in the anal canal, which was left open to heal by secondary intention. Later the procedure was modified to include skin closure (**Figure 18.8**) with an absorbable suture.

The pain that patients experienced associated with a healing wound in the anal canal led Sir Alan Parks in 1967 [49] to recommend a circumanal incision located at the level of the intersphincteric groove. His modification is called a lateral subcutaneous internal anal sphincterotomy (**Figure 18.9**). It avoids an intra-anal incision

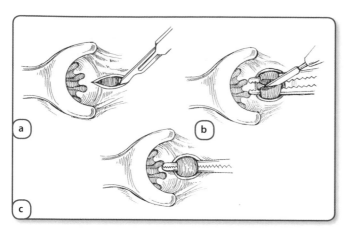

Figure 18.8 Internal anal sphincterotomy. (a) Radial skin incision distal to the dentate line exposing the intersphincteric groove. (b) Elevation and division of the internal anal sphincter. (c) Primary wound closure.

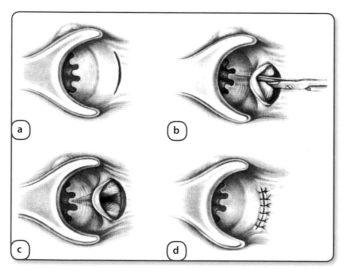

Figure 18.9 Lateral subcutaneous internal anal sphincterotomy. (a) Circumferential skin incision maintaining the integrity of the skin of the anal canal. (b) and (c) Subcutaneous division of the internal anal sphincter. (d) Closure of the incision at the anal verge.

while allowing division of the internal sphincter under direct visualization. A short time later, in 1969, Notaras [50,51] described a technique for blind lateral subcutaneous internal anal sphincterotomy (**Figure 18.10**) in which a scalpel blade (No. 11 Bard-Parker or No. 52 Beaver [**Figure 18.11**]) is inserted through a puncture wound at the anal margin, advanced beneath the anoderm of the anal canal until its tip is at the dentate line, and with a lateral sawing motion divides the internal sphincter. The blade is removed resulting in a very small perianal wound. Hemostasis is obtained by placing digital pressure on the sphincterotomy site for several minutes. In order to avoid inadvertent cutting of the external sphincter, Goligher suggested inserting the blade in the intersphincteric groove and division of the sphincter from lateral to medial (**Figure 18.10d**). In both techniques the resulting puncture

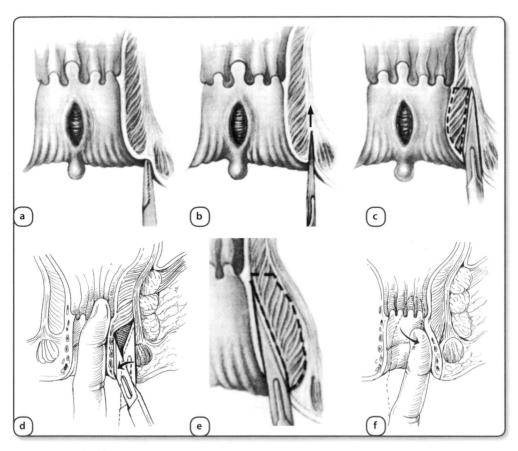

Figure 18.10 Blind lateral subcutaneous internal anal sphincterotomy. (a) Location of the intersphincteric groove (b) Insertion of knife blade in the intersphincteric plane in performing a 'blind' lateral subcutaneous internal anal sphincterotomy. (c, d) Lateral to medial division of the internal anal sphincter by a gentle sawing motion preserving the integrity of the anal skin (Notara's technique). (e) Medial to lateral division of muscle (Goligher's modification). (f) Hemostasis by digital pressure on the sphincterotomy site.

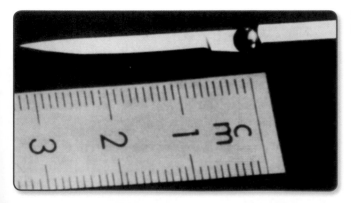

Figure 18.11 No. 52 Beaver blade.

wound does not require closure. The blind technique is particularly amenable to being performed under local anesthesia containing epinephrine [15]. Persistent bleeding or puncture of the anoderm requires that the remaining anoderm overlying the sphincterotomy be opened to obtain hemostasis and prevent the development of a fistula.

Results reported with lateral subcutaneous internal sphincterotomy are excellent (**Table 18.1**). Between 97 and 100% of fissures heal completely. More than 90% of patients are pain free within 48 hours. An occasional patient does experience impairment of fecal continence, which supports the approach of nonoperative management whenever possible. Generally, any impairment of fecal continence is encountered immediately postoperatively and resolves with the passage of time. Of the 1214 patients reported in **Table 18.2**, only two experienced persistent fecal incontinence. Additional complications, including bleeding, hematoma, abscess, fistula, hemorrhoidal prolapse, and pruritus occurred in less than 7% of patients [51–59]. Lateral internal anal sphincterotomy and lateral subcutaneous internal anal sphincterotomy, whether by direct visualization or blind technique, have become the operative procedures of choice for the treatment of anal fissure [60].

Rounds questions

1. What are the symptoms of pruritus ani?
2. What are the major principles for treating pruritus ani?
3. What is the most common anatomic location for idiopathic anal fissures?
4. What are the common symptoms of an anal fissure?
5. What are the differential diagnoses for anal fissures?
6. What is the nonoperative therapy for anal fissure?
7. What topical agents can be used to treat anal fissures?
8. What is the most common operative procedure for anal fissures?.

Table 18.1 Results and complications of internal anal sphincterotomy	
Outcome	Percentage of cases
Complete healing	97–100
Pain free in 48 hours	>90
Healing in 1 month	96
Poor control of flatus	0–18
Soiling	0–7
Fecal incontinence	0–0.17
Other complications	0–7

Table 18.2 Lateral internal anal sphincterotomy

Authors	No. of patients	Healed (%)	Recurrence (%)	Minor defects of anal control (%)			Other complications (%)
				Feces	Flatus	Soiling	
Hawley, 1969 [54]	24	100	0	0	0	0	3
Notaras, 1969 [50]	82	100	0	1.4	2.7	5.5	1.4
Hoffman and Golligher, 1970 [55]	99	97	3	1	6.1	7.1	0
Ray et al, 1974 [56]	21	100	0	0	0	0	4.8
Rudd, 1975 [57]	200	99.5	0.5	0	0	0	0.5
Abcarian, 1980 [52]	150	98.7	1.3	0	0	0	1.3
Bell, 1980 [58]	56	98	1.8	?	?	?	–
Marya et al, 1980 [59]	100	98	2	0	0	0	–
Vafai and Mann, 1981 [60]	300	97	3	0	15	11	–
Oh, 1982 [61]	550	99.6	0.4	?	?	?	6.9
Ravikumar et al, 1982 [62]	60	96.7	3.3	0	0	0	5
Boulos and Arajo, 1984 [53]	28	100	0	0	17.9	?	7.1
Hsu and Mackeigan, 1984 [63]	89	94	5.6	?	?	?	1.1
Jensen et al, 1984 [64]	30	97	3.3	0	0	3.3	–
Gingold, 1987 [65]	86	94	3.6	0	0	0	–
Weaver et al, 1987 [66]	39	95	5.1	2.6	?	?	5.1
Lewis et al, 1988 [67]	350	–	6	–	–	2.6	6
Hiltunen and Metikainen, 1991 [68]	65	–	12.3	0	0	0	12.3
Frezza et al, 1992 [69]	134	–	0.6	0	0	0	0.6
Xynos, 1993 [70]	42	–	4.8	–	–	–	4.8
Leong et al, 1994 [71]	114	–	2.6	0	7.9	?	2.6
Pernikoff et al, 1994 [72]	500	–	3	0.4	2.8	4.4	3
Romano et al, 1994 [73]	44	–	0	4.5	9	4.5	0
Neufeld et al, 1995 [74]	112	–	2.7	0.9	12.5	8.9	2.7
Oh et al, 1995 [75]	1313	–	1.3	–	–	0	1.3
Usatoff and Polglase, 1995 [76]	98	–	3	1	7	11	3
Hananel and Gordon, 1997 (77)	265	–	1.1	0.4	0.4	0.4	1.1

References

1. Smith LE, Henrichs D, McCullah RD. Prospective studies on the etiology and treatment of pruritus ani. Dis Colon Rectum 1982;25:358–63.
2. Smith LE. Idiopathic pruritus ani. In: Gordon PH, Nivatvongs S (eds). Principles and Practice of Surgery for the Colon, Rectum, and Anus. St. Louis: Quality Medical Publishing 1992;281–96.
3. Friend WG. The cause and treatment of idiopathic pruritus ani. Dis Colon Rectum 1977;20:40–2.
4. Alexander-Williams J. Pruritus ani [editorial]. Br Med J 1983;287:159–60.
5. Dailey TH. Pruritus ani. In: Condon RE, (ed). Surgery of the Alimentary Tract, 4th ed, vol IV. Philadelphia: WB Saunders, 1996; 317–21.
6. Alexander-Williams J. Pruritus ani. What to do, what not to do to control this infernal itch. Postgrad Med 1985;77:56–65.

7. Allan A, Ambrose NS, Silverman S, Keighley MR. Physiological study of pruritus ani. Br J Surg 1987;74:576–9.

8. Eyers AA, Thomson JP. Pruritus ani: Is anal sphincter dysfunction important in aetiology? Br Med J 1979;2:1549–51.

9. Hoffmann BA, Timmcke AE, Gathright JB Hicks TC, Opelka FG, Beck DE. Fecal seepage and soiling: A problem of rectal sensation. Dis Colon Rectum 1995;38:746–8.

10. Eusebio EB, Graham J, Mody N. Treatment of intractable pruritus ani. Dis Colon Rectum 1990;33:770–2.

11. Shafik A. A new concept of the anatomy of the anal sphincter mechanism and the physiology of defecation XXIII. An injection technique for the treatment of idiopathic pruritus ani. Int Surg 1990;75:43–6.

12. Finne O. Pruritus ani. In: Beck DE, Wexner SD, Roberts PL, Sacclarides TJ, Senagore A, Stamos M (eds). ASCRS Textbook of Colorectal Surgery. 2nd ed. New York: Springer-Verlag, in press.

13. Corman ML. Colon and Rectal Surgery. Philadelphia: JB Lippincott 1984;74–84.

14. Schouten WR, Briel JW, Auwerda JJ. Relationship between anal pressure and anodermal blood flow. The vascular pathogenesis of anal fissures. Dis Colon Rectum 1994;37:664–9.

15. Timmcke AE, Hicks TC. Fissure-in-ano. In: Condon RE (ed). Surgery of the Alimentary Tract, 4th ed, vol IV. Philadelphia: WB Saunders 1996;322–9.

16. Oh C. Lateral subcutaneous internal sphincterotomy for anal fissure. Mt Sinai J Med 1975;42:596–601.

17. Nothmann BJ, Schuster MM. Internal anal sphincter derangement with anal fissures. Gastroenterology 1974;67:216–20.

18. Hancock BD. The internal sphincter and anal fissure. Br J Surg 1977;64:92–5.

19. Arabi Y, Alexander-Williams J, Keighley MRB. Anal pressures in hemorrhoids and anal fissure. Am J Surg 1977;134:608–10.

20. Mazier WP, De Moraes RT, Dignan RD. Anal fissure and anal ulcers. Surg Clin North Am 1978;58:479–85.

21. Bennett RC, Goligher JC. Results of internal sphincterotomy for anal fissure. Br Med J 1962;2:1500–3.

22. O' Connor JJ. Pediatric proctology. Dis Colon Rectum 1975;18:126–7.

23. Gabriel WB. Treatment of pruritus ani and anal fissure: The use of anesthetic solution in oil. Br Med J 1929;1:1070.

24. Miller LG, Rogers JC, Brown EB, Perkins G. Dicyclomine for medical management of persistent anal fissure with associated spasm of the internal sphincter. Tex Med 1992;88:65–6.

25. Schouten WR. Local ISDN reduces pressure in patients with chronic anal fissure, avoids surgery. Gastroenterology and Endoscopy News. 1996;47:1.

26. Wiley KS, Chinn BT. Anal fissures. Clin Colon Rect Surg 2001;14:193–201.

27. Hyman NH, Cataldo PA. Nitroglycerin ointment for anal fissures: effective treatment or just a headache? Dis Colon Rectum 1999;42:383–5.

28. Dorfman G, Levitt M, Platell C. Treatment of chronic anal fissure with topical glyceryl trinitrate. Dis Colon Rectum 1999;42:1007–10.

29. Manookian CM, Fleshner P, Moore B, et al. Topical nitroglycerin in management of anal fissure: An explosive outcome! Am Surg 1998;64:962–4.

30. Gorfine SR. Treatment of benign anal disease with topical nitroglycerin. Dis Colon Rectum 1995;38:453–7.

31. Watson SJ, Kamm MA, Nicholls RJ, Phillips RK. Topical glyceryl trinitrate in the treatment of chronic anal fissure. Br J Surg 1996;83:771–5.

32. O'Kelly T, Brading A, Mortensen N. Nerve mediated relaxation of the human internal anal sphincter: the role of nitric oxide. Gut 1993;34:689–93.

33. Richard CS, Gregoire R, Plewes EA, et al. Internal sphincterotomy is superior to topical nitroglycerin in the treatment of chronic anal fissure: results of a randomized, controlled trial by the Canadian Colorectal Surgical Trials Group. Dis Colon Rectum 2000;43:1048–58.

34. Brisinda G, Maria G, Betivoglio AR, et al. A comparison of injections of botulinum toxin and topical nitroglycerin ointment for the treatment of chronic anal fissure. N Engl Med 1999;341:65–9.

35. Jost WH. One hundred cases of anal fissure treated with botulin toxin: early and long-term results. Dis Colon Rectum 1997;40:1029–32.

36. Minguez M, Melo F, Espi A, et al. Therapeutic effects of different doses of botulinum toxin in chronic anal fissure. Dis Colon Rectum 1999;42:1016–21.

37. Triggle DJ. Calcium, calcium channels, and calcium channel antagonists. Can J Physiol Pharmacol 1990;68:1474–81.

38. Katoh N, Hiramo S, Kishimoto S, Yasumo H. Calcium channel blockers suppress the contact hypersensitivity reaction (CHR) by inhibiting antigen transport and presentation by epidermal langerhans cells in mince. Clin Exp Immunol 1997;108:302–8.

39. Antropoli C, Perrotti P, Rubiano M, et al. Nifedipine for local use in conservative treatment of anal fissures: preliminary results of a multicenter study. Dis Colon Rectum 1999;42:1011–15.

40. Carapeti EA, Kamm MA, Phillips RK. Topical diltiazem and bethanechol decrease anal sphincter pressure and heal anal fissures without side effects. Dis Colon Rectum 2000;43:1359–62.

41. Recamier JC. Extension, massage et percussion cadencee dans le traitement des contractures musculaires. Rev Medicale Franc 1:74, 1838. (Translated : Classic articles in colonic and rectal surgery. Stretching, massage and rhythmic percussion in the treatment of muscular contractions: Joseph-Claude-Anthelme Recamier (1774–1852). Dis Colon Rectum 1980;23:362–7).

42. Goligher JC. An evaluation of internal sphincterotomy and simple sphincter stretching in the treatment of fissure-in-ano. Surg Clin North Am 1965;42:1299.

43. Lord PH. Diverse methods of managing hemorrhoids: dilatation. Dis Colon Rectum 1973;16:180–3.

44. Watts JM, Bennett RC, Goligher JC. Stretching of anal sphincters in treatment of fissure-in-ano. Br Med J 1964;2:342–3.

45. Gabriel WB. Anal Fissure. In: Principles and practice of rectal surgery, 4th ed. London: HK Lewis, 1948.

46. Eisenhammer S. The surgical correction of chronic internal anal (sphincteric) contracture. S Afr Med J 1951;25:486.

47. Eisenhammer S. The internal anal sphincter: Its surgical importance. S Afr Med J 1953;27:266.

48. Eisenhammer S. The evaluation of the internal anal sphincterotomy operation with special reference to anal fissure. Surg Gynecol Obstet 1959;109:583–90.

49. Parks AG. The management of fissure-in-ano. Hosp Med 1967;1:737.

50. Notaras MI. Lateral subcutaneous sphincterotomy for anal fissure–a new technique. Proc R Soc Med 1969;62:713.

51. Notaras MJ. The treatment of anal fissure by lateral subcutaneous internal sphincterotomy–a technique and results. Br J Surg 1971;58:96–100.

52. Abcarian H. Surgical correction of chronic anal fissure: Results of lateral internal sphincterotomy vs. fissurectomy-midline sphincterotomy. Dis Colon Rectum 1980;23:31–6.

53. Boulos PB, Araujo JGC. Adequate internal sphincterotomy for chronic anal fissure: Subcutaneous or open technique? Br J Surg 1984;71:360–2.

54. Hawley PR. The treatment of chronic fissure-in-ano. A trial of methods. Br J Surg 1969;56: 915–8.

55. Hoffmann DC, Goligher JC. Lateral subcutaneous internal sphincterotomy in treatment of anal fissure. Br Med J 1969;3:673–5.

56. Ray JE, Penfold JCB, Gathright JB, Roberson SH. Lateral subcutaneous internal anal sphincterotomy for anal fissure. Presidential address. Dis Colon Rectum 1974;17:139–44.

57. Rudd WWH. Lateral subcutaneous internal sphincterotomy for chronic anal fissure, an outpatient procedure. Dis Colon Rectum 1975;18:319–23.

58. Bell GA. Lateral internal sphincterotomy in chronic anal fissure-A surgical technique. Ann Surg 1980;46:572–5.

59. Marya SK, Mittal SS, Singla S. Lateral subcutaneous internal sphincterotomy for acute fissure-in-ano. Br J Surg 1980;67:299.

60. Vafai M, Mann CV. Closed lateral internal sphincterotomy without removal of sentinel pile for fissure-in-ano. Coloproctology 1981;3:91–3.

61. Oh C. The role of internal sphincterotomy. Mt Sinai J Med 1982;49:484–6.

62. Ravikumar TS, Sridhar S, Rao RN. Subcutaneous lateral internal sphincterotomy for chronic fissure-in-ano. Dis Colon Rectum 1982;25: 798–801.

63. Hsu TC, Mackeigan JM. Surgical treatment of chronic anal fissure. Dis Colon Rectum 1984;27:475–8.

64. Jensen SL, Lund F, Neilson OV, Tange G. Lateral subcutaneous sphincterotomy vs. anal diltation in the treatment of fissure-in-ano in outpatients: A prospective randomized study. Br Med J 1984;289:528–30.

65. Gingold BS. Simple in-office sphincterotomy with partial fissurectomy for chronic anal fissure. Surg Gynecol Obstet 1987;165:46–8.

66. Weaver RM, Ambrose NS, Alexander-Williams J, Keighley MRB. Manual dilation of the anus vs. lateral subcutaneous sphincterotomy in the treatment of chronic fissure-in-ano. Results of the prospective randomized clinical trial. Dis Colon Rectum 1987;30:420–3.

67. Lewis TH, Corman ML, Prager ED, Robertson WG. Long-term results of open and closed sphincterotomy for anal fissure. Dis Colon Rectum 1988;31:368–71.

68. Hiltunen KM, Metikainen M. Closed lateral subcutaneous sphincterotomy under local anesthesia in the treatment of chronic anal fissure. Ann Chir Gynaecol 1991;80:353–6.

69. Frezza EE, Sander G, Leoni G, Birad M. Conservative and surgical treatment in acute and chronic anal fissure. A study of 308 patients. Int J Colorectal Dis 1992;7:188–91.

70. Xynos E, Tzortzinis A, Chrysos E, Tzovaras G, Vassilakis JS. Anal manometry in patients with fissure-in-ano before and after internal sphincterotomy. Int J Colorectal Dis 1993;8:125–8.

71. Leong AFP, Husain MJ, Seow-Choen F, Goh HS. Performing internal sphincterotomy with other anorectal procedures. Dis Colon Rectum 1994;37:1130–2.
72. Pernikoff MJ, Eisenstat TE, Rubin RJ, Oliver GC, Salvati EP. Reappraisal of partial lateral internal sphincterotomy. Dis Colon Rectum 1994;37:1291–5.
73. Ramano G, Rotondano G, Santangelo M, Esercizio L. A critical appraisal of pathogenesis and morbidity of surgical treatment of chronic anal fissure. J Am Coll Surg 1994;178:600–4.
74. Neufeld DM, Paran H, Bendahan J, Freund U. Outpatient surgical treatment of anal fissure. Eur J Surg 1995;161:435–8.
75. Oh C, Divino CM, Steinhagen RM. Anal fissure 20 year experience. Dis Colon Rectum 1995;38:378–82.
76. Usatoff V, Polglase AL. The longer term results of internal anal sphincterotomy for anal fissure. Aust N Z J Surg 1995;65:576–8.
77. Hananel N, Gordon PH. Lateral internal sphincterotomy for fissure-in-ano revisited. Dis Colon Rectum 1997;40:597–602.
78. Rosen L, Abel ME, Gordon PH, et al. Practice parameters for the management of anal fissure. The Standards Task Force American Society of Colon and Rectal Surgeons. Dis Colon Rectum 1992;35:206–8.

Most authors attribute the first report of pilonidal disease to Anderson in 1847 [1] and the first series of patients to Warren [2] The term pilonidal was first associated with this condition by Hodges in 1880 [3] It was derived from the Latin 'pilus' (hair) and 'nidus' (nest). The term notes the association of trapped hair in this unusual form of natal cleft skin infection.

Etiologic factors

The cause of pilonidal disease has been debated for years and authors have proposed congenital and acquired theories [4,5]. If the congenital theory was true, then removal of all epithelial tracks to the sacral fascia would be curative. However, even when all tissues overlying the sacrum are removed and a rotation flap is constructed from tissue away from the midline, the recurrence rate remains substantial [6]. Congenital theories also cannot account for the lack of intermediate stages between the congenital sinuses or tracks noted in childhood and the pilonidal disease seen in adults. Finally, congenital sinuses are usually located more superiorly over the lumbar area rather than the sacrum, do not contain hair, frequently communicate with the spinal canal, and contain cuboidal epithelium rather than granulation tissue [7, 8].

The congenital theories for pilonidal disease were challenged in 1946, when Patey and Scarff [9, 10] noted that the interdigital pilonidal sinuses of barbers were pathologically identical to postnatal pilonidal sinuses. This has been followed by other reports of hair causing pilonidal disease in the interdigital clefts [11] and periareolar skin of barbers [12]. In addition, pilonidal disease has been associated with loose hairs forming abscesses in the mammary ducts [13], penis [14], axilla [15], and umbilicus [16]. There are even reports of an identical inflammatory process associated with the fur of dogs [17]. The wool from sheep [18], and feathers from bedding material [19]. These types of observations lend credibility to acquired theories of pilonidal disease.

Currently the debate on the cause of pilonidal disease centers around two main theories. One is that pilonidal disease is the result of a foreign body reaction to hairs embedded in the skin, commonly in the midline sacrococcygeal area. Patey and Scarff [9] noted that although pilonidal tracks contain hair, they do not always contain hair follicles. This would suggest that the hair and not the follicle is the source of the disease. Keratin plugs and other debris may contribute to the inflammation of the hair in the midline internatal cleft pits [20]

The inflammation around the hair follows the path of least resistance and often tracks in a cephalad and lateral direction, thus forming secondary tracks and openings.

An alternative theory, proposed by Bascom [21], is that the origin of pilonidal disease is in the hair follicles of the natal cleft. Keratin occludes the follicle, which eventually becomes inflamed and ruptures into the surrounding fat, forming a pilonidal abscess. If the abscess drains, inflammation subsides and the mouth of the follicle reopens. The remnant of the follicle and abscess cavity, now a tube open at two ends, forms a draining pilonidal sinus. Vagrant hairs from the region gather in the gluteal cleft and into the sinus. If the sinus cavity fails to heal promptly, epithelium migrates into the sinus from the edges of the follicle and forms an epithelial lined tube.

Incidence

All forms of pilonidal disease are reported to be more common in men than in women, with a relative frequency ratio of 2.2-4.0:1 [22, 23]. The greatest incidence of pilonidal disease occurs between puberty and 40 years of age [24]. Pilonidal disease was identified in 365 of 31,497 men and 24 of 21,367 women in a study of Minnesota college students [24]. The same study noted an association between pilonidal disease and obesity. Between 1950 and 1955 an average of 411 of every 100,000 Navy personnel were treated at least once for pilonidal disease [25]. One author noted the association of pilonidal disease with hair on the glabella in Navy personnel [26]. During World War II, Buie [27] referred to pilonidal disease as 'Jeep disease' because of its association with mechanized warfare.

Microbiology

A review of the predominant organisms cultured from infected pilonidal sinuses in 75 patients revealed anaerobic bacteria in 77% of aspirate samples, aerobic bacteria in 4%, and mixed aerobic and anaerobic in 19% [28]. The presence of polymicrobial infection does not seem to require antibiotic therapy unless primary closure is anticipated [29].

Classification and physical findings

Pilonidal disease has three common presentations. Nearly all patients have an episode of acute abscess formation. When this abscess resolves, either spontaneously or with medical assistance, many patients will develop a pilonidal sinus. Although most sinus tracts resolve, a small minority of patients will develop chronic disease or recurrent disease after treatment.

Physical examination typically reveals one or more small (1-2 mm) dermal pits at the base of the intergluteal cleft (**Figure 19.1**). Tracking from the pits (usually in a cranial and lateral direction) will appear

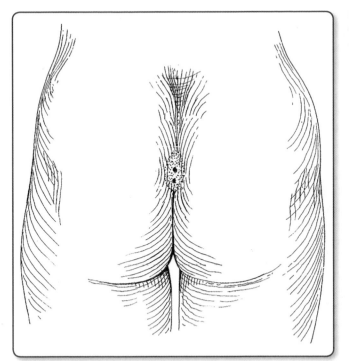

Figure 19.1 Pilonidal cyst disease. Dermal pits associated sinus and abscess.

as areas of induration. With an associated abscess, the diseased area may be tender and erythematous, and draining pus may be evident. The more extensive the disease, the more prominent the findings. Treatment methods vary for each stage in pilonidal disease.

Management

Preoperative preparation

Preoperative preparation is similar to that for other anorectal procedures (Chapter 8). A patient with abscess or associated cellulitis may be given antibiotics in conjunction with drainage. Prophylactic antibiotics are not administered routinely unless wound closure is anticipated. Mechanical preparation of the bowel is not necessary, but some providers administer a small enema before operative intervention to minimize the possibility of a spontaneous bowel movement during anesthesia. The patient should be informed about the chance of recurrence, the importance of proper postoperative wound management, and the length of time that may be required for wound healing [29].

Abscess

Abscesses must be drained. Simple incision and drainage of first-episode acute pilonidal abscesses resulted in an improvement in symptoms in all patients and complete eradication in 58% of patients within 10 weeks of the procedure in one study [30]. Between 20% and 40% of patients develop recurrent disease after this form of treatment. Some authors have recommended adding excision of infected granulation tissue [31], freezing [32], and other techniques to try to decrease the recurrence rate, all without success. Bascom [21] has reported a recurrence rate of only 15% by excising the epithelial pits with small 7 mm incisions 5 days after initial incision and drainage.

Incision and drainage of acute abscesses is readily performed in an office setting using local anesthesia. A solution of 1% lidocaine (Xylocaine HCI) with 1 : 100,000 epinephrine is injected as a field block around the area of inflammation with a 25-gauge needle. In cases of simple abscess with minimal cellulitis, incision, drainage, and curettage of the wall of the cavity will provide definitive treatment. Cultures of the abscess contents are rarely obtained and antibiotics are rarely required. The wound may initially be packed with gauze for hemostasis. However, if an adequate skin incision was created, additional packing is unnecessary to prevent premature closure of the skin over the cavity. The wound is kept clean by irrigating the area twice daily with warm tap water using a shower attachment, sitz bath, or even a Waterpik. It is important keep the surrounding skin dry to avoid maceration. The skin in the gluteal cleft is shaved before drainage and then during weekly office visits. Also during office visits, granulation tissue is cauterized and removed. Success in treatment results from diligent wound care by both the patient and the physician.

Sinus

Up to 40% of acute pilonidal abscesses treated by incision and drainage form a chronic sinus that requires additional treatment [21]. The predominant organisms cultured from pilonidal sinuses are anaerobic and seldom require antibiotic therapy [33]. A prospective randomized trial comparing a single preoperative dose of cefoxitin with no antibiotic prophylaxis in excision and primary closure of chronic pilonidal sinuses failed to show a benefit with antibiotic prophylaxis [34]. The majority of pilonidal sinuses resolve, regardless of treatment option, by age 40 [23]. It is theorized that changes in body habitus (altered and increased fat deposition alters the gluteal cleft) and softening of body hair account for this change with age.

There is debate about the best method of treatment for a nonhealing pilonidal sinus. Many treatments have been reported and then abandoned [35, 36]. A review of articles published in the last 30 years on the treatment of pilonidal disease divided the procedures and analyzed them by broad category (**Table 19.1**) [29, 37]. Closed techniques (injection with phenol or coring out follicles and brushing the tracts) required shaving of the area but could be performed on an outpatient basis. Mean healing time was about 40 days and recurrence rates were slightly higher than other forms of treatment. **Laying open**

Table 19.1 Comparison of techniques by time to healing and recurrence rate based on minimal follow-up in several review articles

Procedure	Number of series	Number of patients	Mean time to healing	Mean recurrence rate (%) < 1 year follow-up	Mean recurrence rate (%) > 1 year follow-up
Debridement of epithelial pit	13	955	44	14	18
Laying open sinus	14	716	48	4	13
Laying open sinus and cauterizing base of sinus	4	630	36	3	13
Excision to fascia	12	572	72	14	13
Excision to fascia and marsupialization of edges	8	538	26	6	4
Primary midline closure	22	872	19	8	15
Primary oblique closure	8	1983	9	1	3
Flap closure	16	536	15	2	8

(unroofing) the tracts with healing by granulation resulted in average healing times of 48 days and required frequent outpatient dressing changes. The incidence of recurrent sinus formation was less than 13% with this technique (**Figure 19.2**). Addition of cauterization of the cavity decreased the average healing time to 36 days and slightly reduced the reported recurrence rates. **Wide and deep excision** of the sinus alone resulted in an average healing time of 72 days and similar recurrent rates as for simple laying open of the sinus with wound granulation (**Figure 19.3**). When partial closure of the wound (marsupialization) is added to wide and deep excision of the sinus, healing time decreases to an average of 26 days (**Figure 19.4**). Excision and primary closure resulted in wound healing within 14 days in successful cases (19 days overall). However, up to 30% of patients failed primary wound healing and the average recurrence rate for these experienced authors was

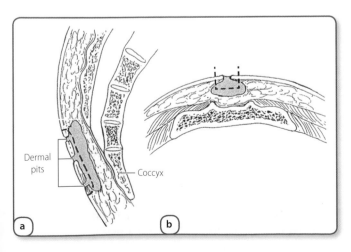

Figure 19.2 Unroofing of sinus removes skin and subcutaneous tissue overlying the cavity. (a) Sagittal section, (b) cross-sectional view.

Dermal pits

Coccyx

a

b

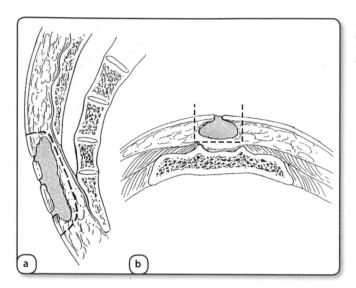

Figure 19.3 Wide and deep excision of sinus to the fascia. (a) Sagittal section, (b) cross-sectional view.

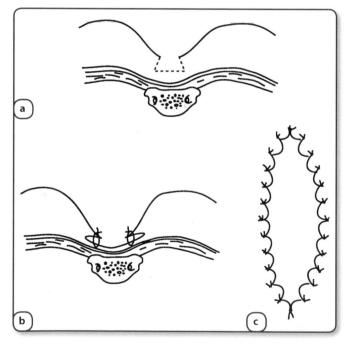

Figure 19.4 Laying-open technique with marsupialization. (a) Overlying tissue is excised. (b) Wound edges are sutured to the base of the wound with absorbable sutures. (c) Appearance of wound at completion of the procedure.

15%. With **excision and primary closure** using oblique or asymmetric incisions the mean healing time dropped to 9 days and the recurrence rate was less than 3%.

Bascom [21] reported less than 10% recurrence with excision of enlarged follicles, with corroborating results by other authors using the same technique [38]. This procedure involved an incision lateral to the midline to scrub the chronic cavity free of hair and granulation tissue (**Figure 19.5a**). Removal of the small midline pits was carried out with small 7 mm incisions (**Figure 19.5b**). When epithelial tubes were present, they were removed through the lateral incision. The lateral wound was then left open but the midline incisions were closed with a removable 4-0 polypropylene subcuticular suture (**Figure 19.5c**).

A nonoperative or conservative approach has been suggested as an alternative to conventional excision [39]. In this approach, meticulous hair control by natal cleft shaving, improved perineal hygiene, and limited lateral incision and drainage for treatment of abscess has resulted in a significant reduction in number of excisional procedures and occupied-bed days. As an added benefit, there is improved patient tolerance and near normal work status during treatment. This concept merits further investigation.

Complex or recurrent disease

Even with proper treatment, a small subgroup of patients are left with persistent, nonhealing wounds. Repeated treatment of complex

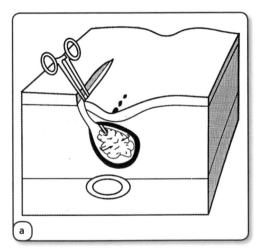

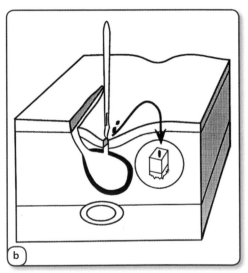

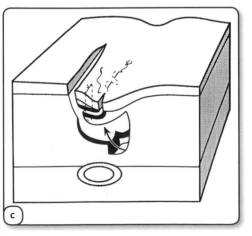

Figure 19.5 Bascom procedure. (a) Lateral incision and debridement of cavity. (b) Removal of a midline pit with a small incision after lateral debridement. (c) Closure of midline wounds without closure of the lateral incision.

or recurrent disease with conventional measures rarely results in satisfactory healing. A number of more aggressive treatments have been described to treat complex or recurrent disease including (but not limited to): wide excision and split thickness skin grafting [40], cleft closure [41], excision and Z-plasty, (**Figure 19.6**) [42–44], modified Z-plasty [45], gluteus maximus myocutaneous flap (**Figure 19.7**) [46], simple V-Y fasciocutaneous flaps [47], rhomboid fasciocutaneous flap [48], multiple flaps [49], U-flap as described by Bascom [50], (**Figure 19.8**) and even reverse bandaging [51]. These **flap techniques** as a group have resulted in primary healing in less than 15 days in 90% of cases [29]. There are, however, disadvantages to these aggressive approaches. Nearly all of these techniques require hospitalization and general anesthesia.

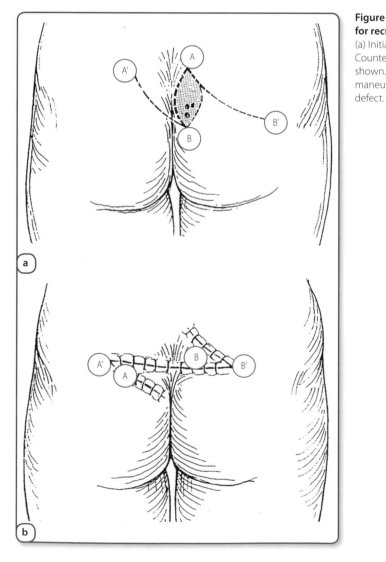

Figure 19.6 Z-plasty technique for recurrent pilonidal disease. (a) Initial excision of the sinus cavity. Counter incisions are created as shown. (b) Flaps are raised and maneuvered as shown to close defect.

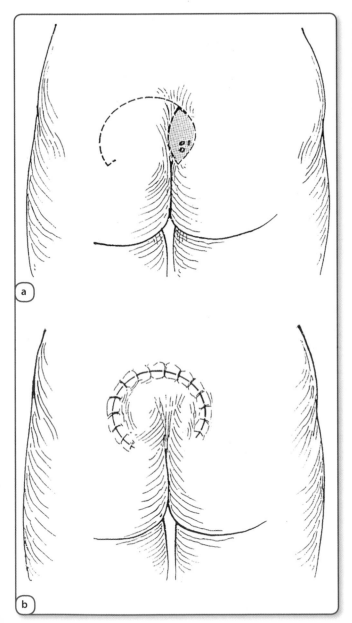

Figure 19.7 Gluteus maximus myocutaneous rotational flap for recurrent disease. (a) Initial excision of the sinus cavity. Skin incisions and division of edge of gluteus muscle create flap as shown. (b) Flap is rotated to close defect.

In addition, up to 50% of those procedures requiring skin flaps for wound coverage or closure develop loss of skin sensation or flap tip necrosis [44].

An extremely rare complication of nonhealing pilonidal disease is squamous cell carcinoma arising from the sinus tract [49, 52, 53]. Most of these tumors are slow growing but with a tendency to aggressive local invasion. Cases typically present after years of long-standing, untreated pilonidal disease. Patients with advanced disease including

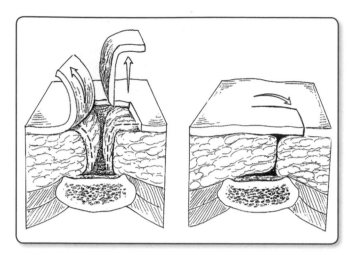

Figure 19.8 U-flap technique as described by Bascom [50] for non-healing midline wounds.

inguinal metastasis had a poor prognosis and most died within 16 months. Long-term survival has been reported in patients treated with aggressive surgical resection and adjuvant radiation therapy and chemotherapy to help reduce local recurrence.

Conclusion

Pilonidal disease has three basic presentations: acute abscess, simple sinus and complex or recurrent disease. Simple incision and drainage of an acute abscess will result in relief of symptoms in nearly all patients. Additional steps at this point may help reduce recurrence rates. Treatment of a simple pilonidal sinus is eventually effective regardless of surgical techniques. Of the many options, wide excision of the sinus tract to the fascia, without flap coverage or marsupialization, should be avoided. This procedure is associated with prolonged healing and comparable recurrence rates when compared with less-morbid procedures. Satisfactory treatment of complex or recurrent disease is possible with good results but often requires an aggressive approach. The use of asymmetric incisions or skin flaps results in reliable primary healing and a low recurrence rate but has a high rate of flap complications.

Rounds questions

1. Is pilonidal disease an acquired or congenital condition?
2. Is pilonidal more common in men or women?
3. How is an acute first-time simple pilonidal abscess treated?
4. What theories explain why pilonidal disease in uncommon after age 40?
5. What types of operative procedures have been used to treat pilonidal disease?

References

1. Anderson AW. Hair extracted from an ulcer. Boston Med Surg J 1847;36:74.
2. Warren JM. Abscess containing hair on the nates. Am J Med Sci 1854;28:112.
3. Hodges RM. Pilo-nidal sinus. Boston Med Surg J 1880;103:485–6.
4. Klass AA. The so-called pilo-nidal sinus. Can Med Assoc J 1956;75:737–42.
5. Franckowiak JJ, Jackman RJ. The etiology of pilonidal sinus. Dis Colon Rectum 1962;5:28–36.
6. Bascom J. Pilonidal disease: Long-term results of follicle removal. Dis Colon Rectum 1983;26:800–7.
7. Goligher JC. Pilonidal sinus. In: Goligher JC (ed). Surgery of the Anus, Rectum and Colon, 4th Ed. London: Bailliere Tindall, 1980;200–14.
8. Powell KR, Cherry JD, Hougen TJ, et al. A prospective search for congenital dermal abnormalities of the craniospinal axis. J Paediatr 1975;87:744–50.
9. Patey DH, Scarff RW. Pathology of postanal pilonidal sinus: Its bearing on treatment. Lancet 1946;2:484–6.
10. Patey DH, Scarff RW. Pilonidal sinus in a barber's hand with observations on postanal pilonidal sinus. Lancet 1948;2:13.
11. Currie AR, Gibson T, Goodall AL. Interdigital sinuses of barbers' hands. Br J Surg 1953;41:278–86.
12. Gannon MX, Crowson MC, Fielding JWL. Periareolar pilonidal abscesses in a hairdresser. Br Med J 1988;297:1641–2.
13. Infection of the breast. In: Hughes LE, Mansel RE, Webster DJT, et al (eds). Benign Disorders and Diseases of the Breast: Concepts and Clinical Management. London: Bailliere Tindall, 1989;149.
14. Griffin SM, McEvilly W, Cole TP. Pilonidal sinus of the penis. Br J Urol 1990;65:422–4.
15. Ohtsuka H, Arashiro K, Watanabe T. Pilonidal sinus of the axilla: Report of five patients and review of the literature. Ann Plast Surg 1994;33:322–5.
16. Sroujieh AS, Dawoud A. Umbilical sepsis. Br J Surg 1989;76:687–8.
17. Banerjee A. Pilonidal sinus of nipple in a canine beautician. Br Med J 1985;291:1787.
18. Bowers PW. Roustabouts' and barbers' breasts. Clin Exp Dermatol 1982;7:445–8.
19. Elliott D, Juyyumi S. A 'pennanidal' sinus. J R Soc Med 1981;74:847–8.
20. Sondenaa K, Pollard ML. Histology of chronic pilonidal sinus. APMIS 1995;103:267–72.
21. Bascom J. Pilonidal disease: Origin from follicles of hairs and results of follicle removal as treatment. Surgery 1980;87:567–72.
22. Sondenaa K, Andersen E, Nesvik I, Soreide JA. Patient characteristics and symptoms in chronic pilonidal sinus disease. Int J Colorectal Dis 1995;10:39–42.
23. Buie LA, Curtis RK. Pilonidal disease. Surg Clin North AM 1952;32:1247–59.
24. Dwight RW, Maloy JK. Pilonidal sinus - experience with 449 cases. N Engl J Med 1953;249:926–30.
25. US Navy. Statistics of Navy medicine: Pilonidal cysts: 1956;12:1950–5.
26. Sebrechts PH. A significant diagnostic sign of pilonidal disease. Dis Colon Rectum 1961;4:56–9.
27. Buie LA. Jeep disease. South Med J 1944;37:103–9.
28. Brook I. Microbiology of infected pilonidal sinuses. J Clin Pathol 1989;42:1140–2.
29. Beck DE. Operative procedures for pilonidal disease. Op Tech Gen Surg: Anorectal Surg I. 2001;3:124–31.
30. Jensen SL, Harling H. Prognosis after simple incision and drainage for a first episode acute pilonidal abscess. Br J Surg 1988;75:60–1.
31. Hanley PH. Acute pilonidal abscess. Surg Gynecol Obstet 1980;150:9–11.
32. O'Connor JJ. Surgery plus freezing as a technique for treating pilonidal disease. Dis Colon Rectum 1979;22:306–7.
33. McLaren CA. Partial closure and other techniques in pilonidal surgery: An assessment of 157 cases. Br J Surg 1984;71:561–2.
34. Sondenaa K, Nesvik I, Gullaksen FP, et al. The role of cefoxitin prophylaxis in chronic pilonidal sinus treated with excision and primary suture. J Am Coll Surg 1995;180:157–60.
35. Schneider IHF, Thaler K, Kockerling F. Treatment of pilonidal sinuses by phenol injections. Int J Colorectal Dis 1994;9:200–2.
36. Feit HL. The use of thorium X in treatment of pilonidal cyst: A preliminary report. Dis Colon Rectum 1960;3:51–64.
37. Allen-Mersh TG. Pilonidal sinus: Finding the right track for treatment. Br J Surg 1990;77:123–32.
38. Mosquera DA, Quayle JB. Bascom's operation for pilonidal sinus. J R Soc Med 1995;88:45–6.
39. Armstrong JH, Barcia PJ. Pilonidal sinus disease: The conservative approach. Arch Surg 1994;129:914–9.
40. Guyuron B, Dinner MI, Dowden RV. Excision and grafting in treatment of recurrent pilonidal sinus disease. Surg Gynecol Obstet 1983;156:201–4.
41. Bascom JU. Repeat pilonidal operations. Am J Surg 1987;154:118–22.

42. Monro RS. A consideration of some factors in the causation of pilonidal sinus and its treatment by Z-plasty. Am J Proctol 1967;18:215–25.
43. McDermott FT. Pilonidal sinus treated by Z-plasty. Aust N Z J Surg 1967;37:64–9.
44. Middleton MD. Treatment of pilonidal sinus by Z-plasty. Br J Surg 1968;55:516–8.
45. Toubanakis G. Treatment of pilonidal sinus disease with the Z-plasty procedure (modified). Am Surg 1986;52:611–2.
46. Perez-Gurri JA, Temple WJ, Ketcham AS. Gluteus maximus myocutaneous flap for the treatment of recalcitrant pilonidal disease. Dis Colon Rectum 1984;27:262–4.
47. Khatri VP, Espinosa MH, Amin AK. Management of recurrent pilonidal sinus by simple V-Y fasciocutaneous flap. Dis Colon Rectum 1994;37:1232–5.
48. Azab AS, Kamal MS, el Bassyoni F. The rationale of using the rhomboid fasciocutaneous transposition flap for the radical cure of pilonidal sinus. J Dermatol Surg Oncol 1986;12:1295–9.
49. Fasching MC, Meland NB, Woods JE, et al. Recurrent squamous-cell carcinoma arising in pilonidal sinus tract-multiple flap reconstructions: Report of a case. Dis Colon Rectum 1989;32:153–8.
50. Bascom J. Pilonidal sinus. In: Fazio V (ed). Current Therapy in Colon and Rectal Surgery. Toronto: BC Decker 1990;32–9.
51. Rosenberg I. The dilemma of pilonidal disease: Reverse bandaging for cure of the reluctant pilonidal wound. Dis Colon Rectum 1977;20:290–1.
52. Jeddy TA, Vowles RH, Southam JA. Squamous cell carcinoma in a chronic pilonidal sinus. Br J Clin Pract 1994;48:160–1.
53. Davis KA, Mock CN, Versaci A, et al. Malignant degeneration of pilonidal cysts. Am Surg 1994;60:200–4.

Sexually transmitted diseases and colorectal infections

Colorectal infections and sexually transmitted diseases (STDs) are important to colorectal surgeons as many of these diseases cause gastrointestinal symptoms and produce lesions in the perineum, anus, and rectum. An explosive growth in the prevalence and variety of STDs has occurred in the past two decades, which can be traced to increases in promiscuity, homosexuality and the use of the anorectum for sexual gratification [1]. Anogenital, oroanal and other anal-based erotic practices have increased, and 4–13% of the adult male population of the United States are predominantly homosexual or bisexual for at least a significant portion of their lives [2,3]. Promiscuity also plays a major role in the transmission of the vast majority of these diseases. It has been estimated that the average homosexual has about 1000 sexual partners during his lifetime [1,2], and other studies suggest that a 'moderately active' homosexual man will have sexual relations with 100 men per year [1].

Sexually transmitted diseases of the anorectum also affect females who participate in anal intercourse. Review of surveys of sexual practices suggests that heterosexual anal intercourse is far more common than generally realized; more than 10% of American women and their male consorts engage in the act with some regularity [1].

The frequent occurrence of STDs (estimated at over 12 million cases a year in the USA) and the gastrointestinal symptoms associated with these infections mandate a high index of suspicion to make an accurate diagnosis [1,4]. Providers must remember that these patients commonly have more than one disease. The diseases presented in this chapter (**Table 20.1**) are divided by etiologic agents. Abscesses and pilonidal infections are covered in other chapters. Medications and dosages are suggested, but clinicians are reminded to consult the full prescribing information before using any medication mentioned in this book.

Viral diseases

Cytomegalovirus

Cytomegalovirus (CMV) is a ubiquitous DNA virus. Positive cultures or serologic studies are very common in immunosuppressed patients.

Table 20.1 Sexually transmitted and infectious organisms that cause anorectal pathology

Organism	Symptoms	Anoscopy and proctoscopy	Laboratory test	Treatment
Viral				
Cytomegalovirus (CMV)	Rectal bleeding	Multiple small white ulcers	Biopsy, viral culture, antigen assay of ulcers	Intravenous ganciclovir foscarnet
Herpes simplex	Anorectal pain, pruritus	Perianal erythema, vesicles, ulcers, diffusely inflamed, friable rectal mucosa	Cytologic examination of scrapings or viral culture of vesicular fluid	Symptomatic: acyclovir, famciclovir, valacyclovir–see text.
Human immunodeficiency virus (AIDS)	See text	See text	Western blot	Nucleoside analogues, non-nucleoside reverse transcriptase inhibitors, protease inhibitors
Human papillomavirus (HPV) (condylomata acuminata)	Pruritus, bleeding, discharge, pain	Perianal warts	Excisional biopsy with viral analysis	Destruction. See text.
Molluscum contagiosum	Painless dermal lesions	Flattened round umbilicated lesions	Excisional biopsy	Excision, cryotherapy
Bacterial				
Campylobacter jejuni	Diarrhea, cramps, bloating	Erythema, edema, grayish-white ulcerations of rectal mucosa	Culture stool using selective media	Erythromycin 500 mg po qid for 7 days
Chlamydia	Tenesmus	Friable, often ulcerated rectal mucosa +/– rectal mass	Serologic antibody titer, biopsy for culture	Doxycycline 100 mg po bid or erythromycin 500 mg po qid for 7 days, azithromycin 1 g po single dose
Lymphogranuloma venereum (LGV)	Enlarged inguinal nodes, fever, malaise, anorexia	Friable, often ulcerated rectal mucosa	Serologic antibody titer, complement fixation test	Doxycycline 100 mg po bid or erythromycin 500 mg po qid for 21 days
Chancroid (Haemophilus ducreyi)	Anal pain	Anorectal abscesses and ulcers	Culture	Erythromycin 500 mg po bid for 7 days, ciprofloxin 500mg po bid for 3 days, single dose ceftriaxone 250 mg IM, single dose azithromycin 1 g PO
Gonorrhea	Rectal discharge	Proctitis, muco- purelent discharge	Thayer – Mayer culture of discharge	Ceftriaxone 125 mg IM for 1 day and doxycycline 100 mg po bid for 7 days

Granuloma inguinale	Perianal mass	Hard, shiny perianal masses	Biopsy of mass	Doxycycline 100 mg po bid, bactrim DS one tab po bid, ciprofloxin 750 mg po bid, erythromycin 500 mg po qid for 21 days – see text
Hidradenitis suppurativa	Pain, discharge from skin	Induration, scarring of subcutaneous tissue, normal rectal mucosa	Culture and biopsy	Complete surgical excision
Mycobacterium avium-intercellulare	Watery diarrhea	Normal	Acid-fast stain of stool; ileal biopsy	Clarithromycin 500 mg po bid or azithromycin 250 mg po qd plus ethambutol 15 mg/kg/day and rifabutin 300 mg po qd – see text
Salmonella	Diarrhea, chills nausea, abdominal pain	Mucosal hyperemia, petechiae	Stool culture	None
Shigella	Abdominal cramps, fever, tenesmus, bloody diarrhea	Erythema, edema, grayish-white ulcerations of rectal mucosa	Stool culture	Trimethoprim-sulfamethoxazole (double strength) po bid for 7 days
Syphilis	Rectal pain	Painful anal ulcer	Dark-field examination of fresh scrapings	Benzathine penicillin 2.4 million units IM
Parasitic				
Amebiasis (*Entamoeba histolytica*)	Bloody diarrhea	Friable rectal mucosa; shallow ulcers with yellowish exudate and ring of erythema	Fresh stool examination (microscopy)	Mitronidazole 750 mg po tid for 10 days, then di-iodohydroxyquin 650 mg po tid for 20 days
Cryptosporidia	Bloody, mucoid diarrhea, dehydration	Normal	Rectal biopsy oocyst	Hydration
Giardia lamblia	Nausea, bloating, cramps, diarrhea	Normal	Fresh stool examination (microscopy)	Mitronidazole 250 mg po tid for 7 days
Isospora	Vomiting, fever, abdominal pain	Normal	Acid-fast stain of stool; endoscopic biopsy	Trimethoprim-sulfamethoxazole (double strength) po bid for 7 days

More than 90% of acquired immunodeficiency syndrome (AIDS) patients develop an active CMV infection [5]. CMV can cause inflammation, hemorrhage, ulceration, or perforation of the gastrointestinal tract. Ileocolitis secondary to CMV is the most common intestinal manifestation of AIDS. Symptomatic CMV proctitis presents with tenesmus, diarrhea, weight loss, melena, or hematochezia. Endoscopic findings vary from submucosal hemorrhage and erythematous patches to multiple wide, deep ulcers. Biopsy helps to confirm the diagnosis. Microscopic findings on biopsy demonstrate vasculitis, neutrophilic infiltration, and large basophilic intranuclear cytomegalic viral inclusions. Viral cultures of the biopsy specimens may also reveal CMV.

Medical treatment of CMV requires either dihydroxypropoxymethyl guanine (DHPG or ganciclovir) or foscarnet [6]. Ganciclovir has a similar formula to acyclovir but is 50 times more effective against CMV [7]. Both ganciclovir and foscarnet are virostatic and must be given intravenously. Relapse of clinical symptoms appears commonly after the drugs are discontinued and thus, life-long therapy may be required. Surgery is required for refractory hemorrhage or perforation. Pathology due to CMV has been a frequent indication for emergency laparotomy in AIDS patients. The most successful results are obtained after subtotal colectomy with end ileostomy. However, these are high-risk procedures in very sick patients and the 30-day mortality exceeds 50% [5].

Herpes simplex

Herpes simplex is a DNA virus that is endemic in the United States population. Two serotypes cause clinical problems. Type 1 (HSV-1) is usually associated with oral lesions and type 2 (HSV-2) is associated with genital infections [1]. However, there is an increasing overlap. Up to 95% of homosexual males have positive serologic tests confirming infection with HSV-2, and 6–30% of homosexual patients with anorectal symptoms will have positive cultures for HSV [1,8]. The Centers for Disease Control and Prevention (CDC) includes chronic mucocutaneous HSV infection in the diagnostic criteria for AIDS [9]. Ulcerative perianal HSV-2 (among other varieties) present for at least one month in a patient with no other identifiable cause of immunodeficiency or who has laboratory-evidenced human immunodeficiency virus (HIV) infection is diagnostic of AIDS.

The virus is transmitted by direct contact to the skin or mucosa and frequently causes symptoms. After a latent period (4–21 days), multiple 1–2 mm vesicular lesions form in infected skin or rectal mucosa (proctitis) [10]. The lesions are painful, contain clear fluid, and may coalesce to aphthous ulcers. The pain associated with proctitis is exacerbated by enemas, intercourse, and bowel movements. Bilateral tender inguinal adenopathy is occasionally seen. Some patients develop a constellation of symptoms associated with lumbosacral radiculopathy (urinary dysfunction, sacral paresthesia, impotence, and pain in the lower abdomen, thighs, and buttocks) [11]. The lesions usually resolve in 1–2 weeks. After the initial lesions resolve, they may recur. In some patients, an inciting factor (e.g. trauma, exposure to sunlight) may be related to the recurrence. Recurrent lesions usually occur in the same dermatome distribution as the initial infection. The disease is highly contagious from the first appearance of the vesicles until re-epithelialization is complete.

Treatment is directed to two areas. First is to provide symptomatic relief of the skin and mucosal lesions. Helpful measures include analgesics, cool compresses, lidocaine ointment, and sitz baths. Hygiene is important to prevent a bacterial superinfection. The second concern is direct treatment of severe active infections or patients with frequent reinfections (more than six per year). Therapy with acyclovir, a synthetic guanine analog, reduces the duration and severity of symptoms, but does not eradicate HSV or cure the disease. The drug does reduce the duration of symptoms and period of viral shedding. Similar results have also been shown with oral famciclovir and valacyclovir [1]. The usual dose of acyclovir is 200–400 mg po five times per day for 10 days. Famciclovir 250 mg po tid or valacyclovir one gram bid may also be used [1]. Suppression therapy is possible with lower doses of these medications.

Human immunodeficiency virus

HIV is an RNA retrovirus that infects human T-lymphocytes [5]. The virus is spread by contaminated body fluids, and after a variable latent period of up to 2 years, it produces diminished immunologic function [12,13]. The incidence of infection with HIV is increasing. The CDC reported more than 540,000 cases of AIDS as of June 1996, with 62% (333,000 patients) having died [14]. Cases have been reported in all states of the United States, and it is estimated that 1–1.5 million American patients have been exposed to the virus. Proctologic conditions are common in HIV patients, and in the absence of routine screening these complaints may be the patient's primary reason for seeking medical help [15, 16]. A systematic approach allows appropriate management of these patients.

The initial evaluation should include a complete history, physical examination, laboratory studies (complete blood cell count [CBC], biochemical profile, serologic tests for common sexually transmitted diseases) and invasive diagnostic procedures (spinal tap). An adequate history is essential to obtain the correct diagnosis for any proctologic complaints. The presenting symptoms should be explored with particular attention given to bowel activity, sexual history, and overall health. A patient's risk for HIV infection or AIDS should be explored with specific questions about sexual preference, intravenous drug usage, and exposure to blood products or to HIV-positive individuals. Alterations in body functions or symptoms may direct the investigations toward specific diseases. In patients who are known to be HIV positive, several systems have been proposed to classify the disease stage. These include the Walter Reed (WR) classification system and that of the CDC (**Table 20.2**). Other articles have discussed these staging systems extensively [17,18]. An essential feature of each system is that early stage patients (WR 1–2 and CDC I–III) have minimal alterations in their gross immunologic or healing ability. Patients with later disease stages (WR 5–6 and CDC IV) have significant immunologic dysfunction, resulting in increased morbidity and mortality. Some authors have attempted to use the absolute T helper cell count to predict healing. Others have not found this helpful [4]. This discrepancy may be explained by the use of newer medications used to treat HIV infection, which may improve a patient's ability to heal despite a low T helper cell count.

In HIV-positive patients with gastrointestinal symptoms, it is essential to evaluate the stool for pathogens by cultures and stains [5,19]. In addition, a biopsy should be performed on any abnormal lesion of the perirectal area or rectal mucosa to complete the evaluation. Since the HIV is transmitted sexually, by use of contaminated needles or by contact with infected body fluids and perhaps tissue, infection control measures are very important. Examiners should observe universal precautions, and any activity with the potential for body fluid contact requires eye and skin protection [2]. Gloves, goggles, mask, and barrier gowns provide the necessary shielding for the examiner. Most patients require only a proctoscopic or anoscopic examination for an adequate evaluation; for convenience, the author uses disposable instruments. Traditional sterilization measures are used should nondisposable instruments be required.

The diseases identified in HIV-positive patients can be grouped into three categories. The first group includes the common proctologic conditions (e.g. hemorrhoids, fissures, pruritus) routinely discovered in the general population [20]. Second are diseases associated with high-risk groups. Diseases associated with homosexuality in males

Table 20.2 CDC classification system for HIV	
Group	Description
I	Acute infection
II	Asymptomatic infection
III	Persistent generalized lymphadenopathy
IV	Other disease
Subgroup A	Constitutional disease
Subgroup B	Neurologic disease
Subgroup C	Secondary infectious diseases
Category C-1	Specific secondary infectious diseases listed in the CDC surveillance definition for AIDS
Category C-2	Other specified secondary infectious diseases
Subgroup D	Secondary cancers, including those within the CDC surveillance definition for AIDS
Subgroup E	Other conditions

Adapted from Classification system for human T-lymphotropic virus type III / lymphadenopathy-associated virus infections. MMWR 1986;35:334–9.

include candidiasis, cryptosporidiosis, cytomegalic inclusion disease, pneumonia (*Pneumocystis carinii*), herpes simplex and herpes zoster, whereas intravenous drug use is associated with hepatitis (hepatitis B virus). The third group are those illnesses associated with HIV infections, such as unusual opportunistic infections, Kaposi's sarcoma, and lymphoma.

The exact incidence of these conditions is not accurately known because of the absence of routine screening and selection biases in the published series. The experience reported by Beck et al [20] in 1990 included 677 HIV-positive patients, most of whom had early stage disease (78% were WR 1 or 2) and were male (95%). Of these patients, 6% had nonsexually related anorectal conditions, whereas more than 60% had at least one other sexually transmitted disease.

Chlamydia and hepatitis were the most common conditions, serology proving positive in 51% and 31%, respectively, followed by anal condylomata (18%). Combining patients with nonsexually related anorectal diseases and those with anal condylomata, 24% had treatable anorectal conditions. Another report of 1117 HIV-positive patients treated at the University of Amsterdam [21] found 7.4% had anorectal disease that required a surgical consultation. Many of these 83 patients had more than one problem, including perianal sepsis (55%), condylomata acuminata (34%), anorectal ulcers (33%), hemorrhoids (17%), invasive anorectal carcinoma (17%), and polyps (11%). Finally, in 1998 Barret et al (22) reported their experience with 260 consecutive human immunodeficiency virus-positive patients with perianal disease between 1989 and 1996. The most common disorders were condyloma (42%), fistula (34%), fissure (32%), and abscess (25%). Neoplasms were present in 7% of patients. Sixty six percent of patients had more than one disorder.

The management of these anorectal conditions in the HIV-positive patient deserves additional comment. Unlike in normal patients, the primary therapeutic goal in HIV-positive patients is to eliminate or reduce symptoms. A secondary goal is resolution of the condition and healing of the wound.

Abscesses with pus usually present with pain and require drainage. Efforts are directed toward keeping the wounds small. Drainage with a latex Pezzer's catheter is very effective [23]. In early stage patients, symptomatic fistulas are treated in the normal fashion (Chapter 13) and can be expected to heal [21]. Late stage patients are treated to minimize symptoms. This usually entails establishing adequate drainage. Performing an extensive procedure to resolve the fistula is contraindicated. These fistulas rarely heal and often result in larger nonhealing wounds.

Anal ulcers (**Figure 20.1**) can be caused by a number of the infectious agents described in this chapter. The ulcers caused by HIV are deep chronic ulcers with overhanging edges. They are often eccentric or multiple, cavitating, and edematous with a bluish-purple hue. It is important to differentiate these HIV anal ulcers from benign

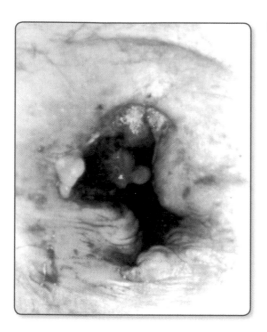

Figure 20.1 Anal ulcer.

anal fissures and neoplasms. Routine anal fissures are either posterior or anterior, accompanied by skin tags, and readily visible when the buttocks are retracted. Anal ulcers usually cause pain when there is 'pocketing' or inadequate drainage of the associated ulcer cavity. Any HIV-positive patient with anal pain should receive an examination under anesthesia to exclude undrained pus. If a deep cavitating ulcer is identified, it should be unroofed to establish drainage; which usually resolves the pain. Gottesman [24] has also recommended injection of a long-acting steroid into the base of the ulcer to relieve symptoms.

HIV patients are afflicated with a variety of neoplastic disorders related to their immunocompromised state [1,24]. Kaposi's sarcoma, non-Hodgkin's lymphoma, and epidermoid anal carcinoma all present as anal masses or ulcers. An incisional biopsy confirms the diagnosis. Unfortunately, the associated immunodeficiency limits therapeutic options, and the prognosis remains poor.

Limited information is available on treatment of the HIV patient. Early studies of HIV-infected patients with perianal disease noted poor healing and high morbidity rates. Recent changes in the systemic treatment of HIV infection and newer drug regimens that include combinations of **protease inhibitors** and nucleoside analogs have greatly improved the prognosis for HIV-infected patients [22]. Certain measures directed at control of infectious organisms are beneficial. Localized infections (e.g. abscesses) require drainage. Previous reports, however, grouped all HIV patients asymptomatic, seropositive, AIDS and AIDS-related complex (ARC) together. Previously cited data reflect findings of markedly altered immunological function associated with advanced disease. These patients had very significant morbidity and mortality, and the results of operative therapy were dismal. The authors have not performed aggressive surgical procedures on late-stage patients. Conservative proctological procedures in early-stage patients have resulted in a good initial outcome, and on follow-up these patients have continued to do well [20, 21].

Treatment of the identified anorectal conditions included stool bulking agents for hemorrhoidal disease and fissures. Abscesses were drained and condylomata, fistulas, or pilonidal disease were treated according to the patient's HIV disease status. Late-stage patients were managed conservatively, whereas early stage patients were offered standard operative procedures as described elsewhere in this book. There were no significant operative complications, and the result of this therapy was similar to that in patients who were not HIV positive.

The published collected experience suggests that 99% of patients who seroconvert (become HIV positive) will eventually progress to clinical AIDS [5]. Early staged patients (CDC I–III) had few complications following anorectal treatment and therapy should be offered if indicated. At present, a vaccine or definitive treatment for the viral infection is not available. Combinations of medications show progress, but investigations are ongoing.

Human papillomavirus

Anal condylomata or condylomata acuminata are the most common STDs seen by colorectal surgeons and result from infection with a human papillomavirus (HPV) (subtypes 6, 11, 16, 18). Subtype 6 is the most common, but subtypes 16 and 18 behave more aggressively and have been more frequently associated with dysplasia and malignant transformation [1]. It is estimated that up to 30–50% of sexually active adults are infected with HPV and it has been found in 40–70% of homosexual men [1, 25]. The highest rates of infection are found in women 19–22 years of age and men 22–26 years of age. Only 1–2% of the infected population have clinically apparent warts of the anogenital region [1]. Ninety percent of patients with anal condylomata admit to anal-receptive intercourse [4].

The natural history of anal condylomata is poorly understood, and occasionally the lesions will spontaneously regress. The lesions can be single or multiple (**Figure 20.2**) and are associated with symptoms of itching, bleeding, discomfort, or difficulty with anal hygiene. Associated genital condylomata are common in 80% of women and 16% of men [1].

Successful therapy requires an accurate diagnosis and eradication of all warts. Multiple types of therapy have included observation, excision, destruction (by a variety of methods-chemicals, fulguration, freezing, laser), and immunotherapy with intralesional injection of d-interferon and other substances [1, 26–28]. Evaluation of each method has been complicated by occasional spontaneous regression of the warts, uncertainty as to whether the warts identified after treatment are true recurrences or reinfection, and the lack of prospective controlled clinical trials. Results of therapy have varied with reported recurrence rates of

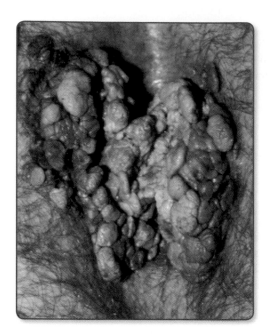

Figure 20.2 Anal condylomata.

50–75% [4]. The method used to destroy the warts appears to be less important than limiting the damage to the surrounding normal skin.

Chemical destruction has been accomplished with two agents. Podophyllin is the resin of podophyllum, an agent which is cytoxic to condylomata and very irritating to normal skin. It is generally applied in either liquid paraffin or tincture of benzoin, the latter adhering best to the warts. Although concentrations of 5–50% have been used, a 25% suspension is readily available and seems optimal. The mixture is carefully applied directly to the condylomata, ensuring that the intervening normal skin bridges are not treated. A sharpened wooden dowel is a good vehicle of delivery. After application, talcum powder is applied to the skin. Six to eight hours later the patient should thoroughly wash the entire area to prevent skin damage.

Because of autoinoculation, multiple treatments are often required. Furthermore, because podophyllin is toxic to skin or mucosa, it cannot be applied to anal canal warts. Local complications include skin necrosis, fistula-in-ano, dermatitis, and anal stenosis. In addition, large doses may result in systemic effects including hepatic, renal, gastrointestinal, respiratory, and neurological problems [1]. Particularly disturbing is the fact that podophyllin causes histological changes in the treated warts that are difficult to distinguish from carcinoma in situ.

Bichloroacetic acid (BCAA) or trichloracetic acid (TCAA) can also be applied to warts in a way similar to applying podophyllin. The major differences are that BCAA or TCAA can be applied to anal canal warts, does not have systemic toxicity, and does not cause histological changes which mimic carcinoma in situ. The recurrence rate is approximately 25% after a mean of five treatments, and up to 13 treatments are necessary to achieve resolution of the condylomata [1]. Treatments can be performed weekly.

Laser destruction of these lesions is expensive and has not offered any advantage over cheaper methods [29]. In addition, concern has been expressed about the presence of viral particles in the smoke produced by the laser [4]. Special filter masks and devices to evacuate the smoke have been used to reduce this hazard. I have found fulguration using electrocautery to be accurate, inexpensive, and effective.

Electrocoagulation requires the use of local or regional anaesthesia. The aim is to produce a white coagulum, which is the equivalent of a superficial second-degree burn. The procedure is best effected with a high current setting. Patients are prepared and positioned as described for excision. The cautery tip is placed near, but not into, the wart and a spark gap is created [1]. A white coagulum is produced which can then be wiped away. If any black eschar appears, a deep second or third-degree burn has been created. This is a major drawback to this procedure, especially in the anal canal. The procedure may also cause intense pain and sphincter spasm, both during and after the procedure. For this reason a general an esthetic may be necessary when a large volume of condylomata are present. Furthermore, an ample quantity of oral analgesics should be given to the patient on discharge home. Obviously anal stenosis is a potential complication. Recurrence rates range from 10–25%.

During operative therapeutic procedures, biopsy samples of several of the condylomata should be sent for pathologic review to confirm the clinical diagnosis and exclude the presence of an invasive squamous cell cancer (Buschke–Lowenstein tumor) that may mimic condylomata. Imiquimod is a topical drug that has an immunomodulatory effect. This treatment is unique from all other recommended therapies for condylomas in that it does not rely on physical destruction of the lesions, but is directed at eradication of the causative agent, HPV. Through immune mechanisms, imiquimod enhances cell-mediated cytolytic activity against HPV. Imiquimod should be applied topically at bedtime, three times per week, for a maximum of 16 weeks. On the morning after application (6–10 hours later), the treated area should be cleansed with soap and water. Warts may clear in 8–10 weeks, or earlier. Several clinical studies have shown improved efficacy and lower recurrence rates with imiquimod, when compared with placebo or other treatment modalities. Local skin reactions including erythema, erosion, excoriation, and flaking are common and are usually mild to moderate in severity. Systemic reactions have not been reported. Imiquimod has not been studied for use during pregnancy, although it is not a teratogen [30].

An unusual problem is the management of condylomata in HIV-positive patients. Beck et al [31] reported on 119 HIV-positive patients with anal condylomata who comprised 18% of the authors' overall HIV patients and whose demographic characteristics and risk factors were similar to those of the other HTV-positive patients. Sixty percent of these patients also had a least one other sexually transmitted disease. Based on their experience, Beck et al recommended that asymptomatic and late stage HIV-positive patients with anal condylomata be observed. Symptomatic patients with warts limited to the anal margin are treated with one to two applications of bichloracetic or trichloracetic acid, and patients with anal canal lesions are offered excision and fulguration with a general or regional anesthetic.

Molluscum contagiosum

Molluscum contagiosum is caused by a virus of the pox group and is transmitted by direct body contact. After an incubation period of 3–6 weeks, 3 mm, painless, flattened, round, umbilicated lesions develop. Biopsy with viral analysis confirms the diagnosis. Although the disease is benign and self-limiting, treatment is used to prevent spread and for cosmetic purposes. Options include local destruction with phenol, surgical removal, and cryotherapy [4]. Antiviral and immunomodulatory therapies include topical imiquimod and cidofovir [1].

Bacterial diseases

Campylobacter jejuni

Campylobacter jejuni is a common cause of enterocolitis or infectious diarrhea. This curved, motile, non-spore-forming gram negative rod can be transmitted by ingestion of infected milk or meat. Sexual transmission is uncertain. The organism infects the small and large bowel and produces endotoxins similar to *Vibrio cholerae* [32]. After an incubation period of 1–5 days, the patient develops crampy diarrhea containing some blood, associated with abdominal pain. These infections are usually self-limited and resolve without sequelae within 1 week. The diagnosis is confirmed by stool culture. If symptoms persist for more than 1 week or if recurrent attacks occur, the patient can be treated with erythromycin, 500 mg qid orally for 7 days.

Chlamydia

Chlamydia are small intracellular organisms, related to bacteria, and have been implicated in a number of clinical syndromes including cervicitis, nongonococcal urethritis and proctitis. Chlamydial infection is currently the most common STD, with over an estimated 3 million cases in the United States [1]. Of the 15 known immuno-types, serotypes D–K are responsible for proctitis.

Symptoms result from inflammation of the infected mucosa, and include fever, malaise, anorexia, headache, joint pain, tenesmus, rectal pain, and a mucoid or bloody rectal discharge. Sigmoidoscopic findings generally include severe non-specific granular proctitis with mucosal erythema, friability, and ulceration. Late findings may include an intraluminal stricture or mass. Treatment includes doxycycline, 100 mg po bid for 7 days or azithromycin 1.0 g po as a single dose. Routine follow-up cultures are not needed, but all sexual partners should be treated simultaneously.

Lymphogranuloma venereum (LGV) is caused by L 1–3 serotypes of *Chlamydia trachomatis*. After a 1- to 4-week incubation period a small vesicular lesion develops. This lesion resolves quickly and the inguinal lymph nodes enlarge. The enlarged nodes progress to an indurated mass with erythema of the overlying skin. This may be associated with malaise, anorexia, fever, headache, and joint pain. Chronic inflammation of the lymph nodes may result in lymphedema, and rectal strictures may occur as a late complication [4,33]. The diagnosis is confirmed by a complement fixation test or the more sensitive microimmunofluorescent antibody titer [4]. Treatment includes tetracycline HCl, 500 mg po qid, for more than 2 weeks or doxycycline hyclate, 100 mg po bid for 14 days.

Chancroid

Chancroid is caused by *Haemophilus ducreyi*, a small, gram negative, nonmotile, non-spore-forming, aerobic bacillus. The infection is characterized by adenopathy, multiple perineal abscesses, and ulcers. The diagnosis is confirmed by culture. Treatment is with erythromycin, 500 mg po bid for 7 days or trimethoprim/sulfamethoxazole, one double-strength tablet po bid for 7 days. The antibiotic susceptibility of this organism varies. If clinical improvement does not occur after the initial course of therapy, another antibiotic should be tried. Resolution of the adenopathy will lag behind resolution of the ulcers [34].

Gonorrhea

Gonorrhea is a common disease with an annual incidence of 3 million cases [35]. The causative organism, *Neisseria gonorrhoeae*, can infect the mucous lining of all body orifices. Up to 55% of homosexual men seen in screening clinics harbor gonorrhea [36]. After a 2- to 5-day incubation period this organism produces an inflammatory response of varying degree. Up to half of anorectal infections may he asymptomatic. When symptoms occur, they consist of discharge and discomfort. Proctoscopy will reveal edematous mucosa with a pus discharge. Ulceration is rare and the abnormal mucosa is usually limited to the rectum.

The diagnosis is confirmed by culture. Swabs of the oral pharynx, urethra, vagina, or rectum should be placed in an aerobic medium (e.g. Thayer–Martin) and rapidly transported to a laboratory. Treatment of this common infection has been complicated by the increasing incidence of resistant strains. Current recommendations for treatment include a single dose of ceftriaxone 250 mg IM plus doxycycline 100 mg po bid for seven days [37]. Other treatment regimens include ceftriaxone and, cefixime plus azithromycin or doxycycline and ciprofloxin plus azithromycin or doxycycline [38]. AS with all other STDs, all sexual contacts must be treated and close follow-up is essential to confirm disease eradication.

Granuloma inguinale

Granuloma inguinale is caused by *Klebsiella granulomatis*, a gram negative bacillus. It produces chronic granulomatous infections that present as hard and shining masses in the perianal area. The diagnosis is confirmed by biopsy. Treatment is doxycycline 100 mg po bid or trimethroprim-sulfamethoxazole, one double strength po bid. Alternative regimens include ciprofloxin 750 mg po bid or erythromycin 500 mg po qid. All of these regimens are administered for a minumim of 3 weeks or until all lesions have healed [1].

Hidradenitis suppurativa

Hidradenitis suppurativa, a common cutaneous condition, results from infection of apocrine skin glands located deep in the subcutaneous tissue and connected to the skin surface via ducts [39, 40]. The highest concentration of these glands occurs in the axilla, neck, groin, and perianal areas, which explains their frequent involvement. Approximately one-third of cases occur in the perianal area. The condition is also related to gland function and thus is uncommon before puberty. Its highest incidence is in early adulthood and is associated with acne. While the exact cause is unknown, stasis of gland secretions is a factor. The retained secretions become infected and abscesses are formed. The abscesses form a tract laterally or toward the skin surface. The natural mechanisms to prevent spread of the infection and to encourage healing result in formation of granulation tissue and fibrosis. Progression of the infectious processes may result in the formation of large, undermined subcutaneous areas, tracts, and sinuses. The organisms commonly cultured include *Staphylococcus* and other skin organisms.

Physical findings will vary with the extent of the disease. Acute early lesions will appear as localized, tender, subcutaneous nodules that may spontaneously resolve or persist and progress to larger lesions.

Treatment requires adequate drainage and removal of granulation tissue, or complete excision of all infected tissue [39–41]. Adequate drainage is obtained by unroofing all subcutaneous cavities and opening all sinuses and fistulas. Removal of the granulation tissue and infected tissue with a curette will allow the area to heal by secondary intention. To speed final closure, skin grafts may be used after the granulation tissue has adequately filled in the defect. This method is effective and minimizes the amount of tissue removed. However, it requires lengthy postoperative wound care [42]. To improve healing, some authors completely excise all involved tissue. As the infection involves only the subcutaneous tissue, dissection can stop at the fascia. The resultant wounds can be closed primarily using flaps or can be allowed to close by secondary intention [43]. Recurrence can occur if all infected tissue is not eliminated. Additional surgery is usually required. Suppressive oral antibiotics have a limited role in selected patients.

Mycobacterium avium-intercellulare

Mycobacterium avium-intercellulare (MAI) are opportunistic microorganisms that produce profuse watery diarrhea, dehydration, and severe abdominal pain [4]. The diagnosis is confirmed by acid-fast stains of the stool or ileal colonoscopic biopsies that demonstrate macrophages filled with acid-fast mycobacteria. Treatment for intestinal MAI is discouraging, because these organisms are usually resistant to standard antituberculosis agents. Newer agents such as clofazimine and ansamycin are being evaluated.

Salmonella

The *Salmonella* species, of which *Salmonella typhi* is the best known, are motile gram negative rods that invade the small bowel and colonic mucosa, produce an endotoxin, and induce an enterocolitis [32]. Transmission is by ingestion of contaminated food or water or through fecal-oral contact. Symptoms develop within 48 hours of ingestion and include diarrhea (usually non-bloody), nausea, vomiting, fever, chills, colicky abdominal pain, and tenesmus. The diarrhea is usually self-limited and resolves in a week. A few patients go on to become asymptomatic carriers. Sigmoidoscopy reveals hyperemia, petechiae, and occasionally ulcerations. Diagnosis is established by stool cultures. Because the disease is self-limited, antimicrobial therapy is not necessary.

Shigella species

Infections with *Shigella* species (gram negative rods) result in a bacillary dysentery. After an incubation period of 1–7 days the patient develops a high fever, colicky abdominal pain, and bloody diarrhea. Arthropy and inflammatory eye changes have been described that accompany the diarrhea. The entire colon may be affected by mucosal edema, hemorrhage, and necrosis. The bacteria remain in the colon and are excreted in high concentrations in the stool.

The diagnosis is suggested by the clinical picture just described and a history of travel to endemic areas or contact with infected individuals. Sigmoidoscopy reveals inflamed, eccymotic, friable, or ulcerated mucosa. Confirmation of the diagnosis is made by isolation of *Shigella* from the stool [32]. Severe cases may require fluid and electrolyte replacement. If clinical symptoms permit, antibiotics are withheld until the diagnosis has been confirmed by culture. The organism is sensitive to treatment with trimethoprim/sulfamethoxazole (one double-strength tablet po bid for 7 days), tetracycline, or ampicillin.

Syphilis

Syphilis, one of the oldest infectious diseases, remains common. The causative agent (*Treponema pallidum*) is a motile spirochete that produces a primary chancre 2–5 weeks after infection at the site of contact [4]. The chancre is a raised 1–2 cm circular indurated lesion that may occur at the anal margin or canal (**Figure 20.3**). The lesions are eccentrically located, multiple or irregular, usually painful, and associated with a discharge and inguinal adenopathy. Chancres heal spontaneously in 2–4 weeks [44]. Proctitis accompanied by tenesmus, mucoid discharge, and rectal pain in the absence of symptoms has also

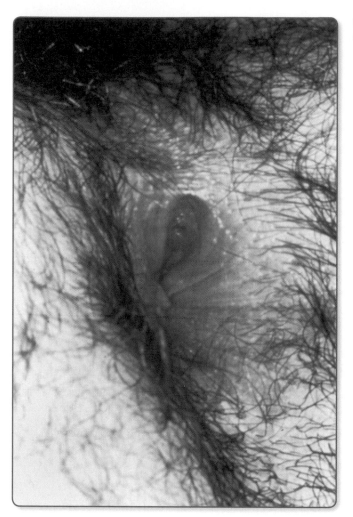

Figure 20.3 Anal chancre (from syphilis).

been reported [4]. The second stage of syphilis appears several weeks later and presents as fever, malaise, lymphadenopathy, anogenital arthropathy, and disseminated cutaneous eruptions that mimic many other skin diseases. In addition, the patient develops multiple, raised, flat lesions (condylomata lata) around the anus that produce an exudate rich in *Treponema*. If syphilis is untreated for several years, the tertiary stage develops, with involvement of the nervous and vascular system and formation of gummata.

The clinical disease can be confirmed in several ways. Dark-field microscopic examination of the exudate from the primary chancre or condylomata lata will demonstrate *Treponema pallidum*. Additional confirmation is provided by serologic tests. The rapid plasma reagin (RPR) and the venereal disease research laboratory slide test (VDRL) are nonspecific screening tests. The RPR can be automated and is used in mass screening of serum. The VDRL also uses serum and has greater specificity. Both tests become positive within 1–2 weeks of infection and may remain positive for long periods even after treatment. The fluorescent treponemal antibody-absorption test (FTA-ABS) is a serum test that uses an indirect immunofluorescence method. It also becomes positive 2 weeks after infection but converts to a negative range after treatment. It is specific and sensitive but more expensive [4].

Because multiple infections are common with sexually transmitted diseases, each patient should be completely evaluated. This includes swabs of the genitourinary tract, oral cavity, and rectum. Treatment for syphilis is guided by the stage of disease. Patients with early syphilis can be treated with benzathine penicillin G, 2.4 million U IM, or erythromycin, 500 mg po qid for 15 days. Patients with late syphilis require benzathine penicillin G, 2.4 million U IM for 3 successive weeks, or tetracycline, 500 mg po qid for 30 days. Patients with syphilis for longer than 1 year or symptoms of neural involvement require a cerebral spinal fluid (CSF) examination. If the CSF is involved, additional therapy is indicated.

Parasitic diseases

Amebiasis

Entamoeba histolytica is a protozoan that commonly infects humans [1]. Transmission is related to sanitation measures, and this organism is endemic in several portions of the world (e.g. Mexico, Russia, rural United States). After amebic cysts contaminating food or drink are ingested, the ameba invades the gut mucosa and submucosa, producing ulcers that may become secondarily infected by bacteria. The ameba may also penetrate the bowel wall and pass through the portal venous system to the liver, where it may produce amebic abscesses.

Following an incubation period of 7–10 days, the disease may take several forms. The most common is an acute infection that produces diarrhea; this may be severe enough to result in dehydration. The attack is usually self-limited and resolves after several days. A more severe colonic infection may progress to a toxic colonic dilatation, which is often fatal. Some patients develop recurrent, intermittent attacks of diarrhea or amebic dysentery. A final pattern is an asymptomatic carrier state that may or may not have been associated with one of the acute presentations. In all forms, amebic cysts are passed intermittently in the stool. The diagnosis can be confirmed by identification of ameba or cysts in stool, pus, or mucosal biopsy Amebic blood titers may also be useful.

Therapy includes metronidazole, 750 mg po tid, plus a luminal amebicide such as diiodohydroxyquin (Iodoquinol), 650 mg po tid for 20 days. Large liver abscesses will usually require drainage and intravenous administration of metronidazole.

Cryptosporidiosis

Cryptosporidia are tiny protozoans that inhabit intestinal microvilli [4]. In immunocompromised patients, they can cause a life-threatening colitis characterized by profuse, bloody mucoid diarrhea. Demonstration of characteristic oocysts with an acid-fast stain of stool or endoscopic biopsy establishes the diagnosis. Treatment is supportive with intravenous hydration and nutrition. Antiparasitic agents have failed to be helpful.

Giardiasis

Giardia lamblia are intestinal flagellates that inhabit the upper small intestine and biliary tract of infected individuals [5]. While they do not infect the lower gastrointestinal tract, they may produce symptoms of diarrhea, flatulence, crampy abdominal pain, steatorrhea, and malabsorption syndromes. The diagnosis can be confirmed by observation of trophozoites or characteristic cysts in stool or jejunal biopsies. Asymptomatic and infected patients should receive metronidazole, 250 mg po tid for 7 days.

Isospora

Isospora beli is an opportunistic protozoan with a lower incidence than *Cryptosporidium*. Symptoms associated with this organism are similar to *Cryptosporidium* (diarrhea, vomiting, fever, and abdominal pain), but the quantity of diarrhea is usually less. Diagnosis is made by a modified acid-fast stain of fresh stool or endoscopic biopsy. Fortunately, this organism is well controlled by trimethoprim/sulfamethoxazole [4].

Rounds questions

1. What effects can cytomegalovirus (CMV) cause to the gastrointestinal tract?
2. What type of viruses are herpes simplex and HIV?
3. How is HIV transmitted?
4. What do HIV anal ulcers look like?
5. What is the causative agent for anal condylomata?
6. What is the most common STD and what diseases does it cause?
7. What type of culture medium is used to grow *Neisseria gonorrhea*?
8. What is hidradenitis suppurativa?
9. What blood tests are used to document syphilis infections?
10. What patterns of disease can *Entamoeba histolytica* cause?

References

1. Beck DE, Ramirez RT. Sexually transmitted diseases and the anorectum. In: Phillips RKS (ed). Colorectal Surgery, 2nd ed. London: Harcourt, 2001;365–95.
2. Willcox RR. The rectum as viewed by the venereologist. Br J Vener Dis 1981;57:1–6.
3. Kinsey AC, Pomeroy WB, Martin LE. Sexual behavior in the human male. Philadelphia: WB Saunders, 1948;650–1.
4. Wexner SD, Beck DE. Sexually transmitted and infectious diseases. In: Beck DE, Wexner SD, (eds). Fundamentals of Anorectal Surgery. New York: McGraw-Hill: 1992;402–22.
5. Wexner SD Beck DE. Acquired immunodeficiency syndrome. In: Beck DE, Wexner SD, (eds). Fundamentals of Anorectal Surgery. New York: McGraw-Hill, 1992;423–39.
6. Modesto VL, Gottesman L. Sexually transmitted diseases and anal manifestations of AIDS. Surg Clin North Am 1994;74:1433–64.
7. Smith LE. Sexually transmitted diseases. In: Gordon PH, Nivatvongs S (eds). Principles and practice of surgery for the colon, rectum, and anus. St Louis: Quality Medical Publishing, 1992;317–36.
8. Goldmeier D. Proctitis and herpes simplex virus in homosexual men. Br J Vener Dis 1980; 56:111–14.
9. Revision of the CDC surveillance case definition for acquired immunodeficiency syndrome. MMWR 1987; 36:1s–15s.
10. Beck DE. Sexually transmitted and infectious diseases. In: Beck DE, Welling DR, (eds). Patient Care in Colorectal Surgery. Boston: Little, Brown, 1991;267–78.
11. Samarasinghe PL, Oates JK, MacLennan IPB. Herpetic proctitis and sacral radiculomyelopathy–a hazard for homosexual men. Br Med J 1974;2:365–6.
12. Ranki A, Valle S-L, Krohn M, et al. Long latency precedes overt seroconversion in sexually transmitted human-immunodeficiency-virus infection. Lancet 1987;2:589–93.
13. Lifson AR, Rutherford GW, Jaffe HW. The natural history of human immnnodeficiencyvirus infection. J Infect Dis 1988;158:1360–7.
14. Massachusetts Medical Society. Morbidity and Mortality Weekly Report. 1995;44;849–53.
15. Dworkin B, Wormser GP, Rosenthal WS, et al. Gastrointestinal manifestations of the acquired immunodeficiency syndrome: A review of 22 cases. Am J Gastroenterol 1985;80:774–8.
16. Gelb A, Miller S. AIDS and gastroenterology. Am J Gastroenterol 1986;81:619–22.
17. Redfield RR, Wright DC, Tramont EC. The Walter Reed classification for HTLV-III/LAV infection. N Engl J Med 1986;314:131–2.
18. Classification system for human T-lymphotropic virus type III/lymphadenopathy-associated virus infections. MMWR 1986;35:334–9.
19. Goldberg GS, Orkin BA, Smith LE. Microbiology of human immunodeficiency virus anorectal disease. Dis Colon Rectum 1994;37:439–43.
20. Beck DE, Jaso RG, Zajac RA. Proctologic management of the HIV-positive patient. South Med J 1990;83:900–3.
21. Consten ECJ, Slors FJM, Noten HJ, et al. Anorectal surgery in human immunodeficiency virus-infected patients. Clinical outcome in relation to immune status. Dis Colon Rectum 1995;38:1169–75.
22. Barrett WL, Callahan TD, Orkin BA. Perianal manifestations of human immunodificiency virus infection: experience with 260 patients. Dis Colon Rectum 1998;41:606–12.
23. Beck DE, Fazio VW, Lavery IC, et al. Catheter drainage of ischiorectal abscesses. South Med J 1988;81:444–6.
24. Gottesman L. Treatment of anorectal ulcers in the HIV-positive patient. Perspect Colon Rectal Surg 1991;419–33.
25. Carr G, William DC. Anal warts in a population of gay men in New York City. Sex Transm Dis 1977;4:56–7.
26. Thomson JPS, Grace RH. The treatment of perianal and anal condylomata acuminata: A new operative technique. J R Soc Med 1978;71:180–5.
27. Swerdlow DB, Salvati EP. Condyloma acuminatum. Dis Colon Rectum 1971;14:226–31.
28. Abcarian H, Smith D, Sharon D. The immunotherapy of anal condyloma acuminatum. Dis Colon Rectum 1976;19:237–44.
29. Billingham RP, Lewis FG. Laser versus electrical cautery in the treatment of condylomata acuminata of the anus. Surg Gynecol Obstet 1982;155:865–7.
30. Brown TJ, Yen-Moore A, Tyring SK. An overview of sexually transmitted diseases. Part II. J Am Acad Dermatol 1999;41:661–77.
31. Beck DE, Jaso RG, Zajac RA. Surgical management of anal condylomata in the HIV-positive patient. Dis Colon Rectum 1990;33:180–3.

32. Whelan RL. Other proctitides. In: Beck DE, Wexner SD (eds). Fundamentals of Anorectal Surgery. New York: McGraw-Hill, 1992;477–500.
33. Goligher JC. Sexually transmitted diseases. In: Goligher JC, (ed). Diseases of the Anus, Rectum, and Colon, 5th ed. London: Bailliere Tindall, 1985;1033–45.
34. Baker DA. Clinical management of sexually transmitted diseases, vol 2. Treatment and management of STDs. Charlotte: Burroughs Wellcome, 1989.
35. Gordon PH, Nivatvongs S (eds). Principles and Practice of Surgery for the Colon, Rectum, and Anus. St. Louis: Quality Medical Publishing, 1992;317–25.
36. Ostrow DG, Shaskey D, Stiffen, et al. Epidemiology of gonorrhea infections in gay men. J Homosex 1980;5:285–9.
37. U.S. Department of Health and Human Services. Sexually transmitted diseases treatment guidelines. MMWR 1993;42(RR-14):1–102.
38. Danielsson D, Johannisson G. Culture diagnosis of gonorrhoea: a comparison of the yield with selective and non-selective gonococcal culture media inoculated in the clinic and after transport of specimens. Acta Derm Venereol 1973; 53:75–80.
39. Karulf RE. Hidradenitis suppurativa and pilonidal disease. In: Beck DE, Wexner SD, (eds). Fundamentals of Anorectal Surgery. New York: McGraw-Hill, 1992;183–91.
40. Mitchell KM, Beck DE. Hidradenitis suppurativa. Surg Clin North Am 2002;82:1187–97.
41. Bascom J. Pilonidal disease: Long-term results of follicle removal. Dis Colon Rectum 1983;26:800–7.
42. Khoury DA. Surgery for pilonidal disease and hidradenitis suppurativa. In: Hicks TC, Beck DE, Timmcke AE, Opelka FG (eds). Complications of Colon & Rectal Surgery. Baltimore: Williams & Wilkins 1996;203–21.
43. Allen-Mersh TG. Pilonidal sinus: Finding the right track for treatment. Br J Surg 1990;77:123–32.
44. Milsom JW. Anorectal veneral infection. In: Fazio VW (ed). Current Therapy in Colon and Rectal Surgery. Philadelphia: BC Decker 1990;52–8.

A polyp is a grossly visible protrusion extending into the colonic lumen from the mucosa or submucosa. Understanding polyps is important because of the symptoms they create as well as their potential to become malignant. Colonic polyps may present as asymptomatic lesions that are discovered during endoscopy or on barium enema, or they may produce symptoms of bleeding, intussusception, or obstruction. The various types of polyps include hamartomas, hyperplastic colonic epithelium, inflammatory polyps, and neoplastic lesions. Neoplastic polyps have the potential to deteriorate into carcinoma. This chapter discusses normal colonic histology, the major classes of polyps, and the polyposis syndromes.

Histopathology

Normal colonic epithelium

The colonic mucosa contains three main elements. The surface of the mucosa is called the colonic epithelium and the majority of colonic polyps arise from this layer. Beneath the epithelium is the lamina propria. Nestled under the lamina propria lies the muscularis mucosa, intertwined with the mucosal lymphatics.

The **normal colonic epithelium** contains straight test tube-shaped (tubular) glands, called crypts of Lieberkuhn, aligned parallel to each other and perpendicular to the muscularis mucosae (**Figure 21.1**). The lower third of the crypts, the normal proliferative compartment, is lined with immature dividing colonocytes. As cells migrate upward along the tubular crypt toward the lumen of the bowel, they differentiate into mature goblet cells or mature absorptive cells [1]. Each crypt is invested by a pericryptal fibroblastic sheath suspended in loose areolar connective tissue, the **lamina propria** [2]. The fibroblasts proliferate in the lowest portion of the crypt and mature as they migrate toward the epithelial lining of the bowel lumen. The lamina propria, which envelops the crypts of Lieberkuhn, is rich in mononuclear cells and capillaries. It contains a few blind ends of lymphatic vessels, reaching upward from the submucosa. The majority of lymphatics are first encountered as a plexus at the level of the **muscularis mucosae**, a narrow band of smooth muscle that marks the anatomic boundary between the mucosa and the submucosa [3]. Invasive carcinoma is declared when the muscularis mucosa is invaded by neoplastic cells.

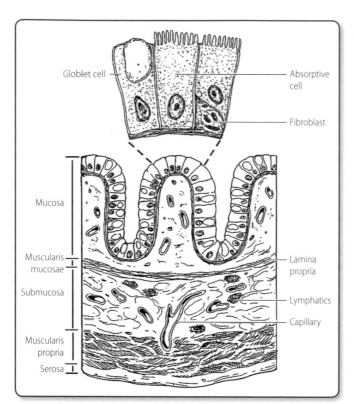

Figure 21.1 Normal histology of the colorectum.

Globlet cell

Absorptive cell

Fibroblast

Mucosa

Muscularis mucosae

Lamina propria

Submucosa

Lymphatics

Capillary

Muscularis propria

Serosa

If abnormalities develop in the colonic epithelium with increased cellular proliferation, polyps develop. Morphologically, polyps are divided into two groups, pedunculated and sessile polyps. **Pedunculated polyps** are attached to the colon by a pedicle or stalk, which consists of an outer layer of colonic mucosa and an inner core of submucosa [2]. **Sessile polyps** have no stalk and are attached directly to the underlying colonic submucosa. Histologically, polyps have been devided into four classes: hamartomas, hyperplastic polyps, inflammatory polyps, and adenomatous polyps.

Hamartomas

Hamartomas are polyps with morphologically normal epithelial cells arranged within an excessive connective tissue stroma in an abnormal location. They are uncommon and occur in three forms: juvenile polyps, in Cronkhite–Canada syndrome, and in Peutz–Jeghers syndrome.

Juvenile polyps

Juvenile polyps are usually found in children under 10 years old [4]. The pattern of age distribution is bimodal. The childhood group peaks at age 4, and the adult group at age 18. In children, males are affected twice as often as females and in adults this ratio expands to 13:1.

Rectal bleeding is the most common presenting symptom. Autoamputation occurs in up to 10% of the cases. Eighty percent of the polyps are located within 20 cm of the anal verge. Juvenile polyps are usually pedunculated and are composed of cystically dilated glands filled with mucus and inspissated inflammatory debris. This hamartoma has no neoplastic potential.

Juvenile polyps can be diagnosed and removed with sigmoidoscopy or colonoscopy. Most patients have a single polyp, but approximately 30% have multiple polyps. Occasionally patients present with multiple juvenile polyps. This is called **juvenile polyposis syndrome**, as described by McColl et al [5]. These patients frequently have a family history of adenoma, polyposis, and colonic carcinoma. The small bowel and stomach may also bear these polyps. Adenomatous polyps, interspersed with juvenile polyps, may be present in this syndrome. Patients with juvenile polyposis coli have a much different clinical course. Patients with massive polyposis develop iron-deficiency anemia, hypoproteinemia, hypokalemia, failure to thrive, and finger clubbing. Juvenile polyposis syndrome is a potentially premalignant condition. Unless the entire colon can be cleared of polyps, a total abdominal colectomy with ileorectal anastomosis or restorative proctocolectomy must be considered.

Cronkhite–Canada syndrome

Cronkhite–Canada syndrome is characterized by gastrointestinal polyposis, hyperpigmentation, alopecia, and nail dystrophy [6]. It is felt to be a variant of juvenile polyposis with ectodermal changes and without evidence of genetic transmission. Diarrhea and malabsorption produce severe vitamin deficiency, hypoproteinemia, and fluid and electrolyte abnormalities. Other symptoms and signs include anemia, rectal bleeding, abdominal pain, weakness, nausea, vomiting, loss of taste, and a variety of neurologic complaints. Hair loss and nail and skin changes may be evident before the gastrointestinal symptoms become apparent.

Pentz–Jeghers syndrome

In this rare disease, polyposis of the alimentary tract occurs in conjunction with pigmented spots in the skin and buccal mucosa. Polyps are found more frequently in the small bowel, particularly in the jejunum, and less often in the stomach and large intestine. These are hamartomatous lesions, with the essential microscopic abnormality being a malformation of the muscularis mucosae. Peutz–Jeghers polyps commonly occur in adolescence and early adulthood. The disease is transmitted in an autosomal dominant fashion.

The most common and troublesome symptom is abdominal pain, often caused by intestinal obstruction, which results from a polyp or intussusception. The other signs and symptoms are rectal bleeding, prolapse of a polyp, passage of a polyp, hematemesis, and anemia. Diagnosis is made by family history, mucocutaneous lesions, gastrointestinal symptoms, and contrast studies.

Controversy surrounds the association of this syndrome with malignancy [7]. In a literature review by Konishi et al [8]. 117 neoplasms were detected in 103 patients. Fifty carcinomas developed in the gastrointestinal tract, the colon and rectum being the most common site. A number of these tumors arose within the Peutz–Jeghers polyps, but many also originated from normal mucosa. On the other hand, the Mayo Clinic [9] did not document a single definite case of malignancy in a median follow-up period of 33 years.

Many of these young patients undergo multiple abdominal operations for obstruction and bleeding. Under these circumstances, if the diagnosis is known, multiple polyps can be removed by enterotomy and polypectomy – not bowel resection. Intraoperative endoscopy or enteroscopy with telescoping the bowel over the endoscope at the time of laparotomy allows endoscopic polypectomy [10]. Multiple large polyps can be removed endoscopically and delivered through one enterotomy site. Massive small bowel resections should be avoided.

Williams et al [11] recommend upper and lower gastrointestinal endoscopy every other year, repeat evaluation if the patient becomes symptomatic, and laparotomy for any small bowel polyp larger than 1.5 cm in diameter. Periodic mammography and ultrasound of the abdomen are useful, since these patients have a higher incidence of breast, ovarian, and pancreatic cancers. The most important issue is to distinguish Peutz–Jeghers polyps from familial polyposis coli, which are adenomatous polyps with high malignant potential.

Hyperplastic polyps

Hyperplastic (metaplastic) polyps are the most common colorectal polyps in adults. These lesions are usually asymptomatic and are invariably smaller than 0.5 cm in diameter [1]. Microscopically, although the proliferative zone within the crypt of Lieberkühn is expanded, the cells lining the individual crypts differentiate and mature. This is truly a hyperplastic process, distinguished from the neoplastic process seen in adenomas. Hyperplastic polyps are usually found in the rectum and sigmoid and are nearly always multiple [12]. Hyperplastic polyps are not neoplasms and do not connote an increased risk for development of tumors. However, small rectosigmoid polyps discovered on flexible sigmoidoscopy or colonoscopy may be hyperplastic or adenomatous polyps. Either polyp type has been associated with proximal colonic adenomas in 30–40% of patients. Significant lesions seen during flexible sigmoidoscopy suggest the need for total colonoscopy [13].

A newly recognized variation of hyperplastic polyps is the serrated adenoma or sessile serrated adenoma [14,15]. There is growing evidence that these lesions have a malignant potential. Features that have been associated with carcinoma include right colon location, large size (>1cm), sessile shape with poor endoscopic circumscription often mimicking a mucosal fold, atypical architecture with exaggerated serration and proliferation features compatible with cytologic dysplasia, and abundant mucin secretion. The diagnosis of sessile serrated adenomas relies mostly on routine histopathologic examination. Management of these lesions should follow guidelines for traditional adenomas. Until more is known, a shorter surveillance interval (1–2 years) may be considered for lesions with evidence of cytologic dysplasia. Careful clinical follow up and possibly prophylactic colectomy has been suggested for patients with hyperplastic polyposis. Additional experience will provide focused recommendations.

Inflammatory polyps

Inflammatory polyps or pseudopolyps are common polyps associated with inflammatory bowel disease. The inflammatory process distorts the colonic epithelium. The crypts branch irregularly and are shortened in height. The entire mucosa is involved in a fibrotic and inflammatory reaction. The surrounding mucosa is uninvolved. The crypt architemre in the neighboring mucosa is normal or minimally distorted. When the colon is inspected endoscopically or during gross examination, the normal mucosa appears elevated as an island of mucosa surrounded by a sea of shortened, inflamed mucosa. This gives the normal mucosa the appearance of a polyp. Biopsy of this tissue reveals normal colonic mucosa. The surrounded area must he biopsied to reveal the underlying inflammatory condition. Inflammatory polyps and pseudopolyps are common in ulcerative colitis [1].

Adenomatous polyps

Adenomatous polyps are neoplasms. Histologically, they can be divided into three types: tubular adenomas, villous adenomas, and tubulovillous adenomas.

Tubular adenoma

Tubular adenomas (adenomatous polyps, polypoid adenomas) are the most common neoplastic polyps, composing 75% of all benign polyps [2]. The lesions may he sessile or pedunculated. Microscopically, polypoid adenomas consist of closely packed epithelial tubules separated by normal lamina propria, which grow and branch horizontally to the muscularis mucosae.

Villous adenoma

Villous adenomas (villous papilloma) tend to be larger than tubular adenomas and are more frequently sessile [16]. The rare McKittrick–Wheelock syndrome is associated with large villous adenomas. It consists of diarrhea, severe hyppokalemia, and dehydration [17]. The syndrome results from the loss of copious amounts of fluid and electrolytes from the mucus-secreting tumor. Microscopically, the villous adenoma consists of fingerlike processes, each made up of a core of lamina propria, covered by epithelial cells growing vertically toward the bowel lumen. In a study from the Mayo Clinic, the median age of patients was 64 years, and one-third of the patients were asymptomatic. The lesions were distributed evenly throughout the colon [18].

Tubulovillous adenoma

Histologically, tubulovillous adenomas (villoglandular adenoma, papillary adenoma, villoglandular polyp, mixed adenoma, polypoidvillous adenoma) contain changes that are intermediate between changes with a villous and polypoid adenoma. In a comprehensive study from St. Mark's Hospital in London, the incidence of the three histologic types was tubular adenoma in 75%, tubulovillous adenoma in 15%, and villous adenoma in 10% [1]. In general, these three types of adenomas are treated similarly. Each adenoma carries malignant potential, but the risk of malignant degeneration increases when the lesion contains a greater villous histologic component than a tubular component. All adenomas require treatment with either fulguration, resection, or a combination of fulguration and resection.

Adenoma–carcinoma sequence

About one in three of all colonic specimens resected for colorectal carcinoma contains one or more adenomas [2]. During follow-up in the series reported by Oommen et al 7% of the group with one or more adenomas as well as a carcinoma in the resected specimen developed a second, or metachronous, tumor in the remaining bowel. This was twice the rate in the group of patients in whom no associated adenomas were found. Seventy-five percent of patients with synchronous colorectal carcinomas have associated adenomas [20]. These statistics indicate that the concurrence of adenomas and carcinomas is not a chance event.

More direct evidence for the adenoma–carcinoma sequence comes from the finding of contiguous benign tumors in carcinomas. Histologic studies of malignant tumors show gradations from the adenoma, with a microscopic focus of invasive adenocarcinoma to the obvious cancer with some residual benign tumor at one edge (**Figure 21.2**).

In a series of malignant tumors examined at St. Mark's Hospital, 14.2% contained varying proportions of adenomatous tissue [21]. Further support for the adenoma-carcinoma sequence comes from a report in which the incidence of a benign component of large bowel carcinoma was related to the extent of spread of the tumor through the bowel wall. Benign tumors contiguous to the adenocarcinoma were found in only 7% of cases in which the cancer had spread through the bowel wall to extramural fat. When spread was limited to the bowel wall, however, an adenomatous component was observed in 20% of cases; with invasion of the submucosal layer, adenomatous tissue was present in only 60% of cases. These findings suggest that as carcinomas enlarge, progressively more of the precursor adenoma is destroyed or transformed into malignant tissue.

Observations on how long it takes for an adenoma to develop malignant change come from patients who had benign tumors and

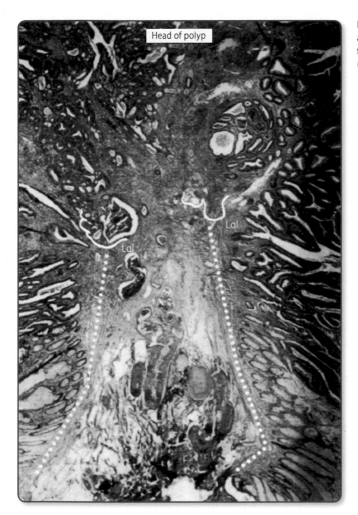

Figure 21.2 Micrograph of adenomatous polyp containing focus of adenocarcinoma (LoI = level of invasion).

refused operations and from patients with familial polyposis coli. With the help of metachronous cancer rate studies and age-distribution curves, it has been estimated that the adenoma–carcinoma sequence is rarely less than 5 years, averages 10–15 years, but it may even cover a normal adult life span. However, cancers are a heterogenous group of lesions and a more rapid progression may occur with other or more numerous genetic changes.

Cancer has a genetic basis. Carcinogenesis is a multistep process, requiring an accumulation of acquired and inherited genetic alterations. With this succession of genetic alterations, cells acquire a growth advantage over surrounding cells [22]. In normal cells, growth and replication is a highly regulated process, and disruption of this regulation at multiple levels is required for clinically relevant cancer to develop [23]. Defects in genes that code for important proteins in the regulation of the cell cycle seem to be critical for carcinogenesis. Hanahan and Weinberg [22] have described six alterations in the regulatory mechanisms that seem constant in most cancers from the several hundred genetic mutations that have been identified in cancer cells (see Figure 22.1).

Although all six alterations are required for the development of clinically significant cancer, the sequence of events and mechanisms are variable. The sequence appears less important than the accumulations of mutations.

Risk of malignancy in colorectal polyps

The overall malignancy rate for tubular adenomas is 5%, compared with 40% for villous adenomas and 22% for the mixed variety of polyps [24]. The malignancy potential for polps under 1 cm is less than 1%. The risk of invasive cancer increases to 10% for polyps between 1 and 2 cm and 35% for polyps larger than 2 cm [24, 25]. With increasing grades of dysplasia, there also seems to be an increasing risk of malignancy [26]. When dysplasia is mild, the chance of malignancy is 6%, compared with 18% for moderate and 35% for severe dysplasia. However, by definition adenomatous polyps have some dysplasia the accuracy and reproducibility of pathologists grading dysplasia is poor.

Management of colorectal polyps

Benign polyps

Fiberoptic colonoscopy has revolutionized the management of colorectal polyps. Even large polyps (greater than 2.5 cm) can be removed by colonoscopic technique if adequate visualization of the pedicle is possible and the head can be ensnared (**Figure 21.3**) [27]. Sessile and submucosal lesions can be removed by endoscopy (**Figure 21.4**), but ulcerated lesions usually harbor a malignancy which usually requires surgical removal. Care must be taken to elevate the mucosa as the snare is tightened. Stripping the mucosa and submucosa with an endoscopic mucosal resection (EMR) or submucosal resection (ESR) is safe, but one must try to leave an intact muscularis propria [28]. If excision is not feasible, the lesion can be biopsied and treated with fulguration or surgically resected.

Bleeding and perforation are the two most serious complications following colonoscopic polypectomy. In a report of 1555 polypectomies, Nivatvongs [18] reported 19 complications, an incidence of 1.2%. Bleeding was the most frequent problem in that series. Hemorrhage can result from several causes, including the polypectomy procedure itself, biopsy, laceration of the mucosa from the instrument, or tearing of the mesentery or spleen. Patients receiving anticoagulants (wafarin or cloprodiginal [Plavix]) are at a higher risk for this complication. Obtaining an adequate history, familiarity with the electrical equipment, use of coagulating current, and the endoscopists clinical experience reduce the risk of this complication (see Chapter 5). If the bleeding

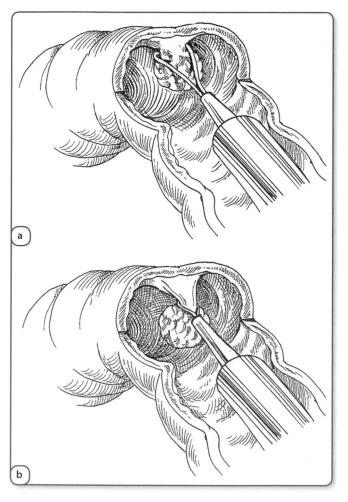

Figure 21.3 Colonoscopic snaring of the pedunculated polyp.
(a) Snare placed around base of polyp. (b) Snare tightened around stalk as cautery is applied.

is recognized at the time of the procedure, the area may be resnared and strangulated for at least 15 minutes, injected with an epinephrine solution, cauterized or clipped. If the bleeding persists, the patient will require resuscitation and hospital observation. Arteriography can identify the hemorrhagic site and embolize or perfuse the selective artery with a vasopressin infusion. If the hemorrhage continues despite medical management, a surgical exploration is warranted. A segmental colectomy encompassing the hemorrhagic site and associated pathology will treat the bleeding and other underlying conditions.

Perforation of the colon with pneumoperitoneum usually becomes manifest almost immediately or within a few hours, and is caused by disease in the colon, excessively rigorous manipulation, or complications from polypectomy. Management depends on the mechanism of perforation, time of recognition, and the state of bowel preparation. If the patient develops peritonitis, the decision to intervene surgically is straightforward. Primary repair can be

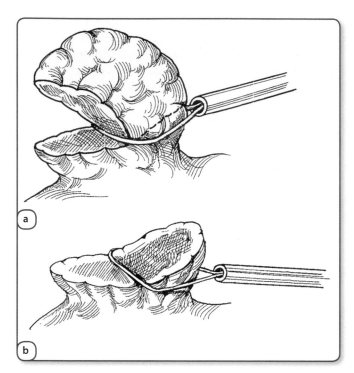

Figure 21.4 Piecemeal snaring of a large sessile polyp. (a) Snare is tightened on a portion of a large polyp. (b) After resection of portion of a polyp, a second application of the snare is applied to remove residual polyp.

achieved if there is minimal contamination and if the perforation is recognized immediately. A diversionary or resectional procedure may be necessary if there is gross contamination or if the diagnosis was delayed. Subcutaneous, retroperitoneal, or mediastinal air without evident peritonitis may he treated conservatively by close observation and antibiotic therapy.

Waye [29] described the postpolypectomy coagulation syndrome. The syndrome consists of localized signs of peritonitis, pain, fever, and leukocytosis, without evidence of perforation on radiologic examination. The symptoms are presumably secondary to transmural thermal injury of the bowel at the polypectomy site. Generally, patients with this syndrome can be managed by in-hospital observation, bowel rest, intravenous fluid therapy, and administration of broad-spectrum antibiotics. Additional discussion on endoscopic complications was provided in Chapter 5.

Malignant colorectal polyps

The management of patients with invasive carcinoma removed by colonoscopic polypectomy remains some what controversial [30–36]. The following findings are considered to be indicators for surgical resection: (1) carcinoma near the polypectomy margin (<2 mm), (2) lymphatic or blood vessel invasion, and (3) poorly differentiated adenocarcinoma. Of these four findings, carcinoma at or close to the resection margin or incomplete resection (<2mm) is the most important indication for subsequent surgery [35]. The distinction between lymphatic and venous invasion is not always easy without using special staining. Therefore, blood vessel invasion is included as a risk factor, although the possibility of preventing blood-borne metastases by colonic resection is uncertain.

Haggitt et al [37] also described a classification system for polyps with invasive carcinomas. The level of invasion was categorized into five levels, as shown in **Figure 21.5**. Based on their experience, this group concluded that the level of invasion should be the major factor in determining prognosis for the management of carcinoma. These authors recommended surgical resection for Level 4 invasion. However, they also confirmed that when one adverse prognostic factor (depth of invasion) was present, several other adverse characteristics were also noted.

Most invasive carcinomas without any of the risk factors described previously can be treated by polypectomy alone [35]. However, one must remember that once carcinoma invades the submucosa, the risk of nodal metastasis increases. Although the risk is assumed to be less than 10%, it is difficult to detect the nodal deposits, if present, without surgery. The criteria mentioned previously form the basis of our current

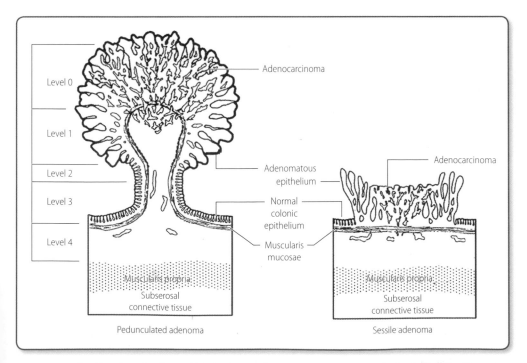

Figure 21.5 Classification of polyps with invasive carcinoma. (From Haggitt RC, Glotzbach RE, Soffer EE, et al. Prognostic factors in colorectal carcinomas arising in adenomas: Implications for lesions removed by endoscopic polypectomy. Gastroenterology 1985;89:328–336. With permission.)

clinical recommendations. However, these recommendations have not been proven with prospective controlled trials (Level 1 evidence). Therefore, it is important to make a clinical decision taking into account lesion characteristics including the site of the lesion and the age and fitness of the patient, as well as the patient's choice. Surgical treatment of a lesion in the lower rectum is a more difficult choice than a lesion in the proximal colon.

Colectomy is recommended for patients with high-risk polyps, as described previously. Using these criteria, Whitlow and colleagues demonstrated a calculated 5 year survival of 85% in patients observed and those who underwent surgical resection [32]. Of note is that approximately 50% of patients who have high risk polyps will have residual colonic or nodal tumor in their surgical specimens [32].

Villous tumors of the rectum

Large benign neoplasms of the rectum, especially villous adenomas, can be challenging management problems. Biopsy results of grossly benign lesions of the rectum can frequently be inaccurate. Taylor et al [38], in a report on preoperative assessment of villous adenomas, found that 44% of the biopsy reports were misleading when compared with the interpretation when the specimen was completely excised. Therefore, the clinical impression gained by palpation and inspection is the best way to determine the appropriate operative approach. If there is no convincing evidence that the lesion contains invasive cancer, every effort should be made to perform a sphincter-saving operation.

The methods employed to remove rectal villous tumors include transanal excision (with or without transanal endoscopic microsurgery [TEM] equipment), transcoccygeal excision (Kraske), trans-sphincteric excision (Mason), and rectal resection with or without restoration of intestinal continuity [35]. Transanal excision is the preferred method if it is possible. The procedure itself may be performed by snare electrocautery, laser therapy, TEM, or by surgical excision. The former two methods have the disadvantage of not procuring the entire intact specimen for histologic study.

Famial adenomatous polyposis syndromes

Our knowledge of polyposis syndromes continues to expand. **Familial adenomatous polyposis (FAP)** is a genetically determined generalized growth disorder which is characterized by the progressive development of hundreds or thousands of adenomatous polyps throughout the entire large bowel [39]. The condition occurs in 1 of 7000 births and has an autosomal dominant expression with a variable penetration [2]. In most families in which a member is diagnosed with an adenomatous polyposis syndrome, the condition's origin is from a spontaneous genetic mutation. Using genetic-linkage analysis, it has been determined that FAP is caused by a mutation in the tumor suppressor gene adenomatous polyposis coli (APC) located on the long arm of chromosome 5q21-22 [40].

Colonic polyps are not present at birth and begin to develop in the early teens. With advancing age, the size and number of polyps increase. If untreated, cancers usually develop by the individual's early thirties. Screening of family members of confirmed polyposis patients is important. Children at risk should be screened starting at age 10; at this age they are large enough to more easily accept flexible sigmidoscopy and mature enough to understand what is being done. It is imperative that the screening examination not be painful: a bad experience will prevent the patient from seeking additional follow-up. Most authors recommend annual flexible sigmoidoscopy for family members at risk [39]. If rectal polyps are identified, additional procedures (biopsy, colonoscopy, and esophagoduodenoscopy) are indicated. Differing combinations of the intestinal and extracolonic manifestations have been grouped into syndromes.

Turcot's Syndrome

Turcot's syndrome is the association of multiple colonic adenomatous polyps with malignant tumors of the central nervous system (medulloblastoma of the cerebellium or glioblastoma of the cerebrum) [39]. The condition is rare and currently is considered a form of FAP or hereditary non-polyposis colorectal cancer (HNPCC). In Turcot's syndrome, the polyps are fewer (20–100) and larger (more than 3 cm), and colonic cancer tends to develop earlier (in the second and third decades of life). If a polyposis patient falls into this category, intracranial investigation should be undertaken at an early date with the hope of identifying the brain tumor at an earlier stage.

Gardner's Syndrome

This syndrome consists of multiple osteomata (usually skull and mandible), cysts, and soft tissue tumors. Other associated conditions include desmoid tumors of the abdominal wall, mesentery, and retroperitoneum; dental abnormalities; thyroid carcinoma; periampullary carcinoma; and gastrointestinal adenwomatosis with or without carcinoma. Pigmented ocular fundus lesions (congenital hypertrophy of the retinal pigment epithelium [CHIRPE]) have been noted in patients with Gardner's syndrome and in some family members [42]. When such lesions are identified in both retinas, they indicate inheritance of the gene for polyposis [43]. Other conditions that may be associated with this syndrome include carcinoid of the small bowel, adrenal cancer, adrenal adenoma, skin pigmentation, and lymphoid polyposis.

Management of polyposis patients

Once the diagnosis is confirmed (multiple adenomatous polyps and family history), three surgical options are currently available: (1) proctocolectomy and ileostomy, (2) total colectomy with ileorectal anastomosis (periodically fulgurating, residual or recurrent rectal polyps), and (3) total colectomy with mucosal proctectomy followed by ileoanal anastomosis with an intervening pouch (restorative proctocolectomy). Total colectomy with ileorectal anastomosis is an operation for selected patients. The cumulative risk of developing cancer in the retained rectum is 3.6%. Thus these patients need to undergo periodic proctosigmoidoscopic evaluation at 6-month intervals. This operation is particularly indicated if there are only a few polyps in the rectum. According to the St. Mark's study [44], polyp regression in the retained rectum seems to take place in the first decade after surgery, but this trend is reversed in the second decade.

Conventional proctocolectomy with ileostomy achieves total ablation of the polyp-bearing area, but at the expense of a permanent stoma. This is a good option for patients who do not wish repeated follow-up examinations and are willing to live with a permanent stoma. Abdominal colectomy with mucosal proctectomy and ileal pouch-anal anastomosis (restorative proctocolectomy) is an operation associated with morbidity even in the hands of experienced surgeons. However, it is the preferred option in young patients with multiple rectal polyps or patients who want the best preventive option for rectal cancer. Additional details of the operation are presented in Chapter 14.

Management of extracolonic manifestations of polyposis coli

Desmoid tumor is one of the most difficult management problems in Gardner's syndrome [45]. Because of the variations in presentation, there is no specific way to manage this problem. Even after aggressive surgical excision, recurrence is likely. For lesions involving the mesentery and causing obstructive symptoms, a bypass procedure may be the safe alternative. Inhibiting prostaglandin synthesis and enhancing the immune response by administration of the nonsteroidal anti-inflammatory drug sulindac, 150 mg bid, has been reported to show diminution in the size of the tumor. The antiestrogen and prostaglandin-inhibitor tamoxifen has also been found useful. Investigations using various chemotherapy agents continue.

Tumors of the stomach and duodenum may be treated by endoscopic removal. The majority of gastric polyps are benign fundic gland polyps and require no therapy. Adenomatous polyps are more frequent in the duodenum. Gastric resection might be necessary for malignant lesions, and pancreatoduodenectomy may be required for periampullary carcinomas.

Polyp follow-up

All polyps managed endoscopically require follow-up [46–49]. Villous adenomas of the rectum frequently recur. When a flat lesion is removed by biopsy or excision, its complete removal cannot be confirmed pathologically. Furthermore, when electrocautery is used, there is often more effect on the remaining tissue than the operator has recognized, so that on repeat examination there may, surprisingly, be no visible residual lesion. It has been recommended that when a sessile lesion larger than 1 cm is removed by biopsy or excision, a repeat endoscopy be done in 3 months and a re-evaluation in 1 year [2].

In the more common scenario of pedunculated adenoma, the approach depends on the rate of metachronous polyp formation as well as the recognized, but not statistically known, incidence of polyps missed at colonoscopy. Most colonoscopists would now recommend colonoscopy in 1–5 years after the index polyp has been removed [50]. The shorter interval would be selected for patients with multiple or larger polyps or those with a technical difficult colonoscopy or poor preparation. The rationale for this is primarily to discover polyps that may have been missed at the time of initial examination. If carcinomas or multiple polyps are found during index examinations, it appears that the incidence of metachronous polyp formation is higher than if a solitary index polyp is found. After the colon has been cleared of adenomatous tissue, new adenomas of medical significance may not appear for an estimated 3–5 years. So once the colon has been 'cleared,' colonoscopy is indicated only once every 5 years [49, 50]. The appropriateness of stopping surveillance when a patient reaches an advanced age or has significant comorbid medical conditions is controversial. At present, this must be an individual decision involving the physician and patient.

Rounds questions

1. Histologically, what are the four classes of polyps?
2. What are the three forms of hamartomas?
3. What are the most common polyps in adults?
4. What are the three types of adenomatous polyps?
5. What is the risk of malignancy in a polyp of less than 1 cm, 1–2 cm, and greater than 2 cm?
6. When is polypectomy adequate therapy for a polyp containing cancer?
7. At what age should children at risk for adenomatous polyposis syndromes begin to be screened?
8. What conditions constitute Gardner's syndrome?
9. What are the surgical options for treating polyposis coli?
10. When should a patient have a follow-up colonoscopy after removal of an adenomatous polyp?

References

1. Fenoglio-Preiser CM. Colonic polyp histology. Semin Colon Rectal Surg 1991;2:234–5.
2. Oommen SC. Polyps. In: Beck DE, Welling DR, (eds). Patient Care in Colorectal Surgery. Boston: Little, Brown, 1991:279–91.
3. Fenoglio CM, Kaye GI, Lane N. Distribution of human colonic lymphatics in normal, hyperplastic and adenomatous tissue. Its relationship to metastasis from small carcinomas in pedunculated adenomas,

with two case reports. Gastroenterology 1973;64:51–66.

4. Roth SI, Helwig EB. Juvenile polyps of the colon and rectum. Cancer 1963;16:468–79.

5. McColl I, Bussey HJR, Veale AMU, Morson BC. Juvenile polyposis coli. Proc R Soc Med 1964;57:896–7.

6. Cronkhite LW Jr, Canada WJ. Generalized gastrointestinal polyposis. An unusual syndrome of polyposis, pigmentation, alopecia and onychotrophia. N Engl J Med 1955;252:1011–5.

7. Linos DA, Dozois RR, Dahlin DC, Bartholomew LG. Does Peutz-Jeghers syndrome predispose to gastrointestinal malignancy? A later look. Arch Surg 1981;116:1182–4.

8. Konishi F, Wyse NE, Muto T, et al. Peutz-Jeghers polyposis associated with carcinoma of the digestive organs: Report of three cases and review of the literature. Dis Colon Rectum 1987;30:790–9.

9. Dozois RR, Judd ES, Dahlin DC, et al. The Peutz-Jeghers syndrome. Is there a predisposition to the development of intestinal malignancy? Arch Surg 1969;98:509–17.

10. Panos RG, Opelka FG, Nogueras JJ. Peutz-Jeghers syndrome. A call for intraoperative enteroscopy. Am Surg 1990;56:331–3.

11. Williams CB, Golblatt M, Delaney PV. 'Top and tail endoscopy' and follow-up in Peutz-Jeghers syndrome. Endoscopy 1982;14:82–4.

12. Opelka FG, Timmcke AE, Gathright JB, et al. Diminutive colonic polyps. An indication for colonoscopy. Dis Colon Rectum 1992;35:178–81.

13. Jass JR. Nature and clinical significance of colorectal hyperplastic polyp. Semin Colon Rectal Surg 1991;2:246–52.

14. Torlakovic E, Skovland E, Snover DC, et al. Morphologic reappraisal of serrated colorectal polyps. Am J Surg Pathol. 2003;27:65–81.

15. Goldstein NS, Bhanot P, Odish E. Hyperplastic-like colon polyps that preceded microsatellite-unstable adenocarcinomas. Am J Clin Pathol. 2003;119:778–96.

16. Chin YS, Spencer RJ. Villous lesions of the colon. Dis Colon Rectum 1978;21:493–5.

17. McKittrick LS, Wheelock FC. Carcinoma of the Colon. Springfield, II: Charles C. Thomas, 1954;61–3.

18. Nivatvongs S. Complications in colonoscopic polypectomy: An experience with 1555 polypectomies. Dis Colon Rectum 1986;29:825–30.

19. Morson BC. President's address: The polyp cancer sequence in the large bowel. Proc R Soc Med 1974;67:451–7.

20. Heald RJ, Bussey HJR. Clinical experience at St. Mark's Hospital with multiple synchronous cancers of the colon and rectum. Dis Colon Rectum 1975;18:6–10.

21. Bussey HJR, Wallace MH, Morson BC. Metachronous carcinoma of the large intestine and intestinal polyps. Proc R Soc Med 1967;60:208–10.

22. Hanahan D, Weinberg RA. The hallmarks of cancer. Cell 2000;100:57–70.

23. Baxter NN, Guillem JG. Colorectal cancer: Epidemiology, etiology, and molecular basis. In: Wolff BG, Fleshman JW. Beck DE, Pemberton JH, Wexner SD (eds). ASCRS Textbook of Colorectal Surgery. Springer-Verlag, New York. 2007;335–52.

24. Muto T, Bussey HJR, Morson BC. The evolution of the cancer of the colon and rectum. Cancer 1975;36:2251–70.

25. Wolfe WI, Shinya H. Endoscopic Polypectomy. Therapeutic and clinopathologic aspects. Cancer 1975;36:683–90.

26. O'Brien MJ, Winawer SJ, Zauber AG, et al. The National Polyp Study. Patient and polyp characteristics associated with high-grade dysplasia in colorectal adenomas. Gastroenterology 1990;98:371–9.

27. Forde KA. Colonoscopic management of polypoid lesions. Surg Clin North Am 1989;69:1287–308.

28. Kantsevoy SV, Adler DG, Conway et al. Endoscopic mucosal resection and endoscopic submucosal dissection. Gastroint Endosc. 2008;68:11.

29. Waye JD. The postpolypectomy coagulation syndrome. Gastrointest Endosc 1981;27:184.

30. Coverlizza S, Risio M, Ferrari A, et al. Colorectal adenomas containing invasive carcinoma. Pathologic assessment of lymph node metastatic potential. Cancer 1989;64:1937–47.

31. Sugihara K, Muto T, Morioka Y. Management of patients with invasive carcinoma removed by colonoscopic polypectomy. Dis Colon Rectum 1989;32:829–34.

32. Whitlow CB, Gathright JB, Hebert JJ, et al. Long term survival after malignant polyps. Dis Colon Rectum 1997;40:929–34.

33. Morson BC. Factors influencing the prognosis of early cancer of the rectum. Proc R Soc Med 1996;59:607–8.

34. Opelka FG, Hicks TC. Management of malignant polyps. Semin Colon Rectal Surg 1991;2:296–304.

35. Katz JA, Nogueras JJ. Management of cancer in a polyp. Clin Colon Rect Surg 2001;14:369–78.

36. Beck DE. Management of the endoscopically removed malignant polyp. Clin Colon Rect Surg 2002;15:121–9.

37. Haggitt RC, Glotzbach RE, Soffer EE, et al. Prognostic factors in colorectal carcinomas arising in adenomas: Implications for lesions removed by endoscopic polypectomy. Gastroenterology 1985;89:328–36.

38. Taylor EW, Thompson H, Oates GD, et al. Limitations of biopsy in preoperative assessment of villous papilloma. Dis Colon Rectum 1981;24:259–62.

39. Jagelman DG. Familial polyposis coli. In: Fazio VW (ed). Current Therapy in Colon and Rectal Surgery, Philadelphia: BC Decker, 1990;284–8.

40. Nivatvongs S. Benign neoplasms of the colon and rectum. In: Gordon PH, Nivatvongs S (eds). Principles and Practice of Surgery for the Colon, Rectum, and Anus, 2nd ed. St. Louis: Quality Medical Publishing 1999;541–73.

41. Itoh H, Ohsato K. Turcot syndrome and its characteristic colonic manifestations. Dis Colon Rectum 1985;28:399–402.

42. Traboulsi EI, Krush AJ, Gardner EJ, et al. Prevalence and importance of pigmented ocular fundus lesions in Gardner's syndrome. N Engl J Med 1987;316:661–7.

43. Chapman PD, Church W, Burn J, Gunn A. Congenital hypertrophy of retinal pigment epithelium: A sign of familiar adenamatous polyposis. Br Med J 1989;298:353–4.

44. Bussey HJR. Familial Polyposis Coli. Baltimore: Johns Hopkins University Press, 1975.

45. Jones IT, Jagelman DG, Fazio W, et al. Desmoid tumors in familial polyposis coli. Ann Surg 1986;204:94–97.

46. Holtzman R, Poulard J, Bank S, et al. Repeat colonoscopy after endoscopic polypectomy. Dis Colon Rectum 1987;30:185–8.

47. Olsen HW, Lawrence WA, Snook CW, Mulch WM. Review of recurrent polyps and cancer in 500 patients with initial colonoscopy for polyps. Dis Colon Rectum 1988;31:222–7.

48. Beck DE, Opelka FG, Hicks TC, et al. Colonoscopy follow-up of adenomas and colorectal cancer. South Med J 1995;88:567–70.

49. Blumberg D, Opelka FG, Hicks TC, et al. The significance of normal surveillance colonoscopy in patients with a history of adenomatous polyps. Dis Colon Rectum. 2000;43:1084–92.

50. Winawer SJ, Zauber AG, O'Brien MJ, et al. Randomized comparison of surveillance intervals after colonoscopic removal of newly diagnosed adenomatous polyps. The National Polyp Study Workgroups. N Engl J Med 1993;328:901–6.

Malignancy of the colon, rectum, and anus

Malignancies of the lower gastrointestinal tract compose a large portion of the practice of colorectal surgery. This chapter describes the anatomy, pathophysiology, evaluation, and treatment of common malignant and premalignant lesions. For ease of understanding, the lesions have been grouped by anatomic location.

Colon and rectum

Anatomy

The general anatomy of the colon and rectum were discussed in Chapter 1. Important oncologic aspects include the segmental blood supply to the colon and rectum and differentiating between the colon and rectum.

Pathophysiology

Incidence and risk factors

The incidence of colorectal cancer varies widely throughout the world. In the United States, adenocarcinoma is the most common malignant lesion of the colon and rectum and will account for approximately 141,219 diagnosed cases and 49,380 deaths in 2011 [1]. Colorectal cancer is the most common visceral cancer; males and females are equally affected. Older patients develop colorectal cancer more often than younger persons, with the incidence rising steadily from 50 years to 80 years of age. The mean age at diagnosis is 67 years of age, and only 6–8% of colorectal cancers are diagnosed before age 40 [2].

Present information suggests multiple etiologic risk factors to include age, heredity, diet, environmental factors, and other diseases or conditions (e.g. inflammatory bowel disease, polyps, breast or gynecologic cancers, ureterosigmoidostomy). The relative importance of these factors allows patients to be divided into high- to low-risk groups (**Table 22.1**).

Adenocarcinoma

Adenocarcinoma is the most common malignant lesion of the colon. According to the polyp cancer theory, these tumors start in the bowel mucosa as adenomatous polyps (see Chapter 21). Our increasing knowledge of genetics and environmental factors is helping to expand our understanding of how these colorectal lesions develop. The genetic changes are summarized in **Figure 22.1**. Colorectal malignancies

Table 22.1 Risk groups for colorectal cancer	
Minimal	**Low**
Age <50 years	Age >50 years
Moderate	**High**
Previous polyp or cancer	Familial polyposis
Family history	Hereditary nonpolyposis cancer syndromes
Gastrointestinal symptoms	No gastrointestinal symptoms
	Ulcerative colitis
	Genetic markers

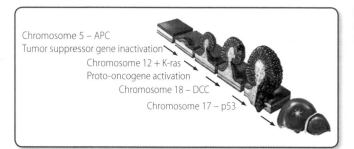

Chromosome 5 – APC
Tumor suppressor gene inactivation
Chromosome 12 + K-ras
Proto-oncogene activation
Chromosome 18 – DCC
Chromosome 17 – p53

Figure 22.1 Genetic changes associated with colorectal malignancies.

other than adenocarcinoma are uncommon. The significant colorectal lesions have been grouped by tissue of origin.

Epithelial tumors

Carcinoid tumors arise from enterochromaffin or Kulchitsky cells, which are located in the crypts of Lieberkühn. The characteristics of these tumors vary depending on the section of the gastrointestinal tract in which the tumors originate. Midgut carcinoids (mid-duodenum to midtransverse colon) are argentaffin and argyrophil positive, frequently multicentric, and often associated with the carcinoid syndrome. Hindgut carcinoids (distal transverse colon to rectum) are rarely argentaffin or argyrophil positive, usually unicentric, and are not associated with the carcinoid syndrome.

The carcinoid syndrome involves symptoms of six organ systems. Episodic manifestations include cutaneous flushing, hyperperistalsis and diarrhea, asthma, and hemodynamic alterations that may result in vasomotor collapse. Permanent manifestations are facial hyperemia, peripheral edema, cutaneous lesions of pellagra, and valvular heart disease. The biochemical aspects of this syndrome are complicated. A major component is serotonin, a biologically active peptide, secreted by Kulchitsky cells. Serotonin is metabolized in the liver to 5-hydroxyindoleacetic acid (5-HIAA), which is biologically inactive and is excreted in the urine. This is the basis for a test of functioning carcinoid tumors [3].

Depending on the practice pattern of the reporting institution, intestinal carcinoids occur most frequently in the appendix (0.26% of appendectomy specimens) or in the rectum [4]. The next most common sites are the small bowel and the stomach. Colonic carcinoids are rare and constitute 2–3% of gastrointestinal carcinoids. Carcinoid tumors develop in women twice as often as in men, and the peak incidence is in the seventh decade of life. They are slow growing. Many patients are asymptomatic at diagnosis, since it is uncommon for these tumors to bleed or form an obstruction; their diagnosis as an incidental finding is common. Early lesions will appear as circumscribed yellowish submucosal nodules.

Microscopically, these tumors contain uniform small round cells with prominent round nuclei and eosinophilic cytoplasmic granules. The incidence of malignancy in carcinoids varies from 8–40% [2]. Microscopic features do not correlate with malignancy. A diagnosis of malignancy usually depends on direct tumor extension or the presence of metastatic disease. The chance of metastatic disease is related to the size of the primary lesion.

Treatment is surgical, and the presence of metastatic disease is not an absolute contraindication to surgical resection. In general, tumors with diameters of less than 2 cm can be managed with local excision (transanal excision for rectal lesions, appendectomy for appendiceal carcinoids, and intestinal resections). Rectal carcinoids greater than 2 cm should be managed with radical resection [4]. Radiotherapy and chemotherapy have not proved to be effective as primary treatment of carcinoids. Streptozocin has a palliative role for symptomatic hepatic metastases. Survival depends on the location of the lesion and the presence of metastatic disease. The average length of survival after resection of colonic carcinoids without metastatic disease is 41 months and with metastatic disease is 26 months. Five-year survival rates for colonic carcinoids has been reported as 52% [5]. The 5-year survival for rectal carcinoids is 92% if there is no metastatic disease, and 7% with distant metastatic disease [6].

Squamous cell carcinoma of the colon is rare, with approximately 100 cases reported [3]. Etiologic factors for this tumor include metaplasia and embryonic rests. Symptoms and treatment are similar to those for adenocarcinomas. If metastatic disease is present, one should consider using a multimodality approach.

Lymphatic malignancies

Primary colorectal lymphomas are unusual and constitute 22% of gastrointestinal lymphomas (preceded by stomach and the small intestine) and only 1.5% of colonic neoplasms [3]. Although intestinal lymphoma is a common presentation of terminal disseminated lymphoma, primary lymphoma of the bowel is diagnosed based on the following criteria

1. there is no evidence of generalized palpable or mediastinal adenopathy

2. leukocyte and differential counts are normal
3. only lymph nodes of intestinal drainage are found to be involved at laparotomy or necropsy
4. the liver and spleen are determined to be free of the disease.

Reported patients range in age from 3–89 years, with an average of 50 years of age. Males are affected twice as often as females. Abdominal pain and weight loss are almost universally associated with a mass on physical examination. Gastrointestinal blood loss presenting as melena or occult blood occurs in 10–50% of patients. Bowel obstruction and intussusception has been reported in up to 25% of cases [2].

Contrast radiographic examination of the intestine is the most commonly used method for preoperative diagnosis of lymphoma, but endoscopy has an increasing role. The predominant site affected is the cecum (more than 75% of patients), followed by the rectum (10%). The remainder have been scattered throughout other portions of the colon. These tumors are usually large, averaging 5–7 cm in diameter on presentation. The prognosis is related to tumor size, nodal involvement, and histologic cell type. The 5-year survival for tumors greater than 5 cm has been reported to be less than 25%, and with nodal involvement it has been less than 20%. According to histiologic type, survival at 5 years has been described as 40% for Hodgkins disease, 35% for mixed tumors, 33% for lymphocytic, and 25% for histiocytic.

Various treatment options (surgery, radiotherapy, and chemotherapy) have been used [7]. The results of individual options or combinations of therapy are difficult to assess, since cases are scarce and treatment strategies have not been standardized. Surgery appears to be the preferred choice for resectable lesions, and there is some evidence to suggest that adjuvant radiotherapy may increase survival. Chemotherapy is of limited value for resectable lesions, but chemotherapy is indicated for disseminated disease.

Gastrointestinal stromal tumors

Gastrointestinal stromal tumors (GISTs) are rare lesions that constitute the majority of mesenchymal tumors of the gastrointestinal tract [8]. Within the colon and rectum, these lesions comprise 0.1% of all cancers and include most tumors that were initially described as leiomyoma, cellular leiomyoma, leiomyoblastoma, and leiomyosarcomas. They can present with a variety of symptoms (obstruction, pain, and bleeding), but are often asymptomatic. Although many lesions may be benign, up to half of these patients develop recurrent disease within a few years. Almost all GISTs contain a mutation in the c-kit tyrosine kinase that leads to its constitutive activation and results in cell proliferation. This discovery has led to the immunostaining of the c-kit antigen (CD117) to distinguish GISTs from other malignancies. Prognostic features include mitotic activity, cellular differentiation, vascular invasion, adjacent organ invasion, and the presence or absence of distant metastases. Radiologic examinations can be helpful in initial diagnosis and staging. Surgery is the best treatment for cure, but recent advances have led to the use of imatinib mesylate, a tyrosine kinase inhibitor, to treat metastatic and/or unresectable disease.

Evaluation and treatment

Diagnosis

Despite improvements in screening, a significant number of colon cancers continue to be diagnosed in symptomatic patients. Symptoms include blood in stool (gross bleeding, melena, or positive stool analysis [e.g. Hemoccult II]), change in bowel habits, obstructive symptoms, obstipation, abdominal mass, weight loss, or pain. The fact that many of these symptoms are nonspecific for carcinomas and may not develop until later stages of the disease explains the high frequency of delayed diagnosis.

The work-up for patients presenting with these symptoms should be individualized and as discussed previously should include an appropriate history, physical examination, colonoscopy, or air contrast barium enema and flexible sigmoidoscopy or proctoscopy. The merits and limitations of these studies have been described in previous chapters. Once a colorectal lesion is identified, a biopsy confirms the malignant nature of the lesion and may assist preoperative counseling in selected patients. The widespread availability of endoscopic photodocumentation and the potential for sampling errors in large lesions has lessened the need for preoperative biopsies. One area in which a preoperative biopsy remains critical is for low rectal lesions. It is often difficult to visually exclude a benign condition such as colitis cystica profunda (the presence of microscopic normal functional epithelial cells deep to the muscularis mucosa) or a squamous cell carcinoma. Both of which are managed differently from an adenocarcinoma. Occasionally, it also may not be possible to obtain a tissue diagnosis. For example, obstructing lesions may produce edematous folds of bowel distal to the obstruction, which limits access to the lesion. Adequate endoscopic access to the lesion may also be prevented by intra-abdominal adhesions from previous surgery.

Treatment

Following an adequate evaluation, therapy is selected. The preferred choice is surgical. Good results depend on preoperative preparation (as described in Chapter 8), performing an appropriate and safe operation, and postoperative care (see Chapter 10). The choice of operation is based on the anatomic location of the lesion. Important operative oncologic principles include early proximal ligation of vessels, accomplishing an anatomic resection, and minimal tumor manipulation.

Surgical treatment

Surgical management of colorectal cancer involves removing a section of bowel proximal and distal to the lesion. The different operations are represented in **Figure 22.2**. Lesions of the right colon are managed with a right hemicolectomy. After the patient is positioned in the supine position, exploration through a vertical midline incision is

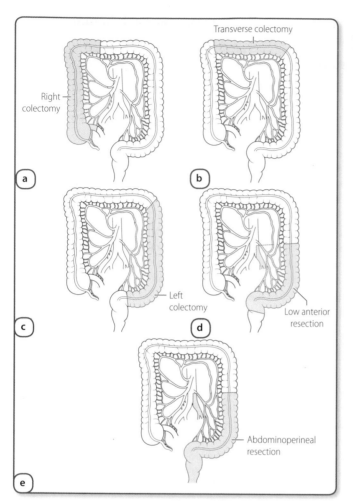

Figure 22.2 Colorectal cancer operations. (a) Right colectomy; (b) transverse colectomy; (c) left colectomy; (d) low anterior resection; (e) abdominoperineal resection.

performed to exclude the presence of metastatic disease. The author prefers, when possible, to use a medial approach with early vascular ligation, accomplished in the following manner (**Figure 22.3**): the small bowel is elevated superiorly by the assistant and the avascular plane between the duodenum and the ileocolic artery is incised. The index and middle finger of the surgeon's right hand (palm up) are inserted between the duodenum and ileocolic artery. By bending these two fingers up, the avascular plane between the right colic and ileocolic artery is identified. The peritoneum is incised with electrocautery. The index and middle finger of the surgeon's left hand then replace the right fingers. After the fingers are bent up, the avascular plane between the ileocolic and superior mesenteric artery is identified. After incision of this mesentery, the ileocolic artery and vein are encircled and the vessels can be thinned. Correct location for division of the ileocolic artery and vein is confirmed and they are clamped, divided, and ligated close to the arterial takeoff from the superior mesenteric artery (SMA). The mesentery cephalad to the ileocolic artery takeoff is then

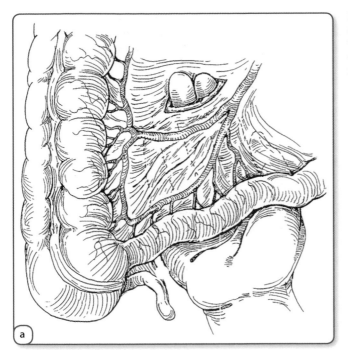

Figure 22.3 Ligation of ileocolic artery and vein. (a) Elevation of the ileocolic artery. (b) Isolation of the ileocolic artery below the superior mesenteric artery.

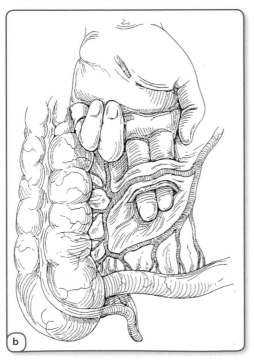

dissected to identify the right colic artery and vein. If present (85% of patients), these are divided and ligated close to their takeoff from the SMA.

The right colonic retroperitoneal attachments are then divided from medial to lateral or lateral to medial. Care is taken to ensure that the dissection remains in the proper avascular plane. If the dissection is performed properly, Gerota's fascia, the ureter, and the gonadal vessels will remain in their anatomic location. The colon, ileum, and associated mesentary are then divided between clamps with the site of division determined by the anatomic location of the lesion and the vascular anatomy.

Anastomotic continuity can be reestablished in several ways. End-to-end, end-to-side, or side-to-side (functional end-to-end) have all been described (**Figure 22.4**). The anastomosis can be performed with staples or sutures (running, interrupted, one or two layers). The method used will vary with the experience and preference of the surgeon. No prospective controlled studies have convincingly demonstrated the superiority of one method over the others. The basic surgical principles of vascular supply, tension, and control of contamination probably play the most important role. After the anastomosis is completed, the mesenteric defect is usually closed to prevent the formation of an internal hernia.

Lesions of the **transverse colon** are managed with a transverse or subtotal colectomy. After the patient is placed in the supine position, exploration is performed through a vertical midline incision. The absence of metastatic disease is confirmed. The lesser sac is entered by division of the gastrocolic omentum just distal to the gastroepiploic vessels. The colon is retracted inferiorly and the peritoneum between the middle colic vessels and the duodenum is incised. The middle colic vessels are identified and ligated at their takeoff from the SMA. Care is taken to prevent avulsion of these vessels during ligation. The corresponding mesentery is divided along with the marginal vessels. The amount of colon resected depends on the location of the lesion and the vascular supply of the colon. If only the transverse colon is resected, the right and left colon are mobilized by incising their lateral peritoneal reflections and the hepatic flexure is moved toward the splenic flexure. An anastomosis is then accomplished, for which I prefer a running sutured one-layer anastomosis. If a tension-free anastomosis cannot be completed, a subtotal colectomy should be performed. The mesenteric defect is then closed to prevent internal hernias.

A lesion located near the **hepatic flexure** may require an extended right colectomy to obtain an adequate margin. If the right colon is resected in addition to the transverse colon, the ileum is anastomosed to the remaining left colon. Lesions near the splenic flexure require removal of the descending branch of the middle colic vessels and the left colic vessels. Bowel continuity is reestablished by the methods described for left colectomies.

Lesions of the **left colon** are managed with either a left or a subtotal colectomy. After the patient is positioned in the modified Lloyd-Davies position (see Figure 3.1), exploration is performed through a vertical

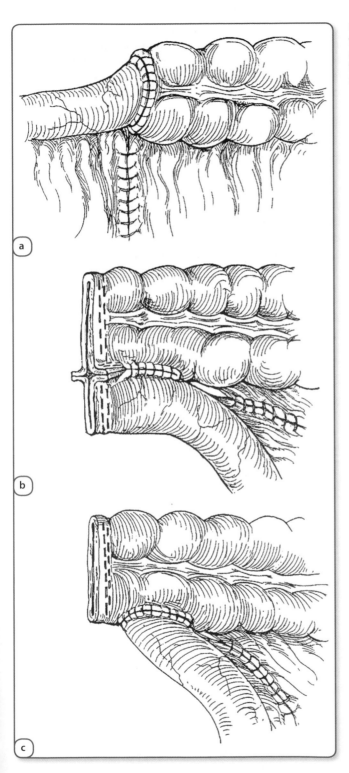

Figure 22.4 Anastomotic techniques. (a) End-to-end anastomosis. (b) Side-to-side functional end-to-end anastomosis, (c) End-to-side anastomosis.

midline incision. Portions of the left colon, proximal to the tumor, are retracted medially and the lateral peritoneal reflection is divided. The dissection is continued in the avascular plane between the colonic mesentery and the retroperitoneum. If the proper plane of dissection is maintained, the gonadal vessels and the ureter will remain in their anatomic location. The dissection is continued until the aorta is reached. While standing on the patient's right side, the surgeon inserts his or her right index and middle finger palm up between the aorta and the inferior mesenteric artery (IMA). Anterior traction and bending of the fingers demonstrates the avascular area on the other side of the IMA. The mesenteric peritoneum is incised, and the surgeon's right fingers are replaced with the left fingers. The peritoneum, fat, and lymphatic tissue around the IMA are incised and the vessel is clamped, divided, and ligated close to the aorta.

The mesentery superior to the IMA is incised until the marginal vessels are identified. These are divided and ligated. Most lesions of the left colon will require mobilization of the splenic flexure to obtain adequate colonic length to make a tension-free anastomosis at the upper rectum. I prefer to mobilize the splenic flexure in the following manner. Gentle inferior and medial traction of the splenic flexure places the splenocolic ligament on slight traction. This thin avascular tissue is incised using the electrocautery. Minimizing traction, keeping in the proper plane, and using an adequate exposure lessen the chances of splenic injury. The most common injury of the spleen is a capsular tear, resulting from excess traction. If this occurs, it can usually be repaired by cautery, hemostatic agents, or suture. To re-establish bowel continuity, the author prefers an end-to-end anastomosis using an intraluminal stapler passed through the anus. To accomplish this a purse-string suture is placed at the proximal line of resection using a purse-string clamp (Purse String device, Davis & Geck, Wayne, NJ, USA) and a 2-0 or 0 nylon or polypropylene suture with a straight needle. A clamp (e.g. Kocher clamp) is placed distal to the purse-string clamp and the bowel is divided. A purse-string suture can also be placed by hand using an appropriate suture with a curved needle (e.g. 2-0 polypropylene with a SH needle).

Mobilization of the colon distal to the lesion is then accomplished. The distal colonic mesentery is incised immediately inferior to the IMA. Keeping the dissection close to the IMA minimizes the chances of injury to splanchnic nerves and major vessels. The distal extent of the resection should be to the upper rectum. The distal sigmoid colon is avoided because the blood supply at this level of the colon may be marginal and the lumen of the sigmoid colon is small. The rectum has a good blood supply and a larger diameter. At the level of the distal extent of resection, branches of the superior hemorrhoidal vessels are divided between clamps and ligated.

A 1 cm section of bowel is cleared of fat and a purse-string suture is applied using a purse-string clamp or placed by hand. The bowel is divided above the clamp or suture and the specimen is handed off the field. As the purse-string clamp is removed, three Babcock clamps are placed on the end of the rectum. The purse-string suture is examined and any defects are repaired. Gaps at the end of the bowel can be corrected using the end of the purse-string suture. Defects at other portions of the purse-string are repaired with interrupted 'pulley sutures' (**Figure 22.5**). An assistant then mildly dilates the anus with two fingers and inserts an intraluminal stapler into the anus. A Fansler or Chelsea-Eaton anoscope may be used to assist the transanal passage of the stapler [9]. The stapler is advanced up the rectum following the curve of the sacrum. As the stapler reaches the top of the rectum, the trocar is extended and the purse-string suture is tightened and tied around the trocar shaft.

Another option to manage the distal portion of the anastomosis is to use a 'double staple' technique. If this option is chosen, the distal portion of the rectum is closed with a linear stapler and the bowel (specimen) is cut proximal to the staple line. A circular intraluminal stapler is then passed through the anus and advanced to the staple line. The stapler trocar is then advanced through the bowel wall adjacent to the staple line. The double staple technique is especially helpful for very low colorectal anastomoses.

To prevent spillage of colonic contents, a tie or noncrushing bowel clamp is placed above the proximal purse-string clamp. This purse-string clamp on the proximal bowel is opened and three small Allis clamps are placed on the edges of the bowel. The purse-string suture is inspected, and any gaps identified are repaired as described previously. Using these clamps for traction, the surgeon carefully maneuvers the detached anvil into the bowel. The clamps are removed and the purse-string suture is tightened and tied (**Figure 22.6**).

The detached anvil (in the proximal bowel) is maneuvered into the pelvis and mated to the stapler trocar. The stapler is then closed completely and fired. The stapler is partially opened and withdrawn. The anastomosis is tested by instillation of a dilute povidone-iodine solution. If leaks are identified, they are repaired with sutures or the anastomosis is reaccomplished. Testing can also be accomplished by filling the pelvis with saline and instilling air into the bowel lumen. The air can be instilled with a bulb syringe or a proctoscope. A leak will result in air bubbles escaping from the anastomosis.

Lesions of the **sigmoid colon** are identified and umbilical tapes are placed proximal and distal to the lesion to lessen the chance of intraluminal spread of tumor during manipulation. Using these tapes for traction, the surgeon incises the peritoneal reflection of the left colon. With continued dissection and retraction, the avascular plane is developed anterior to the gonadal vessels and the ureter until the aorta is reached. The IMA is identified and ligated at the aorta as described for a left colectomy. The mesentery and marginal vessels are divided until the left colon is reached. A portion of the left colon and possibly the splenic flexure are then mobilized. The superior hemorrhoidal vessels

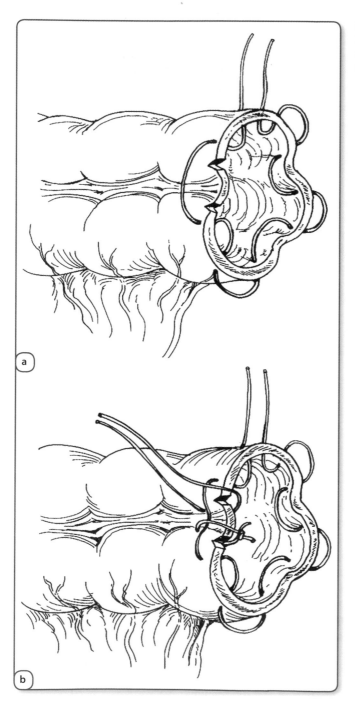

Figure 22.5 Purse-string suture repair. (a) Purse-string suture with gap. (b) Gap closed with 'pulley' stitch.

are divided at the upper rectum and a section of bowel is cleared of fat. Proximal and distal purse-string clamps are placed as described in the previous section. An anastomosis is performed as described for a left colectomy.

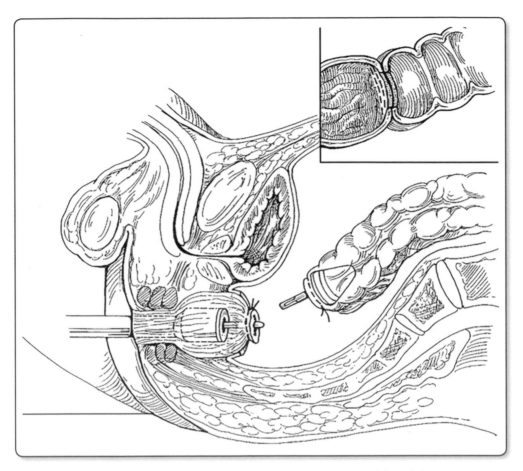

Figure 22.6 End-to-end colorectal anastomosis. An intraluminal stapler is inserted through the anus. Inset: sagittal section of completed anastomosis.

Lesions of the upper and middle **rectum** are managed with an anterior resection. With the patient in the modified Lloyd-Davies position, exploration is performed through a vertical midline incision. The left and sigmoid colon are mobilized as previously described. The IMA is divided proximal or distal to the takeoff of the left colic artery. The site of division will depend on the lesion location and the amount of bowel needed for a safe anastomosis.

The posterior rectum is mobilized by sharp dissection in the avascular plane immediately posterior to the IMA (a dissection described as a total mesorectal excision [TME]). I prefer to open this plane sharply with scissors or electrocautery. Dissection in this plane is continued until Waldeyer's fascia is encountered at the level of the levators. If done properly, the dissection leaves the upper portion of Waldeyer's fascia covering the presacral veins. If Waldeyer's fascia is incised near the sacral promontory, the risk of injuring the presacral veins is increased (**Figure 22.7**). If the presacral veins are damaged, the

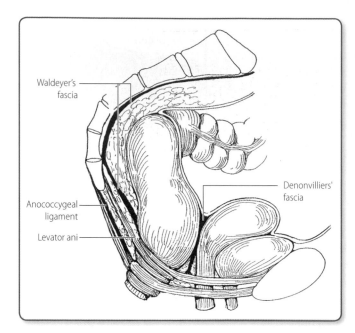

Figure 22.7 Pelvic fascia.

bleeding may be very difficult to stop. Options include tamponade with a specially designed sterile thumbtack (Hemorrhagic occluder pin, Surgin, Tuftin, CA, USA), packing the pelvis with laparotomy sponges, pledgeted sutures, or suturing a piece of rectus muscle against the presacral space. [10]

The lateral dissection involves division of the lateral rectal vessels at the pelvic side wall. Hemostasis is obtained with the electrocautery. Clamping and ligating the vessels before division leaves too much rectal mesentery behind and compromises the cancer operation. The dissection continues in the lateral plane to 2–5 cm below the tumor. It is important to resist dissecting close to the tumor as one proceeds into the pelvis. This 'coning' into the tumor during the dissection has the potential to leave residual tumor at the lateral margins. The minimal acceptable distal margin has been the subject of much discussion. From a scientific standpoint, inadequate information is available to make a definite statement. Pathologic studies have shown that in the absence of a very large or poorly differentiated tumor, the maximal reported microscopic tumor extension in the distal bowel wall is 5 mm. Clinical studies have demonstrated equivalent results with any distal margin greater than 1 cm. Therefore a margin greater than 2 cm appears to be adequate.

The anterior dissection starts at the anterior peritoneal reflection. For a malignant anterior tumor, the appropriate plane of dissection is outside Denonvilliers' fascia (**Figure 22.7**). In males this fascia separates the seminal vesicles from the rectum and in females the vagina from the rectum. The correct dissection will leave the seminal vesicles or the backwall of the vagina exposed. For posterior lesions, many surgeons will perform the anterior dissection in the plane between the fascia propria of the rectum and Denonvilliers'. This does not appear to impact local recurrence and reduces the potential of nerve injury. Whichever plane is used, the dissection is carried down to an appropriate distal margin or to the level of the puborectalis.

After completion of rectal mobilization, a determination is made as to whether an adequate distal margin exists between the levators and the tumor. If the margin is adequate, an anastomosis may be performed with an intraluminal stapler as described above. If an adequate margin does not exist, an abdominoperineal resection (APR) or coloanal pullthrough will be required.

After the low anterior anastomosis is accomplished in a manner similar to that described for a left colon, the anastomosis is tested by instilling a dilute povidone-iodine solution or air into the rectum with a bulb syringe inserted into the anus. Any leak in the anastomosis will be readily identified. A leak can be repaired directly with suture (via the abdomen or the anus), or the anastomosis may be excised and reperformed.

If the anastomosis is created in an extraperitoneal location, a closed suction or sump drain may be placed posterior to the rectum (presacral space). The drain is brought out through a separate stab incision in the lower quadrant of the abdominal wall. When studied prospectively, sump irrigation of these drains has not demonstrated any advantages over simple suction and the actual value of routine drainage has been difficult to prove [11].

Lesions of the **lower rectum** are managed with an APR, coloanal pullthrough, or a transanal excision. The patient is prepared as described in Chapter 8. For an APR, the patient is positioned in a modified Lloyd-Davies position, and exploration is performed through a vertical midline incision. The left and sigmoid colon are mobilized as described above. The upper and middle rectum is mobilized as described for a low anterior resection. The dissection is continued posteriorly and laterally until the levators are reached. Anteriorly, the dissection continues posterior to the prostate to the top of the levators (puborectalis muscle).

An intraoperative decision will usually be required to determine which operation is appropriate. If the lesion is suitable to obtain clear margins (an R0 resection) a **coloanal pullthrough** may be performed. The rectum is mobilized as above to the level of the levators. At this level (which should be below the cancer), the dissection continues along the top of the levators to the rectal wall. The colon is divided at the distal left or proximal sigmoid colon with the site of this division based on the vascular anatomy and the length of bowel required to reach the anus without tension. It is almost always necessary to divide the inferior mesenteric vein (IMV) a second time just below the pancreas to obtain adequate length.

The surgeon then moves to the perineum and accomplishes a mucosal dissection (proctectomy) in a manner similar to the method described for a pouch-anal anastomosis (Chapter 14). After the anal mucosa is stripped to the top of the levator sling, the remaining rectal wall is incised (top of the levators) and the specimen is removed (**Figure 22.8a**). Eight sutures are placed through the anoderm and the distal portion of the internal sphincter muscle. The end of the left colon is brought through the pelvis and out the muscular anal canal. The previously placed sutures are used to perform an anastomosis. Most authors routinely place a drain into the presacral space and perform a temporary diverting loop ileostomy (in the right lower quadrant).

A colonic pouch (e.g. J-shaped pouch) or coloplasty can be incorporated into the procedure. Some evidence suggests that these modifications may reduce the early bowel alterations associated with a conventional ultra-low anterior resection or coloanal pullthrough [12,13]. However, when many of these patients are studies long-term their function seems similar.

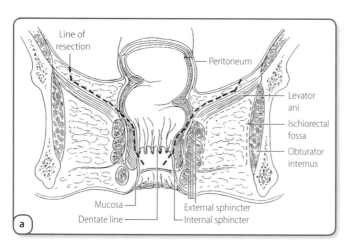

Figure 22.8 The dissection plane for rectal lesions. (a) Coloanal pullthrough. (b) Abdominoperineal resection.

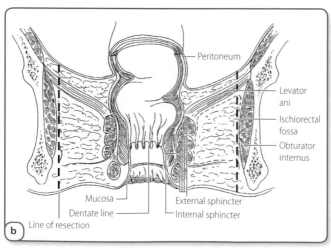

If a coloanal pullthrough is not indicated, an APR should be performed. The rectum is removed as previously described and the entire anus is also excised. The rectum is mobilized as described (**Figure 22.8b**). The perineum is then prepared with a povidone-iodine solution and incisions are made in the perineal skin (**Figure 22.9**).

It is important for the surgeon to picture the dissection in a three-dimensional manner. A straight plane of dissection is used from the pelvis to the top of the levators (**Figure 22.8b**). The correct margins of this dissection include the prostate (anteriorly), the tip of the coccyx (posteriorly), and the pubic rami (laterally). Electrocautery is used to divide the perineal tissue. The levators are then opened posteriorly just anterior to the tip of the coccyx. The remaining levators are divided with electrocautery at the lateral pelvic side walls. The specimen is removed, hemostasis is obtained, and the pelvis is closed. Performing the dissection in the correct manner will leave inadequate levator or perirectal tissue to close the pelvic defect. However, there should be adequate subcutaneous tissue and skin to perform a tension-free closure of the perineum. To eliminate the requirement for suture or staple removal in the perineum, I use absorbable suture to approximate

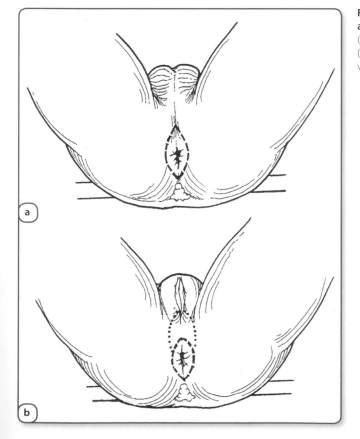

Figure 22.9 Perineal incision for an abdominoperineal resection. (a) Male patient. (b) Female patient. (Dotted line indicates posterior vaginectomy.)

this tissue. An omental pedicle flap is then placed into the pelvis to eliminate dead space and reduce chances for small bowel to fall into the pelvis. This is especially important if the patient will receive radiotherapy in the postoperative period.

For selected lesions, a **transanal excision** is an option. The lesion should be small (2–3 cm in diameter), mobile, and within reach of the anus (5–6 cm from the anal verge) and intrarectal ultrasound uT1-2 N0 (see Table 4.1). The technique involves infiltrating a 1:100,000 epinephrine solution into the submucosal space below the lesion (**Figure 22.10**). This produces hemostasis and delineates the correct surgical dissection plane. The mucosa is then marked at 1 cm out

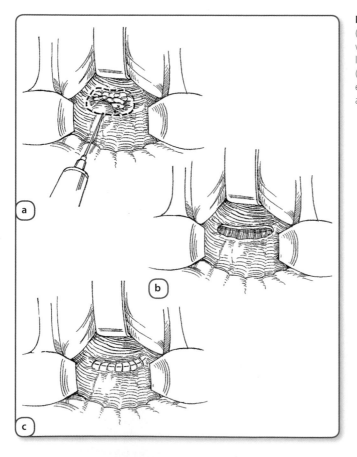

Figure 22.10 Transanal excision. (a) The dissection plane is infiltrated with epinephrine solution and the lesion is excised with a 1 cm margin. (b) Defect after the lesion has been excised. (c) The defect is closed with absorbable suture.

Table 22.2 Submucosal SM classification system (Kikuchi et al, 1995 [14])		
Classification	**Description**	**Submucosal depth**
SM1	Slight submucosal invasion from the muscularis mucosa	200–300 µm
SM2	Intermediary between SM1 and SM3	–
SM3	Carcinoma invasion near the inner surface of the muscularis propria	–

from the lesion using electrocautery. Traction sutures are occasionally helpful.

The lesion is excised using electrocautery, with care taken to keep the lesion and surrounding tissue intact during the excision. Once completely removed, the specimen should be pinned out on a flat surface and placed in fixative solution to allow orientation of the specimen and an accurate assessment of the margins. If the specimen has adequate clear margins and invasion is limited to the submucosa (T1), no additional surgical treatment is needed. To enhance our understanding of the behavior of these early lesions a submucosal (SM) classification has been proposed. (**Table 22.2**) [14].

Many authors recommend adjuvant radiotherapy for T2 lesions [15]. Positive margins require an additional excision, a coloanal pull-through, or an APR. For patients with lesions found to be T3–4 or N1, radical resections are usually recommended.

In order to overcome the technical challenges of transanal excision and facilitate endoluminal dissection, Gerhard Buess developed transanal endoscopic microsurgery (TEM) in Tubingen, Germany in the early 1980s [16]. The equipment was developed by Wolf Surgical Instruments Company (Vernon Hills, Illinois, USA) and is now available through Wolf and Storz (Karl Storz & Co.). The operating rectoscope is 40 mm in diameter and is available in lengths of 12 and 20 cm [17]. The distal end is angled 45° and delivers a light from an external source while rectal insufflation is accomplished with CO_2. A double-ball joint attached to the operative table allows for stability and easy adjustment. The sealing system prevents gas leakage while allowing for instrument introduction through three operative ports.

Patient preparation is similar to transanal excision with special care noting the exact position of the tumor. Postoperative care is also similar to that of local excision. Advantages of TEM include superior visualization with an insufflated and magnified view of the rectum as seen from above the tumor, precise full-thickness dissection with improved lymph node harvest and ability to excise larger tumors, and better access to tumors in the mid- and upper-rectum as well as the distal colon. Disadvantages include cost of the equipment and the learning curve associated with the use of this highly specialized piece of equipment.

As with conventional local excision, proper case selection is critical. Although TEM is technically challenging, the proper use of the equipment allows enhanced visualization and superior access to tumors of the rectum and distal colon. The reported experience suggests a lower recurrence rate compared to traditional transanal excision [17].

One disadvantage of a transanal excision is that it does not allow assessment of the lymph node status, which limits the accuracy of lesion staging. This has led some authors to suggest postoperative radiotherapy. Proponents feel that radiotherapy is associated with low morbidity and possible reduction of local recurrence rates. Opponents argue that many patients who have no residual disease are being treated. In the absence of prospective controlled trials, therapeutic decisions must be individualized, taking into account the lesion's character, experience of the surgeon, and the patient's desires.

Additional local treatment options include electrocauterization and posterior excisions (e.g. Kraske or York-Mason procedures). In appropriately selected patients, good results are possible with either method [4].

Radiotherapy

Radiotherapy for colorectal cancer has been used in several ways [1]. The therapy can be delivered in the preoperative, intraoperative, or postoperative period or a combination of these (e.g. a 'sandwich' method using low-dose preoperative and conventional dose postoperative radiotherapy). It may also be used as primary or adjuvant therapy. Currently the three methods for delivering ionizing radiation to colorectal cancers are external beam, implant, and endocavitary radiation. The amount of radiation delivered is measured in units of Gray (Gy) (1 Gy = 100 rads).

Most external beam therapy is delivered by linear accelerators (4–25 million electron volts [MEV]) or cobalt sources (1.25 MEV). The higher the energy, the deeper the penetration and the lower the skin dose. This form is useful for deep tumors and irradiating larger volumes of tissue, such as the pelvis or inguinal regions. It is the mainstay of adjuvant therapy. External beam therapy can also be administered interoperatively. This requires radiotherapy equipment in the operating room or transporting the anesthetized patient with the abdomen open to the radiotherapy suite.

Brachytherapy involves placing radioactive sources (implants) into close anatomic relationship with a tumor. This minimizes the radiation to distant surrounding tissue, yet delivers very high doses of radiation to the local area. Commonly iridium-192 (^{192}Ir) seeds are placed through hollow needle applicators and later removed, or iodine-131 (^{131}I) seed implants are placed permanently into the tissue. The latter technique is particularly helpful for irradiating the bed of locally excised tumors in those situations where the margins are questionable.

Endocavitary radiation (Papillion technique) is delivered by a hand-held 50 kilovolt peak (kVp) generator introduced transanally [15, 18, 19]. In this fashion, 9 Gy/min of superficial therapy can be delivered. It is used most often as primary therapy for early small anorectal cancers (less than 2 cm in diameter). Unfortunately, only a few of these therapy units currently exist and none are being manufactured.

For colon carcinomas, radiotherapy has limited uses, with no truly defined primary or adjuvant role. Patients who undergo resection for large, locally invasive tumors with microscopically positive margins have undergone palliative irradiation to the tumor bed, using both external beam and brachytherapy, with mixed results. In rectal carcinoma, radiotherapy plays a large role. With the exception of small cancers, radiotherapy in the United States has evolved as an important means of adjuvant therapy and for the treatment of locally recurrent disease.

Adjuvant radiotherapy for rectal cancer assists with local recurrence and resectability. Local (pelvic) recurrence is related to the location, pathologic stage, and differentiation of the primary tumor. Pelvic recurrence rates after 'curative' resections for rectal cancer have ranged from 3–53% [4]. High local recurrence rates have prompted trials of adjuvant therapy. Multiple trials have been performed with varying doses, schedules of radiotherapy, and types of controls. The studies available to date show significant reduction in local recurrence when groups treated with radiotherapy are compared with control groups with a 30% or greater rate of local recurrence. In studies with lower local recurrence rate (5–15%), no statistical improvement in local recurrence rate has been demonstrated with radiotherapy. Additional well-controlled trials are necessary to delineate the appropriate role of adjuvant radiotherapy.

Outside of ongoing protocols, the author prefers using preoperative radiotherapy in patients with questionably resectable rectal lesions (large, fixed, uT3-4 N1, poorly differentiated tumors, and those close to the anal sphincter). Postoperative radiotherapy is offered to rectal cancer patients who did not receive preoperative radiotherapy and were unresectable for cure or those with a pathologically poor prognosis (e.g. Astler-Coller B_2, C_1, or C_2 lesions, [stage III]), those with large bulky tumors whose chances for local recurrence seems inordinately high, and patients with perforated lesions.

Chemotherapy

The role of chemotherapy for colorectal cancer continues to evolve. In patients with metastatic disease it has been used in a therapeutic role, and after 'curative resections' it has been used as adjuvant therapy [15, 20].

In the treatment of metastatic disease, several drugs have consistently produced response rates above 15% (**Table 22.3**). The best of these, 5-fluorouracil (5-FU), has produced an objective response in 10–20% of patients. The optimal dosage schedule and mode of delivery have yet to be defined. Previous trials suggested improved results when 5-FU was combined with leucovorin (LV) (a folic acid agonist) or levamisole (an antihelmintic drug with immunologic or biochemical modulatory activity) [20]. The current standard uses 5-FU, LV, and Oxaliplatin (FOLFOX). Irinotecan has also been approved for first-line therapy in combination with 5-FU and LV. However, other agents are being used and are under study. To date chemotherapy has not produced a clinically significant improvement in overall survival for patients with metastatic disease.

Adjuvant chemotherapy is less defined and results have differed for colonic and rectal carcinomas. Some of these observed differences are explained by the different recurrent patterns of these tumors.

Table 22.3 Chemotherapeutic agents

Therapy	Mechanism of action	Indications	Potential common toxicities
5- fluorouracil (5-FU)	Blocks the enzyme thymidylate synthase (TS), which is essential for DNA synthesis	Multiple uses in combination with other agents, both in the adjuvant (postoperative) and palliative setting	Gastrointestinal (nausea, diarrhea) Myelosuppression Fatigue
Capecitabine	Blocks thymidylate synthase (orally administered prodrug, converted to 5-FU)	Multiple uses in combination with other agents, both in the adjuvant (postoperative) and metastatic setting	Gastrointestinal (nausea, diarrhea) Myelosuppression Fatigue Palmar – plantar syndrome (hand – foot syndrome)
Oxaliplatin	Inhibits DNA replication and transcription by forming inter- and intra-strand DNA adducts/cross-links	Used in combination with 5-FU, leucovorin (LV) (FOLFOX) in the adjuvant (postop) and metastatic setting	Peripheral neuropathy Gastrointestinal (nausea, diarrhea) Fatigue Myelosuppression Hypersensitivity
Irinotecan	Inhibits topoisomerase I, an enzyme that facilitates the uncoiling and recoiling of DNA during replication	Used alone or in combination with 5-FU, LV (FOLFIRI) in the metastatic setting	Cholinergic (acute diarrhea) Gastrointestinal (nausea, late diarrhea) Fatigue Myelosuppression Alopecia
Bevacizumab	Monoclonal antibody which binds to VEGF ligand	Used in combination with either FOLFOX or FOLFIRI in the metastatic setting	Hypertension Arterial thrombotic events Impaired wound healing Gastrointestinal perforation
Cetuximab	Monoclonal antibody to EGFR (chimeric) that blocks the ligand-binding site	Used with irinotecan or as a single agent in the metastatic setting	Acneform rash Hypersensitivity Hypomagnesemia Fatigue
Panitumumab	Monoclonal antibody to EGFR (fully humanized) that blocks the ligand-binding site	Used as a single agent in the metastatic setting	Acneform rash Hypomagnesemia Fatigue
Mitomycin C	Inhibits DNA synthesis	Anal cancer	
Leucovorin	Folic acid	Used with 5-FU	

Local recurrence is a major problem in rectal cancers. The lack of a rectal serosa, extensive blood supply, and difficulty in obtaining wider margins may partially explain this finding. Many patients with colonic and rectal carcinoma do ultimately develop systemic disease in addition to local recurrences. Preliminary evidence suggests that the combination of systemic adjuvant chemotherapy and local radiotherapy improves the disease-free survival and the overall survival of patients with rectal cancer. Chemotherapy alone has yet to show a beneficial effect on survival or local recurrence rates in rectal cancer.

Adjuvant chemotherapy has a role in the treatment of colon carcinoma. An intergroup study reported a lower recurrence rate and improved survival in stage C colon cancer patients who received levamisole plus fluorouracil after curative resections. These advantages were not observed in patients with B_2 lesions. The National Cancer

Institute Consensus Development Conference recommended that Stage II and III rectal cancer patients who are not enrolled in adjuvant therapy protocols receive a sequential regimen of 5-FU and radiation therapy after curative resection of their tumors [21].

Follow-up care

Currently there is no consensus on the appropriate follow-up for cancer [22].

My preference is to see patients every 3–4 months for the first 2 years, every 6 months for the next 2 years, and every year thereafter. On each visit a complete history is obtained, physical examination performed, and serum evaluated for a carcinoembryonic antigen (CEA). If the colon was cleared preoperatively by a colonoscopy or high-quality barium enema, a colonoscopy is done at 1 year postoperatively. If the colon was not cleared for synchronous or metachronous lesions before surgery, a colonoscopy is performed at 3 months postoperatively. Patients with a left-sided anastomosis may be offered a sigmoidoscopic examination between colonoscopies. Other patients with an intact rectum have a colonoscopy during their yearly follow-up and subsequent colonoscopy at 1–3 years, depending on the findings at the first postoperative colonoscopy [23]. This follow-up has recommended by the American Society of Colon and Rectal Surgeons in their published guidelines [24].

If the CEA becomes elevated during follow-up, a CT scan of the abdomen and pelvis and a colonoscopy are obtained. If these tests are negative or suggest resectable tumor, additional studies such as positive emission tomography (PET) scan or immunologic scan (e.g. CEA) can be obtained [25, 26]. If a surgically resectable lesion is identified, exploratory surgery is offered. Patients with unresectable disease are referred for consideration of chemotherapy. If no lesions are found on evaluation, the patient is offered continued follow-up or in very selected patients, an exploratory laparotomy. The benefits (survival or palliation) and risks (morbidity, mortality, and costs) must be evaluated with each patient.

Prognosis and staging

The extent of tumor penetration into the bowel wall, involvement of lymph nodes, and distant metastases all affect outcome. The first two factors can be determined only by pathologic review of surgical specimens. To relate these factors to prognosis, several staging systems have been proposed. Cuthbert Dukes, a pathologist at St. Marks Hospital in London, proposed his original system for rectal cancers in 1932 [27]. As shown in **Figure 22.11**, this system had three categories: **A lesions** were confined to the bowel wall, **B lesions** penetrated the bowel wall, and **C lesions** had positive lymph nodes. In 1949 Kirkland, Dockerty, and Waugh [28] described modifying Dukes' system in several ways. They expanded it to include colon lesions and altered the classes by changing the A category to lesions limited to the mucosa, and splitting the B category into B_1 (confined to the muscularis propria) and B_2 (through the bowel wall).

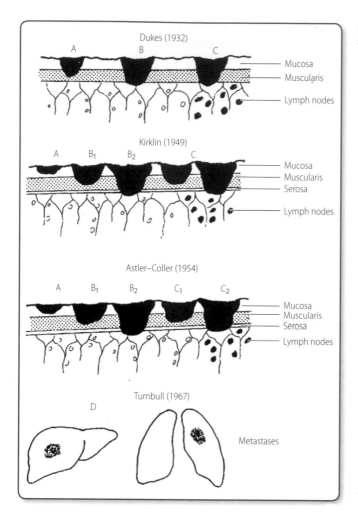

Figure 22.11 Colorectal cancer staging systems.

In 1954 Astler and Coller [29] proposed splitting the C lesions into C_1 (penetration similar to B_1 and tumor in nodes) and C_2 (penetration through bowel wall and positive nodes). In 1967 Turnbull et al [30] proposed a clinicopathologic staging system and described a D category for patients with metastatic disease.

Using these staging systems, ranges of survival figures have been described (**Table 22.4**) [31].

Table 22.4 Survival rates of each stage of colon and rectal carcinoma	
Stage	**5-year survival (%)**
A	90
B	60–80
C	20–50
D	6

The reported variability may be the result of differences in patient groups, follow-up, and classification. The overall survival for all patients with colorectal cancer is 50–60% at 5 years.

A TNM (tumor-node-metastasis) staging system has been proposed for colorectal cancer and subsequently modified:

T   1–Tumor invades submucosa

      2–Tumor invades muscularis propria

      3–Tumor invades through muscularis propria into or through serosa

      4–Tumor invades other organs or structures

N   0–No regional lymph node metastasis

      1–Metastasis in one to three pericolic or perirectal lymph nodes

      2–Metastasis in four or more pericolic or perirectal lymph nodes

      3–Metastasis in lymph nodes along a named vascular trunk

M   0–No distant metastasis

      1–Distant metastasis

Anus

Anal neoplasms are uncommon, with an incidence one twentieth that of rectal adenocarcinoma or 1.5–4% of large bowel cancers [32]. Current statistics indicate that this incidence is increasing, and the management of these tumors has undergone significant changes.

Anatomy

For clinical purposes, the anus can be divided into two areas: the anal canal and the anal margin (see Figure 1.4). The **anal canal** runs from the anorectal junction (top of the anal sphincter muscles) to the intersphincteric groove (approximately 2 cm distal to the dentate line). Thus it corresponds to the internal sphincter. The lining of this portion of the anus is formed by transitional epithelium, which contains elements of both columnar and squamous epithelium above the dentate line and squamous epithelium distal to the dentate line.

The **anal margin** runs from the intersphincteric groove to approximately 5 cm on the perineum. This area is covered by nonkeratinizing squamous epithelium which changes to keratinizing squamous epithelium at the anal margin's outer border with the perineal skin.

Anal canal

Epidermoid carcinoma

Epidermoid carcinomas are the most common forms of anal canal neoplasms [33]. On histologic review of these neoplasms, 70% are found to be squamous cell neoplasms, 25% are basaloid neoplasms, and 5% are mucoepidermoid. Clinically the different histologic types act in a similar manner.

The lymphatic drainage of the anus follows the arterial vessels. Thus metastatic anal disease can spread in three different directions. Superiorly, this includes the pararectal and superior hemorrhoidal nodes, laterally the internal iliac nodes, and inferiorly the inguinal and external iliac nodes. For prognostic purposes, anal canal cancers have been grouped into four stages: Stage 1 tumors are confined to the sphincteric mechanism, Stage 2 have extended into the perirectal fat, Stage 3 have involved lymph nodes, and Stage 4 have distant metastases. Other staging systems have been described. The TNM system has been adopted by the American Joint Committee on Cancer.

T1	Carcinoma: < 2 cm in diameter
T2	> 2 and < 5 cm in diameter
T3	> 5 cm in diameter
T4	invading adjacent organ

N0	No regional node involvement
N1	Metastasis in perirectal lymph nodes
N2	Metastasis in unilateral iliac or inguinal nodes
N3	Metastasis in bilateral iliac or inguinal nodes

M0	No distant metastasis
M1	Distant metastasis

Unfortunately, lymph node involvement is difficult to determine in the absence of surgical specimens.

Diagnosis

Patients with anal cancer usually present with bleeding per rectum and pain. The bleeding is red and usually more constant than that associated with hemorrhoids [3]. The pain is less severe than with an acute fissure and also more constant. An occasional patient will also complain of an ulcerated or mass lesion of the anus. Additional questions help to evaluate these symptoms and exclude other differential diagnoses.

The physical examination is helpful in making the diagnosis and is essential to determine the clinical stage of disease. Anal cancers are within reach of the examining finger and are hard, irregular, and usually ulcerated (**Figure 22.12**). The exact location and size of the lesion must be documented. This includes the vertical and horizontal diameter of the lesion, as well as the height above the anal verge. The anatomic location (e.g. anterior versus posterior and right or left) should also be noted. An assessment of the lesion's fixity, relation to other structures, and the status of the sphincteric muscles completes the perineal examination. In addition to an evaluation of the lesion, the patient should be examined for the presence of inguinal adenopathy.

Direct visualization of the anus and rectum is essential to exclude other lesions and allows biopsy of the lesion to confirm the clinical diagnosis. Anoscopy provides good exposure and is the least expensive method to examine the anal canal. After identification, the lesion should undergo biopsy. Several specimens should be obtained from the edges of the lesion. A local anesthetic is usually not required.

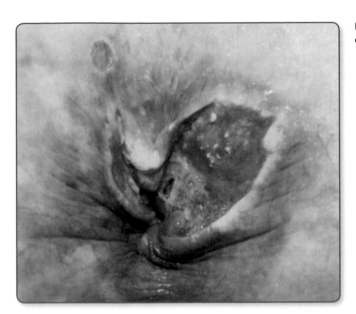

Figure 22.12 Anal squamous cell carcinoma.

To assist in clinical staging, several modalities are currently available. The details of each diagnostic procedure were discussed in Chapter 4. Anal or rectal ultrasound is being used with increased frequency and is helpful in assessing the depth of anal tumors and in identifying the presence and characteristics of lymph nodes. The difficulty remains with the identification of suspicious nodes. The quality of the examination depends on the operator, and further widespread experience is necessary.

CT and MRI scans help assess the extent of the primary tumor and the presence of enlarged lymph nodes. A scan can determine the size and location of lymph nodes but again cannot accurately determine if the nodes contain tumor. This study can also evaluate the liver to exclude the presence of large hepatic metastases (greater than 1 cm). therapy, and combinations of these modalities.

Treatment

Anal cancer has been treated by surgery, radiation, chemotherapy, and combinations of these modalities.

Surgical options include APR and transanal excision. The standard surgical therapy for anal cancer before 1974 was APR. An APR performed for anal cancer is similar to that described for rectal cancer, with the exception that a slightly wider margin of perineal skin is removed. The 5-year survival rate after this form of treatment averaged 50%, with a published range of 30–70% [34, 35].

An **APR** is a major intra-abdominal operation to remove the rectum and results in significant morbidity and a permanent stoma. The perioperative mortality after an APR is 2–14%, and the local (pelvic) recurrence rate is 11–40% [4].

For early lesions **local excision** (transanal excision) is a valid consideration but must be limited to lesions that are well differentiated, less than 2 cm in diameter, and located in the distal anal canal. The procedure is similar to that described for early rectal cancers. Using this procedure in selected patients, the reported 5-year survival has ranged from 45–100% [34, 36].

Anal carcinomas are radiosensitive tumors, and chemoradiotherapy is the current treatment of choice. As surgery or radiotherapy alone produced suboptimal results, Dr Nigro and colleagues at Wayne State University proposed initial chemotherapy and radiotherapy followed by APR. In 1974, they reported initial results using 5-FU, mitomycin-C, and radiotherapy (3000 rads), followed by an APR [37]. Additional experience and longer follow-up were reported by the same group in 1983 [38]. Summarizing the early published reports reveals a local recurrence rate of 10–25% and a toxicity of 20–30%.

Experience at two major center helps describe the management of these uncommon tumors. At Wilford Hall USAF Medical Center, from 1981–1991, 35 patients with epidermoid anal canal carcinoma were treated with a combination of chemotherapy and radiotherapy [33]. Mitomycin-C and 5-FU were administered as suggested by Nigro et al [38]. The radiotherapy was delivered in 2 Gy doses in apposed fields and averaged 40 Gy (30–60 Gy). In the initial seven patients, an APR was performed following the combined therapy. In the first six patients treated by this method, no tumor was found in the pathologic specimens. Based on this finding and reports of Nigro and other authors, the tumor sites of later patients were examined 6 weeks after initial therapy. Any abnormal lesions underwent biopsy. Only one patient was found to have a persistent tumor, which was treated with an APR. Of the remaining 29 patients who did not receive an APR, five had moderate problems with continence and one required a diverting colostomy for incontinence. Follow-up ranged from 4 months to 12.9 years (mean 5.2 years). There were two pelvic recurrences, and three patients developed distal metastasis. Eight patients died during follow-up, including three with recurrent or persistent disease. The 5-year survival rate using life-table analysis was 89%.

At the Ochsner Clinic Foundation, 51 patients with epidermoid were treated from 1979–2000 with chemoradiation [39]. The average dose of radiotherapy was 57 Gy. The average tumor size was 3.9 cm and 12 patients had clinically positive nodes. With mean follow-up of 5.6 years 96% of the patients retained a functional anus. However 29% of the patients complained of bowel or bladder incontinence at some point during follow-up and three patients had severe complications in the form of acute respiratory distress syndrome (ARDS), severe neutropenia, or the development of leukemia. Although chemoradiation is currently the standard of care for epidermoid carcinoma of the anus, it caries numerous acute and late complications that may be life-threatening.

Several studies have evaluated various chemotherapy regimens and compared chemoradiotherapy to radiotherapy alone [40–42].

Chemoradiotherapy with 5-FU and mitomycin-C was better in terms of local control, preservation of anorectal function and survival. The reported experience with multimodality treatment for anal carcinoma continues to expand [37]. The low incidence of epidermoid cancer necessitates multicenter prospective controlled trials to study these issues.

Chemoradiotherapy for anal cancer entails 30–60 Gy (given over 3–5 weeks) using apposed fields with: 5-FU (1000 mg/m^2/day) on days 1–5 and days 31–35 and mitomycin C (15 mg/m^2) on day 1. Using an anoscope, the lesion site is inspected 6–8 weeks after the radiotherapy is completed and a biopsy is performed on any abnormalities. Some providers will allow additional time after therapy to confirm complete clinical regression of the tumor before embarking on additional therapy. An APR, local excision, or additional chemoradiotherapy is offered to patients with residual disease following combined therapy.

Melanoma

Anorectal melanomas are rare; they account for 1% of all melanomas and 0.25–1% of anorectal tumors [43]. The mean age of occurrence is in the fifth decade; females are affected more frequently than males. The most frequent presenting symptom is bleeding, followed by an anal mass or pain. The lesions are usually elevated and 34–75% will be pigmented.

These tumors are locally invasive and have a high metastatic potential. Because many patients present late, the reported 5-year survival rates range from 0–12%. The prognosis is related to tumor size, thickness, and clinical stage. Evaluation should include a biopsy and a search for metastatic disease (by CT of the abdomen, pelvis, and chest; liver function tests; chest X-ray evaluation; and bone scans). Special stains or electron microscopy may be required to confirm the diagnostic biopsy.

Surgery provides the only hope for cure. However, both the small chance for cure and the limited experience have led to controversy about the appropriate procedure. Reports comparing APR with local excision have shown little difference in the mean survival rates following either procedure [4]. Therefore, if the lesion can be excised with clear margins, local excision is recommended. APR is reserved for larger lesions in which a clear margin can still be obtained. Prophylactic lymphadenectomy is not indicated for clinically negative nodes but is helpful for clinically suspicious nodes. Radiotherapy and chemotherapy have demonstrated little benefit in this disease.

Anal margin

Premalignant lesions

Premalignant lesions of the anal margin are uncommon and include **highgrade squamous intraepithelial lesion (HSIL)**, formally knows as Bowen's disease, and Paget's disease. HSIL or Bowen's disease, an intraepithelial squamous cell carcinoma, is named after John T. Bowen, who in 1912 described two patients with atypical epithelial proliferation of the skin. The first perianal case of Bowen's disease was reported by Vickers in 1939, and to date a few hundred cases have been reported in the literature [44]. Increased experience has demonstrated that infection by human papilloma virus (HPV) is a necessary but not sufficient cause for the development of this lesion [45].

Paget's disease is an even rarer intraepithelial adenocarcinoma. It was named for Sir James Paget, who described 15 patients with a characteristic breast lesion in 1874. The extramammary variety can be found wherever apocrine glands are located. The first case of perianal disease was reported in 1893 by Darier and Coulillaud. Since then, approximately 200 cases of perianal disease have been reported in the surgical literature [44]. Patients with perianal Bowen's or Paget's disease commonly present with nonspecific complaints of anal itching, burning, or bleeding. Examination of the perineum in symptomatic patients usually reveals raised, irregular, scaly, brownish-red plaques with eczematoid features in perianal Bowen's disease. In Paget's disease the lesions are well demarcated eczematoid plaques that are either ulcerative and crusty or papillary. Less commonly, these lesions may have a gross appearance similar to other diseases (e.g. leukoplakia, squamous cell cancer, condylomata acuminata, dermatitis, eczema, downward spread of rectal carcinoma, or prolapsed hemorrhoids), making the diagnosis by inspection alone difficult. A significant percentage of patients will be diagnosed after pathologic evaluation of operative specimens.

The microscopic appearance of these perianal lesions is characteristic and readily confirms the diagnosis. HSIL demonstrates a disordered epidermal hyperplasia with parakeratosis and hyperkeratosis in the superficial surface layers. The malpighian cells also reveal a disordered hyperplasia, with atypism and malignant dyskeratotic cells. Large atypical cells with haloed large hyperchromatic nuclei (bowenoid cells) are present and are negative for a periodic acid-Schiff (PAS) stain. Mitotic figures are present in all layers [46]. On cytologic examination (anal 'pap smears'), abnormal cells are identified that have been referred to as anal intraepithelial neoplasia (AIN). Cells are graded from 1 to 3, with Grade 3 lesions corresponding to HSIL.

Perianal Paget's disease is characterized by large, faintly basophilic or vacuolated cells located in the epidermis. The nuclei are vesicular and demonstrate little mitotic activity [47]. In contrast to bowenoid cells, the Paget cells become highlighted with a PAS stain because of the high mucin content of these cells. They also stain with a CEA immunofluorescence stain.

An accurate diagnosis is important for prognostic and therapeutic reasons. The clinical course of HSIL has been relatively benign, with progression toward invasive carcinoma in 2–6% of cases. In Paget's disease, progression into an invasive carcinoma has been reported to be as high as 40% in untreated lesions. However, the small number of reported patients with these perianal lesions has limited our understanding about prognosis.

In addition to concern about progression to an invasive cancer, a relationship of these epithelial lesions to nonepithelial malignancies has been proposed. Early reports described such a relationship. However, a re-examination of the methods and analyses used in these published studies by Arbesman and Ransohoff [48] demonstrated several flaws and led to the conclusion that the evidence was insufficient to confirm a relationship between HSIL and the subsequent development of internal malignancies. In addition, a recent collective survey of experience with perianal HSIL found the incidence of subsequent nonsquamous malignancy to be low at 4.7% [49].

In Paget's disease the association with cancer has been much stronger. The incidence of associated malignancies in the reported series averaged 50–73% and the mortality was high from this cancer despite aggressive therapy. There are several differences in patients with Bowen's disease and those with Paget's disease [50]. Patients with Bowen's disease are younger (average 48 years of age) than those with Paget's disease (average 66 years of age). The sex distribution is equal for Paget's disease patients, whereas in HSIL there is a higher proportion of women. The incidence of an associated invasive malignancy is higher with Paget's disease and the prognosis is worse [43].

Patients with anal lesions that appear suspicious or fail to respond to conventional therapy within a month should undergo a biopsy. An adequate biopsy is essential both to confirm the diagnosis and to exclude an invasive carcinoma. A proper biopsy technique entails three or four full-thickness biopsies (i.e. including subcutaneous tissue) from the central portion and edges of the lesion. This can be easily accomplished with local anesthesia, a sharp punch biopsy, and fine-pointed scissors or a scalpel. If pathologic evaluation identifies a pre- or potentially malignant lesion, the patient should undergo an evaluation to exclude an associated invasive cancer.

If evaluation demonstrates an invasive carcinoma without metastases, an aggressive approach is warranted to improve the historically poor prognosis associated with these diseases. For adenocarcinoma of the lower rectum, I recommend an APR, and for an epidermoid anal cancer, chemoradiotherapy is suggested.

In the absence of invasive cancer, a local excision with clear margins is indicated. Adequate, microscopically clear margins are important for Paget's and less critical for HSIL. In both conditions abnormal cells may extend beyond the gross margins of the lesion. To ensure a complete excision, 'lesion mapping' has been used by some authors [44]. Biopsies are obtained 1 cm from the edge of the lesion and in all four quadrants of the perineum. Two to 3 mm biopsy specimens are taken at the dentate line, anal verge, and the perineum (approximately 2–3 cm from the anal verge). With this mapping as a guide, a wide local excision of the lesion is accomplished. Following removal of the specimen, the margins of resection may be examined by frozen section techniques to ensure complete excision. In the absence of this the lesion is oriented on cardboard to allow the pathologist to accurately identify any involved margin.

The wound defect is either closed primarily, covered with a split-thickness skin graft (either at the initial operation or 3–4 days later), or allowed to heal by secondary intention. The low recurrence rate in patients treated by wide local excision supports this therapy as the appropriate method. Wide excision of lesions, especially very large ones, can produce significant morbidity. As experience has increased, some authors have stressed balancing the morbidity of large wide excisions against the low incidence of cancer development in patients who are monitored closely. In selected patients, especially HSIL, there may be a role for excision of gross lesions followed by close follow-up [51].

Long-term follow-up is recommended to prevent recurrence of both perianal HSIL and Paget's disease. However, the limited experience with this disease has hindered the development of a standardized follow-up regimen. A complete physical examination, anoscopy, and punch biopsy of any new lesion are performed on a 3–12 monthly basis. If a recurrence is found, it is excised with adequate clear margins using the methods described above.

Malignant lesions

Squamous cell carcinoma of the anal margin acts in a manner similar to that of lesions occurring in other cutaneous areas of the body. The lesions appear as raised hard flat masses that may ulcerate. The appropriate therapy is wide local excision with clear margins.

Basal cell cancers of the anal margin are rare and appear as ulcerated masses. Nonspecific complaints include bleeding and pruritus. Wide local excision with clear margins is the treatment of choice [51].

Rounds questions

5. What is the most common visceral cancer?
6. From what cells do carcinoid tumors arise?
7. What is the primary method to treat colorectal cancer?
8. What are the names of important fascial planes anterior and posterior to the rectum?
9. Who was Dukes?
10. In what stage would a colonic tumor that penetrates through the bowel wall without lymph node involvement be classified as?
11. Which colon cancer patients should receive adjuvant therapy?
12. Which rectal cancer patients should receive adjuvant therapy?
13. What is a CEA test?
14. Define the anatomic boundaries of the anal canal.
15. What is the primary treatment for epidermoid carcinoma of the anal canal?
16. What is HSIL? What is Paget's disease?

References

1. http://www.cancer.org/Cancer/
   ColonandRectumCancer/DetailedGuide/
   colorectal-cancer-key-statistics. March 28, 2011.
2. Beck DE. Malignant lesions. In: Beck DE, Welling
   DR (eds). Patient Care in Colorectal Surgery.
   Boston: Little, Brown, 1991;293–318.
3. Beck DE, Wexner SD. Anal neoplasms. In: Beck
   DE, Wexner SD (eds). Fundamentals of Anorectal
   Surgery. New York McGraw-Hill, 1992;222–37.
4. Jetmore AB, Ray JE, Gathright JB, et al. Rectal
   carcinoids: The most frequent carcinoid tumor.
   Dis Colon Rectum 1992;35:717–25.
5. Gordon PH. Malignant neoplasms of the colon.
   In: Gordon PH, Nivatvongs S (eds). Principles
   and Practice of Surgery for the Colon, Rectum,
   and Anus. St. Louis: Quality Medical Publishing,
   1992;501–90.
6. Gordon PH. Malignant neoplasms of the rectum.
   In: Gordon PH, Nivatvongs S (eds). Principles
   and Practice of Surgery for the Colon, Rectum,
   and Anus. St. Louis: Quality Medical Publishing,
   1992;591–653.
7. Henry CA, Berry RE. Primary lymphoma of the
   large intestine. Am Surg 1988;54:262–6.
8. Reddy RM, Fleshman JW. Colorectal
   gastrointestinal stromal tumors: A brief review.
   Clinics Colon Rectal Surgery 2006;19:69–77.
9. Khoury DA, Opelka FG. Anoscopic-assisted
   insertion of end-to-end anastomosing staplers.
   Dis Colon Rectum 1995;38:553–4.
10. Perry WB. Management of perioperative
    hemorrhage. Clinics Colon Rectum Surg
    2001;14:49–56.
11. Galandiuk S, Fazio VW. Postoperative irrigation-
    suction drainage after pelvic colonic surgery. A
    prospective randomized trial. Dis Colon Rectum
    1991;34:223–8.
12. Farid A, Margolin DA. Low colorectal and
    coloanal anastomosis. Clinics Colon Rectal Surg
    2001;14:33–40.
13. Fazio VW, Mantyh CR, Hull TR. Colonic 'coloplasty.'
    Novel technique to enhance low colorectal
    or coloanal anastomosis. Dis Colon Rectum
    2000;43:1448–50.
14. Kikuchi R, Takano M, Takagi K, et al. Management
    of early invasive colorectal cancer. Dis Colon
    Rectum 1995;38:1286–95.
15. Orkin BA. Rectal carcinoma: Treatment. In:
    Beck DE, Wexner SD (eds). Fundamentals of
    Anorectal Surgery. New York: McGraw-Hill,
    1992;260–369.
16. Buess GF, Raestrup H. Transanal endoscopic
    microsurgery. Surg Oncol Clin N Am
    2001;10:709–31.
17. Geiser DP. Local treatment for Rectal Cancer.
    Clinics Colon Rectum Surgery 2007;20:182–9.
18. Kuske RR Jr. Acute and late toxicity of radiation
    therapy in rectal cancer. In: Hicks TC, Beck DE,
    Opelka FG, Timmcke AE (eds). Complications of
    Colon & Rectal Surgery. Baltimore: Williams &
    Wilkins, 1996;382–404.
19. Papillon J. New prospects in the conservative
    treatment of rectal cancer. Dis Colon Rectum
    1984;27:695–700.
20. Moertel CG, Fleming TR, Macdonald JS, et al.
    Levamisole and fluorouracil for adjuvant therapy
    of resected colon carcinoma. N Engl J Med
    1990;322:352–8.
21. National Cancer Institute Clinical Announcement
    on Adjuvant Therapy of Rectal Cancer, US.
    Department of Health and Human Services,
    Public Health Service, National Institutes of
    Health, Bethesda, 1999;14.
22. Vernava AM III, Long WE, Virgo KS, Coplin
    MA, Johnson FE. Current follow-up strategies
    after resection on colon cancer. Results of a
    survey of members of the American Society of
    Colon and Rectal Surgeons. Dis Colon Rectum
    1994;37:573–83.
23. Khoury D, Opelka FG, Beck DE et al. Colonoscopy
    surveillance after colorectal cancer surgery. Dis
    Colon Rectum 1996;39:252–6.
24. Anthony T, Simmang C, Hyman N, et al.
    Standards Practice Task Force. The American
    Society of Colon and Rectal Surgeons. Practice
    parameters for the surveillance and follow-up of
    patients with colon and rectal cancer. Dis Colon
    Rectum 2004;47:807–17.
25. Falk PM, Gupta NC, Thorson AG, et al. Positron
    emission tomography for preoperative staging
    of colorectal carcinoma. Dis Colon Rectum
    1994;37:153–6.
26. Divgi CR. Status of radiolabeled monoclonal
    antibodies for diagnosis and therapy of cancer.
    Oncology 1996;10:939–58.
27. Dukes C. The classification of cancer of the
    rectum. J Pathol Bacteriol 1932;35:323–32.
28. Kirklin JW, Dockerty MB, Waugh JM. The role
    of the perineal reflection in the prognosis of
    carcinoma of the rectum and sigmoid colon.
    Surg Gynecol Obstet 1949;88:326–31.
29. Astler VB, Coller FA. The prognostic significance
    of direct extension of carcinoma of the colon and
    rectum. Ann Surg 1954;139:846–52.
30. Turnbull RB, Kyle K, Watson FR, Spratt J. Cancer
    of the colon: The influence of the no-touch
    isolation technic on survival rates. Ann Surg
    1967;166:420–7.

31. Glass RE, Fazio VW, Jagelman DG, et al. The results of surgical treatment of cancer of the colon at the Cleveland Clinic from 1965–1975: Classification of the spread of colon cancer and long-term survival. Int J Colorect Dis 1986;1:33–9.

32. Localio SA, Eng K, Coppa GF. Anorectal Presacral and Sacral Tumors: Anatomy, physiology, and management. Philadelphia: WB Saunders, 1987;46–67.

33. Beck DE, Karulf RE. Combination therapy for epidermoid carcinoma of the anal canal. Dis Colon Rectum 1994;37:1118–25.

34. Frost DB, Richards PC, Montague ED, Giaco GG, Martin RG. Epidermoid cancer of the anorectum. Cancer 1984;53:1285–93.

35. Nivatvongs S. Perianal and anal canal neoplasms. In: Gordon PH, Nivatvongs S (eds). Principles and Practice of Surgery for the Colon, Rectum, and Anus. St. Louis: Quality Medical Publishing, 1992;401–17.

36. Gordon PH. Current status-perianal and anal canal neoplasms. Dis Colon Rectum 1990;33:799–808.

37. Nigro ND, Vaitkenicius VK, Considine B. Combined therapy for cancer of the anal canal: A preliminary report. Dis Colon Rectum 1974;17:354–6.

38. Nigro ND, Seydel HG, Considine B, Vaikevicius UK, Leichman L, Kinzie JJ. Combined preoperative radiation and chemotherapy for squamous cell carcinoma of the anal canal. Cancer 1983;51:1826–9.

39. Nguyen W, Mitchell K, Hawkins T, et al. Risk factors associated with requiring a stoma for management of anal cancer. Dis Colon Rectum 2004;47:843–6.

40. Cummings BJ, Keane TJ, O'Sullivan B, Wing ES, Cotton CN. Epidermoid anal cancer: Treatment by radiation alone or by radiation and 5-flurouravil with and without mitomycin C. Int J Radiat Oncol Biol Phys 1991;21:1115–25.

41. Allal A, Kurtz JM, Pipard G, et al. Chemoradiotherapy versus radiation therapy alone for anal cancer: A retrospective comparison. Int J Radiat Oncol Biol Phy 1993;27:59–66.

42. UKCCCR Anal Cancer Trial Working Party. Epidermoid anal cancer: Results from the UKCCR randomized trial of radiotherapy alone versus radiotherapy, 5-flurouracil and mitomycin. Lancet 1996;348;1049–54.

43. McNamara MJ. Melanoma and basal cell cancer. In: Fazio VW (ed). Current Therapy in Colon and Rectal Surgery. Philadelphia: BC Decker, 1990; 62–3.

44. Beck DE. Paget's disease and Bowen's disease of the anus. Semin Colon Rectal Surg 1995;6:143–9.

45. Welton ML, Raju N. Anal cancer. In: Beck DE, Wexner SD, Roberts PL, Sacclarides TJ, Senagore A, Stamos M (eds). ASCRS Textbook of Colorectal Surgery, 2nd ed. New York: Springer-Verlag, 2011; In press.

46. Beck DE, Fazio VW. Perianal Paget's disease. Dis Colon Rectum 1987;30:263–6.

47. Beck DE, Fazio VW, Jagelman DG, Lavery IC. Perianal Bowen's disease. Dis Colon Rectum 1988;31:419–22.

48. Arbesman H, Ransohoff DF. Is Bowen's disease a predictor for the development of internal malignancy? A methodological critique of the literature. JAMA 1987;257:516–8.

49. Marfing TE, Abel ME, Gallagher DM. Perianal Bowen's disease and associated malignancies. Results of a survey. Dis Colon Rectum 1987;30:782–5.

50. Beck DE, Fazio VW. Premalignant lesions of the anal margin. South Med J 1989;82:470–4.

51. Beck DE, Timmcke AE. Anal margin lesions. Clinics Colon Rectal Surgery 2002;15.

Other conditions: colonic volvulus, ischemia, radiation injury and trauma

This chapter discusses a number of important colorectal conditions that have not been covered previously: colonic volvulus, ischemic colitis, radiation bowel injuries, and colorectal trauma.

Colonic volvulus

Volvulus is the axial torsion or twisting of the bowel on its mesentery to a degree sufficient to cause symptoms. Symptoms result from the partial or complete obstruction of the lumen and associated vascular compromise. If the volvulus is not reduced, the circulatory impairment and increased interluminal pressure may lead to gangrene and perforation. The incidence of large bowel obstruction from chronic volvulus varies worldwide. In the United States, Ballantyne [1] found that chronic volvulus accounted for 3.4% of intestinal obstructions and 9.6% of chronic obstructions. Certain populations in Africa, Western Europe, and Iran have reported an increased frequency of volvulus. This increased frequency is felt to result from a long, redundant colon acquired because of the presence of a high degree of coarse vegetable fiber in the diet (see p. 442). The incidence of volvulus in these areas averages 20–30%, with highs of 85% in Northern Iran and 54.2% in Ethiopia [2]. The distribution of chronic volvulus is 80% in the sigmoid colon, 15% in the cecum, 3% in the transverse colon, and 2% in the splenic flexure [3]. Each type of volvulus will be discussed in detail.

Sigmoid volvulus

The average age at which sigmoid volvulus occurs varies according to geographic region. Although it has been reported in infants and children, the average onset in Western countries is 60–65 years of age [4]. In developing countries onset often occurs earlier between the fourth and sixth decades of life. Sigmoid volvulus is more common in men by a 2 : 1 ratio, and in the United States, two-thirds of patients are black. The development of sigmoid volvulus has been associated with patients residing in long-term care facilities such as mental health institutions or nursing homes. The condition has been linked with numerous neural psychiatric disorders such as chronic schizophrenia, Parkinson's disease, dementia, and multiple sclerosis. Elderly patients with serious cardiovascular or pulmonary disease that leads to inactivity also represent an identifiable risk group.

Etiologic factors

The cause of sigmoid volvulus depends on congenital or acquired predisposing anatomic factors. The most consistently found congenital feature is a long, redundant, mobile sigmoid associated with a large and freely mobile mesentery [5]. Another frequent anatomic factor is a narrowed mesenteric attachment with close endpoint fixation, which brings the limbs close together. The most important acquired etiologic factor is an elongated sigmoid megacolon. A diet very high in residue fiber can lead to chronic sigmoid fecal loading, elongation of the sigmoid colon and its mesentery, and chronic constipation. Megacolon has also been associated with other diseases, including ischemic colitis, celiac sprue, diabetes mellitus, peptic ulcer disease, Chagas' disease, and hypokalemia. Chronic constipation is often associated with patients who are bedridden, taking psychotropic medications, or laxative or enema dependent.

In sigmoid volvulus the mesentery usually twists in a counter-clockwise direction [6]. If the torsion reaches 180°, a significant closed loop obstruction occurs. If the obstruction becomes complete and the ileocecal valve is competent, a second closed loop obstruction occurs between the ileocecal valve and the point of the sigmoid obstruction. Although the sigmoid colon can tolerate more interluminal pressure without vascular compromise than other intestinal segments, it eventually reaches a point at which the interluminal pressure exceeds the vascular pressure necessary for bowel viability. With high degrees of angulation, venous occlusion precedes arterial occlusion which in turn results in mesocolic thrombosis and infarction. The resultant gangrene leads to perforation and concomitant peritonitis.

Presentation and diagnosis

Sigmoid volvulus may present as an acute or subacute intestinal obstruction. In the acute form, symptoms include intermittent, crampy lower abdominal pain, absence of flatus, progressive marked abdominal distention, obstipation, nausea, vomiting, and dehydration. Frequently patients are in a toxic state when initially seen, with tachycardia and respiratory depression. The respiratory embarrassment may be secondary to the extreme abdominal distention, pain, and elevation of the diaphragm. Some patients relate similar episodes in the past that have spontaneously resolved with the passage of large amounts of flatus and stool. In the subacute form, the onset is more gradual, with abdominal distention but minimal abdominal tenderness. Patients with the subacute form are generally older and have a more benign course.

The diagnosis of volvulus is usually confirmed by plain abdominal radiographs (see Figure 4.5). Classic films reveal a markedly dilated sigmoid colon with both ends of the loop in the pelvis and the bow below the diaphragm ('bent inner tube' or 'ace of spades' sign). Gas is usually absent from the rectum. Plain films are diagnostic in 61–93% of cases. When the diagnosis is in doubt, a water-soluble contrast enema may be useful (**Figure 23.1**). The contrast column may demonstrate complete retrograde obstruction to flow at the level of the torsion, producing the pathognomonic twisted 'bird's beak' or 'ace of spades' deformity. Colonoscopy may also be used to confirm the diagnosis and serve as a therapeutic maneuver. The torsion may be visualized as a narrowing, and if there is an area that can be safely passed, passage of a great amount of flatus or fluid confirms the diagnosis.

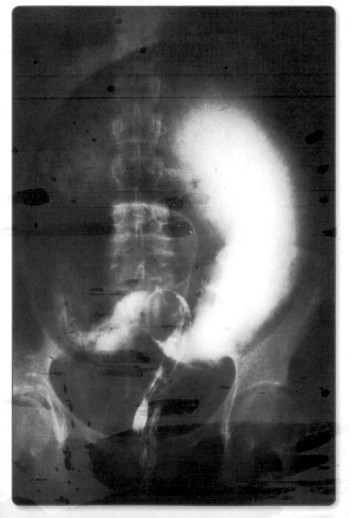

Figure 23.1 Contrast radiograph demonstrating sigmoid volvulus.

Treatment

The treatment of sigmoid volvulus requires a two-part strategy: first is the treatment of the acute episode; second is definitive management of the mobile sigmoid. For patients with acute abdominal findings (strangulated bowel), a laparotomy is mandated. Therapeutic options include resection with a proximal stoma, resection with an anastomosis, or a proximal stoma. A morbidity rate of 33–80% is associated with strangulated sigmoid volvulus with gangrene [7–9].

The approach to nonstrangulated volvulus is nonoperative detorsion followed by an elective resection (in the same hospitalization); the initial nonoperative maneuver focuses on stabilizing the patient with nasogastric decompression, intravenous hydration, and correction of electrolyte abnormalities. This is followed by nonoperative reduction of the volvulus using a rigid proctoscope and a rectal tube. Successful reduction results in an explosive passage of liquid stool and gas. The endoscopist then looks for signs of strangulation such as mucosal ulceration, sloughing, or the presence of dark blood, which would demand emergent operative intervention. If signs of strangulation are not present, a soft rectal tube may be passed through the scope beyond the obstructing twist and secured to the buttocks with tape or suture. The tube remains for 2–5 days, allowing the bowel to decompress. In rare instances in which a proctoscope cannot reach the obstruction (greater than 25 cm), a colonoscope can be used for detorsion. A limitation of using a colonoscope is the inability to simultaneously pass a rectal tube. Successful endoscopic decompression is possible in 77–91% of patients, with a mortality rate of 1–5% [10–12]. Volvulus recurs in up to 50–90% of patients after detorsion. Because the surgical mortality is higher after a recurrent episode than after the initial episode, surgical correction of the megasigmoid is recommended during the same hospitalization, after adequate resolution of the presenting episode [13]. The definitive procedure includes resection of the megasigmoid, with primary anastomosis in viable bowel.

Results

Mortality associated with sigmoid volvulus depends on the therapy selected and on the patient population. Reported rates vary from 0–42%. The higher mortalities were related to patients with gangrenous bowel.

Cecal volvulus

Cecal volvulus accounts for 1% of all intestinal obstructions [14]. It occurs much less commonly than does sigmoid volvulus, which accounts for 25–40% of all colonic volvulus. Cecal volvulus patients range in age from 40–60 years, with women affected 1.5–7 times more frequently than men [15].

Etiologic factors

Cecal volvulus is associated with a consistent congenital anatomic variant – incomplete peritoneal fixation of the right colon to the right abdominal wall (posterior peritoneal) – resulting in an abnormally mobile right colon. Cadaver studies confirm this anatomic variant to be present in 10–22% of the population [16]. When these features are present, two clinical sequelae can occur: the right colon and terminal ilium may undergo an axial torsion (usually clockwise), leading to intestinal obstruction with potential vascular compromising gangrene, or the cecum may fold anterior to the ascending colon, forming an obstruction (cecal bascule). The precipitating factors for cecal volvulus include adhesions from previous surgery, congenital bands, distal colonic obstruction, alteration of the cecal position by pregnancy or a pelvic mass, and hypermotility states.

Presentation and diagnosis

The most frequent clinical presentation mimics that of a small bowel obstruction. Laboratory values are rarely helpful except in patients who have an acute fulminant picture. Abdominal X-ray examination establishes the diagnosis in 40–90% of cases [17,18]. A plain abdominal film demonstrates a dilated cecum with a single air-fluid level (usually located in the left upper quadrant), an empty right iliac fossa, associated with the picture of a small bowel obstruction and a collapsed distal colon (**Figure 23.2**). The dilated cecum is positioned with its convex surface facing the left lower quadrant. A barium enema will demonstrate a classic finding of a 'bird's beak' deformity at the site of torsion without visualization of the cecum. In patients with free air in the abdomen or acute abdominal findings of peritonitis or ischemia, a barium enema is precluded. The role of colonoscopy for diagnosis and decompression of cecal volvulus remains to be defined.

Treatment

Patients presenting with gangrene or perforation require right colon resection with primary anastomosis or ileostomy and mucous fistula.

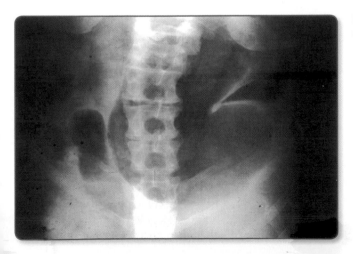

Figure 23.2 Radiograph demonstrating cecal volvulus.

Patients with viable bowel and no perforation are candidates for simple colopexy and/or tube cecostomy. The preference for nonresectional therapy is supported by its equivalent low long-term recurrence rate and lower morbidity [15,19].

Results

In Todd and Forde's series of 151 patients [20], the overall mortality rate associated with cecal volvulus was reported to be 22%. Patients with gangrene or perforation (29 patients) demonstrated a 41% mortality rate, whereas in patients with viable bowel (117 patients), the mortality rate was only 14%.

Transverse colon volvulus

Volvulus of the transverse colon is rare, with only 71 cases reported in the literature to date. In the United States, it accounts for about 4% of colonic volvulus [21]. Women are affected twice as often as men [22].

Etiologic factors

The transverse colon is usually protected from volvulus formation because of its short mesocolon and the wide points of fixation of the hepatic and splenic flexures. Factors that promote volvulus of the transverse colonic include congenital bands, 'hypermobile' colonic flexures, chronic constipation, prior abdominal surgery, pregnancy, and distal colonic lesions.

Presentation and diagnosis

The clinical features of transverse volvulus mimic other causes of large bowel obstruction with two clinical patterns: the acute fulminant presentation and the subacute presentation. Patients with an acute fulminant condition present with acute abdominal symptoms indicating ischemia, and their condition rapidly deteriorates; patients with a subacute condition present with a more gradual onset, with crampy abdominal symptoms compatible with a distal small bowel obstruction. The diagnosis of bowel obstruction is usually made clinically and confirmed by radiographs. A supine abdominal film usually shows a grossly dilated colonic loop with distention of the proximal right colon; the distal colon will contain little or no gas. An erect film frequently shows two fluid levels in the twisted loop and a third in the right colon. The diagnosis of transverse volvulus is most frequently made at operation.

Treatment

Because of the paucity of reported cases, the optimal treatment for transverse volvulus remains controversial. Colonoscopic detorsion and decompression have been reported and may play a role in patients with evidence of viable bowel [23]; however, there is no universal agreement regarding this approach. Definitive therapy always requires a laparotomy with bowel resection – a segmental colectomy or an extended right hemicolectomy. The surgeon must decide on a case-by-case basis whether to perform a primary anastomosis or to use a diversion after completion of the resection. The decision should be made with consideration for the patient's condition, the viability of the bowel, and the presence of abdominal contamination. Fixation procedures (colopexy) have been described, but the high recurrence rate after this procedure makes it an unreliable alternative to resection.

Results

In 1969 Kerry and Ransom [21] reported a 33% mortality rate with transverse colon volvulus. In a series of 45 patients, Zinkin et al [24]. reported only five deaths (11%), none of which was related to the volvulus or type of procedure. Early diagnosis and appropriate therapy are paramount to an optimal outcome.

Ischemic colitis

Although the colon has a generous overlapping blood supply, any interruption in blood flow produces ischemia. Anatomic locations that have the potential to be vulnerable to ischemic disease include: Griffith's point at the splenic flexure (junction of the superior mesenteric artery [SMA] and the inferior mesenteric artery [IMA]), Sudeck's critical point at the mid-sigmoid colon (junction of the IMA and hypogastric vasculature), and the cecum (distal distribution of SMA).

Etiologic factors and pathophysiology

As outlined in **Table 23.1**, interruption of flow in large vessels can occur in several ways. The incidence of colonic ischemia (endoscopic or clinical) following aortic surgery varies from 1–2% for elective cases to as high as 60% during emergency aneurysmectomy [25, 26]. During aneurysmectomy and aortobifemoral reconstruction for occlusive disease, the IMA is routinely ligated. Sigmoid or left colonic ischemia

	Table 23.1 Classification of ischemic colitis	
I.	Interruption of flow in large vessels	
	A. Following ligation during aortic surgery	
	B. Injury secondary to angiographic, blunt, or penetrating trauma	
	C. Spontaneous thrombosis of large vessels	
II.	Intrinsic small vessel disease	
III.	Low-flow state in the critically ill	
IV.	Spontaneous ischemic colitis without demonstrable vessel occlusion	
	A. Self-limiting without sequelae	
	B. With subsequent stricture formation	
V.	Miscellaneous	
	A. Secondary to luminal obstruction	
	B. Young adults	
	C. Renal allograft recipients	

occurs in these circumstances if the collateral circulation from the SMA via the marginal artery is insufficient to supply the oxygen demands of the left colon. The adequacy of colonic circulation can also be compromised by large fluid shifts and the use of various vasoactive drugs in these cases. Measurement of the IMA stump pressure in patients with a patent IMA, identification of Doppler signals on the bowel surface, and measurement of intraluminal pH have all been used to predict which patients are at highest risk for developing ischemia following IMA ligation [27, 28]. Sudden occlusion of the IMA can also occur as a result of angiographic trauma with subintimal dissection or as a result of either blunt or penetrating abdominal trauma.

Atheromatous narrowing or occlusion of the IMA is not unusual. However, in most cases this occurs gradually, and the collateral circulation from the SMA can compensate for the decrease in flow through collateral circulation via the marginal artery. If the IMA becomes acutely thrombosed or occluded with an embolus and collateral circulation is inadequate, the clinical picture will be similar to that found after IMA ligation during aortic surgery.

Any of the connective tissue diseases that produce inflammation in the small arteries (**intrinsic small vessel disease**) can also result in colonic ischemia. This has been described in polyarteritis nodosa, systemic lupus erythematosus, rheumatoid arthritis, dermatomyositis, primary amyloidosis, and Degos' disease. These diseases can cause ischemia in the small and large bowel. Colonic ischemia resulting from small vessel disease has also been described in patients with diabetes mellitus and chronic renal failure.

Ischemic colitis has also been reported in approximately 1% of renal allograft recipients. Another variant of ischemic colitis occurs in patients who are severely ill with conditions that cause hypotension, decreased cardiac output, or peripheral vasoconstriction, with a decreased flow to the end organ (**low-flow states**). This group of patients appears to have a higher incidence of full-thickness necrosis than do those with spontaneous ischemic colitis who were previously well. Also noticed is the preponderance of patients with right-sided colonic involvement. The mortality associated with colonic infarction in these patients who are severely ill from another disease process is extremely high. In the group of 17 such patients reported by Sakai et al the mortality rate was 57% [29]. One must have a very high index of suspicion for full-thickness necrosis in this group of patients and be ready to intervene early.

Over the five-year period from 1995–2000, 48 patients with ischemic colitis were hospitalized at the Ochsner Clinic Foundation hospital [30]. Ten of these patients required operative management. Eight were women and the mean age was 71.4 years (range 43–85 years). Presenting symptoms included abdominal pain (9/10), diarrhea (5/10) and fecal blood (4/10).

At operation 3 patients had total colonic ischemia, while 7 had segmental ischemia (4, right; 2, sigmoid; 1, left). Six of the patients had severe ischemia, 4 had gangrene, and 3 had perforations. Eight of the patients had resections (5, segmental and 3, total colonic) and one had repair of a perforation. Six patients had stomas (5, ileostomies and 1, transverse colostomy) and a primary anastomosis was performed in three. Mean operating time was 135 (range, 60–220) minutes and mean hospital stay was 13 (range, 4–28) days. Major or minor complications occurred in 7 patients.

With a follow-up of 1–48 months (mean = 17.4 months), there was one postoperative death due to multiple organ failure and a second patient died one month after discharge of gastrointestinal bleeding and multiple organ failure. Only two of the six patients with a stoma had closure during follow-up.

Spontaneous ischemic colitis in individuals who were previously well was described in the 1960s by Boley et al [31] and Marston et al [32]. The ischemia occurs without any demonstrable vessel occlusion on angiography. The pathologic changes seen in the colon are identical to those reproduced in the laboratory with vessel occlusion; the presumption is that this entity is caused by a decreased flow to the colon. The spectrum of disease varies from mild submucosal edema to frank full-thickness necrosis. Most cases are the milder, self-limiting variety that is typically seen in middle aged or elderly patients often following episodes of dehydration.

In younger patients the clinical syndrome is identical to that of the spontaneous ischemic colitis seen in the older age group, and since the majority of these reported cases occur in women, some authors have proposed an association between this type of ischemic colitis and the use of oral contraceptives [33].

Diagnosis

Colonic ischemia usually presents in one of two ways. The milder cases are manifest by diffuse and/or bloody diarrhea. Patients with frank colonic infarction frequently develop acidosis, glucose intolerance, renal failure, obvious sepsis, and abdominal distention or tenderness. The diagnosis of postoperative ischemia can be made with flexible sigmoidoscopy done at the bedside. If the symptoms are not explained by flexible sigmoidoscopy, a colonoscopy may occasionally be required to rule out more proximal disease. The endoscopic appearance of colonic ischemia may range from submucosal edema with hemorrhage and ulceration to the dusky blue color of the mucosa of infarcted bowel. Frank gangrene mandates immediate surgery and resection. The colon with just mucosal edema and hemorrhage may be watched closely. The endoscopy is repeated in 24 hours, and surgery is recommended if the lesion appears to be progressive. This approach should enable the surgeon to intervene before perforation occurs. Some authors suggest that flexible endoscopy be done routinely after aortic surgery because endoscopic findings may precede the development of symptoms [34]. The hope is that early recognition can facilitate more effective and timely treatment of this condition, which is associated with a 40% mortality rate.

Patients with spontaneous ischemic colitis typically present with a sudden onset of usually mild, crampy lower abdominal pain, mostly on the left side. Often the patient will have bloody diarrhea within 24 hours of the onset of pain. There is often some accompanying fever or tachycardia. On physical examination the left lower quadrant is tender to palpation. The diagnosis can be made with endoscopy or CT scan. Endoscopy is preferred because it can be done in the office or at the bedside and the pathologic state can be viewed directly. A CT scan ill show colon wall thickening (**Figure 23.3**).

A barium enema study performed soon after the onset of the pain will show a typical thumbprinting pattern (**Figure 23.4**) that is the result of submucosal edema and hemorrhage. However, a barium enema is contraindicated if the patient has peritoneal signs, is septic, there is a strong suspicion of bowel necrosis, or performance of an angiogram is contemplated. Fortunately, this serious clinical picture is unusual.

There are three possible outcomes of ischemic colitis:

1. **Resolution** of the process is the most common clinical course. Typically the symptoms will subside over a few days or occasionally a week or so, and the patient will fully recover without any sequelae. Repeat episodes are rare.

2. Progression to **full-thickness necrosis** is unusual, especially if there is no evidence of gangrenous bowel at the first examination. In the experience of Marston et al [32], it occurred only twice in 174 patients.

3. The condition may evolve to an ulcerative stage, which may eventually result in **stricture** formation. During the ulcerative stage the endoscopic and radiographic findings may mimic Crohn's disease. Occasionally the early phases of this disease will go unnoticed or undiagnosed, and the patient will present

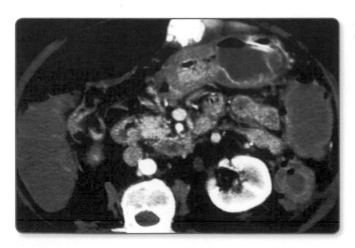

Figure 23.3 CT scan demonstrating ischemia.

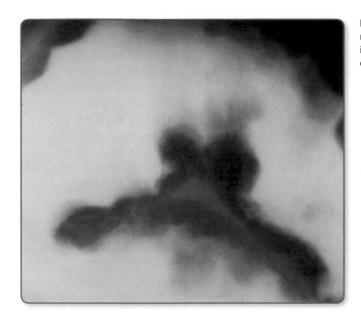

Figure 23.4 Barium contrast radiograph demonstrating ischemic colitis (thumbprinting of mucosa).

with a stricture. The differential diagnosis of a chronic stricture also includes inflammatory bowel disease or malignancy. If the strictured area can be adequately examined, is found to be asymptomatic and biopsies are taken to rule out malignancy, nothing else need be done. If it cannot be completely examined endoscopically or it is causing symptoms, a resection is indicated.

Ischemic colitis may also be associated with a complete or partial bowel obstruction. In the series by Boley et al [31], 10% of patients with colonic ischemia had an associated carcinoma and another 10% had some other condition that potentially interfered with colonic motility. When ischemic colitis occurs in association with tumor, the ischemic area is usually proximal to the tumor and may or may not be associated with obstruction. These investigators and other colleagues speculated that colonic blood flow could be decreased as a consequence of increased intraluminal pressure, hyperperistalsis with increased muscular spasm, and resultant diminution in blood flow in the colonic wall, or a decrease in aortic blood pressure and vena caval return with straining in obstructive lesions [35]. Knowledge of this association is of obvious importance to avoid using ischemic bowel for an anastomosis.

Treatment

If the diagnosis of ischemic colitis is made early, conservative therapy is warranted. Mild cases can be managed on an outpatient basis with a clear liquid diet, close observation, and possibly antibiotic therapy [36]. More serious cases require hospitalization, bowel rest, and optimizing blood flow to the mucosa (intravenous hydration and optimization of cardiac output). If the patient is receiving digitalis, a serum level should be checked because toxic digitalis levels can have a marked vasoconstrictive effect on visceral circulation. Parenteral antibiotics (such as a second- or third-generation cephalosporin) are used by some surgeons because of the suggestion that colonic ischemia may allow colonic bacterial transmigration [37]. Patients with ischemia resulting from arteritides may respond to corticosteroid treatment.

Specific indications for surgery include peritonitis, perforation, sepsis, and failure of nonoperative therapy [37]. At operation a wide resection of nonviable colon is performed. Primary anastomosis is usually unsafe because of the potential for postoperative progression of the ischemia. A double-barrel stoma or end stoma and separate mucous fistula is safer and allows assessment of the bowel viability in the postoperative period.

The mortality rate for ischemic colitis among renal transplant patients is 70%. Diagnostic maneuvers should be initiated at the first suspicion of ischemia in these high-risk patients, and surgery should be aggressive once the diagnosis is made (resection of any compromised bowel with an end stoma). Primary anastomosis after resection is ill-advised in these cases.

Radiation injury

Radiation therapy was first used in 1899. With continued technical advances and improved basic science understanding, radiation therapy has now become a therapeutic option for nearly 50% of cancer patients [38]. Despite these advances, radiation injury to normal tissue remains a significant clinical problem. The small bowel, colon, and rectum frequently receive serious injury from this form of therapy. The injury may be acute, with nonspecific inflammatory symptoms, or may be a chronic problem for up to 20 years after radiation therapy, long after the patient has been cured of the cancer.

Pathophysiology

Radiation injury is any injury to cellular tissue or organ resulting from the use of ionizing radiation. At the cellular level, ionizing radiation produces free radicals from intracellular water; the free radicals produce DNA injury and eventual cellular death. Important factors that affect potential tissue injury include: (1) a dose administered to the target area, (2) a lapsed time dose, (3) the dose fractionation size, and (4) proliferated activity of the tissue (more proliferative equals more sensitive) [39]. Other factors that can increase tissue susceptibility to radiation therapy leading to possible injury are: (1) low-flow states, (2) thin patients (who are more prone to radiation injury), (3) previous abdominal surgery, (4) treatment with radiation-sensitizing drugs such as 5-hydroxyfluorouracil, (5) diabetes, (6) hypertension, and (7) inflammatory bowel disease [40]. Radiation therapy for gynecologic malignancies is the most common cause of radiation enteritis. The terminal ilium is the most radiosensitive organ within the abdominal cavity.

Early injury from radiation therapy occurs in 40–75% of patients receiving treatment to the pelvis, usually appearing within the first 3 months of treatment [41,42]. Fortunately, only 20% of this group will have symptomatology requiring cessation of treatment [43]. Late radiation-induced injury from treatment to the abdomen or pelvis ranges from 1–17% [44,45]. Less than 5% of this group will develop injury severe enough to require operative therapy [46,47].

Early injury from radiation therapy presents as an acute inflammatory process, with histologic changes most prominent 14 days after completion of the initial treatment. The focus of injury in the bowel is the mucosal crypt cell. As crypt cell injury progresses from atrophy to death, mucosal edema and ulceration are present, as is an inflammatory exudate [48]. The resulting diarrhea arises from the loss of absorptive area and from anomalies in small bowel motility from direct radiation damage to the myenteric plexus [49].

Late radiation injury arises from ischemia. Tissues suffer from obliterative endarteritis. The ischemia produces the deposition of collagen and subsequent fibrosis [50]. This irreversible change is seen primarily in the bowel submucosa and serosa. Grossly chronic radiation injury appears as thickened bowel with a greyish serosa. Fistula formation and obstructive strictures are common.

Diagnosis

The diagnosis of early radiation injury is usually made in the 2- to 8- week period following completion of therapy. The principal symptoms include abdominal cramping, nausea and vomiting, diarrhea, and malaise. CT scans or contrast studies may confirm hypotonic loops, spasm, and thumbprinting. Radiation proctitis will mimic the symptoms of inflammatory bowel disease. These include bleeding, tenesmus, mucous discharge, and increased frequency of stools. Endoscopic examination may reveal edema, ulceration, decreased distensibility, and bleeding. Absorption studies (i.e. lactose, D-xylose) may be abnormal. The key differential diagnosis for radiation injury symptoms is infectious diarrhea. The appropriate cultures and microscopic evaluations are necessary to exclude infection as a nidus of the symptomatology.

Treatment

Initial management of early radiation injury is focused on supportive measures.

This includes adequate hydration and correction of any electrolyte abnormalities. Symptomatic diarrhea can be treated with anticholinergic agents, opiates, or nonprescription medications. Anti-inflammatory agents (nonsteroidal), antispasmodics, and a mild sedative are also helpful. Severe cases require hospitalization with bowel rest, intravenous hydration, and parenteral nutrition. A decision must be made for each case on whether to discontinue therapy or to use a hyperfractionation technique [51].

Patients with radiation proctitis present with urgency and rectal bleeding.

Initial therapeutic options include steroid retention enemas, 5-ASA enemas, a low residue diet, stool softeners, and sulfasalazine [52]. If isolated bleeding sites can be identified, point fulguration with silver nitrate may be effective. Laser application (Nd:YAG) to bleeding sites has also been used [53]. Instillation of 30 mL of a 4% formalin solution or Dab application of 10% formalin has been reported [54, 55]. If other treatment modalities are unsuccessful, a diverting loop colostomy may be used. Success with this has varied because the rectal bleeding may continue, but a stoma is often helpful for severe symptoms of tenesmus and uncontrollable diarrhea.

Patients with severe radiation injuries often develop complications that require surgical intervention. The appropriate surgical management for affected small bowel remains controversial as to whether to resect or bypass the damaged bowel. In theory, resecting the small bowel may lead to increased anastomotic complications and potential bowel fistulization. However, bypassing a problematic section of intestine leaves a diseased segment that is vulnerable to fistula formation, a possible blind loop syndrome, or a neoplasm. In a series of 244 patients who required surgical intervention for radiation-induced small bowel injury, Swan et al [56] concluded that bypass was as effective a therapy as resection but carried a much lower operative morbidity rate. Primary anastomosis is reserved for cases in which minimal small bowel resection is necessary and normal small bowel and colon are available for an ileocolic anastomosis. Enterolysis is associated with grave consequences such as perforation and fistula formation. The surgeon must exercise a high level of clinical judgment and extreme technical skill in dealing with radiated small bowel.

When small bowel fistulas develop, an initial course of bowel rest and total parenteral nutrition is instituted. A contrast study of the fistula is obtained to identify the primary source of the fistula and to rule out distal obstruction. For cases requiring surgical intervention, total exclusion of the involved segment is performed and one limb of this excluded segment is brought to the skin as a mucous fistula.

Radiation-induced rectal injury also includes stenosis and the formation of rectovaginal fistulas. Conservative therapy may allow some resolution of stenosis, but perforations and rectovaginal fistulas require surgical therapy. The most conservative surgical approach is simple fecal diversion. This successfully treats obstruction, decreases the discomfort resulting from fistulas, and may ameliorate chronic pain. If a colostomy is performed, it is advisable to use nonirradiated descending or transverse colon and to bring it through nonirradiated skin to avoid stomal necrosis and mucocutaneous separation. Low anterior resection using an omental pedicle to protect the anastomosis has been used for rectal stenosis, with minimal leak rates (2 of 31 patients). An abdominosacral approach with low colorectal anastomoses has also been successfully used. Bricker et al [57] advocated using the proximal colon as a pedicle graft to treat patients with rectal stenosis or rectovaginal fistula. They reported satisfactory functional results in 18 of 19 patients.

A third technique, applicable to patients with rectovaginal fistulas and severe proctosigmoiditis, is a rectal mucosectomy and pull-through coloanal anastomosis. This operation avoids extensive pelvic dissection and preserves anal sphincter function. The functional results of this operation demonstrate that continence is satisfactory. However, urgency and frequency of defecation remain a problem for many of these patients. A temporary diversion measure (e.g. loop ileostomy) is advised after performance of all surgical procedures in this group.

Radiation injuries are always difficult problems, and the surgeon must also deal with postirradiation necrosis and the possibility of recurring pelvic malignancy. Therefore meticulously performed biopsies are required to exclude recurrent tumor while avoiding perforation or creation of fistulas. It is also important to know that the radiation injury is progressive, and even if present repairs or surgical manipulations are successful, they must be monitored as the initial results are not always sustained in the long-term.

Colorectal trauma

Etiologic factors

Colorectal trauma can occur from a variety of causes and remains a significant cause of death and major morbidity [58, 59]. Most colorectal injuries (96%) are caused by penetrating injuries [60]. Although stab wounds may penetrate the bowel, projectile (e.g. gunshot) wounds account for most injuries. Projectiles may cause injury by direct penetration of the bowel, blast effect, or secondary penetration from fragmented bone [61]. The latter mechanisms are especially important in high-velocity wounds associated with military-type weapons. A rectal impalement injury occurs from a fall on a penetrating object. Because of the protected location of the anus and rectum, anorectal injuries are infrequent with blunt trauma and usually are associated with pelvic fractures. Blunt trauma counts for only 4% of colorectal injuries with motor vehicle accidents being the most frequent cause [60]. Falls and crush injuries compromise most of the remaining blunt trauma.

Iatrogenic injuries of the colon may occur from endoscopic perforation, barium enema, or during other abdominal procedures [57]. Iatrogenic injuries of the rectum and anus are uncommon and may result from barium enema, cleansing enemas, thermometers, proctosigmoidoscopy and colonoscopy, radiation necrosis, and chemical burns. Sexually related trauma can cause significant injury to the anorectum [62]. A great variety of rectal foreign bodies are used for sexual gratification and have the potential for serious injury [63]. Most causes of anorectal trauma in children are related to child abuse.

The surgeon's challenge in treating the individual patient with colorectal trauma is to select an approach that provides the best clinical outcome with the least morbidity. To optimize decision making, Moore et al [64] and Flint et al [65] each described an injury severity scale to quantify the effects of the degree of intra-abdominal organ injury and the presence of associated injuries, shock, and delay in treatment. Factors found to be significant in contributing to colon injury morbidity include shock, fecal spillage with evidence of peritonitis, additional organ injury, treatment delay greater than 4 hours, abdominal wall loss, extensive colon damage, and hemoperitoneum of greater than 1000 mL. These investigators noted that no single variable determines outcome; thus the surgeon is obligated to consider a myriad of factors before selecting the appropriate clinical approach.

Diagnosis

The colon's intra-abdominal location often precludes the physician's making an accurate diagnosis of colon injury through an external examination [58]. Colon injury is most frequently diagnosed during exploratory laparotomy undertaken for trauma criteria (e.g. peritonitis, positive diagnostic peritoneal lavage, intra-abdominal gunshot wound, or hemodynamic instability). Patients who are candidates for a selective workup for colonic injury include those with stab wounds and blunt trauma who are hemodynamically stable and do not meet the criteria for trauma exploratory laparotomy; these patients can be observed and selectively evaluated for colon injury. Patients with trauma to the retroperitoneal or the extraperitoneal portion of the rectum can usually be evaluated by abdominal and pelvic CT with oral and rectal contrast media [66,67]. The possibility of rectal injury must be considered if a projectile crosses the pelvis or if it enters through the midline. A finding of blood on digital rectal examination should make one suspect a rectal injury and mandates a proctosigmoidoscopy, which will accurately diagnose perforation in the rectum in more than 90% of injuries [68].

Treatment

Preoperative considerations

A systemic approach (**Figure 23.5**) with simultaneous evaluation and resuscitation is recommended by the American College of Surgeons Advanced Trauma Life Support (ATLS) program [69]. All patients with abdominal trauma who are to undergo an exploratory laparotomy should receive preoperative antibiotics that cover colon-related bacterial flora (aerobes and anaerobes) [70]. Single-agent antimicrobial therapy with broad-spectrum coverage (e.g. cefoxitin, cefotetan, ampicillin/sulbactam) is appropriate, although some surgeons prefer multiple-drug therapy (e.g. an aminoglycoside such as gentamycin or tobramycin combined with clindamycin, metronidazole, ticarcillin disodium/clavulanate potassium (Timentin or ampicillin). The presence of a colon or rectal injury is the most important determinant of infectious

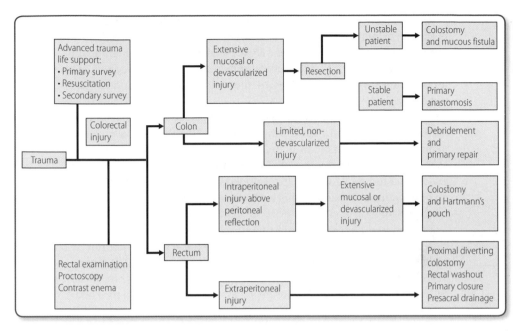

Figure 23.5 Algorithm for management of colorectal trauma.

complication [70]. Jones et al [71] of Parkland Hospital in Dallas observed an infection rate of 36% in 96 patients with penetrating colon injuries.

Operative treatment

Colon injuries

Treatment options for colon injuries include exteriorization of the injured segment, resection with or without anastomoses, closure of the injured segment with a proximal protecting colostomy, or primary closure of the colonic injury [58].

A significant number of colon injuries may be primarily closed. No distinction is currently made in this group between right and left injuries or between mesenteric or antimesenteric injuries [58,65,72,73]. These injuries may be closed in one or two layers. There are, however, several situations in which primary closure is not advisable [58,73]: (1) in a patient who is or has been in shock (systolic pressure lower than 80 mmHg); (2) when the interval between the original colon injury and the discovery at laparotomy is greater than 4–8 hours; (3) if more than one organ system is significantly injured; (4) if there is massive colon destruction (a defect greater than 2 cm in the colon wall after adequate debridement); (5) if there is massive contamination (the presence of gross feces more than 5 cm away from the colonic defect); (6) if associated injuries will require the use of prosthetic material for repair; or (7) if the colon is injured in two different anatomic locations (e.g. the hepatic flexure and sigmoid).

Simple **exteriorization** of the colon injury as a colostomy has been described. Unfortunately, this is not an optimal option, because it requires a second operation for the closure (associated with a significant morbidity of 8–50%), and few bowel injuries are small enough or are located in appropriate sections of the colon to accommodate this option [58,74].

To avoid these problems, it has been suggested that the injured colon be repaired and then exteriorized [75]. This theoretically would allow the exteriorized repair to be returned to the abdomen during the same hospitalization (generally 14 days after the original repair). In two major studies, 34–50% of exteriorized repairs failed (leaked or had an obstruction). Because of these poor results, this technique is rarely used [59,75].

Injuries to the lower sigmoid that do not fulfill criteria for primary closure present a special problem. Frequently these injuries cannot be brought up to the abdominal wall for exteriorization or as a colostomy despite adequate mobilization of the sigmoid colon [58]. In these cases, the injury is closed in two layers and is protected by a proximal colostomy or loop ileostomy. The bowel distal to the stoma must be irrigated to wash out residual stool.

In colonic injuries in which there is extensive loss of tissue (e.g. gunshot wounds), the entire injured and devitalized segment should be resected, and the proximal colon brought out as a colostomy in the distal segment, managed as a mucous fistula. Simple injuries to the cecum that fulfill the criteria for **primary closure** can be closed in one or two layers. With more complex injuries, cecal resection is advocated. Once the cecum is resected, a primary anastomosis can be created or an ileostomy and a long Hartmann's closure of the distal bowel can be performed.

Rectal injuries

The mortality rate for rectal injuries decreased from 67% during World War I to 45% during World War II, with the addition of routine diverting colostomies, prececal drainage, antibiotics and blood transfusions [66,76]. During the Vietnam era, surgeons added distal rectal washouts to limit further contamination of the pelvis through the rectal injury site [77]. These advances, along with improved antibiotics and rapid evacuation of the wounded, reduced the mortality rate to 14% [78]. The lessons learned from war time surgery in concert with civilian experience with low- and high-velocity injuries to the rectum have shaped the treatment of rectal injuries [58].

It is mandatory that rectal injuries be confirmed by endoscopy before the surgeon begins an exploratory laparotomy. A proctoscopic examination should be carried out to at least 20 cm in patients who present with penetrating pelvic trauma, complex pelvic fractures, and blood on rectal examination [58]. It is preferable that the operating surgeon perform this examination to prevent confusion as to whether any abnormal mucosal findings were iatrogenically produced during a proctoscopic examination by another physician.

A middle or high rectal injury requires formal operative intervention with a diverting proximal sigmoid colostomy. It is also important to place a large Silastic sump drain into the presacral space. For lower injuries, the presacral space is drained via incisions made between the anus and the tip of the coccyx; Penrose drains can be inserted into the prececal space through the perineal skin incision. Any feces retained in the rectum and sigmoid colon distal to the colostomy should be removed, either through proctoscopic examination or by irrigation through the distal limb of the colostomy or via a transrectal approach [79]. The skin edges of both entry and exit wounds should be carefully debrided to remove any contamination (i.e. bullet material, clothing). Skin closure following significant contamination in trauma patients has produced a 40% to 50% incidence of wound infections [80]. For this reason, the wound should be treated in an open fashion [73]. Sterile dressings should be changed three times daily.

Anal injuries

A variety of traumatic events can lead to anal and perineal trauma. The most common injury is iatrogenic obstetric trauma [80]. An extensive episiotomy or puerperal anal injuries from third and fourth degree tears create anal sphincter damage [81]. For the best clinical outcome, these injuries, when identified, should be repaired immediately. Undetected sphincter injuries frequently lead to delayed diagnosis of incontinence; therefore the sphincter function of all patients should be documented on the initial physical examination. In a patient with acute trauma, it is often not possible to perform appropriate studies of sphincter function or suspected sphincter injuries. Once the patient has recovered from the acute phase of injuries, electromyography and intra-anal ultrasonography may provide important prognostic information [57]. The primary goal of treatment for anal injuries is debridement of necrotic tissue and open drainage to prevent perineal sepsis. Attempts are then made to restore the contractile competence of the sphincter by identification, mobilization, and reapproximation of severed muscular components, with recreation of the perineal body. Antibiotics are used to assist in control of local wound infections. In stable patients, significant sphincter injuries are managed by meticulous reapproximation of tissue without tension [81]. Sphincter injuries are rarely life threatening in an unstable patient and are best managed with a diverting stoma, drainage, and delayed repair.

Rounds questions

1. What is colonic volvulus?
2. In which part of the colon is volvulus most likely to occur?
3. How is sigmoid volvulus managed initially?
4. What three areas of the colon are especially vulnerable to ischemia?
5. What techniques can help to predict patients at risk for ischemia during aortic surgery?
6. How does colonic ischemia present?
7. What are the outcomes of ischemic colitis?
8. What is the most common cause of a colorectal injury?
9. What are the surgical treatment options for management of colonic trauma?
10. What causes most anal injuries?

References

1. Ballantyne GH. Review of sigmoid volvulus: Clinical patterns and pathogenesis. Dis Colon Rectum 1982;25:823–30.
2. Johnson LP. Recent experience with sigmoid volvulus in Ethiopia; its incidence and management by primary resection. Ethiop Med J 1965;4:197–204.
3. Sgambati SA, Ballantyne GH. Management of volvulus. In: Wexner SD, Vernava AM, (eds). Clinical Decision Making in Colorectal Surgery. New York: Igaku-Shoin, 1995;315–20.
4. Northeast ADR, Dennison AR, Lee EG. Sigmoid volvulus: New thoughts on the epidemiology. Dis Colon Rectum 1984;27:260–1.
5. Harper SG. Colonic volvulus. In: Mazier WP, Levien DH, Luchtefeld MA, Senagore AJ (eds). Surgery of the Colon, Rectum and Anus. Philadelphia: WB Saunders, 1995;657–69.
6. Gordon PH, Nivatvongs S (eds). Principles and Practice of Surgery for the Colon, Rectum, and Anus. St. Louis: Quality Medical Publishing, 1992;800–14.
7. Shepherd JJ. Treatment of volvulus of sigmoid colon: A review of 425 cases. Br Med J 1968;1:280–3.
8. McDonald CC, Boggs HW. Volvulus of the sigmoid colon. South Med J 1975;68:55–8.
9. Scott GW. Volvulus of the sigmoid flexure. Dis Colon Rectum 1965;8:30–4.
10. Drapanas T, Stewart JD. Acute sigmoid volvulus: Concepts in surgical treatment. Am J Surg 1961;101:70–7.
11. Arnold GJ, Nance FC. Volvulus of the sigmoid colon. Ann Surg 1973;177:527–37.
12. Bruusgard C. Volvulus of the sigmoid colon and its treatment. Surgery 1947;22:466–78.
13. Moseson DL, Lindell T, Brant B, Krippachre W. Sigmoid volvulus. Am Surg 1976;42:492–7.
14. Anderson MJ, Okike N, Spencer RJ. The colonoscope in cecal volvulus: Report of three cases. Dis Colon Rectum 1978;21:71–4.
15. Anderson JR, Welch GH. Acute volvulus of the right colon: An analysis of 69 patients. World J Surg 1986;10:336–42.
16. Wolfer JA, Beaton LE, Anson BJ. Volvulus of the cecum: Anatomical factors in its etiology. Report of a case. Surg Gynecol Obstet 1942;74:882–93.
17. Tejler G, Jiborn H. Volvulus of the cecum: Report of 26 cases and review of the literature. Dis Colon Rectum 1988;31:445–9.
18. Burke JB, Ballantyne GH. Cecal volvulus: Low mortality at a city hospital. Dis Colon Rectum 1984;27:737–40.
19. O'Mara CS, Wilson TH, Stonesifer GL, Cameron JL. Cecal volvulus: Analysis of 50 patients with long-term follow-up. Ann Surg 1979;189:724–31.
20. Todd GJ, Forde KA. Volvulus of the cecum: Choice of operation. Am J Surg 1979;138:632–4.
21. Kerry RL, Ransom HK. Volvulus of the colon: Etiology, diagnosis and treatment. Arch Surg 1969;29:78–85.
22. Anderson JR, Lee D, Taylor TV, Ross AHM. Volvulus of the transverse colon. Br J Surg 1981;68:179–81.

23. Joergensen K, Kronborg O. The colonscope in volvulus of the transverse colon. Dis Colon Rectum 1980;23:357–8.

24. Zinkin LD, Katz LD, Rosin JD. Volvulus of the transverse colon: Report of case and review of the literature. Dis Colon Rectum 1979;22:492–6.

25. Hagihara PF, Ernst CB, Griffen WO. Incidence of ischemic colitis following abdominal aortic reconstruction. Surg Gynecol Obstet 1979;149:571–3.

26. Johnson WC, Nabseth DC. Visceral infarction following aortic surgery. Ann Surg 1974;180:312–8.

27. Buckley GB, Zuidema GD, Hamilton SR, et al. Intraoperative determination of small bowel viability following ischemic injury: A prospective, controlled trial of two adjuvant methods Doppler and fluorescein compared with standard clinical judgment. Ann Surg 1981;193:628–37.

28. Erust CB, Hagihara PF, Daugherty ME, Griffen WO. Inferior mesenteric artery stump pressure: A reliable index for safe IMA ligation during abdominal aortic aneurysmectomy. Ann Surg 1976;187:641–6.

29. Sakai L, Keltner R, Kaminski D. Spontaneous and shock-associated ischemic colitis. Am J Surg 1980;140:755–60.

30. Beck DE, Aguilar-Nascimento JE. Surgical management and outcome in acute ischemic colitis. The Ochsner Journal 2011; 11:282–5.

31. Boley SJ, Schwartz S, Lash J, Stemhill V. Reversible vascular occlusion of the colon. Surg Gynecol Obstet 1963;116:53–60.

32. Marston A, Pheils M, Thomas ML, Morson BC. Ischaemic colitis. Gut 1966;7:1–15.

33. Stamos MJ. Intestinal ischemia and infarction. In: Mazier WP, Levien DH, Luchtefeld MA, Senagore AJ (eds). Surgery of the Colon, Rectum and Anus. Philadelphia: WB Saunders, 1995;685–718.

34. Ernst CB, Hagihara PF, Daughtery ME, Sachatello CR, Griffen WO. Ischemic colitis incidence following abdominal aortic reconstruction: A prospective study. Surgery 1976;80:417–21.

35. Boley SJ, Brandt LJ, Veith FJ. Ischemic disorders of the intestines. Curr Probl Surg 1978;15:57–9.

36. Bubrick MP. Mesenteric vascular diseases. In: Gordon PH, Nivatvongs S, (eds). Principles and Practice of Surgery for the Colon, Rectum, and Anus. St. Louis: Quality Medical Publishing, 1992;817–33.

37. Harford FJ. Miscellaneous colorectal conditions. In: Beck DE, Welling DR, (eds). Patient Care in Colorectal Surgery. Boston: Little, Brown, 1991;319–29.

38. DeVita VT. Principles of chemotherapy. In: DeVita VT, Hellman S, Roseberg SA (eds). Cancer: Principles and Practice of Oncology, 2nd ed. Philadelphia: JB Lippincott, 1985;257–85.

39. Wiseman JS. Radiation enteritis. In: Mazier WP, Levien DH, Luchtefeld MA, Senagore AJ (eds). Surgery of the Colon, Rectum and Anus. Philadelphia: WB Saunders, 1995;670–7.

40. Fonkalsrud EW, Sanchez M, Zerubauel R, Mahoney A. Serial changes in arterial structure following radiation therapy. Surg Gynecol Obstet 1977;145:395–400.

41. Gilinsky NH, Burns DG, Barbezat GO, et al. The natural history of radiation-induced proctosigmoiditis: An analysis of 88 patients. Q J Med 1983;52:40–53.

42. Hatcher PA, Thomson HJ, Ludgate SN, Small WP, Smith AN. Surgical aspects of intestinal injury due to pelvic radiotherapy. Ann Surg 1985;201:470–5.

43. Joslin CAF, Smith CW, Mallik A. The treatment of cervix cancer using high activity ^{60}Co sources. Br J Radiol 1972;45:257–70.

44. Bourne RG, Kearsley JH, Grove WD, Roberts SJ. The relationship between early and late gastrointestinal complications of radiation therapy for carcinoma of the cervix. Int J Radiat Oncol Biol Phys 1983;9:1445–50.

45. Roswit B, Malsky SJ, Reid CB. Severe radiation injuries of the stomach, small intestine, colon and rectum. Am J Roentgenol Radium Ther Nucl Med 1972;114:460–75.

46. Cram AE, Pearlman NW, Jochimsen PR. Surgical management of complications of radiation-injured gut. Am J Surg 1977;133:551–3.

47. Morgenstern L, Thompson R, Friedman B. The modern enigma of radiation enteropathy: Sequelae and solutions. Am J Surg 1977;134:166–72.

48. Marks G, Mohiudden M. The surgical management of the radiation-injured intestine. Surg Clin North Am 1983;63:81–96.

49. Stearner SP, Devine RL, Christian EJB. Late changes in the irradiated microvasculature: An electron microscopy study of the effects of fission neutrons. Radiat Res 1976;65:351–70.

50. Earnest DL, Trier JS. Radiation enteritis and colitis. In: Sleisenger MH, Fortran IS, (eds). Gastrointestinal Disease: Pathophysiology, Diagnosis, Management, 5th ed. Philadelphia: WB Saunders, 1989;1257–70.

51. Hauer-Jensen M. Late radiation injury in the small intestine. Clinical, pathophysiologic and radiobiologic aspects. A review. Acta Oncol 1990;29:401–15.

52. Sherman LF, Prem KA, Mensheha NM. Factitial proctitis: A restudy at the University of Minnesota. Dis Colon Rectum 1971;14:281–5.

53. Ahlquist DA, Gostout CJ, Viggiano TR, Pemberton JH. Laser therapy for severe radiation-induced rectal bleeding. Mayo Clin Proc 1986;61:927–31.

54. Rubinstein E, Ibsen T, Rasmussen RB, Reimer E, Sorensen BL. Formalin treatment of radiation-induced hemorrhagic proctitis. Am J Gastroenterol 1986;81:44–5.

55. Biswal BM, Lal P, Rath GK et al. Intrarectal formalin application, an effective treatment for grade III haemorrhagic radiation proctitis. Radiotherapy & Oncology 1995;35:212–5.

56. Swan RW, Fowler WC, Boronow RC. Surgical management of radiation injury to the small intestine. Surg Gynecol Obstet 1976;142:325–7.

57. Bricker EM, Johnston WD, Patwardhan RV. Repair of post irradiation damage to colorectum: A progress report. Ann Surg 1981;193:555–64.

58. Opelka FG, Beck DE. Colorectal trauma. In: Hicks TC, Beck DE, Opelka FG, Timmcke AE (eds). Complications of Colon & Rectal Surgery. Baltimore: Williams & Wilkins, 1996;446–67.

59. Abcarian H, Barrett JA. Complications of surgery for trauma to colon and rectum. In: Ferrari ET, Ray JE, Gathright JB (eds). Complications in Colon and Rectal Surgery. Philadelphia: WB Saunders, 1985;143–55.

60. Abcarian H, Lowe R. Colon and rectal trauma. Surg Clin North Am 1978;58:519–37.

61. Lung JA, Turk RP, Miller RE, Eiseman B. Wounds of the rectum. Ann Surg 1970;172:985–90.

62. Sohn N, Weinstein MA, Gonchar J. Social injuries of the rectum. Am J Surg 1977;134:611–2.

63. Hicks TC, Opelka FG. The hazards of anal sexual eroticism. Perspect Colon Rectal Surg 1994;7:37–57.

64. Moore EE, Cogbill TH, Malangoni MA, et al. Organ injury scaling, II: Pancreas, duodenum, small bowel, colon, and rectum. J Trauma 1990;30:1427–29.

65. Flint LM, Vitale GC, Richardson JD, Polk HC. The injured colon. Relationships of management to complications. Ann Surg 1981;193:619–23.

66. Marcet JE, Gottesman L. Anorectal trauma and necrotizing infections. In: Beck DE, Wexner SD, (eds). Fundamentals of Anorectal Surgery. New York: McGraw-Hill, 1992:440–52.

67. Himmelman RG, Martin M, Gilkey S, Barrett JA. Trial-contrast CT scans in penetrating back and flank trauma. J Trauma 1991;31:852–5.

68. Mangiante EC, Graham AD, Fabian TC. Rectal gunshot wounds. Management of civilian injuries. Am Surg 1986;52:37–40.

69. Committee on Trauma, American College of Surgeons. Advanced Trauma Life Support. Chicago: The College, 1981.

70. Rowlands BJ, Ericsson CD, Fischer RP. Penetrating abdominal trauma: The use of operative findings to determine length of antibiotic therapy. J Trauma 1987;27:250–5.

71. Jones RC, Thal ER, Johnson NA, Gollihar LN. Evaluation of antibiotic therapy following penetrating abdominal trauma. Ann Surg 1985;201:576–85.

72. Thompson JS, Moore EE, Moore JB. Comparison of penetrating injuries of the right and left colon. Ann Surg 1981;193:414–8.

73. Stone HH, Fabian TC. Management of perforating colon trauma. Randomization between primary closure and exteriorization. Ann Surg 1979;190:430–6.

74. Beck DE, Opelka FG. Pelvic and perineal trauma. Perspect Colon Rect Surg 1993;6:134–56.

75. Lou MA, Johnson AP, Atik M, et al. Exteriorized repair in the management of colon injuries. Arch Surg 1981;116:926–9.

76. Trunkey D, Hays RJ, Shires GT. Management of rectal trauma. J Trauma 1973;13:411–5.

77. Ganchrow MI, Laverson GS McNamara JJ. Surgical management of traumatic injuries of the colon and rectum. Arch Surg 1970;100:515–20.

78. Lavenson GS, Cohen A. Management of rectal injuries. Am J Surg 1971;122:226–30.

79. Lowe RJ, Boyd DR, Folk FA, Baker RJ. The negative laparotomy for abdominal trauma. J Trauma 1972;12:853–61.

80. Tancer ML, Lasser D, Rosenblum N. Rectovaginal fistula or perineal and anal sphincter disruption, or both, after vaginal delivery. Surg Gynecol Obstet 1990;171:43–6.

81. Hambrick E. Sphincteroplasty/perineoplasty for traumatic anal sphincter injuries. Perspect Colon Rect Surg 1989;2:91–8.

Section 4

Appendixes

Appendix I

Preoperative orders

1. Service: _____
2. Diagnosis: _____
3. Procedure: _____
4. Condition: _____
5. Allergies/unfavorable effects: _____
6. Vital signs: per routine
7. Activity: ad lib
8. Diet: NPO except medications
9. Intravenous fluids: _____
10. Bowel preparation: _____
11. Preoperative medications: _____
    Antibiotics: _____
    Heparin
    Motility agents: _____
12. Labs: CBC, electrolytes
    Type and match
13. Sequential compression stockings
14. Studies: EKG

Postoperative orders

Perineal cases

1. Diagnosis: _____
2. Vital signs: q 15 min until stable, then q 4 h
3. Ambulate: ad lib; out of bed every shift
4. Diet: Advance to regular as tolerated
5. Intake and output: q 8 h
6. Sitz baths tid after dressing removed
7. Medications: stool softener, pain, preoperative
8. Call MD if temperature >101°F (39°C) and/or urine output <100 mL/4 h

Abdominal cases

1. Diagnosis: _____
2. Condition: _____
3. Vital signs: q 15 min until stable, then q 4 h
4. Ambulate: ad lib; out of bed every shift

5. Drains: Foley, abdominal, pelvic
6. Dressings: _____
7. Diet: Clear liquids
8. Intake and output: q 8 h
9. Intravenous fluids: _____
10. Allergies: _____
11. Medications: Pain, preoperative, heparin, steroids
12. Lab tests:
13. Notify stoma therapist if patient has a stoma
14. Call MD if temperature >101°F (39°C), pulse >110/min, blood
    pressure (systolic) <90 or >120 mmHg, or urine output <250 mL/8 h

Discharge instructions

Abdominal operations

1. Regular or usual diet (avoid spicy or greasy foods, raw vegetables
   or fruits, and carbonated drinks for the first month unless
   instructed otherwise). Try eating six small meals a day.
2. Alcoholic beverages are okay in moderation. Do not combine with
   pain medication.
3. Exercise, walking, and climbing stairs are okay. Avoid any activity
   that causes pain. Avoid lifting weights greater than 13 kg until
   cleared by your physician. Avoid physical exercise that puts a
   strain on the abdominal muscles – for example, sit-ups, push-ups,
   jogging – for 2–3 months.
4. Driving: you may drive in 10–14 days. Do not go alone for the first
   time and do not drive while on pain medication.
5. Daily baths or showers are okay and recommended.
6. Dressings: keep your incision clean and dry, or dress the wound as
   directed by your physician.
7. Medications:
   a. Pain: Darvocet N-100, Lortab, or Percocet by mouth, one to two
      orally every 4–6 hours as needed for pain.
   b. Vitamins: vitamins are permitted.
   c. Resume any medications that your own physician has
      prescribed unless otherwise instructed.
8. Bowel Function:
   a. Avoid any foods that cause diarrhea or gas.
   b. If you were given antidiarrheal medication in the hospital, the
      dosage may need to be adjusted if you experience diarrhea or
      constipation.
   c. It is normal to have more gas or gas cramps after discharge from
      the hospital. Avoid those foods that cause gas.
   d. With respect to diarrhea, it is normal to have some good days
      and some not-so-good days. It takes your body time to adjust
      after surgery.

9. If your follow-up appointment has not been arranged prior to discharge, call the office to schedule an appointment.
10. If you experience any problems, call or contact your physician as directed.

Anal-rectal surgery

1. Regular or usual diet.
2. Alcoholic beverages are okay in moderation. Do not combine with pain medication.
3. Full activity is okay in moderation. Avoid straining or lifting heavy objects or sports activities for the next 4–6 weeks.
4. You may sit on a soft foam cushion or flat pillow. Avoid sitting on doughnuts or rubber rings.
5. You may drive when directed by your physician (usually 1–2 days). Do not go alone the first time and do not drive while on pain medication.
6. Continue sitz baths two to three times a day for 20 minutes and especially after each bowel movement.
7. Use soft damp tissue or cotton balls when wiping, pat the area, and gently dry. Avoid excessive or vigorous wiping. It may help to place soft tissue or cotton pad between the buttocks to keep the cheeks separated and to absorb any moisture.
8. Do not take an enema unless this is discussed first with your physician. Enemas may cause serious damage or injury. Do not give yourself an enema.
9. Pink staining and a few spots of blood may be seen from the anus. If heavy bleeding occurs or if you have any problems, call your physician.
10. Medications:
    a. Darvocet N-100 by mouth, one to two every 4–6 hours as needed for pain.
    b. Vitamins are permitted.
    c. Stool normalizers: Metamucil or Konsyl, 1–2 teaspoons by mouth, as directed by your physician, mixed with an adequate amount of fluid.
    d. Resume all medications that your own physician has prescribed.
    e. If a follow-up appointment has not been scheduled prior to discharge, call your physician to schedule an appointment.
    f. If you experience any problems or have questions, contact your physician as directed.

Common colorectal medications

The medications and their dosages listed below are provided to assist the clinician. Medications commonly used by colorectal surgeons are listed and the list is not meant to be complete. Although reasonable efforts have been made to insure accuracy, providers are reminded to consult prescribing information to ensure accuracy.

Table key

bid	twice a day
h	hours
hs	bedtime
IM	intramuscular
IV	intravenously
mg	milligrams
OTC	over the counter
po	per os, by mouth, orally
pr	per rectum
q	every
qd	every day
tid	three times a day
UC	ulcerative colitis
$	least expensive
$$$$$	most expensive

Table A1 Antimicrobials and medications for infectious diseases

Generic Name	Trade Name	Dosage	Comments	Cost
Acyclovir	Zovirax	200 mg po q4h	Antiviral (Herpes simplex)	$$$
Ampicillin	Omnipen	250–1000 mg po q6h 500 mg–2 g IV q6h	Gram (+) except *S. aureus, Shigella, Salmonella, E. coli, H. influenzae, N. gonorrhoeae, N. meningitidis, P. mirabilis*	$
Ampicillin/Sulbactam	Unasyn	1.5–3 g IV q6h	*S. pneumoniae, S. pyogenes, S. aureus, E. coli, H. influenzae, Klebsiella, B. fragilis*	$$$
Amoxicillin	Amoxil	250–500 mg po q8h 3 g po (SBE protection)	Similar to ampicillin, enterococci	$
Aztreonam	Azactam	1–2 g IV or IM q8–12h	Gram (–) aerobic bacilli	$$
Cefazolin	Ancef	500 mg–1 g IV 8h	Gram (+) streptococci and staphylococci, Gram (–) *E. coli, P. mirabilis, Klebsiella*	$
Cefotetan	Cefotan	1–2 g IV q1–2h	Similar to cefoxitin	$$
Cefoxitin sodium	Mefoxin	1–2 g IV q6–8h	Adds Enterobacteriaceae, *B. fragilis*	$$
Ciprofloxacin	Cipro	250–500 mg po bid 400 mg IV q 12h	*P. aeruginosa, Serratia, Enterobacter* spp, enteric pathogens, *S. aureus*	$$$$
Clindamycin phosphate	Cleocin	150–500 mg IV q6–8h 250–500 mg po q6–8h	*S. pneumoniae, S. pyogenes, S. aureus*, anaerobic spp, *B. fragilis, Fusobacterium* spp	$$$
Doxycycline	Vibramycin	50–100 mg po q12 h	Many Gram (+) and (–), anaerobes, PID	$
Erythromycin base		1 g po at 1, 2, 11 pm the day before a 7:30 case	Gram (+), *M. pneumoniae, S. pneumoniae*, some *S. aureus, Chlamydia, Mycoplasma, Campylobacter* spp	$
Fluconazole	Diflucan	20–200 mg po qd	Antifungal agent	$$$$$
Ganciclovir	Cytovene	5 mg/kg IV q12h for 7–21 days	Synthetic guanine derivative active against cytomegalovirus	
Gentamicin	Garamycin	3 mg/kg /day divided q8h	Gram (–) bacilli , Pneumococci, streptococci, some staphylococci	$
Imipenem & cilastatin	Primaxin	500–1000 mg IV q6h	Gram (–) bacilli, *Enterobacter*	$$$$$
Metronidazole	Flagyl	250–500 mg po q6–8h 250–500 mg IV q6–8h	*Bacteroides* spp	$
Neomycin sulfate	Neomycin	1 g po at 1, 2, 11 pm the day before a 7:30 case	*K. pneumoniae, Proteus, E. coli, E. aerogenes*	$
Nystatin	Mycostatin	30 mL swish and swallow tid cream or powder to skin	Antifungal (*Candida*)	$$
Piperacillin & Tazobactam	Zosyn	3.3 g IV q6h	Gram (–) and (+) organisms	$$$
Trimethoprim & sulfamethoxazole	Septra Bactrim	10–20 mg/kg/day IV Divided q6–12h 1 po bid	*E. coli, Klebsiella, Enterobacter, Proteus, Serratia*	$
Ticarcillin/clavulanate	Timentin	3.1 g IV q4–6h	*S. aureus*, Gram (+) bacteria, *Klebsiella* spp, *Proteus* spp, *Pseudomonas, E. coli, B. fragilis*	$$
Vancomycin HCl	Vancocin	500–1000 mg IV q6h 500 mg po q6h	Staphylococci (methicillin resistant), enterococci, *Clostridia*, antibiotic-associated colitis	$$$
Zidovudine (AZT)	Retrovir	100 mg po q4h 1 mg/kg IV q4h	Pyrimidine analogue active against HIV	

Table A2 Anti-inflammatory medications

Generic Name	Trade Name	Dosage	Comments	Cost
Budesonide	Entocort	9 mg po qd	Treat moderate to severe colitis or Crohn's disease	$$$$
Hydrocortisone acetate	Cort Enemas (10%)	1 (100 mg) enema per day (hs)	Proctitis : treat for up to 21 days	$$$$$
Hydrocortisone acetate	Cort Foam (10%)	1 applicator in rectum q12-24h × 2–3 weeks then qod	Proctitis	$$$
Hydrocortisone acetate	Proctocream (1%) Analpram (1, 2.5%) Proctofoam (1%)	Apply thin film q6–8h One applicator pr q6–8h	Pruritus ani, anal fissure 30 g tube	$$
Hydrocortisone	Solu-cortef	25–150 mg IV q6–12h	Treat severe ulcerative colitis (UC)	
Mesalamine	Asacol	800 mg po q8h	Mild to moderate UC, tablets release at pH ≥ 7; 400 mg tablets	$$$
Mesalamine	Pentasa	1 g po q6h	Mild to moderate UC;250 mg controlled release capsule	$$$$
Mesalamine	Lialda	2.4–4.8 mg po qd	Mild to moderate UC; controlled release capsule	$$$$$
Mesalamine enema	Rowasa	1 (4 g) enema qd (hs) 1 (500 mg) suppository q12h	Proctitis: treat 3–6 weeks	$$$$$
Methylprednisolone	Solu-medrol	30 mg/Kg q4–6h	Potent anti-inflammatory steroid with less sodium and water retention	
Olsalazine sodium	Dipentum	500 mg po q12h	Mild to moderate UC	$$$
Prednisone	Deltasone	2.5–60 mg po qd	Moderate to severe UC	$
Sulfasalazine	Azulfidine	350 mg–1 g po q6h	Mild to moderate UC Treat for over 1 month	$

Table A3 Antispasmodic medication

Generic Name	Trade Name	Dosage	Comments	Cost
Chlordiazepoxide & clidinium bromide	Librax	1–2 po qid (before meals and hs)	For irritable bowel disease (IBD) Withdrawal symptoms may occur	
Dicyclomine HCl	Bentyl	20–40 mg po q6h	10–20 mg capsules for 2 weeks	$$
Phenobarbital, atropine scopolamine	Donnatal	1–2 po q6-8h	IBD, cramps	$$
Hyoscyamine sulfate	Levsin, Symax, NuLev	1–2 tablets po q12h 1 tablet sublingual	For abdominal cramps or spastic colitis	$$$$

Table A4 Bowel Preparations and laxatives

Generic Name	Trade Name	Dosage	Comments	Cost
Polyethylene glycol electrolyte lavage	Golytely Colyte, Nulytely	240 mL po q 10 minutes until diarrhea is clear	Oral lavage preparation Prescribe 4 L	$$
Polyethylene glycol electrolyte lavage	Half Lightly	240 mL po q 10 minutes until diarrhea is clear	Oral lavage preparation 2 L and Dulcolax	$$
Polyethylene glycol electrolyte lavage and ascorbic acid	Movie Prep	2 doses diluted in 480 mL of water	Oral lavage preparation	$$
Sodium sulfate, potassium sulfate and magnesium sulfate	SurPrep	2 doses of 170 mL diluted in 480 mL of water	Oral lavage preparation	$$
Sodium phosphate	Visacol	28–32 tablets as directed	Cathartic preparation	$$$
Magnesium citrate	Evac Q Kwick	284 mL po	Cathartic preparation	$
Senna	Senna X-Prep	70 mL po × 2	Colonic stimulant	$
Bisacodyl	Dulcolax	2–3 tablets (5 mg) po 1 suppository ; OTC	Colonic stimulant	
Sodium phosphate enemas	Fleet enemas	133 mL PR × 2; OTC	Preparation for flexible sigmoidoscopy	

Table A5 Antineoplastic and immunosuppressant agents

Generic Name	Trade Name	Dosage	Comments	Cost
Azathioprine	Imuran	50–100 mg po q 12–24 h 100 mg IV	Derivative of 6-mercaptopurine Immunosuppressive	$$$
Fluorouracil	5-FU	12 mg/kg or 100 mg/m^2	Dukes' C colon cancer antimetabolite	
Leucovorin		150 mg po q6h	Diminish toxicity of folic acid antagonists	
Levamisole HCl	Ergamisol	50 mg po q8h for 3 days q 2 weeks	Adjuvant chemotherapy in Dukes' C colon cancer	
Mercaptopurine (6-MP)	Purinethol	50–200 mg/day	Purine analog which interfers with nucleic acid biosynthesis Useful in refractory Crohn's disease	
Methotrexate	Rheumatex	12 g/m^2	Antimetabolite	
Mitamycin	Mitomycin-C	20 mg/m^2	Antitumor activity	
Sandimmune	Cyclosporin		Immunosuppressive Experimental treatment for ulcerative colitis	

Table A6 Fiber products and stool normalizers

Generic Name	Trade Name	Dosage	Comments	Cost
Calcium polycarbophyll	Fibercon	1–6 capsules po qd	OTC, stool bulking agent	$$$$
Carboxy methyl cellulose	Citracel Citracel fiber tablets	1–2 tbsp po qd 1–2 tablets q6–8h	OTC, stool bulking agent	$$$
Ducusate calcium	Surfak	50–100 mg po bid	Docusate sodium; OTC	$$
Docusate sodium	Colase	50–100 mg po bid	Wetting agent to soften stool	$$
Lactulose	Enulose, Cephilac	15 mL po q12–24h	Nonabsorbed sugar	$$
Polyethylene glycol 3350	Miralax	17 g (1 capful) in water qd	Nonabsorbed osmotic agent	$$
Psyllium	Metamucil Konsyl Perdeum Fiber	1–4 tbsp po qd	OTC	$
Psyllium and senna	Perideum	1–2 tbsp po qd	Fiber with mild stimulate; OTC	$$
Sorbitol	Sorbitol		Nonabsorbed sugar	$

Table A7 Anti-diarrheal medications

Generic Name	Trade Name	Dosage	Comments	Cost
Bismuth	Pepto-Bismol	2 tbsp or tablets q1h up to 8 doses/day	OTC	$
Codeine sulfate		30–60 mg po tid	May cause sedation	$
Diphenoxylate HCl & atropine sulfate	Lomotil	1–2 po qid (before meals & HS)	Limit to 8 doses/day	$
Kaolin-pectin suspension	Kayopectate	3–6 tbsp po	OTC	$$
Loperamide HCl	Immodium	1–2 po qid (before meals & HS)	Limit to 8 doses/day; OTC	$$$
Morphine elixir	Roxanol	5–20 drops qid	Constipating, schedule II Dispense 125–250 mL	$$
Tincture of opium		5–20 drops qid	Very constipating; difficult to obtain	$$

Table A8 Motility agents

Generic Name	Trade Name	Dosage	Comments	Cost
Cisapride	Propulsid	10–20 mg po q6h	Prokinetic agent Only available on protocol	$$
Metoclopramide	Reglan	10–15 mg po q6h 10–20 mg IV q6h	Stimulates upper gastrointestinal motility	$

Table A9 Sedatives and reversal agents

Generic Name	Trade Name	Dosage	Comments	Cost
Alprazolam	Xanax	0.25–0.5 mg po tid	Anti-anxiety	
Diazepam	Valium	5–10 mg po, IV, IM	Sedative	
Diphenhydramine	Benadryl	25–50 mg po q4–6h 10–50 mg IV or IM	Antihistamine	
Chloral hydrate		500 mg po or pr hs	Sedative	
Flumazenil	Romazicon	0.2–1 mg IV	Benzodiazepine receptor antagonist	$$$
Flurazepam	Dalmane	15–30 mg po hs	Sleep medication	$
Haloperidol	Haldol	0.5–5 mg po q8h 2–5 mg IM q1–8h	Major tranquilizer	$
Lorazepam	Ativan	0.5–2 mg po tid	Anti-anxiety	
Midazolam HCl	Versed	0.5–5 mg IV	Sedative	
Naloxone HCl	Narcan	0.2–2 mg IV 0.2 mg IM	Narcotic antagonist	
Temazepam	Restoril	7.5–15 mg po hs	Benzodiazepine hypnotic agent	$
Triazolam	Halcion	0.125–0.25 mg po hs	Sleep medication	$$$
Zolpidem tartrate	Ambien	5–10 mg po hs	Sleep medication	

Table A10 Pain medication

Generic Name	Trade Name	Dosage	Comments	Cost
Acetaminophen & codeine	Tylenol # 3	1–2 po q4–6h	Moderate pain	$
Belladonna and opium suppositories	B&O #16 A	1 pr q8h	For rectal spasm	$$
Fentanyl	Duragesic (transdermal)	2.5–10 mg patch q72h	Potent opioid analgesic	$$$$
Hydrocodone bitartrate & acetaminophen	Vicodin	1–2 po q4–6h	Severe pain	$$
Ibuprofen	Motrin Advil, Motrin IB	200–800 mg po q 6h	Nonsteroidal anti-inflammatory, OTC	$
Ketorolac tromethamine	Toradol	60 mg IM 30 mg IV 10–20 mg po q4–6h	Nonsteroidal inflamatory agent	
Meperidine HCl	Demerol	25–150 mg IM q3–4h	Severe pain	
Morphine	Astramorph	1–2 mg IV q1–2h 5–15 mg IM q3–4h	Opium alkaloid	
Morphine	MS Contin MSIR	15, 30, 60, 100 mg po bid 15 or 30 mg po q 4 h	Potent analgesic	$$
Oxycodone & acetaminophen	Percocet 5-10/325 Tylox	1–2 po q4–6h	Severe pain Semisynthetic narcotic analgesic	$$
Oxycodone	Oxycontin	10–160 mg po bid	Controlled release opium analgesic	$$
Propoxyphene napsylate & acetaminophen	Darvocet-N-100	1–2 po q4–6h	Mild to moderate pain	$
Tramadol HCl	Ultram	50–100 mg po q4–6h	Centrally acting analgesic	$$

Table A11 H₂ Blockers, proton pump inhibitors and antacids, etc.

Generic Name	Trade Name	Dosage	Comments	Cost
Aluminum hydroxide & magnesium hydroxide	Mylanta, Maalox	30 mL po q2h prm	Antacid, OTC	$
Cimetidine	Tagamet	400–800 mg po hs 300 mg q6–8h	H₂ blocker, OTC	$
Famotidine	Pepcid	40 mg po qd 20 mg IV q12h	H₂ blocker, OTC	$$
Nizatidine	Axid	150 mg po bid	H₂ blocker	$$$
Omeprazole	Prilosec	20 mg po qd	Suppress gastric acid via proton pump	$$
Pantoprazole sodium	Protonix	40 mg po qd	Suppress gastric acid via proton pump	$$
Rabeprazole sodium	Aciphex	20 mg po qd	Suppress gastric acid via proton pump	$$$
Ranitidine HCl	Zantac	150 mg po bid 50 mg IV q8–12h	H₂ blocker, OTC	$
Esomeprazole magnesium	Nexium	20 mg po qd	Suppress gastric acid	$$$$$$
Sucralfate	Carafate	1 gm po q6h	Local protection of ulcer site	$$$$

Table A12 Miscellaneous

Generic Name	Trade Name	Dosage	Comments	Cost
Podophyllin in benzoin	Podocon-25	Apply to lesion	Cytotoxic agent (condylomata)	
Pramoxine HCl	Prax lotion	Apply topically	Topical anesthetic	
Hyaluronidase	Wydase	150 units sq	Reduces edema and swelling	
Fibrin sealant	Tissel	2–5 mL		
Botulinum toxin A	BoTox	10–50 units IM	Paralyzes muscle for 3 months	

References

1. Meyers BR. Antimicrobial therapy guide. Newton: Antimicrobial Prescribing 1991.
2. Physicians Desk Reference. Montvale: Medical Economics Company 2002.
3. Sanford JP, Gilbert DN, Sande MA. Guide to antimicrobial therapy. Dallas: Antimicrobial Therapy, Inc., 1996.

Appendix III

Answers to rounds questions

Chapter 1

1. There are three taeniae: the taenia mesocolica, the taenia omentalis, and the taenia libera (p. 4–5).
2. The rectum is larger in diameter, has no taeniae, sacculations, or appendices epiploicae, and lacks a posterior mesentery (p. 7).
3. The anal canal starts at the anorectal junction located at the palpable upper edge of the anal sphincter mechanism (junction of puborectalis and anal sphincter). The anal canal ends at the intersphincteric groove (approximately 2 cm distal to the dentate line) (p. 7).
4. The cecum is supplied by the ileocolic artery (p. 8–9).
5. The splenic vein (p. 9).
6. Columnar epithelium (p. 11).
7. The submucosa (p. 11).
8. S 2–4 (p. 10)

Chapter 2

1. The function is to mix the colonic contractions to improve absorption (p. 14).
2. The midtransverse colon (p. 14).
3. Temporary impairment of intestinal motility after operation (p. 16).
4. A profound ileus without evidence of mechanical obstruction (p. 17).
5. The colon absorbs water, sodium, and chloride and secretes potassium and bicarbonate (p. 18).
6. The internal sphincter (p. 20).
7. Transient relaxation of the upper part of the internal sphincter, which allows the rectal contents to come into contact with the sensory epithelium of the proximal anal canal (p. 22).
8. Hirschsprung's disease (p. 24).

Chapter 3

1. False; abdominal pain is usually ill defined and is often referred to areas on the surface removed from the site of pathology (p. 29).
2. True; this symptom may also be seen with inflammatory conditions or following pelvic irradiation (p. 30).
3. False; melena may be from the right colon and although bright red bleeding is usually anal, a more proximal source may need to be excluded (p. 30).

4. True; a family history in a first-degree relative increases the patient's risk of colorectal cancer (p. 31).
5. False; if peritonitis is detected by gentle percussion, further vigorous palpation only hurts the patient and adds nothing to the clinical picture (p. 32).
6. True; atypical lateral fissures may indicate inflammatory bowel disease, malignancy, or infectious diseases (p. 35).
7. True; when correctly done, the anorectal examination is no more stressful than any other part of the examination and may yield vital information about the patient's condition (p. 35).

Chapter 4

1. 3 cm (p. 41).
2. 5.5 cm (p. 41).
3. Small polyps and mucosal changes of inflammatory bowel disease (p. 45).
4. Because retained stool may result in an inconclusive examination or be mistaken for a small polyp (p. 45)
5. Intravenous administration of glucagon (p. 47).
6. Answers (a) and (c) (p. 45, 48).
7. Answer (c) (p. 48).
8. For an abdominal ultrasound, the patient should be NPO for at least 4–8 hours. For an intrarectal ultrasound, the patient should receive two Fleets type enemas. (p. 51–52).
9. An ultrasonographically detectable abnormality that indicates bowel wall thickening. The pattern simulates the appearance of the kidney. It is seen in any abnormality that causes bowel wall thickening, such as neoplasm, inflammatory bowel disease, diverticulitis, and appendicitis (p. 49).
10. True (p. 53).
11. A water-soluble contrast medium (Hypaque or Gastrografin) (p. 53).
12. False; the intravenous contrast agents used in MRI do not contain iodine (p. 55).
13. False; both intraoperative liver ultrasound and CT arterial portography are more sensitive. MRI is, of course, less invasive than intraoperative ultrasound and CT arterial portography (p. 55).
14. All of the above (p. 58–62).
15. Answer (d) (p. 58).
16. A nuclear medicine bleeding study (p. 61).
17. Nuclear medicine = 0.2 mL/min; conventional angiography = 1.0 mL/min (p. 61).
18. Four days (p. 62).
19. In normal subjects, 80% of markers are passed in 5 days and 100% in 7 days (p. 62–63).

Chapter 5

1. 17–20 cm (p. 68).
2. During withdrawal (p. 70).
3. The patient feels faint and light-headed, and the skin will be cool and diaphoretic (p. 71).
4. No; enemas do not remove enough of the explosive gas contained in the colon (p. 73).
5. If it is performed too vigorously, the bowel may be perforated (p. 75).
6. Narcan, 0.2 mg IV and 0.2 mg lM for the meperidine, and Romazicon, 0.2–1.0 mg lV for the midazolam (p 77).
7. Pulse oximetry and automated blood pressure (p. 77).
8. In the 6 o'clock position (p. 78).
9. Bleeding, perforation, and transmural burn (p. 79–80).

Chapter 6

1. The cosmetic results are better (p. 83).
2. Gravity (p. 83).
3. The same as for open colorectal procedures (p. 88)
4. Yes, they are inversely related (p. 99).
5. If untreated or uncompensated, it will lead to acidosis (p. 100).
6. The patient is placed in a left lateral and head down position, 100% oxygen is administered, and aspiration of the gas from the right ventricle may be attempted using a central venous line (p. 101).

Chapter 7

1. A stoma should be located within the rectus muscle, at a site that is free of scars, can be seen by the patient, and does not abut any bony prominences (p. 107).
2. Leakage (p. 114).
3. Stenosis, ischemia, retraction, abscess, and hernia (p. 114).
4. Valve slippage (p. 116–117).
5. No (p. 117).
6. It is more common after a colostomy (p. 122).
7. Stomas shrink considerably in the first 8 postoperative weeks (p. 123).
8. Patients who had less than two formed stools per day before surgery (p. 124).

Chapter 8

1. 1900 mL (p. 133).
2. Replace mL for mL with 1/2 normal saline solution plus 20 mEq/L (p. 134).
3. Protein 1 g/kg/day; carbohydrate 50–100 g/day (p. 134).
4. No (p. 141).
5. No, as long as the drugs are used properly and have an appropriate bacterial spectrum (p. 142).
6. Calf swelling and discomfort, distal venous engorgement, and pain on dorsiflexion of the foot (Homan's sign) (p. 143).

Chapter 9

1. ASA III (p. 151).
2. No, unless the patient has an intestinal obstruction or a long procedure (more than 3 or 4 hours) is anticipated (p. 152).
3. Lidocaine: 5 mg/kg plain; 7 mg/kg with epinephrine. Bupivacaine: 2 mg/kg plain; 4 mg/kg with epinephrine (p. 153–154).
4. Epinephrine prolongs the effect of local anesthetic by preventing diffusion and uptake. It also provides hemostasis secondary to vasoconstriction. Bicarbonate will alter the solution pH and reduce the pain associated with injecting the solution (p. 153).
5. No decreased cardiac risk; greatly reduced pulmonary risk (p. 153).
6. Continuous epidural with light sedation, which gives the added advantage of postoperative pain control (p. 154).
7. Naloxone (Narcan); flumazenil (Romazicon) (p. 158).
8. None; a pulmonary artery catheter only helps identify silent events and helps with intraoperative and postoperative fluid management (p. 158).
9. 630 mL/h (p. 158–159).
10. Peroneal nerve compression (foot drop) (p. 159).

Chapter 10

1. Use of PCA results in lower medication requirements (p. 163).
2. An inhibition of bowel motility (p. 164).
3. No, 90% of postoperative patients do well without a nasogastric tube (p. 165).
4. Psyllium is a hydrophilic grain product (p. 166).
5. It inhibits bowel peristaltic activity by direct action on all muscles of the intestinal wall (p. 166–167).
6. No (p. 168).
7. It may be closed primarily, packed open for delayed primary closure, or allowed to heal by secondary intention (p. 169).
8. Signs include skin erythema, warmth, edema, and increasing incisional pain (p. 170).
9. A urine output of at least 0.5–1 mL/kg/h (p. 170).
10. HIV, hepatitis B and C, syphilis (p. 172).

Chapter 11

1. As an intestinal obstruction in the newborn or as constipation in an older patient. It can occasionally present as enterocolitis (p. 183).
2. The absence of ganglion cells on rectal or bowel biopsy (p. 184).
3. Genitourinary anomalies (in up to 90% of patients with high lesions and up to 30% with low lesions (p. 192).
4. Proximal sigmoid colostomy (p. 194).
5. Diabetes (p. 198).
6. Necrotizing enterocolitis (p. 199).

Chapter 12

1. Constipation is frequently defined as less than three bowel movements in a 7-day period, excessive straining (more than 25% of the time) at stool, or impacted hard stools (p. 205).
2. Inadequate fiber or water intake, constipating medications, colonic inertia and megacolon, and pelvic floor obstruction (p. 205–6).
3. Take a history and perform a physical examination and endoscopy to rule out life-threatening or significant causes of constipation (p. 207).
4. It should include colonic transit times, defecography and balloon expulsion to differentiate colonic inertia, internal intussusception, and a nonrelaxing puborectalis muscle as the cause of the problem (p. 208).
5. The patient may be considered for a total colectomy and ileorectal anastomosis (p. 209).
6. Stop all constipating agents; consider epidural anesthesia, neostigmine, Hypaque enemas, colonoscopic decompression or surgery (p. 209–210)
7. The inability to control the release of rectal contents until a socially acceptable time and place (p. 211–212).
8. Etiologic factors include (1) altered anal sphincter function (mechanical injury or neurogenic problems) and (2) altered colorectal function (irritable bowel syndrome, diminished rectal capacity, idiopathic causes) (p. 212).
9. The complete objective evaluation of the anal canal includes anal manometry, measurement of pudendal nerve terminal motor latency (PNWL) with electromyographic techniques, and endoluminal ultrasound of the anal sphincter (p. 214–215).

Chapter 13

1. Colonic diverticula are false diverticula of the colonic mucosa that protrude through the colonic musculature alongside the taeniae (p. 223).
2. The sigmoid colon (p. 223).
3. Factors that appear to predispose to colonic diverticula include decreased colonic wall strength, increased intraluminal pressure, decreased stool bulk, and lack of dietary fiber (p. 224).
4. Pressure is related to wall tension and inversely related to the radius (p. 224).
5. Left lower quadrant pain and tenderness, fever, and elevated white blood cell count (p. 226)
6. With CT- or ultrasound-guided percutaneous drainage and antibiotics (p. 227).
7. A colovesical (colon to bladder) fistula is the most common (p. 228).
8. Cystoscopy is the most sensitive and will demonstrate bullous edema at the site of the fistula (p. 229).

9. A hysterectomy (p. 229).

10. (1) Exteriorization, (2) resection, end colostomy, mucous fistula, (3) resection, end colostomy, oversew rectum (Hartmann's), (4) resection, primary anastomosis, (5) resection, primary anastomosis, diverting colostomy or ileostomy. (p. 230).

11. Three or more attacks of diverticulitis in a good-risk patient, one major attack of diverticulitis with complications (abscess, fistula) or in a patient younger than 40 years of age (p. 231–232).

12. The distal line of resection should be healthy rectum; the proximal limit is soft, pliable, uninvolved left or transverse colon (p. 232).

Chapter 14

1. Ankylosing spondylitis and sclerosing cholangitis (p. 248).

2. Either a total proctocolectomy with ileostomy or a restorative proctocolectomy (colectomy with ileoanal reservoir and mucosectomy) (p. 249, 253).

3. Subtotal colectomy with ileostomy and Hartmann's pouch (p. 249).

4. Pouchitis, confirmed on pouchoscopy with biopsy. It is treated with hydration and oral administration of metronidazole or ciprofloxacin (p. 258).

5. He was chairman of the Department of Gastroenterology at Mount Sinai Hospital in New York in the 1930s (p. 260).

6. Metronidazole. Its potential side effects include a metallic taste, nausea, peripheral neuropathy, and an antabuse effect when mixed with alcohol (p. 263).

7. Separate the fistula, perform a segmental bowel resection, and drain the bladder with a Foley catheter for at least 5 days (p. 265).

8. These fistulas are classified as complex and require an advancement flap for repair. Note that the rectum must be pliable and not severely diseased. Alternatives include a transvaginal approach, sphincteroplasty, muscle flaps (such as gracilis), and proctectomy (p. 268).

9. Extent and duration of disease (p. 269).

Chapter 15

1. Redundant sigmoid colon, deep pouch of Douglas, patulous anal sphincter, diastasis of the levator ani, and loss of normal attachments of the rectum (p. 277–278).

2. Protrusion of the rectum with straining or spontaneously, constipation, incontinence, tenesmus, rectal bleeding, and pain (p. 278).

3. Ripstein procedure (mesh rectopexy), Wells procedure (Ivalon sponge rectopexy), anterior resection, and suture rectopexy with or without resection (p. 283–287).

4. The Altemeier procedure is a perineal rectosigmoidectomy. A full-thickness bowel resection is performed, in contrast to the Delorme procedure, which involves removal of the mucosa only (p. 288).
5. The Thiersch procedure is an anal encirclement operation. Many different materials have been used for the anal encirclement, including steel, nylon, Silastic, and silicone (p. 292).

Chapter 16

1. The blood is arterial (p. 299).
2. No; both conditions are common but are not related (p. 300).
3. External hemorrhoids are located in the distal third of the anal canal (distal to the dentate line) and are covered by anoderm or skin that is sensitive to touch, temperature, stretch, and pain. Internal hemorrhoids are located proximal to the dentate line and covered by mucosa (p. 301).
4. Grade 1 hemorrhoids protrude into but do not prolapse out of the anal canal; grade 2 hemorrhoids prolapse out the anal canal with bowel movements or straining, but spontaneously reduce; grade 3 hemorrhoids prolapse during the maneuvers described above and must be manually reduced by the patient; grade 4 hemorrhoids are prolapsed out the anus and cannot be reduced (p. 301).
5. The patient may have postband sepsis and should be examined by anoscope and antibiotics should be administered intravenously (p. 304).
6. The additional complications include rectovaginal or rectourethral fistulas, rectal leaks, abscesses, sepsis of bleeding (p. 313).

Chapter 17

1. 90% are thought to arise from non-specific cryptoglandular infection (p. 317).
2. This theory suggests that anorectal suppuration results from obstruction of the anal glands and ducts (p. 317).
3. They are classified according to the existence of potential anorectal spaces as perianal, ischiorectal, intersphincteric, and supralevator (p. 318).
4. Patients present with disproportionate pain in the absence of physical findings. Urinary symptoms may also be a presenting feature (p. 319).
5. With incision and drainage or catheter drainage (p. 319–322).
6. Intersphincteric, trans-sphincteric, suprasphincteric, and extrasphincteric (p. 324).
7. An opening seen posterior to a line drawn transversely across the perineum will originate from an internal opening in the posterior midline. An anterior opening will originate in the nearest crypt (p. 326).

8. Identification of the primary opening (p. 327).
9. A nonabsorbable suture or elastic inserted into the fistula tract following division of the skin and overlying internal sphincter, the ends of which are tied securely. It is used for high- level fistulas, in Crohn's disease, in complicated and simultaneous fistulas, and in patients with weakened sphincter muscles (p. 328–329).
10. The rectal mucosal advancement flap (p. 330).

Chapter 18

1. Intense perianal itching or burning (p. 338).
2. Keep the perianal area dry, avoid further trauma, avoid irritating foods and drinks, maintain regular bowel habits, and avoid all proprietary creams, lotions, and emollients (p. 340).
3. Posterior (p. 342).
4. Tearing anal pain associated with bright blood from the rectum (p. 343).
5. Inflammatory bowel disease, infections, and malignancy (p. 344–346).
6. Bulk stool softeners, increased oral fluid intake, and warm sitz baths (p. 346).
7. Lidocaine, Nitroglycerin, Diltiazem (p. 347–348).
8. Lateral internal anal sphincterotomy (p. 349).

Chapter 19

1. It is acquired (p. 357).
2. It is more common in men (2.2–4:1) (p. 358).
3. It is treated with incision and drainage (p. 359).
4. Changes in body habitus (altered and increased fat deposition alters the gluteal cleft), and softening of hair are associated with aging (p. 360).
5. Debridement of the epithelial pit; laying open the sinus; excision to fascia; excision and marsupialization; excision and closure; and excision and flap closure (p. 360–366).

Chapter 20

1. CMV can cause inflammation, hemorrhage, ulceration, or perforation of the GI tract (p. 372).
2. Herpes is a DNA virus, whereas HIV is an RNA retrovirus (p. 372–373).
3. It is transmitted by contact with contaminated body fluids (through sexual contact, needle sticks, blood products, and so on) (p. 372).
4. HIV ulcers are deep ulcers with overhanging edges; they are often eccentric, cavitating, and edematous with a bluish-purple hue (p. 375).
5. Anal condylomata are caused by the human papilloma virus (p. 377).
6. Chlamydial infection is the most common STD and causes cervicitis, urethritis, and proctitis (p. 380).

7. An anaerobic medium such as Thayer–Martin (p. 381).
8. A common cutaneous condition that results from infection of apocrine skin glands located deep in the subcutaneous tissue and connected to the skin surface via ducts. The highest concentration of these glands occurs in the axilla, neck, groin, and perianal areas (p. 382).
9. Rapid plasma reagin (RPR), the venereal disease research laboratory slide test (VDRL), and the fluorescent treponemal antibody-absorption test (FTA-ABS) are used in syphilis (p. 384).
10. An acute diarrheal infection; toxic colonic dilatation; a symptomatic carrier state (p. 385).

Chapter 21

1. Hamartomas, hyperplastic polyps, inflammatory polyps, and adenomatous polyps (p. 389).
2. Juvenile polyps, Cronkhite–Canada syndrome, and Peutz–Jefhers syndrome (p. 390).
3. Hyperplastic polyps (p. 392).
4. Tubular adenomas, villous adenomas, and tubulovillous adenomas (p. 393).
5. 1%, 10%, and 50% (p. 396).
6. Polypectomy is adequate if the resection margin is clear (greater than 2 mm), there is no blood vessel or lymphatic invasion, and the cancer is not poorly differentiated (p. 398).
7. At age 10 (p. 401).
8. Familial polyposis coli, with multiple osteomata, cysts, and soft tissue tumors (p. 401).
9. Proctocolectomy and ileostomy, total colectomy with ileorectal anastomosis, and restorative proctocolectomy (p. 401).
10. In 1–3 years (p. 403).

Chapter 22

1. Colorectal cancer (p. 407).
2. Carcinoid tumors arise from enterochromaffin or Kulchitsky cells, which are located in the crypts of Lieberkühn (p. 408).
3. Surgery is the primary treatment; radiotherapy and chemotherapy are useful in an adjuvant role (p. 411).
4. Waldeyer's fascia is posterior to the rectum and Denonvilliers' fascia is anterior (p. 419–420).
5. Cuthbert Dukes, a pathologist at St. Marks Hospital in London in the 1930s, proposed a staging system, A through C, for rectal cancer (p. 429).
6. It would be a Dukes' B, an Astler-Coller B2, or a T3 N0 MO (p. 430).
7. Current recommendations suggest that Dukes' C patients (node positive) should receive adjuvant chemotherapy (p. 428).

8. The National Cancer Institute Consensus Development Conference recommended that Stage II and III rectal cancer patients not enrolled in adjuvant therapy protocols receive a sequential regimen of 5-FU and radiotherapy after curative resection of their tumors (p. 429).
9. Carcinoembryonic antigen (CEA) is a protein made by cells near colorectal tumors. Many surgeons use it as a follow-up test for colorectal cancer (p. 429).
10. The anal canal runs from the anorectal junction (top of the anal sphincter muscles) to the intersphincteric groove (approximately 2 cm distal to the dentate line). It essentially corresponds to the internal anal sphincter muscle (p. 431).
11. Chemoradiotherapy similar to that described by Nigro (p. 434).
12. HSIL is an intraepithelial squamous carcinoma, whereas Paget's disease is an intraepithelial adenocarcinoma (p. 435).

Chapter 23

1. It is the axial torsion or twisting of the colon on its mesentary (p. 441).
2. The sigmoid colon (p. 441).
3. The patient is stabilized with nasogastric decompression, intravenous hydration, and correction of electrolyte abnormalities. This is followed by nonoperative reduction of the volvulus using a rigid proctoscope and a rectal tube (p. 444).
4. Sites potentially vulnerable to ischemic disease include Griffith's point at the splenic flexure (junction of the SMA and IMA), Sudeck's critical point at the midsigmoid colon (junction of the IMA and hypogastric vasculature) and the cecum (distal SMA) (p. 447).
5. Measurement of IMA stump pressure in patients with a patent IMA, identification of Doppler signals on the bowel surface, and measurement of intraluminal pH have all been used (p. 448).
6. The milder cases are manifest by diffuse and/or bloody diarrhea. Patients with frank colonic infarction frequently develop acidosis, glucose intolerance, renal failure, obvious sepsis, and abdominal distention or tenderness (p. 449).
7. Resolution of the process, progression to full thickness necrosis, or evolution to an ulcerative stage, which may eventually result in stricture formation (p. 450).
8. Penetrating trauma (p. 455).
9. Treatment options for colonic injuries include exteriorization of the injured segment, resection with or without anastomoses, closure of the injured segment with a proximal protecting colostomy, or primary closure of the colonic injury (p. 457).
10. Iatrogenic obstetric trauma (p. 459).

Index